OB/GYN

Curry:

    CH: 21, 22, 23, 24

    Hen

      CH: 13, 15, 17, 14, 18,
           19, 20, 25, 22, 32
           16, 23, 24

SONOGRAPHY

Introduction to Normal Structure and Function

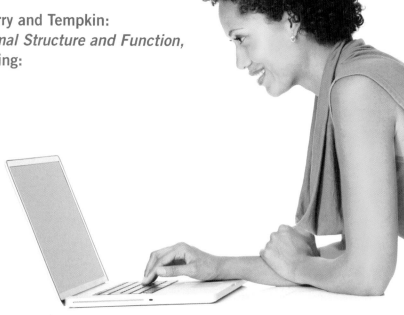

SONOGRAPHY

Introduction to Normal Structure and Function

FOURTH EDITION

Reva Arnez Curry, PhD, RT(R), RDMS

Vice-President, Instruction and Learning Services
Delta College
University Center, Michigan

Betty Bates Tempkin, BA

Ultrasound Consultant
Formerly Clinical Director of the Diagnostic Medical Sonography Program
Hillsborough Community College
Tampa, Florida

I will pass on anything I ever wanted if it cost me my dignity.

ELSEVIER

ELSEVIER

3251 Riverport Lane
St. Louis, Missouri 63043

Previous editions copyrighted 2011, 2003, and 1995.

Library of Congress Cataloging-in-Publication Data
Sonography (Curry)
  Sonography : introduction to normal structure and function / [edited by] Reva Curry, Betty Bates
Tempkin.—4th edition.
      p. ; cm.
  Includes bibliographical references and index.
  ISBN 978-0-323-32284-3 (hardcover : alk. paper)
  I. Curry, Reva A., editor.   II. Tempkin, Betty Bates, editor.   III. Title.
  [DNLM: 1. Ultrasonography.   2. Anatomy. WN 208]
  RC78.7.U4
  616.07'543—dc23
                                                                                    2015029187

Executive Content Strategist: Sonya Seigafuse
Content Development Manager: Laurie Gower
Content Development Specialist: John Tomedi, Spring Hollow Press
Publishing Services Manager: Julie Eddy
Senior Project Manager: Mary Stueck
Marketing Manager: Kristin Conrad
Manufacturing Supervisor: Debbie Larocca
Design Direction: Ashley Miner

Printed in Canada

Last digit is the print number: 9   8   7   6   5   4   3   2   1

Working together
to grow libraries in
developing countries

www.elsevier.com • www.bookaid.org

My efforts with this textbook would not have been possible without the love, encouragement, and support from my husband, Dwight, and my family: Tiana, Serena, Jeremy, and Omar. To Mom and Dad, thank you for showing me that age is just a number. I dedicated the third edition to feisty little Lena, my first grandchild, born 3 months early. You have taught me the meaning of resilience and strength, and will start kindergarten this year! I now dedicate the fourth edition to your little brother, Princeton, born full-term and healthy. Thank you Dr. Joshua Elgibor for your loving care of Lena. A special thank you to Dr. Jerome Cunningham, my first teacher in ultrasound, and Dr. Barry B. Goldberg, who has been unfailing in his support for sonographers for many, many years. Betty, it's been over 20 years—you are amazing! Thank you.

R.A.C.

Dedicated to David and Max for always sharing the best of themselves with me and making me the luckiest person on the planet! And to my long time affiliation and friendship with Reva Curry. A consummate professional: dedicated, caring and witty. It is always a pleasure!

B.B.T.

Contributors

Jill Beithon, RT, RDMS, RDCS, RVT
Owner
Just Wright Ultrasound Consulting, LLC
Fergus Falls, Minnesota
Fetal Echocardiography

Peggy Ann Malzi Bizjak, MBA, RDMS, RT(R)(M), CRA
Radiology Manager, Ultrasound Division
University of Virginia Health System;
Adjunct Faculty, Diagnostic Medical Sonography
    Program
Piedmont Virginia Community College
Charlottesville, Virginia
Introduction to Ergonomics and Sonographer Safety

Myka Bussey-Campbell, MEd, RT(R), RDMS
Program Coordinator, Diagnostic Medical
    Sonography Program
Department of Therapeutic and Therapeutic Sciences
Radiologic Sciences Degree Program
Armstrong Atlantic State University
Savannah, Georgia
*The Abdominal Aorta; The Inferior Vena Cava; The Portal
Venous System*

Reva Arnez Curry, PhD, RT, RDMS, FSDMS
Vice-President of Instruction and Learning Services
Delta College
University Center, Michigan
*Embryology; Introduction to Laboratory Values; The
Abdominal Aorta; The Inferior Vena Cava; The Portal
Venous System; The Biliary System; The Pancreas;
The Urinary and Adrenal Systems; The Spleen;
The Neonatal Brain*

Tiana V. Curry-McCoy, PhD
Assistant Professor, Medical Laboratory Science
Georgia Regents University
Augusta, Georgia
Introduction to Laboratory Values

Kacey Davis, BSRS, RDMS
Program Director, Diagnostic Medical Sonography
Darton State College
Albany, Georgia
The Spleen

Yonella Demars, MS, RDMS, RVT
Staff Sonographer/Clinical Preceptor
University of Virginia Medical Center
Charlottesville, Virginia
The Biliary System

Vivian G. Dicks, PhD, MPH, RDCS
Assistant Professor and Environmental Health
    Coordinator
Master of Public Health Program
Georgia Regents University
Augusta, Georgia
Pediatric Echocardiography

Kathryn A. Gill, MS, RT, RDMS
Program Director
Institute of Ultrasound Diagnostics
Mobile, Alabama
*Before and After the Ultrasound Examination; First
Scanning Experience*

Michael J. Kammermeier, RDMS, RVT, RDCS
America's Clinical Product Specialist
Voluson Ultrasound Education Manager,
    GE Healthcare
Venore, Tennessee
*The Male Pelvis: Prostate Gland and Seminal Vesicles
Sonography; Scrotal and Penile Sonography*

Zulfikarali H. Lalani, RDMS, RDCS, APS
Alta Bates Summit Medical Center
Department of Ultrasound
Merritt Pavilion
Oakland, California
*The Male Pelvis: Prostate Gland and Seminal Vesicles
Sonography; Scrotal and Penile Sonography*

Robbi R. King, BS, RDMS, RVT
Staff Sonographer
Winn Army Community Hospital
Fort Stewart, Georgia
*First Trimester Obstetrics (0 to 12 Weeks); Second and
Third Trimester Obstetrics (13 to 42 Weeks)*

Alexander Lane, PhD
Coordinator of Anatomy and Physiology
Triton College
River Grove, Illinois
Anatomy Layering and Sectional Anatomy

Wayne C. Leonhardt, BA, RDMS, RVT
Staff Sonographer
Mayo Clinic Hospital
Phoenix, Arizona;
Clinical Instructor, Diagnostic Medical
    Sonography Program
Gurnick Medical Academy
San Mateo, California
The Thyroid and Parathyroid Glands

Vivie Miller, BA, BS, RDMS, RDCS
Ultrasound Consultant and Clinical Specialist
Hephizabah, Georgia
Pediatric Echocardiography

Marsha M. Neumyer, BS, RVT, FSVU, FAIUM, FSDMS
International Director, Vascular Diagnostic
    Educational Services
Vascular Resource Associates
Harrisburg, Pennsylvania
Abdominal Vasculature; Vascular Technology

Timothy L. Owens, RDMS, RT(R), MBA
Staff Sonographer
Fossil Creek Care
San Antonio, Texas
*The Male Pelvis: Prostate Gland and Seminal Vesicles
Sonography; Scrotal and Penile Sonography*

J. Charles Pope III, PAC, RDCS, RVS
Echocardiology Clinical Coordinator
University Heart and Vascular Institute;
Assistant Clinical Professor, Allied Health Department
Georgia Regents University
Augusta, Georgia
Adult Echocardiography

Marilyn Dickerson Prince, MPH, RDMS, RVT
Vascular Ultrasound Supervisor Technologist
Emory University Hospital
Department of Radiology
Atlanta, Georgia
The Liver, The Gastrointestinal System, The Female Pelvis

Angie Rish, RDMS
Assistant Sonography Lab Instructor, Diagnostic
    Medical Sonography Program
Department of Diagnostic and Therapeutic Sciences
Armstrong Atlantic State University
Savannah, Georgia
The Neonatal Brain

Lisa Strohl, BS, RT(R), RDMS, RVT
Master Clinical Applications Specialist
GE Healthcare Ultrasound
Wauwatosa, Wisconsin
*Before and After the Ultrasound Examination; Ultrasound
Instrumentation: "Knobology," Imaging Processing, and
Storage; Breast Sonography*

Betty Bates Tempkin, BA
Ultrasound Consultant
Formerly Clinical Director of the Diagnostic Medical
    Sonography Program
Hillsborough Community College
Tampa, Florida
*Before and After the Ultrasound Examination;
General Patient Care; Interdependent Body Systems;
Anatomy Layering and Sectional Anatomy; First Scanning
Experience; Embryology; The Portal Venous System;
The Biliary System; The Pancreas; The Urinary and
Adrenal Systems, First Trimester Obstetrics (0 to 12
Weeks); Second and Third Trimester Obstetrics (13 to 42
Weeks); High-Risk Obstetric Sonography; The Neonatal
Brain; Interventional and Intraoperative Ultrasound*

Avian L. Tisdale, MD, FAAP
Division Director, Nemours Inpatient Pediatrics
    at *Inspira*
Vineland, New Jersey;
Clinical Assistant Professor of Pediatrics
Rowan University School of Osteopathic Medicine
Stratford, New Jersey
Embryology

Cheryl A. Vance, MA, RT, RDMS, RVT
Chief Executive Officer
C&D Advance Consultants, LLC
San Antonio, Texas
3-D/4-D Sonography

Reviewers

John B. Cassell, RT(R), RDMS, RVT, BS
Medical Sonography Program Coordinator
Forsyth Technical Community College
Winston-Salem, North Carolina

Marcia J. Cooper, MSRS, RT(R)(M)(CT)(QM), RDMS, RVT
Clinical Coordinator, Diagnostic Medical
    Sonography Program
Morehead State University
Morehead, Kentucky

Susanna Ovel, RT, RDMS, RVT
Senior Sonographer Instructor, Sutter
    Medical Foundation
Mint Medical Education
Sacramento, California

Catherine E. Rienzo, MS, RT(R), RDMS, FSDMS
Professor and Program Director, Diagnostic Medical
    Sonography Program
Northampton Community College
Bethlehem, Pennsylvania

Angela Smith, BS, RDMS
Director, Diagnostic Sonography,
    Department of Health Sciences
Parker University
Dallas, Texas

Kimberly Strong, BA, AS, RDMS, RVT
Program Director, Diagnostic Medical Sonography
Gwinnett Technical College
Lawrenceville, Georgia

Gloria Michelle Winings, RT, ARDMS
Program Director, USAF Diagnostic Medical
    Sonography Program
United States Air Force/Community College of
    the Air Force
Fort Sam Houston, Texas

Preface

Welcome to the fourth edition of *Sonography: Introduction to Normal Structure and Function*. This revision updates and expands upon all the elements that have made this title a success with students for over 20 years, presenting a thorough overview of normal ultrasound anatomy and physiology, delivered in a student-friendly manner—with easy-to-understand text, images, charts, tables, and study questions.

Our philosophy toward ultrasound education hasn't changed. The more comfortable the new sonographer is with normal anatomy and physiology and normal ultrasound appearance, the easier it is to recognize pathophysiology and differentiate abnormal ultrasound appearances. Hence, we spend a lot of time presenting multiple normal images with correlative gray scale illustrations to help the student understand sectional anatomy and its sonographic presentation.

Our learning strategy is a two-part repetition approach: first, repetition *within* each chapter through key words, various images, and detailed illustrations. Second, repetition *between* the textbook and the laboratory manual, where students are given another opportunity to study and work with keywords, objectives, un-labelled images, and additional assignments. The laboratory manual is strengthened though elements from the popular Bloom's Taxonomy cognitive learning strategy: memorization of key words, comprehension and application of objectives and related material, image analysis, and chapter evaluation. We feel the dual repetition approach combined with the Bloom's Taxonomy emphasis in the Workbook is an effective method to help students process what they have learned, from short-term into long-term memory. The end result, we hope, is improved didactic and clinical student performance from having studied and worked with our textbook and laboratory manual.

New to this Edition

For the fourth edition, we've made every effort to enhance our students' learning experience, while strengthening the features that have made previous editions of *Sonography* so effective. New features of the fourth edition include the following.

- **Three new chapters**—All new content is included in chapters on Ergonomics, Laboratory Values, and Fetal Echocardiography. The first introduces students to the importance of injury prevention as a practicing sonographer; the Laboratory Values chapter serves as a reference for normal, high, and low lab values; and Fetal Echocardiography discusses the anatomy and physiology of the fetal heart along with the imaging considerations necessary for its evaluation.
- **Brand new design**—A full, 4-color design presents the subject matter in an appealing way, and helps highlight important points within each chapter. Color images are placed upon mention within the appropriate chapter, rather than in a color plates section at the front of the book.
- **Updated sonograms and illustrations**—We have included 200 new drawings and images from state-of-the-art ultrasound equipment, demonstrating the latest and best images from the newest equipment, including 3D and 4D images.
- **Expanded test bank**—New questions for each chapter have increased the size of the test bank, providing over 1000 questions on the material for student assessment.
- **Review questions**—Over unique 500 review questions available to students on the companion Evolve site for extra practice with the chapter concepts.

Workbook and Lab Manual for Sonography: Introduction to Normal Structure and Function

Workbook and Lab Manual for Sonography: Introduction to Normal Structure and Function, a separate for-sale product, is a reinforcement and review tool for the information taught in the text. It supports and completes the text by providing an excellent introduction to sonography and in preparing students for the pathology to will encounter in their other textbooks later in their programs. For the fourth edition we have updated the images to match the text, and added extra review questions for students to test their knowledge. Lab exercises follow Bloom's taxonomy and promote critical thinking, a very important skill for future sonographers.

For the Instructor

The following resources are available at http://evolve.elsevier.com/Curry/sonography.

- PowerPoint slides for each chapter
- The test bank, available in Word or Examview, includes over 1000 questions
- The image collection can be downloaded in Power-Point or as jpeg files

We are honored to have prepared this fourth edition for you and hope you are as excited as we are about the end product. We believe sonographic learning is a journey that stretches our growth in the cognitive, affective, and psychomotor domains. We hope this textbook helps you accomplish this goal and thank you for including us in your educational journey. We also want to extend a special thank you to our contributors. Some have been with us since the beginning and others have joined us to give our very best to you. Without our contributors, this edition would not have been possible.

• • •

In closing...

Best wishes to didactic and clinical instructors; we hope this textbook and laboratory manual help you help your students be the very best you know they can be.

For sonography students, we extend to you warm regards and encouragement as you work to excel in exceptional patient care, superb diagnostic imaging and accurate technical observations. May you grow in wisdom and stature in the sonography profession.

Reva Arnez Curry and Betty Bates Tempkin

Contents

Clinical Applications

CHAPTER 1

Before and After the Ultrasound Examination

LISA STROHL, KATHRYN A. GILL, AND BETTY BATES TEMPKIN

OBJECTIVES

List the information that should be included on the ultrasound request form.

Explain the roles of the sonographer and sonologist/ radiologist.

Describe the importance of reviewing the patient's chart/ EMR (electronic medical record) prior to the examination.

Contrast technical observation against the interpretive report.

KEY WORDS

Assessment Notes — Results of the physical examination, including a listing of the patient's symptoms.

Differential Diagnoses — Multiple pathologic conditions that may be indicated by the ultrasound findings and reported as such by the interpreting physician.

Electronic Medical Record (EMR) — A computer-based version of a patient's medical information.

Hepatitis B (HBV) — Bloodborne pathogen that requires Standard Precautions to reduce exposure risk. Health care workers can protect themselves with the hepatitis B vaccine, which requires 3 shots over 6 months and is offered at most health care facilities.

Human Immunodeficiency Virus (HIV) — Bloodborne pathogen that requires Standard Precautions to reduce exposure risk.

Virus may lead to AIDS, a deficiency of the autoimmune system that in many cases is terminal.

Interpretive Report (Final Report) — Sonologist's (radiologist, physician) formal, legal, interpretive report of the ultrasound findings.

Occupational Safety and Health Administration (OSHA) — An agency within the United States Department of Labor. OSHA standards are designed to protect health care workers from major bloodborne diseases.

Patient Chart — Compilation of patient information, including medical history, results of physical examination, patient's symptoms, and laboratory test results.

Sonographer — Ultrasound professional responsible for performing and recording ultrasound studies for physician interpretation.

Sonologist/Radiologist — Physician responsible for providing the final, legal, interpretive report (which may include differential diagnoses) of ultrasound findings.

Standard Precautions — Treating all patients as if they may have HBV/HIV or other bloodborne disease, meaning that engineering, workplace, and housekeeping controls are in place to ensure safety.

Technical Observation — Sonographer's written summary of ultrasound findings using sonographic terminology. Never a diagnosis, as it is not considered justified (level of education, training, experience) or legal.

Ultrasound Request Form — Patient identification data, clinical symptoms, the examination requested, and the reason why.

Sonographers enter the allied health field of diagnostic medical sonography through several avenues. Programs may be hospital based or in vocational-technology institutes, the military, colleges, and universities. Curriculum includes courses in cross-sectional anatomy, ultrasound physics and instrumentation, physiology, pathology, patient care, and medical ethics. Most programs prefer that applicants have previous health care experience or a science background. In some cases, high school graduates and liberal arts students are accepted based on grade point average and completed levels of science and math. Most employers prefer sonographers trained in accredited programs and certified by registry. The American Registry of Diagnostic Medical Sonography (ARDMS) credential is by written examination based on professional standards. Certification can be earned in multiple sonography specialties, including abdominal sonography, obstetric and gynecology sonography, neurosonography, breast sonography, adult and pediatric echocardiography, and vascular technology. The sonographer is also required to take the Sonography Principles and Instrumentation (SPI) exam at the time of certification. At present, there is no assessment of scanning ability.

Sonographers work with ultrasound imaging equipment to produce cross-section images of anatomy and diagnostic data. Specific responsibilities include the following that will be discussed in greater detail in later chapters:

- Good communication skills
- Ability to obtain and record patient data pertinent to the ultrasound study
- Proper use of ultrasound machinery
- Provide quality patient care
- Acquire, analyze, modify, and select images to record and present to the interpreting physician for diagnosis
- Use ultrasound terminology to prepare a written (or oral) technical summary of the ultrasound findings, which are presented to the interpreting physician
- Assist with ultrasound-guided invasive procedures
- Knowledge of Standard Precautions

Sonographers have a high level of responsibility in the ultrasound diagnostic process, and when performed at the highest level they become an essential part of patient evaluation.

BEFORE THE ULTRASOUND EXAMINATION
Understanding Standard Precautions

Increased concern for health care workers becoming infected with bloodborne diseases through accidental needle sticks and spills was the impetus for the Occupational Safety and Health Administration (OSHA) to issue a standard designed to protect these workers. The major bloodborne diseases that health care providers may be exposed to on the job include the various forms of hepatitis, such as hepatitis B (HBV), and syphilis, malaria, and human immunodeficiency virus (HIV). Of these, HBV and HIV are the two most significant. These diseases can be transmitted in body fluids such as blood, saliva, semen, vaginal secretions, amniotic fluid, and cerebrospinal, synovial, and pericardial fluid. Other sources of transmission could include dental procedures, handling unfixed tissues or organs from living or dead humans, handling cell or tissue cultures contaminated with HIV/HBV, as well as organ cultures and culture mediums or similar solutions. Research workers must also be careful when handling blood, organs, or tissues from HIV-/HBV-contaminated experimental animals. Health care workers must use caution when handling blood, organs, or tissues from known HIV/HBV patients. Health care workers can protect themselves with the hepatitis B vaccine, which requires 3 shots over 6 months and is offered by most health care facilities. See Table 1-1 for a summary of sources of transmission and how transmission can occur.

There are many ways these diseases can be transmitted. Accidental injuries from contaminated sharp objects—such as needles, scalpels, broken glass, and exposed dental wires—are among the most common. Exposure can occur from open cuts and skin abrasions, including dermatitis and acne, and via mucous membranes of the mouth, nose, and eyes. Touching contaminated surfaces and transferring the infectious material to the mouth, nose, or eyes is a more indirect means of transmission. Health care workers must be aware that work surfaces can be heavily contaminated without visible evidence. Surface contamination is a major mode of transmission for HBV, especially in hemodialysis units. It is known that HBV can survive dried on surfaces at room temperature for a week!

■ ■ ☐ **Table 1-1** Sources of HBV/HIV Transmission and How Transmission Occurs

Sources of Transmission of HBV/HIV	How Transmission Can Occur
Blood, saliva, vaginal secretions	Accidental injuries from contaminated sharp objects
Amniotic, cerebrospinal, synovial, pericardial fluids	Sharp objects such as needles, scalpels, broken glass, dental wires
Dental procedures, inappropriate handling of human tissues from living or dead sources, and organ cultures or mediums	Exposure from open cuts and skin abrasions, including dermatitis and acne and transfer to mucous membranes
Handling infected blood, tissues, and/or organs from known infected animals	Touching contaminated surfaces and transferring contaminants to eye, nose, and/or mouth

Since we cannot know, with certainty, every patient carrying or infected with a bloodborne disease, Standard Precautions require treating all patients as if they were known to be infected with HIV/HBV, or other bloodborne disease. OSHA guidelines provide five major tactics to reduce risks of exposure (Table 1-2) that include the following:

- Establishing engineering controls
- Employee work practices
- Housekeeping protocols
- Providing personal protective equipment
- Offering vaccination against hepatitis B

Engineering controls involve things such as the utilization of autoclaves and sterilization methods, self-sheathing needles, and the use of biosafety cabinets and proper disposal methods.

Work practice protocols include wearing protective gear such as gowns, face shields, and gloves and concentration on personal hygiene, such as frequent handwashing. Handwashing with soap and water should be performed for at least 30 seconds before and after the ultrasound examination is performed.

Housekeeping controls include keeping equipment clean and contaminant free as well as disposing of sharps and laundry into the appropriate containers.

Last, vaccination against hepatitis B is optional and is provided at no cost to health care employees if their jobs put them at risk for exposure. The vaccine is administered over a 6-month period, in three injections, and is 85% to 97% effective for 9 years or longer. Those who should not be vaccinated include individuals whose antibody test indicates they are immune, those who have already received the complete vaccination series, or those with a specific medical reason. Although the vaccination does not reduce exposure to the disease, it does protect the health care worker if exposure occurs.

Medical facilities are now required to offer an in-service to employees regarding the OSHA requirements and guidelines. Check with the Human Resources or Infection Control departments for scheduled in-services at individual facilities.

Sonographers must be well trained in how to reduce exposure to bloodborne pathogens for themselves and others before actually examining patients. Once Standard Precautions are mastered, entry-level sonographers should turn their attention to the essential documents for ultrasound studies. These include the ultrasound request form, patient chart, technical observation, and final interpretative report.

Reviewing the Ultrasound Request Form and Patient Chart

A sonographer is responsible for acquiring patient information pertinent to the ultrasound study before the examination procedure.

This process begins when the sonographer reviews the ultrasound request form and patient chart before the ultrasound examination is performed. An ultrasound request form should include patient identification data, clinical symptoms, type of examination requested, and reason for the examination.

A sample ultrasound request form is shown in Figure 1-1. This form includes four main sections:

Section One
- Space to record patient identification
- Information needed to report preliminary results
- Check box for "stat" or portable procedures
- Check box for patients who require isolation precautions

Section Two
- Requesting physician's or clinic's name, address, and contact number(s)
- Essential clinical data explaining reason the examination has been requested

Section Three
- For additional patient history
- Bar code for computerized entry into the department's data system
- Space for requesting physician's signature and contact number(s)

Section Four
- Check boxes for the type of examination ordered
- Space for sonographer identification and where the procedure was performed

■ ■ ■ **Table 1-2** Strategies to Reduce Exposure to Bloodborne Pathogens

Strategy to Reduce Exposure to Bloodborne Pathogens	Description/Examples
Engineering controls	Medical instruments or practices that reduce the risk of exposure such as autoclaves and sterilization methods, self-sheathing needles, biosafety precautions
Work practice protocols	Gloves when handling blood or bodily fluids, additional protective gear, including gowns, may be indicated; proper and frequent handwashing is essential
Housekeeping controls	Keeping equipment clean and contaminant free; disposal of sharps and laundry in appropriate containers
Hepatitis B vaccination*	3 doses over 6-month period recommended for health care workers at risk

*Does not reduce exposure, but does protect the health care worker should exposure occur.

ULTRASOUND REQUEST
THOMAS JEFFERSON UNIVERSITY HOSPITAL
DEPARTMENT OF RADIOLOGY
DIVISION OF DIAGNOSTIC ULTRASOUND

MEDICAL
RECORD #
NAME

ADDRESS

AGE

BIRTH

PHONE NO.

☐ STAT

☐ PORTABLE

CALL PRELIMINARY REPORT TO:

DOCTOR

LOCATION

PHONE NO

ISOLATION PRECAUTION ☐ YES

REFERING PHYSICIAN/CLINIC (NAME & ADDRESS)   PHONE NO.

ESSENTIAL CLINICAL FACTS • (MUST BE COMPLETED BEFORE EXAMINATION IS PERFORMED)

REASON FOR EXAMINATION

RELEVANT MEDICAL HISTORY

A 3 4 1 4 7 6

PHYSICIAN'S SIGNATURE & BEEPER#   DATE

ABDOMEN	PELVIS	GYNECOLOGY
ABDOMEN COMPLETE	**RENAL TRANSPLANT**	**PELVIS COMPLETE**
LIVER	URINARY BLADDER	UTERUS
GALLBLADDER	PROSTATE	OVARIES
SPLEEN	RECTUM	FOLLICLE SIZE
ASCITES	SCROTUM	IUD LOCALIZATION
PALPABLE MASS	DOPPLER	DOPPLER
DOPPLER	**HEAD AND NECK**	**OBSTETRICAL**
RETROPERITONEUM	BRAIN	**FETAL COMPLETE**
RETROPERITONEUM COMPLETE	URINARY BLADDER	FETAL COMPLETE (INTERNAL GROWTH)
PANCREAS	URINARY BLADDER	OBSTETRIC DOPPLER
KIDNEYS	**HEART**	AMNIOCENTESIS
ADRENALS	**COMPLETE ECHOCARDIOGRAM**	SPECIAL (SPECIFY)
AORTA/IVC	M-MODE & 2D ECHOCARDIOGRAM	**SUPERFICIAL**
LYMPH NODES	DOPPLER ECHOCARDIOGRAM	BREAST
DOPPLER	**VASCULAR**	PALPABLE
CHEST	CEREBROVASCULAR COMPLETE	JOINT/TENDON/MUSCLE
MEDIASTINUM	PERIPHERAL VASC. (ARTERIAL)	**INTERVENTIONAL**
PLEURAL EFFUSION	PERIPHERAL VASC. (VENOUS)	BIOPSY (SPECIFY AREA BELOW)
THORACENTESIS	☐ IMAGING ☐ IPG	ASPIRATION (SPECIFY AREA BELOW)
	NOT LISTED	ABSCESS DRAINAGE
	(SPECIFY)	INTRAOPERATIVE GUIDANCE
		AREA:

EXAM.

TECH.

ROOM

DATE

FIGURE 1-1   **Radiology Department Request Form.** (Modified from Pinkney N: *A review of concepts of ultrasound physics and instrumentation,* ed 4, Copiague, NY, 1992, Sonicor, Inc.)

The request form in Figure 1-1 stresses information needed in that particular tertiary care center. Notice the effort to accommodate requesting physicians by providing a checklist of the different types of ultrasound procedures offered and the request to receive a preliminary reading from the interpreting physician (sonologist/radiologist). Check your institution's request form to see where the information listed here is located.

Another document that sonographers review before an inpatient examination is the **patient chart** or **Electronic Medical Record (EMR)**. Box 1-1 provides the

---

■ ■ □ BOX 1-1 PATIENT CHART

ROUTINE INPATIENT CHART
1. Diagnosis worksheet
2. Admission form
3. Consent for routine examination and treatment
4. Patient authorizations
5. Consent for operations, procedures, etc.
6. Consent for anesthesia
7. Release form
8. Living will
9. Preadmission forms
10. Physician's orders for admission
11. Discharge summary
12. Discharge summary sheet
13. Emergency room record
14. Patient care plan
15. Acute dialysis unit patient care plan
16. Patient problem list
17. Nursing transfer summary
18. History, physical progress notes
19. Social work evaluation and social work notes go in date order within progress notes
20. Respiratory care department, patient care record
21. Patient teaching record
22. Discharge planning record
23. Discharge planning assessment
24. Home IV therapy performance checklist
25. Instructions to patient
26. Discharge summary note
27. Consultations
28. Cardiac catheterization reports:
    Preoperative nursing record, cardiac catheterization nursing report, preliminary catheterization report Catheterization report
29. Operative reports: Perioperative nursing record
30. Preoperative anesthesia summary
31. Operative notes
32. Pathology
33. OR sponge/instrument count
34. Postanesthesia record
35. Recovery room record
36. Cardiopulmonary perfusion record
37. Endoscopy report
38. Fiberoptic bronchoscopy
39. Data mount
40. Clinical laboratory summary sheets
41. Medical Respiratory Intensive Care Unit (MRICU) blood gas laboratory report
42. Radiology reports
43. Ultrasound reports
44. ECG/EKG rhythm strips
45. EEG
46. Nuclear medicine
47. Pulmonary function test
48. Request for blood components and testing
49. Antibody ID report
50. Blood component-ID tag
51. Miscellaneous
52. Energy expenditure/nutrition department
53. Cardiopulmonary resuscitation record
54. Transfer order sheet
55. Adult total nutrient admixture physician's treatment sheet
56. Acute dialysis unit treatment sheet
57. Physician's treatment sheets: *Precatheterization order, postanesthesia physician's treatment sheets*
58. Physician's order sheet for antimicrobial agents
59. Assessment notes:
    Assessment guidelines/falls risk potential, assessment guidelines/pressure sore potential, nursing assessment, daily assessment
60. Medication administration record
61. Nursing Kardex
62. Nursing care record
63. Critical care flow sheet
64. Flow sheet
65. Neurologic assessment sheet
66. Neurologic checklist
67. Diabetes control chart
68. Intake-output chart
69. Graphic record

OB CHART
1. Diagnosis worksheet
2. Admission form
3. Consent forms
4. Obstetric discharge summary
5. Prenatal: *Initial pregnancy profile, health history summary, prenatal flow record*
6. Perinatal database
7. Patient care plan
8. Progress notes
9. Discharge instruction sheet
10. Operative notes
11. Delivery room count record
12. Labor unit prep room assessment
13. Hollister forms: *Obstetric admitting record, labor progress chart, labor and delivery summary, postpartum progress notes*
14. Laboratory test results
15. Radiology
16. ECG/EKG

Continued

■ ■ ■   **BOX 1-1** PATIENT CHART—cont'd

17. Obstetric ultrasound
18. Antenatal evaluation center form
19. Physician's treatment sheets
20. Medication sheets
21. Nursing Kardex
22. Nursing care record
23. (Antenatal unit) pad count
24. Intake-output chart
25. Graphic record

BABY CHART
1. Diagnosis worksheet
2. Admission form
3. Birth certificate
4. Consent forms
5. Newborn discharge summary
6. Pediatric admission nursing assessment and discharge planning
7. Patient care plan
8. Progress notes
9. Discharge instructions
10. Hollister forms: *Obstetric admitting record, labor and delivery summary, labor progress chart, initial newborn profile, newborn flow record*
11. Footprints
12. MicroBase
13. Laboratory test results
14. Newborn maturity rating and class
15. Growth record for infants
16. Audiologic record
17. Impedance measurement
18. Neonatal neurosonography
19. Pulmonary evaluation and diagnostic system
20. Neonatal test report
21. Physician's treatment sheets
22. Nursing Kardex

23. Flow sheet
24. IV therapy record
25. Apnea and bradycardia record

REHAB CHART
Same order as medical chart except for the following forms:
1. Patient discharge/readmission form: before discharge summary
2. Assessment/treatment/plan/goals form: before progress notes. Department of Rehabilitation Medicine progress note. Sheet: behind progress notes
3. Interdisciplinary conference summary and discharge plan form: after progress notes
The following forms are placed in the miscellaneous section of the chart in the order listed:
4. Neurologic examination
5. Record of patient visits
6. Occupational therapy section form
7. Physical therapy section, general rehabilitation in-patient summary form

PSYCHIATRY ASSEMBLY ORDER CHART
1. Application for involuntary emergency examination and treatment forms are placed behind consent forms
2. Psychiatric database form: after ER sheets
3. 12-hour treatment plan: after psychiatric database
4. Creative arts therapies form: after 72-hour treatment plan
5. Psychiatric database, corresponds to admissions
6. Crisis medication sheet: before medication administration sheets
7. Seclusion/restraint observation record: behind flow sheets
8. Observation checklist for patients in seclusion or on suicide precautions form: behind seclusion/restraint observation record

different information that may be included. The most important items in a patient's chart for sonographers to review are assessment notes, laboratory test results, and reports from any correlating image modality studies (i.e., CAT scan). **Assessment notes** include results from the patient's physical examination, a list of his or her symptoms, and any other notable findings.

Outpatient charts usually stay in referring physician's offices; hence, the sonographer may not have access to it. Therefore, it is essential that the ultrasound request contain the patient's clinical symptoms and reason for the ultrasound study being ordered.

Additionally, many ultrasound departments require sonographers to take a brief medical history from the patient before conducting the examination. In lieu of a detailed history provided on the request form, this may be the only means of obtaining pertinent information for outpatient examinations.

AFTER THE ULTRASOUND EXAMINATION
The Sonographer's Technical Observation
The responsibilities of a sonographer include collecting pertinent clinical information before the examination, providing patient care during the examination, documenting representative images of the ultrasound findings to provide the sonologist/physician with the information necessary to arrive at a diagnosis, and describing the ultrasound findings, using sonographic terminology, to the interpreting physician.

In addition, after a study is completed, most institutions require sonographers to complete a worksheet (an examination data sheet) to accompany the images. The data generally include the information a sonographer gathered from patient charts, the request form, and/or the patients themselves:
• Medical history
• Clinical symptoms

FETAL AGE

DIAGNOSIS

Findings compatible with complete spontaneous abortion, ectopic pregnancy, or very early intrauterine pregnancy.

COMMENT

Real-time ultrasound of the pelvis was performed using transabdominal and endovaginal technique. No previous studies are available for review. The patient has a positive urine pregnancy test by history.

The uterus measures 10.2 × 4.2 × 5.0 cm. No intrauterine gestational sac is identified on transabdominal or endovaginal scan.

The left ovary is enlarged, measuring 4.2 × 2.9 × 3.6 cm. A cystic structure measuring less than 1 cm is seen in the left ovary.

The right ovary measures 2.6 × 1.1 × 2.8 cm. There are no right adnexal masses.

There is no free fluid in the cul de sac.

In light of the history of positive urine pregnancy test, the differential diagnosis for the above findings includes complete spontaneous abortion, ectopic pregnancy, or, less likely, very early intrauterine pregnancy. Correlation with serial beta-HCGs is advised.

Survey views of both kidneys reveal no hydronephrosis.

FIGURE 1-2 **Example of Radiologist/Sonologist's Final Interpretive Report.** (Modified from Pinkney N: *A review of concepts of ultrasound physics and instrumentation*, ed 4, Copiague, NY, 1992, Sonicor, Inc.)

• Pertinent laboratory test results
• Any reports from other imaging tests or procedures

Some institutions may also require sonographers to provide a technical observation. A **technical observation** is a summary of the ultrasound findings, written by the sonographer using sonographic terminology. Written documentation of any type almost always becomes part of a patient's medical record. For this reason, a sonographer's technical observation should be documented in a way as to not be legally compromising.

Technical observations should be confined to descriptions of the ultrasound findings based on echo pattern and size (see Chapter 7 for further detail). The origin or location, number, size, and composition are also included for descriptions of abnormal findings. Sonographers should *never* provide diagnoses (interpretive results or technical impressions) because it would be unjustified (according to a sonographer's level of education, training, and experience) and potentially legally compromising. Only physicians are justified (according to level of education, training, and experience) to render diagnoses.

A sonographer who has individual knowledge and experience can obviously draw his or her own conclusion based on the ultrasound findings. Even so, a sonographer's conclusion regarding an ultrasound examination should *never* be part of the technical observation. The sonographer should comply with the heading "technical observation" by simply **describing what is seen in sonographic terms**. Note that describing the sonographic appearance of abnormal ultrasound findings does not depend on knowledge of diseases and their sonographic presentations. This will be discussed in further detail in Chapter 7.

■ ■ ■ **CLINICAL CORRELATION**

Writing technical observations requires restraint and the careful selection of appropriate sonographic terminology. Keep in mind that technical observations are a summary of a sonographer's findings that may serve as a reference for the interpreting physician; however, it is the documented images provided by the sonographer that the physician uses to render a diagnosis. If a sonographer fails to make an accurate description in the technical observation but demonstrates the findings on the images, he or she has performed **within the legal guidelines of the scope of practice for diagnostic medical sonographers**. The final interpretation of the ultrasound examination will always be the responsibility of the physician. By virtue of education, training, and legal parameters, physicians exclusively render diagnoses.

Chapter 7 provides examples of how to describe abnormal ultrasound findings or pathology.

Interpretive Report

When the ultrasound examination is completed, the sonologist (usually a radiologist; always a physician) provides an **interpretive report (final report)** that includes a detailed description and diagnosis of the ultrasound findings. The rendered diagnosis may be a definitive diagnosis or a **differential diagnosis** that includes multiple possible pathologic conditions indicated by the ultrasound findings (Figure 1-2).

A copy of the final report is sent to the requesting physician; a copy goes in an inpatient's chart or EMR, and a copy is kept in the patient's ultrasound file.

- # CHAPTER 2

Ultrasound Instrumentation: "Knobology," Imaging Processing, and Storage

LISA STROHL

OBJECTIVES

Explain why it is important to learn the "knobology" of the ultrasound system.

Compare and contrast the functions of the keyboard controls: primary imaging controls, calculation controls, and additional controls.

Demonstrate the steps to operate the ultrasound system.

Describe the differences between PACS, HIS, and RIS.

Discuss the functions of the electronic "Worklist" program.

KEY WORDS

Additional Controls — Imaging controls such as body pattern, Doppler, power Doppler, pulsed wave, M Mode, and screen monitor controls.

Alphanumeric Keyboard — Keyboard on the ultrasound system that allows alphabetic and numeric characters to be entered for the patient's examination.

Calc Key — Appropriate calculations package based on imaging preset.

Clinical Applications Specialist — Customizes imaging settings and measurements; demonstrates proper use of ultrasound system.

HELP Menu — Accesses reference manual for ultrasound system.

Hospital Information System (HIS) — Electronic system that stores patient demographic information and medical records.

Knobology — Ultrasound system controls including (1) primary imaging, (2) calculation, and (3) additional controls.

PACS — Acronym for Picture Archiving and Communications System. PACS enables improved image resolution as images are stored in digital format and manipulated by software controls.

Primary Imaging Controls — Controls such as imaging preset, frequency, depth, and time-gain compensation (TGC) that directly affect image quality.

Radiology Information System (RIS) — Electronic, radiology-specific network that supports imaging, reporting, and relevant patient data. RIS is generally a subsystem of HIS.

Teleradiology — Radiologists consult for imaging diagnoses using PACS to view images transmitted from site of origin.

Ultrasound Field Service Engineer — Performs installation of ultrasound system at imaging site.

Ultrasound System — Software-based control system for image settings and measurements.

This chapter describes ultrasound system controls and explains how to operate them along with image processing and storage. Ultrasound systems are software-based units that need to be configured correctly before some controls will appear on the ultrasound system's touch panel or function as expected on the operator control panel. An ultrasound field service engineer performs the initial configuration at the installation of the ultrasound system. The clinical applications specialist then demonstrates the proper use of the system and customizes imaging settings and measurements for use by the facility.

Although hospitals around the world employ different types of ultrasound systems, the basic "knobology" is the same. Some common control buttons and their functions are explained in this chapter. Sonographers must master these controls in order to produce optimal images and retrieve diagnostic information from the ultrasound examination.

ALPHANUMERIC KEYBOARD

The alphanumeric keyboard controls allow the sonographer to enter the patient's name, ID number, and full-screen annotation (although some software programs like "Worklist" will enter patient data automatically once the correct patient is selected). The keyboard may also include specific function keys, as indicated in Table 2-1.

Some systems employ a HELP Menu to access and provide a quick reference manual to the system usage.

■ ■ ■ **Table 2-1** Keyboard Controls and Functions

Keyboard Controls	Function	Comments
Annotation On/Off or Comments On/Off	Allows annotation or comments to be entered on the screen	Many systems have a library of preprogrammed, commonly used annotations based on the imaging preset selected
Erase/Clear/Clear Screen	Erases all user-entered annotations from where the cursor is located	
Backspace	Erases the last character to the left of the cursor	
New Patient Key/End Current Patient	Clears current patient ID, graphics, stored images, and comments	Allows new information to be entered

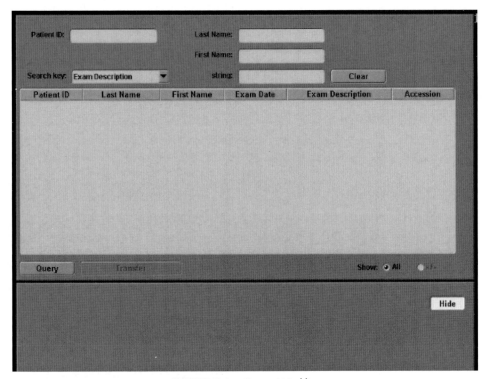

FIGURE 2-1   Query Worklist.

This is often accessed through a HELP key located directly on the keyboard, or it is a function key located on the top row of the keyboard. Information to be input into the system can be taken off the patient request form. Many hospitals and imaging centers now use an electronically driven program referred to as "Worklist." Patient information is electronically transferred to the ultrasound system via Worklist. Sonographers are able to "query" Worklist from their ultrasound system through a dedicated computer network (Figure 2-1). Detailed pertinent patient information such as full name, date of birth, referring physician, medical record number, and type of study are then populated into a patient information page on the ultrasound system (Figure 2-2). Sonographers may also input their initials on examinations they perform. This type of program facilitates department tracking of procedures and helps maintain quality control.

PRIMARY IMAGING CONTROLS

Primary imaging controls directly affect imaging quality. The clinical application specialist will encourage staff sonographers to experiment with the controls to see the varying effects on the resulting images. An experienced sonographer will be able to quickly learn how to manipulate the controls so the images will be of optimal

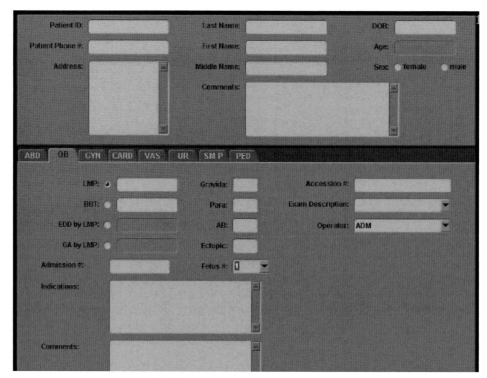

FIGURE 2-2   Patient Information Page.

diagnostic quality. Students need more time, not only to locate the controls but also to understand the effect each control has on an image. First, students should be encouraged to study the system manual, then locate and manipulate the system controls, and, finally, observe the effect each control has on the resulting image. Table 2-2 lists the primary imaging controls.

Based on imaging preset, the appropriate calculations package is activated by the Calc key. Specific measurement keys sonographers use frequently are listed in Table 2-3.

Table 2-4 shows additional controls that are used to complete the knobology necessary for optimal imaging.

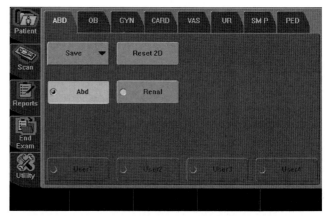

FIGURE 2-3   Imaging Presets for Ultrasound Facility.

■ ■ ■ **Table 2-2**   Primary Imaging Controls and Functions

Primary Imaging Control	Sonographers Use This To...	Comments
Transducer/Probe Button	Select different transducers/probes	
Imaging Preset/Model	Select an appropriate imaging preset or model as a starting point for preprogrammed imaging parameters (Figure 2-3)	This is the starting point from which the examination will be performed.
Frequency	Select imaging frequency based on patient anatomy and type of examination	Better tissue resolution of superficial structures is attained with higher frequencies. Lower imaging frequency is used for deeper structures, but image definition for more superficial structures will be lost.
Depth	Select imaging depth of 2-D and overall gain (for most examinations)	Adjusts image size.

■ ■ ■ **Table 2-2** Primary Imaging Controls and Functions—cont'd

Primary Imaging Control	Sonographers Use This To...	Comments
Time-Gain Compensation (TGC)	Equalize differences in received echo amplitudes due to reflector depth	Returning echoes from deep in the body are amplified so information on deeper structures can be received.
TGC Curve	Display TGC information (Figure 2-4, A and B)	TGC curve is located vertically on the right side of the ultrasound image on the screen. Shape of the TGC curve is affected by the TGC setting.
Focal Zone Position and Focal Number	Position the focal zone to the desired scan depth (Figure 2-5, A and B)	Adds or removes additional focal zones.
Dual Image and/or Left/Right Key	Display two images side by side for comparison	Image measurements can be compared.
Image Direction	Reverse the scan direction of the displayed image	Image will change from either a right to left direction or up and down direction.
Freeze Key	"Freeze" image and suspend real time. Press button again to unfreeze image and resume real time	After image is stored, measurements and calculations can be performed.
Cine Loop	Store recently scanned image frames into system memory before freeze key is depressed	Images can be reviewed by sonographer using this control.
Print/Store Key	Activate programmed storage device to store frozen image	The system will remain in "freeze" until image is stored.
Trackball	1. Guide cursor on the screen 2. Position measurement cursors during freeze mode 3. Change the scan area for the sector size and color box size for Doppler and color Doppler application	A "set" or "enter" key allows sonographer to set the selection made through the trackball function. In systems with cine loop, 2-D images can be scrolled in real time. Trackball can serve additional functions depending on the system.

2-D, Two-dimensional.

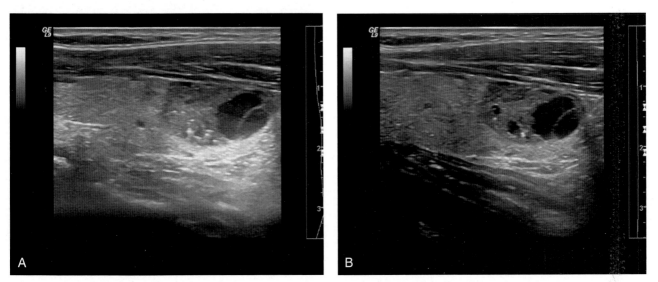

FIGURE 2-4 **A,** Incorrect time-gain compensation (TGC) control placement. **B,** Correct TGC control placement.

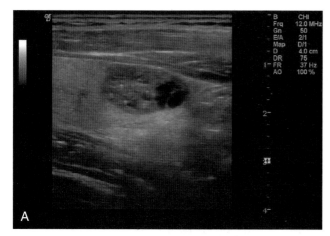

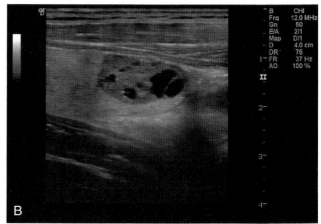

FIGURE 2-5 **A,** Incorrect focal zone. The focal zone is too low in this thyroid examination; thus the thyroid mass cannot be accurately assessed. Observe the focal zone indicator on the right side of the screen. **B,** Correct focal zone. Proper focal zone placement in the same patient. Notice that the focal zone indicator is at the same level as the mass. Now the internal components of the mass can be accurately assessed.

Table 2-3 Measurement Keys and Functions

Measurement Keys	Function
Distance	Place cursors for distance measurements (Figure 2-6).
Trace/Ellipse	Outline for curve or circumference measurements (Figure 2-7).
Measure	Complete measurements and display results to calculate volume measurements (Figure 2-8).
Off	Erase cursors, outlines, and measurement results.

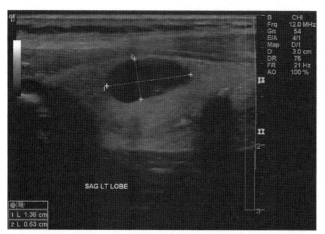

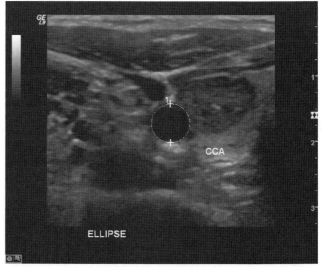

FIGURE 2-6 **Distance Measurement.** Note (1) calibers as shown on the screen measure 1.36 cm in length, and (2) calibers taken perpendicular to the first set of calibers measure 0.63 cm anteroposteriorly.

FIGURE 2-7 **Circumference Measurement.** The trace/ellipse key is used to outline the circumference and calculate the measurement of this axial section of the common carotid artery.

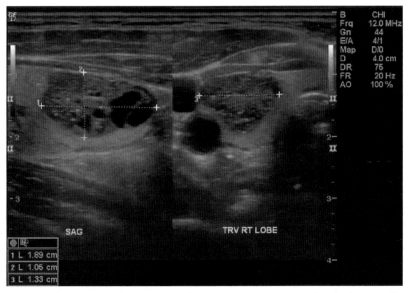

FIGURE 2-8 **Volume Measurement.** Complete measurements using the dual image feature to measure an abnormal mass in the right lobe of the thyroid gland. Three sets of measurements are taken: two in a longitudinal section of the mass, (1) long axis and (2) depth measurements; and (3) a width measurement in an axial section of the mass. Thus, three dimensions of the mass are obtained and a volume measurement can be calculated: L × W × D = Volume.

■ ■ ■ **Table 2-4** Additional Controls and Functions

Additional Controls	Functions	Comments
Body Pattern	Displays body pattern to indicate patient positioning (Figure 2-9).	Pattern is displayed on the monitor screen and on images.
Color Doppler/Power Doppler/Power Angio/ Pulsed Wave/M Mode	Activates color or power Doppler, pulsed-wave, and/or M mode imaging (Figures 2-10 to 2-13).	Imaging and trackball will change based on which imaging mode is activated.
Monitor Controls	Controls on the system monitor that can be adjusted to improve visualization of images. Brightness and contrast controls are two main controls on the display monitor.	Brightness control: adjusts light output for the image. Contrast control: adjusts the difference in light and dark parts of the image. Note: maintaining a very high–contrast level display setting can eventually damage the monitor screen. Avoid using high-contrast settings for extended periods. See the system manufacturer's guidelines for recommended contrast, brightness, and temperature settings.

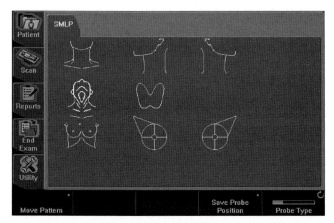

FIGURE 2-9 **Body Pattern Display.** Various body parts can be shown on the imaging screen and on the images.

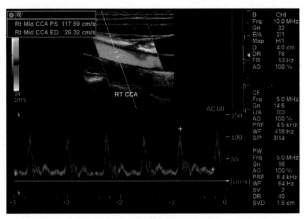

FIGURE 2-10 Color flow Doppler and pulsed wave imaging of a longitudinal section of the common carotid artery with pulsed wave with measurements.

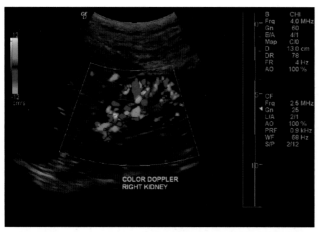

FIGURE 2-11   Color flow Doppler of a longitudinal section of the right kidney.

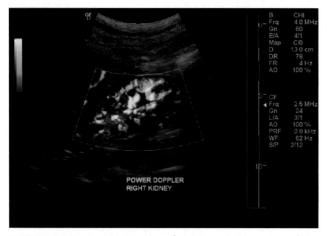

FIGURE 2-12   Power Doppler of a longitudinal section of the right kidney.

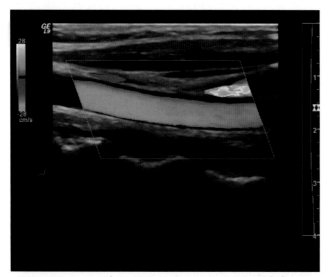

FIGURE 2-13   Longitudinal section of the common carotid artery with color flow Doppler box steered to the right or toward the feet.

BASIC OPERATIONS OF AN ULTRASOUND SYSTEM

Use the following steps when operating the ultrasound system:

1. Enter Patient Name and ID:
   - Either select "new patient" soft key or "query" the Worklist to select the current patient.
   - The "query" function will update a list of current patients in the Radiology Information System (RIS). Note: RIS is discussed in the next section.
2. Select Appropriate Transducer and Scanning Preset:
   - See Box 2-1 for types of transducers.
3. Place transducer on the patient with a generous amount of coupling gel.
4. Adjust TGC until the desired image is obtained.
5. Adjust focal zones to cover the area of interest in the image.
6. Adjust image size using depth control.

Proper use of these controls must be coupled with appropriate transducer selection, as seen in Box 2-1.

Table 2-5 lists specialized transducers that are available to help view specific areas of the body or for ultrasound-guided special procedures.

IMAGE PROCESSING AND STORAGE

Technology has rapidly moved image processing into the twenty-first century. Many hospitals and practices employ a range of image storage techniques, from the very basic to the most technologically advanced.

Most hospitals and imaging centers currently run filmless by using a computer technology system called **PACS**, an acronym for Picture Archiving and

---

■ ■ ■   **BOX 2-1** TRANSDUCERS

TRANSDUCERS AVAILABLE WITH MOST UNITS
Linear array
Matrix array
Curved or convex array
Electronic phased array
Vector or sector array

SMALL-FOOTPRINT TRANSDUCERS
Small parts/superficial Imaging
10 MHz, 12 MHz, 14 MHz, 15 MHz, 18 MHz (i.e., to scan the thyroid gland, scrotum, musculoskeletal, etc.)

■ ■ ■   **Table 2-5**   Specialized Transducers and Functions

Specialized Transducers	Functions
Endocavitary	Transvaginal and transrectal
Intraoperative and laparoscopic	Performed under surgical conditions
Endoluminal	Imaging within vessels

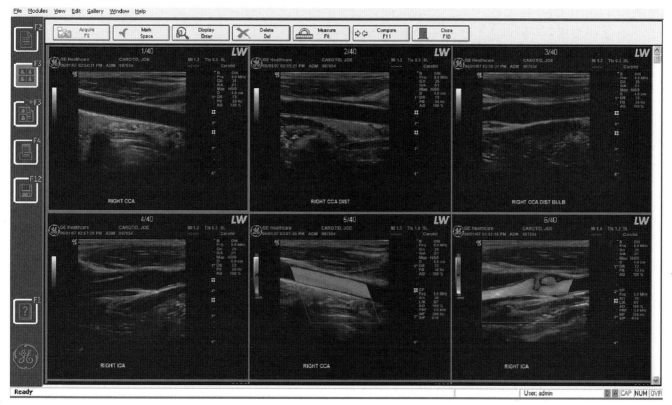

FIGURE 2-14   **PACS Image Viewer.** (Courtesy GE Healthcare.)

Communication System. This computer technology allows for improved image resolution as images are stored in a digital format and are software controlled.

Ultrasound images are acquired digitally and are viewed and stored on a computer and/or network server (Figure 2-14). This system can be dedicated to the ultrasound department or used on a larger scale throughout the entire radiology division and hospital. PACS can communicate with outside hospitals and imaging centers located anywhere in the world that are also equipped with PACS capabilities.

PACS's ability to interface with other computer systems within the hospital allows the sonographer to communicate with the Hospital Information System (HIS) to capture the demographic information of the patient and the patient's medical record. It also may have the ability to interface with the Radiology Information System (RIS). Advantages of RIS include its ability to integrate with other information systems, patient scheduling, digital dictation, and ability to use worklists. Communicating with RIS via PACS provides the sonographer with images and reports from other imaging examinations that the patient may have had previously. Some of the main advantages of PACS are that it allows for quick and reliable retrieval of images and can send images to external locations for interpretation

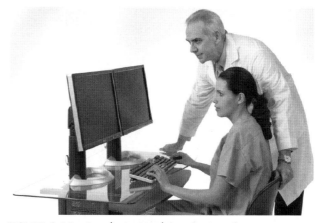

FIGURE 2-15   **Sonologist Workstation.** Area for image review and interpretation. (Courtesy GE Healthcare.)

and consultation. Radiologist consultation that allows remote image viewing, retrieval, and digital dictation has modernized teleradiology.

PACS works by capturing the ultrasound image, storing it locally on a hard drive, and then sending it to the computer workstation. The images may then be interpreted at the workstation by a radiologist or sonologist (Figure 2-15). The images are then digitally stored, with or without a report, on a hospital server,

GE Healthcare

ViewPoint
Connect, Report, Relax

Med. Record No.: 37259
Reference No.:   12
Date of Exam: 10/02/2011
Date of Print: 11/06/2011

Obstetrical Ultrasound Report

Patient name: Julie Anderson
Patient's DOB: 02/04/1985 (age: 26 years)
Patient's address: 114 Pleasant St., Boston, MA 02110
Referring physician: Dr. Will Smith, 13 Park Ave., Boston, MA 02110

02110 Indication: Anatomy survey, unknown dates second or later pregnancy.

History: Age: 26 years. LMP not sure.

Dating:

LMP:	05/05/2011	EDC: 02/09/2012	GA by LMP:	21w3d
Current scan on:	10/02/2011	EDC: 02/09/2012	GA by current scan:	22w4d
Best overall assessment:	10/02/2011	EDC: 02/09/2012	Assessed GA:	22w4d

The calculation of the gestational age by current scan was based on EPO, HC, AC, FL, and HJML
The best overall assessment is based on the ultrasound examination on 10/03/2011.

General Evaluation:
Fetal heart activity: present. Fetal heart rate: 140 bpm.
Presentation: cephalic.
Amniotic fluid: normal. AFI: 9.5 cm.
Cord: 3 vessels.

Anatomy Scan:
Biometry:

BPD	55.2	mm	-	22w8d	(22w2d to 23w3d)
HC	204.5	mm	-	22w4d	(21w1d to 24w0d)
AC	172.8	mm	-	22w2d	(21w1d to 22w6d)
FL	39.5	mm	-	22w5d	(20w8d to 24w4d)
HUM	38.2	mm	-	22w3d	
EFW (lbs/oz)	1 lbs	2 ozs			
EFW (g)	507	g	38th%		

Fetal Anatomy:

	Normal	Abnormal	Not visualized		Normal	Abnormal	Not visualized
Head	x	0	0	Abdominal Wall	x	0	0
Brain	x	0	0	GI Tract	x	0	0
Face	0	x	0	Kidneys	x	0	0
Spine	x	0	0	Bladder	x	0	0
Neck/Skin	x	0	0	Extremities	x	0	0
Thoracic	x	0	0	Skeleton	x	0	0
Heart	x	0	0	Genitalia	c	0	x

Details: Face: cleft lip right side.

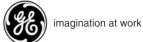 imagination at work

GE Healthcare
Wauwatosa, WI USA
877 644 3114
www.gehealthcare.com

FIGURE 2-16 Simulated Ultrasound Report With Images. Obstetric ultrasound report that includes sample images from the study. (Courtesy GE Healthcare.)

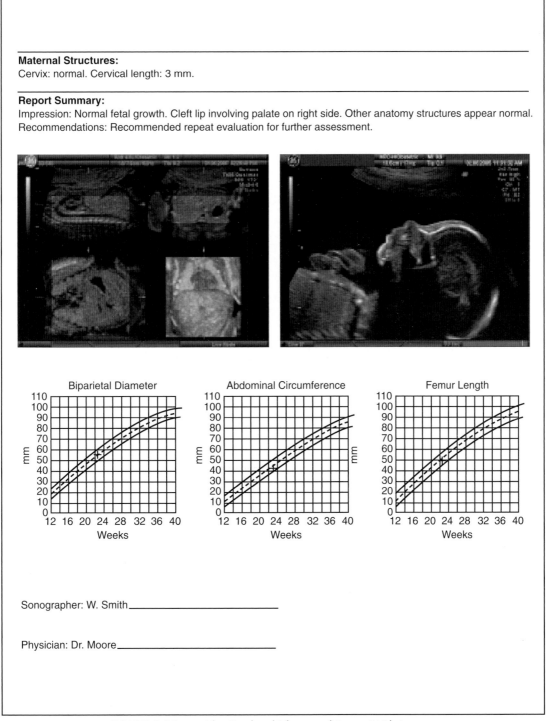

Maternal Structures:
Cervix: normal. Cervical length: 3 mm.

Report Summary:
Impression: Normal fetal growth. Cleft lip involving palate on right side. Other anatomy structures appear normal.
Recommendations: Recommended repeat evaluation for further assessment.

Sonographer: W. Smith_____

Physician: Dr. Moore_____

FIGURE 2-16, cont'd   Simulated Ultrasound Report With Images.

a computer that controls the storage and transfer of imaging studies, patient data, and reports (Figure 2-16).

Sonographers have a wide range of technological support at their disposal: from ever-advancing ultrasound systems to electronically connected patient data and physician workstations. Therefore it is important for sonographers to possess superb technological skills to ensure the proper handling of the ultrasound system and additional electronic data systems at their disposal. Well-educated sonographers advance patient care and the ultrasound profession through the proper use of technology and their assistance to sonologists.

CHAPTER 3

General Patient Care

BETTY BATES TEMPKIN

OBJECTIVES

Describe effective interpersonal skills.

Describe a "patient-ready" ultrasound examination room.

Describe the sonographer's responsibilities regarding patient care.

Describe specific practices required for aseptic technique.

KEY WORDS

Asepsis — A germ-free condition.

Aseptic Technique — Protects patients from infection and prevents the spread of pathogens.

Invasive Procedure — Process of inserting something into or operating on the body through a needle puncture, an incision, or a natural orifice.

Every patient deserves your undivided attention, consideration, and care. All patients feel vulnerable, whether they appear to be ill or not; therefore every effort should be made to gain their confidence and put them at ease.

During an ultrasound examination the well-being of the patient is the sonographer's responsibility. The use of interpersonal skills helps to establish a good rapport with patients, and utilizing proper patient care techniques ensures their safety.

INTERPERSONAL SKILLS

Developing proficient interpersonal skills makes it easier to interact with patients. Putting patients at ease and establishing a good rapport with them are essential to gaining their confidence and cooperation. When patients feel comfortable, they become more focused and receptive. Subsequently, the sonographer's job becomes more efficient, less time consuming, and ultimately more enjoyable.

Dress should be professional and include a visible, easy-to-read source of personal identification. To develop a good rapport with patients, greet them with a smile and make eye contact (Figure 3-1). Address patients by using their first and last name, along with Ms., Mrs., or Mr., as applicable. Introduce yourself to the patient using your first and last name as well. Adjust the tone and expression of your voice to convey a sense of

genuine interest in the patient. Conversation should be informal but respectful and professional.

It is standard practice to obtain a brief medical history from the patient or his or her representative if the patient is unable to communicate. Begin by gathering all available information about the patient, either from the inpatient chart or outpatient ultrasound study request form (see Chapter 1). This eliminates unnecessary questions.

Avoid using medical terms that a patient may not understand and asking questions that require only a yes or no answer. Many patients will not admit that they do not comprehend a question and will typically answer yes or no when given that option. Therefore questions should be open-ended to obtain more accurate and specific details. Events should be kept in the proper time sequence as patients relate their past history and current problem(s). If patients wander too far off the subject, gently lead them back to the reason for the question without appearing disinterested in their other concerns. Never insist that patients talk about more than they are comfortable discussing. The interpreting physician can follow up with any unanswered questions.

Learn to be a good listener and pay close attention to the patient's answers. Some answers may prompt you to ask additional questions that elicit information that will affect the focus of the ultrasound examination and ultimately aid the interpreting physician's diagnosis.

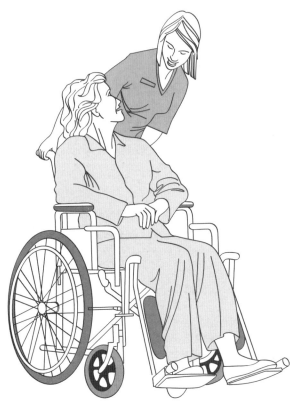

FIGURE 3-1 Greeting patients with a smile and making eye contact, addressing them by their first and last name, and introducing yourself are all gestures that help to establish a good rapport.

ULTRASOUND EXAMINATION ROOM

A "patient-ready" ultrasound examination room should exemplify a well-equipped medical examination room; it must be clean and organized and convey a professional atmosphere. The room should be free of clutter and all personal items except modestly framed ultrasound training and registry certificates. The room obviously requires an examination table or stretcher, a handled step stool, and an ultrasound machine (Figure 3-2). The ultrasound examination room should also be stocked at all times with items listed in Box 3-1.

PATIENT CARE DURING THE ULTRASOUND EXAMINATION

To provide your patients with the best possible care, you should be aware of your institution's Standard Precautions and isolation policies (see Chapter 1, Standard Precautions) and "Code" procedures for incidences of heart failure. Also, most clinical institutions offer cardiopulmonary resuscitation (CPR) classes and require employees to be certified to administer CPR. Diligent practice of these policies and practices benefits and protects the patient as well as the sonographer.

Before the examination, make sure you have the correct patient. Patients have been known to answer to the wrong name. Check the patient's identification bracelet (or patient number) against the patient's chart; ask outpatients to repeat their name back to you.

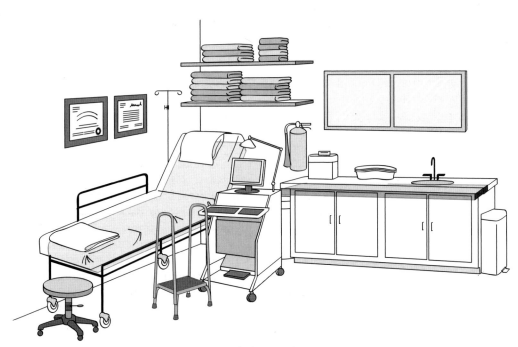

FIGURE 3-2 Typical ultrasound examination room.

■ ■ ■   **BOX 3-1** ULTRASOUND EXAMINATION ROOM STOCK ITEMS

■ Patient examination gowns
■ Scanning gel (bottles and refill containers)
■ Towels and washcloths
■ Blankets
■ Drapes
■ Packaged alcohol swabs
■ Wrapped tongue blades (in case of seizures)
■ Covered dirty laundry bin
■ Fire extinguisher
■ Betadine
■ Angled sponges (for patient positioning)
■ Antibacterial cleaning solution
■ Saline
■ Prepared sterile packages for ultrasound-guided procedures

■ Paper pillow covers
■ Bottle warmers
■ Sheets
■ Examination gloves
■ Emesis basins
■ Alcohol
■ Covered waste container(s)
■ Needle and sharp object disposal container
■ Crash cart
■ Sterile gauze pads of various sizes
■ Hand sanitizer
■ Surgical masks
■ Cotton balls
■ Variety of needles, syringes, and tubing

Depending on the ultrasound study, some outpatients will need to put on a hospital gown. Patients should be told how to put on the gown and instructed to leave on undergarments. Ask patients whether they need assistance disrobing, offering your help if necessary. If patients do not need assistance, give them their privacy and adequate time to change into the gown.

Assist patients with medical equipment attachments such as IV poles (metal poles holding bags of intravenous medications) or oxygen (Figure 3-3). Before a patient gets on or off the examination table or stretcher, make certain it is stationary with the brakes set. Always have a handled step stool available for shorter patients or those who require a little more assistance (see Figure 3-2). When helping a patient out of a wheelchair (or before seating a patient in the chair), make certain that both brakes are locked and the leg- and footrests are pushed out of the way. If the patient is already on a stretcher, avoid bumping into the walls when wheeling the stretcher into the examination room. After the stretcher is situated, set the brakes. Patients who are confused, upset, or uncooperative should not be left unattended.

See that the patient is kept as comfortable as possible during the examination; provide blankets or additional pillows as necessary. If a patient is not comfortable or able to lie flat, adjust the angle of the head of the stretcher or examination table. If a patient requests something to drink or eat, check the chart or ultrasound request form to see whether the patient is allowed to have fluids or food; they may be scheduled for another examination that requires them to be fluid-/food-restricted, so it is essential to check all available patient information and/or contact the referring physician, floor nurses, or the outpatient's physician's office to find out.

Instruct the patient in a slow, clear, and concise manner. Briefly explain the examination process, including the following, and then offer to answer any questions:

• Ultrasound does not hurt or require radiation.
• The lights must be dimmed to see the images on the computer monitor.
• With all due respect, certain areas of the body will be draped and others exposed.
• A warm, gelatinous scanning couplant will be applied to the exposed area to facilitate imaging.
• An imaging transducer will be placed on the gel and moved in various positions and directions to visualize the area(s) of interest (Figure 3-4).
• You may be asked to change your position to facilitate imaging.
• You may be asked to hold your breath or exhale.

An **invasive procedure** is the process of inserting something into or operating on the body through a needle puncture, incision, or a natural orifice. Such ultrasound procedures—for example, ultrasound-guided biopsies and aspirations (see Chapter 34 for further details) or endocavital (e.g., endovaginal, endorectal; see Chapters 20 and 21)—are considered invasive and therefore require informing patients about the details of the procedure and obtaining their signed informed consent before the procedure can take place. If a patient is incapacitated and cannot sign or speak, a patient representative, such as a family member or the referring physician, can grant permission for the study to be performed.

In an effort to protect the interests of the sonographer and the patient, it is recommended that endocavital procedures be witnessed by another healthcare professional. The sonographer's and witness's initials both should be recorded on the ultrasound images and on any permanent written record of the examination.

Most transabdominal female pelvis studies require the patient to have a full urinary bladder to facilitate visualization of pelvic structures. Because this can cause

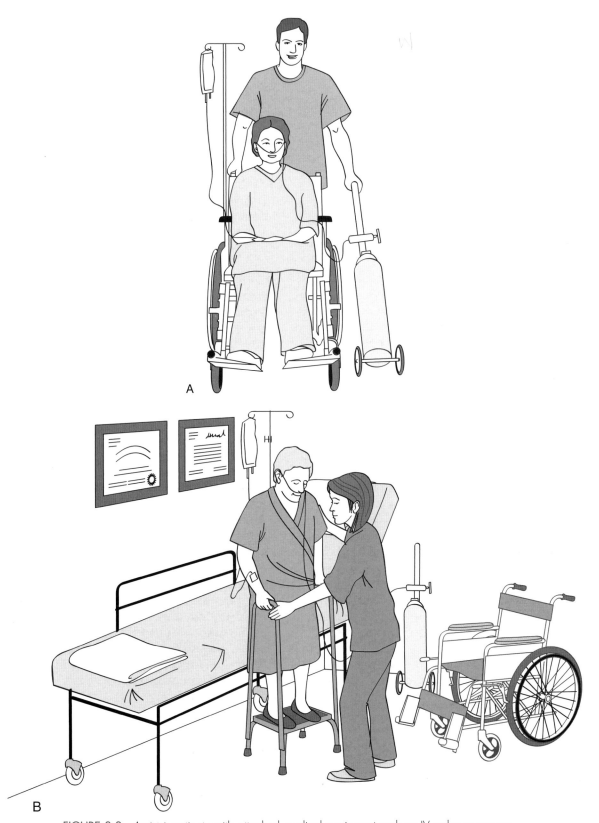

FIGURE 3-3 Assist inpatients with attached medical equipment such as IV poles or oxygen.

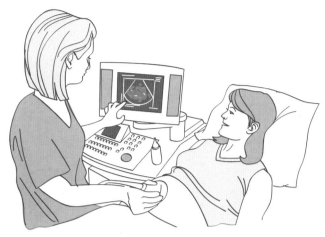

FIGURE 3-4 Ultrasound transducers are placed on the surface of the skin over various areas of interest. A water-soluble gel serves as a scanning couplant to reduce air between the transducer and skin surface, thus facilitating the imaging process.

the patient discomfort, every effort should be made to scan quickly and prudently.

Conversations should be kept to a minimum, and facial expressions should be guarded during the ultrasound examination; never show surprise, shock, or confusion because this could alarm the patient. Be prepared for some patients to ask, "What you are looking at?" or "What do you see?" It is acceptable to briefly point out a structure(s). It is *not* acceptable to point out abnormal echo patterns or give a patient your opinion of the ultrasound findings. Explain to patients that you do not make diagnoses but provide the images to an interpreting physician, who in turn provides an interpretive report to the patient's referring physician. Providing anything beyond that is not sensible, responsible, or legal, unless you are willing to assume the same liability that a physician does. By virtue of their education and training experience, only physicians can legally render a diagnosis. Physicians have the credentials to assume legal liability; sonographers do not.

Most institutions require that items such as stretcher railings, step stool handles, etc., be wiped down with an antibacterial solution between patients. Follow the manufacturer's guidelines for cleaning and disinfecting ultrasound transducers. Dispose of examination table or stretcher coverings and replace these with fresh ones.

ASEPTIC TECHNIQUE

Ultrasound is routinely used for invasive percutaneous needle-guided biopsies, aspirations, and drainage procedures, as well as interventional and intraoperative procedures (see Chapter 34). To adequately assist the physician in an ultrasound-guided percutaneous procedure and to protect the patient from obtaining a possible infection during the procedure, a sonographer must be adept at implementing asepsis technique. Asepsis is defined as a germ-free condition. Aseptic technique is the procedures and practices used in any clinical setting to protect patients from infection due to germs. All patients are susceptible to infection, particularly those with excessive burns or immune disorders that disturb the body's natural defenses. Patients undergoing invasive procedures can be infected through contact with the environment, equipment, or personnel.

Aseptic technique encompasses the following:
- **Sterile equipment.** This includes sterile gloves, gowns, face masks, and eye shields.
- **Patient preparation.** The skin encompassing the area where the procedure will be performed must be cleaned with an antibacterial solution poured onto sterile sponges or gauze held by forceps. The accepted practice is to clean the site using a circular motion, starting in the center of the site and moving outward. Any long hair around the site should be clipped short.
- **Sterile field.** A sterile field is created by placing prepackaged sterile drapes around the cleaned site. All packages containing sterile items should be opened in such a way that the contents do not touch nonsterile surfaces or items. Areas below the level of the sterile drapes are outside the field and are not sterile. To maintain a sterile field, all items that enter the sterile field must be sterile.

CHAPTER 4

Introduction to Ergonomics and Sonographer Safety

PEGGY ANN MALZI BIZJAK

OBJECTIVES

Define *ergonomics* and discuss its history as it relates to Sonography and the Occupational Safety and Health Administration Act's (OSHA's) involvement.

List the types of patient injuries most likely to occur while scanning.

Explain the causes and risk factors that influence work-related musculoskeletal disorders (WRMSDs) and musculoskeletal injuries (MSI).

Learn how the industry has changed over the years to counteract injury, and describe the various practice changes made.

Describe what comprises a stress-free and safe, injury-free scanning environment and how that environment is managed.

KEY TERMS

Abduction — Extension of the shoulder and arm away from the body.

Burnout — Result of chronic stress over time.

Bursitis — Inflammation of the bursa.

Carpal Tunnel Syndrome (CTS) — Entrapment of the median nerve as it runs through the carpal bones of the wrist.

De Quervain's Disease — A specific type of tendonitis involving the thumb, believed to be a result of repeated gripping of the transducer.

Ergonomics — The science or study of work.

Occupational Safety and Health Act (OSHA) — The 1970 U.S. law that ensures safe and healthful working conditions for the nation's workforce.

Presbyopia — Blurred vision.

Spinal Degeneration — Intervertebral disc degeneration that results from awkward and static postures, bending, and twisting while scanning.

Tendonitis — Inflammation of the tendon.

Work-Related Musculoskeletal Disorder (WRMSD) — An injury that results in restricted work or time away from work or that involves symptoms that last for 7 days or more and injuries that include the muscles, tendons, and joints.

ERGONOMICS DEFINED

Ergonomics is the science or study of work. The application of ergonomics is important for improving performance and the general well-being of workers. Ergonomics is proactive in that it removes barriers to productivity, fosters safety, and promotes comfort when performing repetitive tasks. It is a human-centered approach to the design of products, workplaces, and systems wherever people are involved.

There are a few important goals of the use of ergonomics in the workplace. These include:

• Improving performance and quality
• Reducing injuries
• Reducing absenteeism and turnover

ERGONOMICS IN SONOGRAPHY

In the 1980s, the most common work-related complaint among sonographers was shoulder pain and discomfort in the scanning arm. The predominant equipment used at the time was a static scanner with an articulated arm. As the industry moved toward real-time scanning, shoulder pain was not reported as much, but another, even more bothersome, issue arose. With this new technology, the transducer was no longer fixed to an arm but connected to a long and heavy cable. By the mid-1990s, sonographers began to complain of muscle strain in the wrist and base of the thumb, as well as shoulder pain. Neck and back problems became much more frequent. Additional movements, including

■ ■ ■ **Table 4-1** Common Injuries and Disorders Among Sonographers

Condition	Explanation
Bursitis	Inflammation of the bursa
Carpal tunnel syndrome (CTS)	Entrapment of the median nerve as it runs through the carpal bones of the wrist
De Quervain's disease	A specific type of tendonitis involving the thumb, thought to be caused by repeated gripping of the transducer
Tendonitis	Pain, swelling, numbness, and muscle weakness that lead to tendonitis (the inflammation of tendons in the extremities) epicondylitis, trigger finger, and general discomfort
Plantar fasciitis	Inflammation of the fascia on the sole or plantar surface of the foot
Rotator cuff injury	Torn tendons of the rotator cuff muscles
Spinal degeneration	Intervertebral disc degeneration

twisting and bending of the neck and torso, abduction (extension) of the shoulder, and applying pressure to the transducer, appear to contribute to further musculoskeletal pain and discomfort. A 2000 study by the Society of Diagnostic Medical Sonography stated that work-related musculoskeletal disorder (WRMSD) incidents—those injuries resulting from or caused by workplace activities—were reported by almost 80% of respondents. A follow-up study reported incidents among almost 90% of respondents.

Types of Injuries

Ergonomic disorders concern the muscles, tendons, and joints in the body and can be aggravated by long-term issues, which should be addressed. Table 4-1 is a list of the types of injuries that sonographers and sonologists can develop over time. These are due to repeated motions of the scanning hand, arm, and wrist; awkward and static postures; and bending and twisting of the torso while scanning.

The Occupational Health and Safety Act (OSHA)

The Occupational Safety and Health Act (OSHA) was passed by Congress in 1970. The purpose of OSHA is to ensure safe and healthful working conditions for the nation's workforce. One of its provisions addresses ergonomic disorders. According to OSHA, an occupational injury can be classified into the following groups:

- Repetitive motion injury (RMI)
- Repetitive strain injury (RSI)
- Musculoskeletal strain injury (MSI)

Work-Related Musculoskeletal Disorders (WRMSDs)

WRMSDs are injuries that result in restricted work. This includes injuries that result in time away from work; injuries that involve symptoms lasting for 7 days or more; and injuries that include the muscles, tendons, and joints.

The following are important signs and symptoms of developing a WRMSD:
- Cramping of the hand/wrist
- Loss of grip
- Pain
- Stiffness
- Tingling
- Swelling
- Spinal degeneration

The upper extremities and the neck appear to be the areas with the highest percentage of injury. Repetitive motion, forceful strain, awkward or uncomfortable body positions, frequent reaching, and static postures requiring considerable length of time needed to complete the examination all contribute to WRMSDs and RSIs. It is the employer's responsibility to provide working conditions that reduce and eliminate the chance of injury from WRMSD.

Contributing Causes and Risk Factors of Workplace Injury

Valuable information has been obtained from surveys of sonographers and sonologists regarding the number of occurrences of musculoskeletal symptoms, with 80% of sonographers suffering from some form of WRMSD. Of those, 20% will experience a career-ending injury.

Workplace activities or conditions that can cause WRMSD and MSI injuries include, but are not limited to:
- Workspace design
- Infrequent breaks or rest periods
- Incentives for overtime and on-call shifts
- Delayed injury reporting
- Improper cable management
- Improper sitting height of chair
- Improper height of monitor, causing flexion of the neck
- "Pinch grip" of the transducer
- Air-quality factors such as heat, cold, humidity
- Poor posture
- Increase in the number of portable ultrasound examinations
- Sustained shoulder abduction
- Aging workforce
- Staffing shortages
- Higher workloads due to advances in technology (Table 4-2)

Table 4-2 Number of Scans in a Typical Workday	Average	Median
Total scans per day	17.1	12.0
Cardiac (adult)	9.3	7.0
OB/GYN	7.8	5.0
Vascular	6.7	4.0
Abdomen	5.7	4.0
Breast	4.9	3.0
Cardiac (pediatric)	4.3	2.0
Cardiac (fetal)	3.5	2.0
Neurosonography	2.1	1.0
Musculoskeletal	1.9	1.0

Sonographers frequently perform scans in various positions each day. The total number of scans performed in a typical workday averaged 17.1, with a median of 12.0 scans. The highest average number of scans per day is in the Adult Cardiac specialty (9.3), followed by OB/GYN (7.8). *Courtesy of SDMS.*

The data in Table 4-2 were taken from the 2013 Sonographer Salary and Benefits Survey from the Society of Diagnostic Medical Sonography (SDMS). The full survey is available free to SDMS members.

Factors that contribute to stressful conditions in the workplace include the following:
- Environmental stress such as physical working conditions
- Vision problems such as eyestrain and eye fatigue
- Cluttered and/or crowded scanning rooms
- Generalized stress, self-imposed or otherwise

Environmental stress factors include air quality, lighting, and scanning room design. A room that is too hot or too cold, or one that lacks good air exchange, can lead to sonographer ailments and general dissatisfaction with working conditions. A room that is too bright and without light dimming capabilities can cause eyestrain, possible degradation of the image on the monitor, or display screen glare.

Eyestrain is a concern for the sonographer. Over time, a focusing issue known as presbyopia can develop. Increased fatigue is possible because of this deficiency. Resting between patients or following the *20-20-20 rule* helps. The rule states that for every 20 minutes of scanning, sonographers should focus their gaze 20 feet away for 20 seconds. Although this may sound like a simple strategy, it is difficult to manage without behavioral modification techniques and practice.

Crowded scanning rooms remain an issue. Sonographers and employers must work together to ensure department scanning rooms are large enough to maneuver equipment, such as scanning tables and stretchers, and have enough storage space. When scanning outside of the laboratory, it may not be possible to avoid clutter. Sonographers and supervisors should work with other health care members to move furniture and equipment out of the way to make room for the sonographer to work as safely as possible.

Stress for the sonographer in the workplace takes many forms. The following situations are also some additional factors that can cause generalized stress:
- Not enough resources available to do the job, such as lack of sufficient training on new equipment
- Overload of patient schedule
- Unsure of basic expectations from management
- Disregard of the sonographer's expertise
- Unmet basic needs, which can create nonparticipation in important work-related discussions
- Communication issues
- Ethical and legal conflicts

As a result of these common stressors, the sonographer can develop either physical symptoms or psychosocial stress-related symptoms—with either short-term or long-term stress—that may increase the susceptibility of illness or injury. Physical signs of stress include fatigue, headaches, high blood pressure, insomnia, or a general feeling of being "stressed out." Psychosocial symptoms include withdrawal, low self-esteem, feelings of failure, and frustration.

Continuation of these stressors without some positive or compassionate intervention can eventually lead to *burnout*. **Burnout**, which is a result of chronic work-related stress, in and of itself can be prevented. Possessing a positive attitude, not taking yourself too seriously, getting a restful night's sleep, and exercising can benefit the sonographer immensely. Simple strategies such as treating yourself to something special, talking to friends, and going to see a movie all have a positive effect on the sonographer and are proactive ways to address workplace stress. Sonographers should take responsibility for their own actions and behaviors by allowing mini rest periods, especially when performing portable examinations, and determining best practices to reduce the potential for WRMSDs. Sonographer awareness of stress and possible coping mechanisms are key to maintaining a healthy and stress-free workplace. Learning what types of injuries can occur on the job and how to prevent them is a crucial component for maintaining sonographer safety. Awareness of the potential for injury and awareness of stress-related workplace issues cannot be overstated.

CREATING A SAFE ENVIRONMENT

Over the years, the sonography industry has made significant and necessary changes as a result of increased awareness and research into the causes of WRMSDs and the ways to reduce injuries. A multidisciplinary approach among sonographers, sonologists, equipment companies, and employers can assist in developing solutions to these occupational injuries.

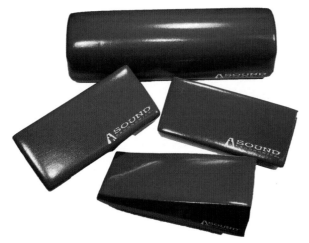

FIGURE 4-1 **Ergonomic Cushions.** (Courtesy Sound Ergonomics, LLC.)

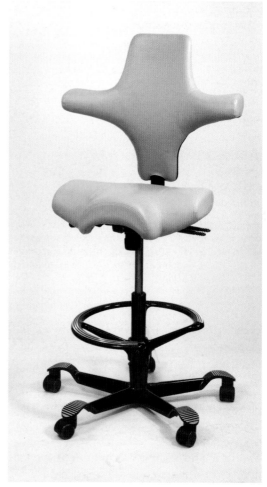

FIGURE 4-2 **Ergonomic Chair.** (Courtesy Sound Ergonomics, LLC.)

Equipment manufacturers have made the most significant changes in the industry. They continue to develop ergonomically designed ultrasound systems that decrease twisting and turning. In addition, they have created lighter transducers and transducer cables. Moreover, sonographers and sonologists must take responsibility in advocating for an ergonomically sound work environment and for maintaining their own health and well-being by eating right, getting enough sleep, and exercising frequently to strengthen and stretch muscles. Employers must increase their awareness of WRMSDs and understand the costs of employee occupational injury. Worker's compensation, hiring temporary staff, retraining staff, loss of productivity, and quality issues all must be examined and considered in developing solutions and managing risk for injury. The following steps to avoid or lessen the risk for injury are strongly encouraged:

- Be aware of work conditions and habits that increase the potential for physical injury.
- Modify behavior as a way to address repetitive stress activities.
- Make frequent breaks mandatory during the scanning day.
- Improve posture while sitting or standing. Ergonomic devices can provide assistance (see Figures 4-1 and 4-2).
- Evaluation by a physical therapists with corrective behaviors, including massage, should be incorporated regularly.
- Work closely with management to revise the layout of scanning rooms and purchase ergonomically designed ultrasound scanning equipment, support cushions, and chairs to lessen the potential for injury (see Figures 4-1 and 4-2).

The Society of Diagnostic Medical Sonography introduced Industry Standards for the Prevention of WRMSD Injuries in *Sonography* in May 2003. Those industry standards have been updated and are important in keeping the sonography scanning environment stress free and safe. Through the pioneering work of Joan Baker and other leading sonographers, strategies to prevent WRMSDs and improve sonographer workplace safety remain an important focus in scanning laboratories.

Time and effort are required to educate hospital management, equipment manufacturers, sonography program instructors, and practicing sonographers that the profession is at high risk for injury from repetitive movements and that the incidence of these injuries can be reduced. Becoming aware of the potential for injury through education and being willing to make the necessary changes to create a safe scanning workplace environment that promotes healthy scanning practices is the ultimate goal.

Ergonomics create a safe scanning environment for the sonographer and sonologist, but the prevention of injury in the workplace must center on manufacturer, sonographer, and employer awareness. Actions to reduce the risk for injury include adopting the basic industry standards for the prevention of WRMSDs regarding equipment control measures, administrative control measures, and professional control measures, as follows:

- Manufacturers make state-of-the-art and ergonomically designed ultrasound systems with adjustable monitors and keyboards. Make more ergonomically designed transducers and lighter cables that minimize strain. Voice recognition allows hands-free scanning, a very creative tool.
- Employers provide adjustable examination tables and chairs, which provide necessary support for the sonographer while scanning. Purchase ergonomically designed scanning equipment. Conduct risk assessments and ensure that equipment is maintained and in good order. Consider scheduling and workload factors so that sufficient quick breaks can happen. Establish stats for the number of scans performed and the amount of time needed to scan.
- Sonographers adopt good posture habits while scanning. Take brief rest breaks during the scan time. Stretch during the day to control stiffness. Get proper rest and exercise, and maintain good eating habits to combat the stressful situations of your day.

Everyone can follow these best practices solutions to prevent injury; the alternative can be costly. Awareness, prevention, and sharing of workable, effective solutions within our industry are essential.

Sonographic Approach to Understanding Anatomy

CHAPTER 5

Interdependent Body Systems

BETTY BATES TEMPKIN

OBJECTIVES

Explain how the body systems maintain homeostasis.
Describe the interdependent nature of body systems and why it is significant to sonographers.

Explain the interrelationship of the various hormone-producing organs.

KEY WORDS

Aorta — Main artery leaving the heart to supply body structures with the nutrient- and oxygen-rich blood they require.

Appendicular Skeleton — The bones of the skeleton that form the appendages; the framework for the arms and legs.

Arteries — Thick-walled blood vessels that transport oxygenated blood away from the heart.

Arterioles — Tiny branches of arteries.

Atria — Two upper chambers of the four-chamber heart.

Atrioventricular (AV) Node — Transfers electrical impulses emitted by the sinoatrial node down to the ventricles to initiate their contraction.

Axial Skeleton — The skull, spine, and ribs portion of the skeleton.

Capillaries — Thinnest and most numerous of the blood vessels, providing a connection between arterioles and venules.

Cardiac Ventricles — Two inferior chambers of the four-chamber heart.

Central Nervous System (CNS) — Consists of the brain and spinal cord.

Corpus Luteum — Cystic glandular mass formed from an empty ovarian follicle after ovulation. Releases the hormones estrogen and progesterone.

Diaphragm — Muscular partition separating the thoracic and abdominopelvic cavities.

Diastole — Filling or relaxing phase of the heart.

Erythropoietin — Hormone released by the kidneys when inadequate oxygen levels are detected in the blood; notifies the bone marrow to increase production of red blood cells.

Gametes — Sexual reproductive cells produced by the male and female gonads. Male spermatozoa and female ova whose union is necessary to produce new life.

Gonads — The male testes and female ovaries. Primary reproductive organs that produce reproductive cells (male spermatozoa and female ova), which are the basis of producing new life.

Homeostasis — The equilibrium of the body's normal physiologic condition.

Hormones — Chemical "messengers" that transfer instructions from one set of cells to another. Manufactured and secreted into the bloodstream by various endocrine glands throughout the body.

Inferior Vena Cava — One of the two major veins transporting deoxygenated blood into the right atrium of the heart from structures of the body that lie below the level of the heart.

Joints — Articulations. Where bones of the skeleton are joined to one another. Either immovable, slightly movable, or freely movable. Also called *articulations*.

Ligaments — Long, elastic connection between the bones of freely movable joints.

Lymph — Interstitial fluid consisting of digested fats, water, protein, white blood cells, and tissue waste.

Lymph Node — Concentration of tissue containing white blood cells—primarily lymphocytes—that filter lymph of foreign material.

KEY WORDS—cont'd

Lymphocyte — Type of white blood cell whose main function is to protect the body from disease-causing microorganisms.

Metabolism — The chemical reactions that occur in the body to maintain life.

Micturition — Process by which the bladder expels urine through the urethra and discharges it from the body. Commonly called *urination.*

Myocardium — Heart muscle.

Ovarian Follicle — Encasement containing an immature ovum (egg cell).

Ovulation — Discharge of a mature ovum from its ovarian follicle.

Peripheral Nervous System (PNS) — Composed of all the nerves and nerve cells outside of the central nervous system.

Peristalsis — Wormlike motion that forces contents through the alimentary tract.

Pleura — Double-walled sac surrounding the lungs.

Pulmonary Circulation — Transports blood from the heart to the lungs and back again.

Renin — Enzyme secreted by the kidneys to help control blood pressure.

Sinoatrial (SA) Node — The heart's natural pacemaker. Emits regular electrical impulses initiating contraction of the atria.

Skeletal Muscle — The only voluntary muscle type in the body; one of three muscle types. Gives form and stability to the skeleton and enables it to move.

Superior Vena Cava — One of the two major veins transporting deoxygenated blood into the right atrium of the heart from structures of the body that lie above the level of the heart.

Systemic Circulation — Transports blood from the heart to all parts of the body (except the lungs) and back again.

Systole — Pumping or contracting phase of the heart.

Tendons — Bands of tough, fibrous, flexible tissue that connect muscles to bones.

Urine — Filtered waste from the blood that passes through the kidneys. Contains products such as ammonia, bilirubin, drugs, and toxins.

Veins — Thin-walled vessels that transport oxygen-depleted blood to the heart.

Venules — Tiny branches of veins.

The purpose of this chapter is to serve as a reference for general information regarding body systems and their relationship(s) to one another (Table 5-1). Although each body system has a unique, primary function, the function may:

- Also relate in kind to another body system with the exact same function. Systems that share the same function can replace each other if one system's performance fails.
- Act as an accessory function to another body system.

With this understanding, it becomes obvious how affiliated body systems can share pathologic conditions. For a sonographer, this knowledge may be the determining factor that leads to further investigation of related body systems during a sonographic examination.

The following body systems work independently and together to maintain homeostasis, the equilibrium of the body's normal physiologic condition:

- Nervous system
- Endocrine system
- Cardiovascular system
- Lymphatic system
- Musculoskeletal system
- Reproductive system
- Excretory systems:
  - Urinary system
  - Digestive system
  - Respiratory system

Text continued on p. 34

■ ■ ■ **Table 5-1** How Body Systems Relate

Body System	Function(s)	Associated Organs	Related Body System(s)
Nervous System	■ Controls a majority of functions throughout the body via voluntary and involuntary muscle signaling. Controls sensory areas (sight, hearing, smelling, touch) and regulatory areas (hypothalamus and pituitary control the endocrine system) ■ Interprets electrical signals and makes decisions about what to do	Brain Spinal cord Eyes Ears	All body systems are assisted by the nervous system either directly or indirectly. Some examples include the following: **Endocrine system:** ■ Is assisted by the nervous system when the hypothalamus of the brain controls the endocrine "master gland," the pituitary gland, which in turn, controls the other endocrine glands ■ Assists the nervous system when hormones are released via the reproductive system to initiate brain development **Respiratory system:** Assisted by the nervous system when the brain regulates the respiratory rate and monitors respiratory volume and blood gas levels **Digestive system:** Assisted by the nervous system when the brain receives signals from sensory receptors located throughout the digestive tract affecting appetite and the muscles that assist eating and the elimination of waste **Urinary system:** Assisted by the nervous system when the brain receives signals from sensory receptors in the urinary bladder and regulates urination **Lymphatic system:** Assisted by the nervous system when the brain initiates the defense against infection **Cardiovascular system:** Assisted by the nervous system when the brain controls blood pressure and heart rate **Musculoskeletal system:** ■ Assisted by the nervous system when the brain receives signals about body position from sensory receptors located in joints; the brain controls the muscles that affect movement ■ Assists the nervous system when bones provide calcium, which is essential for the nervous system to function properly
Endocrine System	■ Secretes hormones directly into the bloodstream to help maintain homeostasis by regulating reproduction, growth and development, metabolism, blood glucose levels, stress response, and ovulation	Hypothalamus gland Pituitary gland Thyroid and parathyroid glands Thymus gland Adrenal glands Pancreas gland Ovaries Testes	**Nervous system:** Assists the endocrine system when the hypothalamus of the brain controls the endocrine "master gland," the pituitary gland, which in turn controls the other endocrine glands **All body systems:** Assisted by the endocrine system either directly or indirectly when hormones are released that influence the body's function (see Table 5-2)

■ ■ ■ **Table 5-1** How Body Systems Relate—cont'd

Body System	Function(s)	Associated Organs	Related Body System(s)
Cardiovascular System	■ Brings oxygen, nutrients, hormones, and white blood cells to body structures and takes toxins away—by pumping blood	Heart Blood vessels (arteries, veins)	**Respiratory system:** Assisted by the cardiovascular system when it accepts the inhaled oxygen **Urinary system:** ■ Assists the cardiovascular system by maintaining blood pressure equilibrium when systemic pressure changes ■ Assists the cardiovascular system by filtering waste and toxins from the blood **Nervous system:** Assists the cardiovascular system when the brain controls blood pressure and heart rate **Musculoskeletal system:** Assists the cardiovascular system when muscle contractions move blood up through the veins against the effects of gravity **Lymphatic system:** Assists the cardiovascular system when lymph reenters the bloodstream to help maintain the fluid level in the blood **Digestive system:** ■ Assisted by the cardiovascular system when it receives and transports the nutrients and minerals from digested food ■ Assisted by the cardiovascular system when it receives and transports the water from indigestible materials to help maintain the body's fluid level
Lymphatic System	■ Transports excess fluid from tissues back into the blood ■ Absorbs fat from the villi in the small intestine and transports it to the bloodstream ■ Protects the body from infection	Lymph nodes Spleen Bone Marrow Thymus gland	**Nervous system:** Assists the lymphatic system when the brain initiates the defense against infection **Cardiovascular system:** Assisted by the lymphatic system when lymph reenters the bloodstream to help maintain the fluid level in the blood **Musculoskeletal system:** Assists the lymphatic system when muscle contractions move lymph up through the lymphatic vessels against the effects of gravity

Continued

■ ■ ■ **Table 5-1** How Body Systems Relate—cont'd

Body System	Function(s)	Associated Organs	Related Body System(s)
Musculoskeletal System	■ Together, the bony skeleton and muscles: • Provide support and protection for internal organs • Allow movement Bone: ■ Marrow produces blood cells ■ Stores minerals such as calcium and phosphorus, then releases them as the body needs them Muscle: ■ Contracts the heart ■ Contracts when walking, moves the blood up through veins against the effects of gravity ■ Moves food through the gastrointestinal tract ■ Helps maintain body temperature by generating heat	Bones (femur, ribs, cranium, vertebrae) Muscles (cardiac, smooth, skeletal)	**Urinary system:** Assists the musculoskeletal system when bone marrow cannot replace dying red blood cells due to disease or severe radiation exposure—the urinary system takes over the production of red blood cells **Circulatory system:** Assisted by the musculoskeletal system by the muscle contractions that move blood up through the veins against the effects of gravity **Lymphatic system:** Assisted by the musculoskeletal system by the muscle contractions that move lymph up through the lymphatic vessels against the effects of gravity **Nervous system:** ■ Assists the musculoskeletal system when the brain receives signals about body position from sensory receptors located in joints; the brain controls the muscles that affect movement ■ Assisted by the musculoskeletal system when bones provide calcium, which is essential for the nervous system to function properly **Respiratory system:** Assisted by the musculoskeletal system when the diaphragm and rib muscles contract for inhalation and relax for exhalation
Reproductive System	■ Produces new life	Vagina Cervix Uterus Ovaries Fallopian (uterine) tubes Prostate gland Testes Vas deferens	**Endocrine system:** Assists the reproductive system when hormones are released to initiate puberty, facilitate reproduction, and facilitate new life

■ ■ ■ **Table 5-1** How Body Systems Relate—cont'd

Body System	Function(s)	Associated Organs	Related Body System(s)
Digestive System	■ Metabolizes ingested food, transfers nutrients, and eliminates waste	Mouth Salivary glands Esophagus Stomach Small bowel Large bowel Anus Liver Gallbladder Pancreas	**Nervous system:** Assists the digestive system when the brain receives signals from sensory receptors located throughout the digestive tract that affect appetite and the muscles that assist eating and the elimination of waste **Musculoskeletal system:** Assists the digestive system with eating and the elimination of waste **Cardiovascular system:** ■ Assists the digestive system (jejunum and ileum) by receiving and transporting the nutrients and minerals from digested food ■ Assists the digestive system (large bowel) by receiving and transporting the water from indigestible materials to help maintain the body's fluid level
Urinary System	■ Maintains the body's chemical and water balance ■ Filters out waste products	Kidneys Ureters Urinary bladder Urethra	**Musculoskeletal system:** Assisted by the urinary system; if bone marrow in the musculoskeletal system cannot replace dying red blood cells, the urinary system steps in and produces new red blood cells **Nervous system:** Assists the urinary system when the brain receives signals from sensory receptors in the urinary bladder and regulates urination **Cardiovascular system:** ■ Assisted by the urinary system's kidneys when they help maintain blood pressure when systemic pressure changes ■ Assists the urinary system by filtering wastes and toxins out of the blood
Respiratory System	■ Supplies oxygen to the blood and eliminates carbon dioxide	Pharynx Larynx Trachea Bronchi Lungs	**Nervous system:** ■ Assists the respiratory system when the brain regulates the respiratory rate ■ Assists the respiratory system when the brain monitors respiratory volume and blood gas levels **Cardiovascular system:** Assisted by the respiratory system when it inhales oxygen and exhales carbon dioxide

NERVOUS SYSTEM

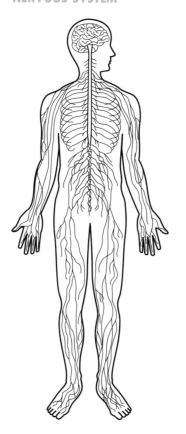

The nervous system monitors and controls almost every organ system in the body (see Table 5-1). It is divided into central and peripheral portions. The brain and spinal cord comprise the central nervous system (CNS). The peripheral nervous system (PNS) is composed of thousands of nerves that connect the CNS with the rest of the body (muscles, glands, and sensory organs). Together, these systems control the majority of functions throughout the body via voluntary and involuntary muscle signaling. They also control sensory areas (sight, hearing, smelling, touch) and regulatory areas (hypothalamus and pituitary gland control of the endocrine system).

The nervous system serves as the body's "computer," responsible for processing data to and from the brain, thus controlling everything from pain sensation to coordination, from high-level cognitive processing to hypothalamic control of the endocrine system. This is all made possible by the billions of neurons (nerve cells) comprising the nervous system; they have the unique ability to send and receive electrical signals so that they can communicate with each other and with other parts of the body.

Central Nervous System

The central nervous system is the processing area of the nervous system. It is responsible for receiving, interpreting, and responding to electrical signals from the peripheral nervous system.

The brain and spinal cord of the CNS are well protected by the cranial vault and spinal column (vertebrae) of the skeleton, which surround these structures like protective armor. Additionally, they are covered by the meninges, three protective layers of connective tissue:

- **Pia mater:** innermost layer
- **Arachnoid:** middle layer
- **Dura mater:** outer layer; located against the inner surface of the cranium and vertebra

Further, the space between the pia mater and arachnoid is filled with cerebrospinal fluid (manufactured in the ventricles of the brain), forming a protective cushion.

Peripheral Nervous System

The main function of the peripheral nervous system is to connect the CNS with the limbs and organs—to relay information from the brain and spinal cord to the rest of the body, as well as from the body to the spinal cord and brain.

The PNS consists of 31 pairs of spinal nerves that branch off from the spinal cord to supply every part of the body except the head and neck, which are served by 12 pairs of cranial nerves that emerge from the brain.

The peripheral nerves carry out voluntary and involuntary actions that are divided into the somatic and autonomic systems:

- **Somatic nervous system:** All conscious awareness of our external environment (voluntary) and all movement (through skeletal muscle)

- **Autonomic nervous system:** Not under conscious control (involuntary). Monitors our internal environment and the function of the glands and organs. Also controls the contraction of smooth muscle. Has two subdivisions that usually exert opposite effects on the same organs, resulting in a balance between the two forces:
  - ○ **Sympathetic division:** Responds to stress or impending danger. Known as the "fight or flight" system. Sympathetic signals cause the adrenal glands to release adrenaline in the bloodstream, which stimulates all cells of the body in preparation for an emergency. Physiologic changes occur, such as increases in heart rate, breathing rate, and blood pressure, along with shunting of the blood to the muscles—all to help the body cope with high-stress situations.
  - ○ **Parasympathetic division:** Maintains and restores the body's energy. Follows sympathetic stimulation (after the "danger" has passed) and works to return body functions to normal. Parasympathetic signals reduce the output of adrenaline, decrease the heart and breathing rates, and lower blood pressure. Even when there is no crisis to recover from, the parasympathetic signals promote a calm state of being.

ENDOCRINE SYSTEM

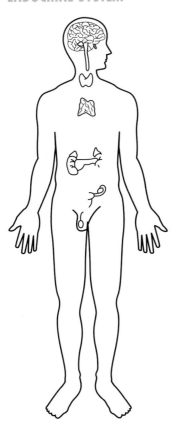

The endocrine system is a collection of glands that secrete **hormones** (chemical "messengers") directly into the bloodstream to arrive at target organs. Unlike the nervous system's precise short-term coordination of responses to stimuli, the endocrine system utilizes long-term coordination of chemical signals to help maintain homeostasis by regulating body functions that include reproduction, growth and development, metabolism, blood glucose levels, stress response, and ovulation.

"Neuro" Endocrine System

The endocrine system is often referred to as the *neuroendocrine system* because the *hypothalamus* of the brain directs and monitors endocrine functions. The hypothalamus communicates directly and exclusively with the "master gland" of the endocrine system, the pituitary gland (also known as the *hypophysis*), which is also located in the brain. The pituitary is a pea-sized gland that sits in a small, bony depression of the skull called the *sella turcica* ("Turkish saddle") directly below the hypothalamus. It is connected to the inferior portion of the hypothalamus by a stalk, through which it receives instructions from the hypothalamus on how to regulate the hormonal activity of the other endocrine glands located throughout the body (Table 5-2).

Pituitary Anatomy

The pituitary is composed of two parts:

- **Anterior pituitary** *(adenohypophysis):* Gland composed primarily of cells that secrete protein hormones
- **Posterior pituitary** *(neurohypophysis):* Actually an extension of the hypothalamus forming the connection or stalk between the hypothalamus and anterior pituitary gland. Composed primarily of axons of hypothalamic neurons that extend inferiorly behind the anterior pituitary

■ ■ ■ **Table 5-2** Endocrine Glands: Location, the Hormones They Secrete, and Their Functions

Gland	Location in the Body	Hormone(s)	Function
Anterior pituitary gland	Brain	Follicle-stimulating hormone (FSH)	Assists in ovarian follicle development in females and sperm maturation in males.
		Luteinizing hormone (LH)	
		Thyrotropin (TSH)	Thyroid gland–stimulating hormone.
		Adrenocorticotropin (ACTH)	Adrenal gland–stimulating hormone.
		Growth hormone (GH)	Stimulates growth in general.
		Prolactin	Initiates and maintains milk secretion in females.
		Melanocyte-stimulating hormone	Melanin formation and deposition in the body.
Posterior pituitary gland	Brain	Oxytocin	Uterine-contracting and milk-releasing actions.
		Vasopressin	Constricts blood vessels, raising the blood pressure and increasing peristalsis; has some influence over uterine contractions; influences resorption of water by kidney tubules; used as an antidiuretic.
Thyroid gland	Neck	Thyroxine (T_4)* Triiodothyronine (T_3)*	Responsible for assisting in metabolism of lipids, proteins, and carbohydrates. Their presence can increase the body's need for oxygen, which leads to increased heat production (body temperature elevation) that will influence most tissues.
		Calcitonin	Responsible for removing calcium via absorption. This causes calcium to be removed from the blood and sent to the bones for storage.
Parathyroid glands	Neck	Parathyroid hormone (PTH)	Basic antagonist for calcitonin. PTH sends a signal, causing bone reabsorption. If the body is low in calcium, it will take what it needs from the bones, adding calcium to the bloodstream.
Adrenal glands	Mid-hypogastrium	Epinephrine	Causes blood glucose levels to elevate. The heart races and major vessels dilate. It also causes ACTH to be released from the pituitary.
		Norepinephrine	Causes diastolic and systolic blood pressure to increase. It is also a vasoconstrictor and causes peripheral vessels to constrict.
		Mineralocorticoids	Control sodium and potassium levels.
		Glucocorticoids	Control glucose use by conserving consumption (ACTH controlled).
Pancreas	Mid-hypogastrium	Insulin	Controls the uptake/use of glucose to prevent glycogen breakdown within the liver; responsible for decreasing the blood glucose level. Glucagon antagonist to glucocorticoids; it increases the blood glucose level.
Ovaries	Pelvic cavity	Estrogen	Responsible for female secondary sex characteristics. Released during the menstrual cycle to prepare the uterus for possible implantation.
		Progesterone	Released during the menstrual cycle to prepare the uterus for possible implantation.
Testes	Scrotum	Testosterone	Responsible for male sex characteristics.
Pineal gland	Brain	Melatonin	Weakly modulates wake/sleep patterns.
Thymus gland	Thoracic cavity	Thymosin	Promotes development of antibodies. Stops working after puberty.

Note: The number in parentheses indicates the number of attached iodine cells (e.g., thyroxine + 4 iodine cells).

System Functions

Hormones transfer instructions from one set of cells to another. Although many different hormones circulate throughout the bloodstream, each one affects only the cells that are genetically programmed to receive and respond to its message.

The hypothalamus secretes hormones that the blood transports directly to the anterior pituitary gland. In response, the anterior pituitary releases its own hormones that travel via the bloodstream to stimulate the other endocrine glands to release their hormones, which control specific body functions to help maintain homeostasis. The posterior pituitary is stimulated by the hypothalamus as well, to release the hormones it stores (see Table 5-2).

Receptors within the hypothalamus monitor blood levels of hormones within the body. When the hypothalamus receives a signal that there is a rise or fall of an organ's hormone level, it sends a message to the pituitary gland, which in turn releases either an inhibiting or releasing hormone into the bloodstream that travels to the organ and causes it to either stop releasing its hormones or to release more of its hormones to maintain equilibrium in the body.

CARDIOVASCULAR SYSTEM

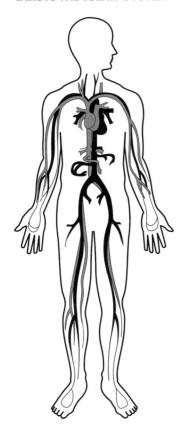

The heart and circulatory system make up the cardiovascular system. The heart works as a pump that pushes blood through a network of arteries and veins. These arteries and veins are responsible for delivering blood, oxygen, and nutrients to every cell and for removing the carbon dioxide and waste products made by those cells. The cardiovascular system has two specific functions:

- **Pulmonary circulation**, which transports blood from the heart to the lungs and back again
- **Systemic circulation**, which transports blood from the heart to all parts of the body (except the lungs) and back again

Arteries and Veins

The vascular components of the cardiovascular system are the arteries and veins. **Arteries** are thick-walled blood vessels that transport oxygenated blood away from the heart. There are two exceptions: the umbilical arteries in the fetus and the pulmonary artery (see Pulmonary Circulation below); both transport oxygen-depleted blood. Arterial walls are three layers thick, which allows them to carry blood under high pressure. The **aorta** is the main artery leaving the heart. It is a massive artery extending from the heart to the lower abdominal cavity. Along its course, it gives off branches throughout the body that supply body structures with the oxygen and nutrients they require.

Except for the pulmonic and aortic valves, arteries do not have valves. The thick, muscular wall in the arteries squeezes the blood forward.

Veins are thin-walled vessels that transport oxygen-depleted blood to the heart. There are two exceptions: the umbilical veins in the fetus and the pulmonary veins (see the section on Pulmonary Circulation below); both of these transport oxygen-rich blood. Venous blood throughout the body ultimately ends up in either of the two major veins (depending on location), the **superior vena cava** (from areas above the heart) or the **inferior vena cava** (from areas below the heart). These large vessels empty the deoxygenated blood into the right atrium of the heart.

Blood in the legs would stagnate were it not for the presence of valves within the veins and skeletal muscle contractions to help move the venous blood up through the veins against the effects of gravity.

Pulmonary Circulation

The venous blood transporting carbon dioxide and cellular waste products must get to the lungs and exchange these for oxygen. The oxygen-depleted blood returns first to the heart via the superior and inferior vena cavae that enter the right atrium. The coronary sinus empties the heart's veins directly into the right atrium. When the deoxygenated blood enters the right atrium, pulmonary circulation has begun. The deoxygenated blood is then pumped through the tricuspid valve into the heart's right ventricle and flows from there through the pulmonary semilunar valve into the main pulmonary artery (note the exception of an artery carrying oxygen-depleted blood). The main pulmonary artery bifurcates into right and left branches, which carry the deoxygenated blood to each respective lung, where the red blood cells exchange the carbon dioxide and waste for oxygen. The now oxygen-rich blood leaves the lungs through pulmonary veins, which transport it to the left atrium, ending pulmonary circulation. The blood is pumped from the left atrium through the bicuspid (or mitral) valve into the left ventricle. When the oxygenated blood leaves the left ventricle, it enters systemic circulation.

Systemic Circulation

Oxygen-rich blood is pumped from the left ventricle through the semilunar aortic valve to enter the aorta, thus beginning the systemic circulation cycle. The aorta arches superiorly to give off branches to supply the upper body before descending through the thoracic cavity and piercing the *diaphragm* to enter the abdominopelvic cavity. The abdominal branches of the aorta supply the lower body structures with nutrient- and oxygen-rich blood. The major branches of the aorta give off their own branches, and those branches in turn may give off branches, with all decreasing in size to small arterioles and ultimately capillaries. **Capillaries** are the thinnest and most numerous of the blood vessels. They provide a connection between **arterioles** (tiny branches of arteries) and tissues for delivery of nutrient- and oxygen-rich blood to the cells, and also between tissues and **venules** (tiny branches of veins). Venules then transport the deoxygenated blood and waste to larger veins that in turn transport it to the superior or inferior vena cavae, which empty the blood into the heart's right atrium, subsequently ending the systemic circulation cycle.

Atypical Blood Flow

As previously discussed, the typical pattern of systemic blood flow in organs and body structures is as follows:

$$\text{Artery} \rightarrow \text{Arteriole} \rightarrow \text{Capillary} \rightarrow \text{Venule} \rightarrow \text{Vein}$$

However, there are two unique areas in the body where this pattern does not apply:
- In the liver, the unusual circumstance is that there is simultaneously free mixing of portal venous blood (oxygen-depleted with cellular waste) and hepatic arterial blood (oxygen-rich with nutrients) in hepatic sinusoids before exiting the liver in the hepatic vein.
- The kidney is unique because it contains two sets of capillary beds rather than a single set, as is the case in all other areas of the body. The additional capillary bed enables the kidneys to assist the cardiovascular system, if necessary, by maintaining a state of blood pressure equilibrium even when the systemic pressure changes. This is an example of independent, yet related, body systems sharing functions and providing protective back-up assistance if the primary system's function fails (see Table 5-1).

The Heart

The heart consists of four chambers, two at the top, called atria, and two at the bottom, the cardiac ventricles. The heart is a specialized muscle, the myocardium, which contracts continuously, pumping blood to the body and the lungs. Each time the heart pumps blood, an intricate coordination of events takes place.

The pumping action of the heart is not controlled by the brain; rather, it is caused by a flow of electricity through the heart that is triggered by the heart's sinoatrial (SA) node—the heart's natural pacemaker. The SA node emits regular electrical impulses from the right atrium that cause both atria to contract and pump blood into the ventricles. The electrical impulse then travels to the ventricles through the atrioventricular (AV) node (which serves as the heart's circuit breaker in case the SA node impulse comes too quickly), causing the muscle to contract and pump blood from the right ventricle into the lungs and from the left ventricle into the body.

In a relaxed state, the normal heart rate is 70 to 90 beats a minute. Heart rate is a measure of both sides of the heart contracting at the same time, then relaxing and filling, then contracting again. The pumping, or contracting, phase is termed systole. The filling, or relaxing, phase is diastole.

The heart beats faster during exercise or states of stress or excitement in response to the body's need for more oxygen. Chemicals circulating in the blood are released by nerves that regulate the heart rate, altering the speed of the SA node and the force of the pumping action.

LYMPHATIC SYSTEM

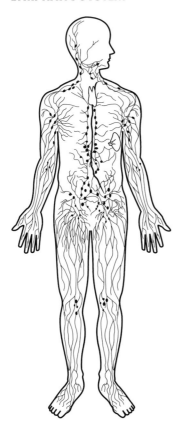

Components of the lymphatic system are lymph, lymphatic vessels, lacteals, lymph nodes, and organs that include the spleen, bone marrow, and thymus gland. The main functions of the lymphatic system include:

- Collection and transportation of excess fluids from interstitial spaces of the body back into the veins in the bloodstream
- Absorption of fats from the small intestine, which are then transported to the liver
- Immune system functions that utilize lymphoid tissue and organs to produce the cells that fight and dispose of foreign material

Collection and Transportation of Fluid

Lymphatic fluid, or lymph, is interstitial fluid consisting of digested fats, water, protein, white blood cells, and tissue waste. Small capillaries drain lymph from the head, abdominopelvic cavity, organs, and the extremities into the lymphatic vessels, which transport the lymph to its destination in the thorax. Along its path, the lymph passes through chains of small, oval-shaped lymph nodes, where the fluid is filtered of foreign material. Once in the thorax, lymph is emptied into large veins at the base of the neck and also just superior to the heart. Lymphatic fluid reentering the bloodstream is essential to the cardiovascular system for maintaining the correct fluid levels within the blood (see Table 5-1).

Fat Absorption

Lacteals are lymphatic vessels located in the gastrointestinal tract lining. They are predominant in the small intestine, where they pick up fats (lipids) that are transported via the lymphatic vessels directly back into the bloodstream. Other nutrients in the small intestine are absorbed into the bloodstream and transported to the liver for processing.

Immune Function

As noted, immune system functions utilize lymphoid tissue and organs to produce the cells, which fight and dispose of foreign material.

- **Lymphoid tissue** is composed of connective tissue and a variety of white blood cells, primarily lymphocytes. It is responsible for immune function, defending the body against infection and disease. Lymph nodes are areas of concentrated lymphocytes and macrophages (types of large phagocytic cells that engulf and ingest foreign bodies).
- **Lymphoid organs** include the thymus gland and bone marrow that produce and store lymphocytes (B cells, T cells), monocytes, and leukocytes until they are mature enough to be transported to the lymph nodes, tonsils, adenoids, and the blood, where they look for foreign material to destroy. B cells are produced by and mature in bone marrow. They provide the body with its best response to bacterial invasion. The spleen filters or purifies blood and lymph.

MUSCULOSKELETAL SYSTEM

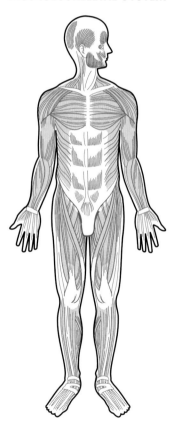

The musculoskeletal system serves as the framework of our body. It is composed of the skeleton (206 adult bones), skeletal muscle, tendons, ligaments, joints, connective tissue, and cartilage. The skeleton is characterized as *axial* and *appendicular*. The skull, spine, and ribs form the axial skeleton. The appendicular skeleton consists of the bones that form the appendages, the framework for the arms and legs.

Skeletal muscles give form and stability to the skeleton and enable it to move voluntarily. When you want to walk across a room, the brain commands the skeletal muscles to move the bones and you walk; it is voluntary. Skeletal muscle is the only voluntary muscle in the body. Smooth muscle, located in the walls of the digestive tract and blood vessels, and cardiac muscle, found only in the heart, are involuntary muscles.

Skeletal muscle is also called *striated muscle* because of its appearance under a microscope. Specifically, skeletal muscle cells are referred to as muscle fibers due to their long, thin appearance. In the body, skeletal muscle cells are arranged into multiple bundles or fascicles that comprise a skeletal muscle. Within each fascicle, a delicate *connective tissue*, the *endomysium*, surrounds each muscle fiber and interconnects surrounding muscle fibers to each other. The *perimysium*, also a connective tissue fiber, divides each skeletal muscle into a series of compartments, each containing a fascicle. In addition to collagen and elastic fibers, the perimysium contains blood vessels and nerves that maintain blood flow and innervate each fascicle. The perimysium and fascicles are enclosed by a dense layer of collagen fibers called the *epimysium*. The epimysium surrounds the entire muscle, separating it from adjacent tissues and organs.

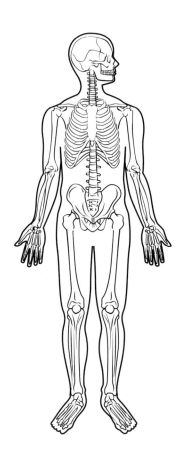

At the end of each skeletal muscle, the collagen fibers of the endomysium, perimysium, and epimysium come together to form a bundle known as a **tendon**, or a broad, flat sheet called an *aponeurosis*. The tendons and aponeuroses generally attach skeletal muscles to bones. Where a tendon attaches to a bone, its fibers actually extend into the bone matrix, providing a firm connection. Consequently, any contraction of the skeletal muscle will exert a pull on its tendon and thereby on the attached bone(s).

Different parts of the skeleton are joined to one another at connections termed *articulations* or **joints**. Joints are categorized as immovable, slightly movable, or freely movable. Articulations of the bones in the skull are immovable with adjacent margins almost touching. They are separated by only a thin, fibrous membrane. The bony surfaces of slightly movable joints, such as the vertebrae, are connected by a layer of fibrocartilage. Adjacent surfaces of a freely movable joint, such as the hip and shoulder joints, are not as close, allowing for a greater range of motion. These margins are separated by cartilage that covers the ends of the bones, which are enclosed by a fibrous tissue or capsule called the bursa. The interior lining of the bursa, the synovial membrane, secretes a fluid that lubricates the joint and reduces friction between the movable surfaces. Further, freely movable joints are made strong and held in position by **ligaments**, which connect the bones to each other. They are tough bands of elastic fibers that extend between the bones. Ligaments can be stretched to gradually lengthen and increase flexibility. To help prevent injury, most athletes perform stretching exercises that lengthen their ligaments to make their joints more supple.

The muscles and skeleton work together to provide the body with vital functions that include movement, protection, hematopoiesis, and mineral homeostasis.

- **Movement:** Movement is produced when skeletal muscles contract to bend the skeleton at movable joints. Contraction starts when an electrical impulse from the brain reaches a motor nerve attached to each muscle fiber. The electrical impulse is transmitted in both directions along the muscle fiber, causing the different strands (myosin and actin) to shorten and slide past each other, producing a contraction. During contraction, the origin (proximal tendon attachment) of the muscle remains stationary and the insertion (distal tendon attachment) moves.
- **Protection:** Bone and muscle provide protection from external forces. They form a protective covering for the vital organs, such as the bony calvarium over the brain and the bony rib cage surrounding the heart and lungs.
- **Hematopoiesis:** Hematopoiesis, or blood cell production, occurs within the marrow of bones. Blood cells usually function for only 120 days before wearing out, at which time they break down into amino acids and other proteins and must be replaced with new blood cells. If the bone marrow is unable to replace the dying blood cells, as in cases such as leukemia or severe radiation damage, death would be certain if the urinary system did not provide an accessory function to the musculoskeletal system by assisting with the production of blood cells and secretion of the hormone erythropoietin, which stimulates bone marrow stem cells to manufacture more cells. This demonstrates how independent yet interrelating body systems support one another (see Table 5-1).

- **Mineral homeostasis:** When various parts of the body need certain minerals to maintain homeostasis, hormones are released that cause a chemical breakdown of bone, allowing it to pass calcium, sodium, and potassium into the bloodstream and thus transport the minerals to the necessary site(s).

REPRODUCTIVE SYSTEM

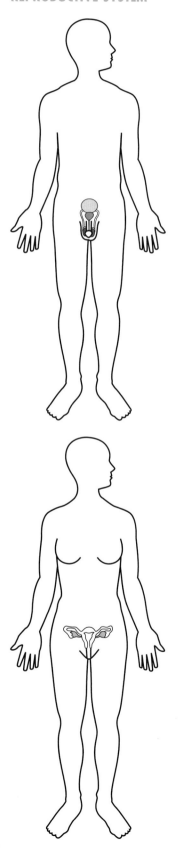

The reproductive system is composed of primary and accessory male and female reproductive organs. In both, the gonads (male testes, female ovaries) are the primary organs. The main responsibility of the reproductive system is for the gonads to produce gametes, or reproductive cells (male spermatozoa, female ova), whose union is the basis of producing new life.

The reproductive system differs from the previously described body systems because it does nothing to directly contribute to the survival of the human body. It does, however, contribute to the survival of the human race. In a process called *fertilization*, the male and female gametes unite to form a zygote, which ultimately provides new life and perpetuation of the human species.

Male Gamete Production and Maturation

Sperm (spermatozoa) are continually produced in the testes of the male reproductive organs. The *pituitary gland* releases luteinizing hormone to stimulate the testes to release the hormone testosterone, which stimulates the production of sperm (see Table 5-1). Each testicle contains several hundred tubules where sperm production occurs. Testosterone is also the hormone responsible for male sex characteristics. The accessory organs of the male reproductive system are the sites of sperm maturation and transport:

- **Epididymis:** A long, coiled tube located next to each testis, where spermatozoa mature and receive nourishment.
- **Vas deferens:** An extension from the epididymis joined by the seminal vesicle before becoming the ejaculatory duct; serves to transport sperm from the epididymis to the urethra.
- **Ejaculatory duct:** The site where sperm mixes with nourishing, suspending fluids secreted from the seminal vesicles to form semen. The semen is transported through the prostate gland, where it receives more secretions, promoting sperm motility, and then joins the prostatic urethra and exits the penis via the urethra.
- **Scrotum:** The exterior sac of skin containing the testes. It is capable of protraction and retraction to maintain a constant temperature, which aids spermatozoa production; the scrotum moves away from the body if the temperature is too high and retracts closer to the body if the temperature is too low.

Female Gamete Production and Maturation

Ova are produced in the ovaries of the female reproductive organs during the *first half* of the menstrual cycle or approximately every 28 days, when the pituitary gland releases follicle-stimulating hormone (FSH). FSH stimulates the ovaries to produce ovarian follicles (encasements, each containing an immature ovum) and to release estrogen to prepare the endometrium of the uterus for potential zygote implantation. The uterus is the normal organ site for a fertilized ovum to implant itself and where the developing embryo and fetus are nourished. It is located between the urinary bladder (anteriorly) and rectum (posteriorly). It is muscular and hollow, with its cavity opening into fallopian/uterine tubes bilaterally and into the vaginal cavity inferiorly. The accessory organs of the female reproductive system are the sites of ovum maturation and transport:

- **Ovarian follicles:** The site of ova maturation.
- **Pituitary gland:** Releases *luteinizing hormone (LH)* during the *second half* of the menstrual cycle, or approximately 14 days after follicle formation, to initiate ovulation and the formation and maintenance of the corpus luteum; typically, only one egg, or ovum, will become mature enough for ovulation.
  - Ovulation occurs when the follicle bursts and releases the mature ovum.
  - The corpus luteum, a glandular mass, forms from the now empty ovarian follicle. It begins releasing the hormone progesterone and a small amount of estrogen to further prepare the uterus for possible implantation by a zygote.
- **Fallopian/uterine tubes:** long, slender tubes that extend bilaterally from the uterus toward the ovary on the same side; they are descriptively divided into the *isthmus, ampulla, infundibulum,* and *intramural* portions (see Chapter 21 for further details). The fallopian tubes transport the released mature ovum toward the uterine cavity. Along the ovum's course through the fallopian tube, fertilization may or may not occur.
- If fertilization *does not* occur (no sperm and ovum encounter or union), the ovum degenerates and the hypothalamus of the brain instructs the pituitary gland to stop releasing LH. This disrupts maintenance of the corpus luteum; no more progesterone or estrogen is produced, and menstruation (the sloughing off of the nonimplanted endometrial lining) begins.
- If fertilization *does* occur, the corpus luteum continues to be maintained and menstruation is suppressed. As the pregnancy progresses, the corpus luteum takes on a cystic composition. The hormone BhCG, or beta human chorionic gonadotropin, can now be detected via blood or urine for pregnancy testing.

Fertilization

Fertilization usually takes place within 1 day of ovulation in the ampulla portion of the fallopian tube and is considered complete when the ovum and sperm fuse to form a zygote. The zygote repeatedly divides to form a cluster of cells called the *morula,* which exits the fallopian tube into the endometrial (uterine) cavity. Endometrial fluid enters the morula, creating a blastocyst that implants itself into the prepared endometrial lining of the uterine cavity. Eventually, the blastocyst embeds itself within the uterine myometrium, completing implantation (see Chapter 22 for further details).

After implantation and organization of blastocyst cells, an embryo is formed. Over several weeks the embryonic cells multiply and undergo the beginnings of structural development. By the ninth week, organs are formed and limb buds begin to enlarge to form the fetus. Development of body systems continues along with growth. The respiratory system is the last system to finish development, which continues through the eighth month, just prior to birth.

■ ■ ■ The Excretory Systems

Digestive System–Urinary System–Respiratory System

The body takes nutrients from the food we eat and uses them to maintain functions throughout the body, such as self-repair and energy restoration. Waste products are left behind in the blood and intestines after the body takes what it needs. The digestive, urinary, and respiratory systems work together to maintain the balance of water and chemicals in the body by excreting the waste.

DIGESTIVE SYSTEM

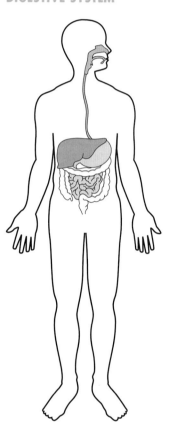

The digestive system includes the gastrointestinal (GI) tract, or alimentary canal, and several accessory organs. The GI tract is basically a series of long tubes that begin with the mouth, followed by the pharynx, esophagus, stomach, small bowel, large bowel, rectum, and anus. The liver, gallbladder, and pancreas provide functions that aid the digestive process.

The main function of the digestive system is to convert ingested food into substances the body uses to maintain **metabolism**, the chemical reactions that occur in the body to maintain life.

The mouth, esophagus, stomach, small bowel, and large bowel work together in the breakdown and absorption of food. Inside the *mouth*, the teeth, tongue, and salivary glands begin the process of breaking down food into smaller particles. The tongue pushes the particles through the pharynx and into the esophagus. The *esophagus* is a thick, muscular tube approximately 10 inches long. It regularly contracts to push the food particles down and into the stomach. The stomach normally holds about a quart of contents. Its walls consist of folds called rugae that allow expansion and contraction. Between the rugae are glands that secrete acid and mucus, which help break down or digest the solid food particles. The *stomach* churns to mix the food particles with the acidic gastric juice, and in 3 to 5 hours the food leaves the stomach and enters the small bowel as a thick liquid called chyme.

The *small bowel* is approximately 23 feet long and is composed of three parts: duodenum, jejunum, and ileum. It is responsible for completing the digestive process through the release of its own digestive enzymes and absorbing substances such as nutrients and minerals across its surface area.

The digestive process in the duodenum is assisted by the introduction of bile and pancreatic enzymes. The liver continually produces bile, a thick fluid that aids digestion by neutralizing stomach acid and breaking down fats. Bile is transported along the biliary tract to the gallbladder for storage, then on to the duodenum, where it meets with the pancreatic duct (carrying pancreatic enzymes) to enter the duodenum, through the *ampulla of Vater*, a small opening in the duodenum, and release the bile and pancreatic enzymes to assist in the digestive process. Digestion is completed in the duodenum and jejunum. Absorption of the nutrients and minerals from the digested food takes place in the jejunum and ileum and enters the bloodstream, which transports it to the liver. The remaining indigestible material is primarily fiber, cellulose, and a large volume of water. **Peristalsis**, a wormlike motion, moves the contents into the large bowel.

The *large bowel*, or colon, is wider and shorter than the small bowel. It has five parts: cecum, ascending colon, transverse colon, descending colon, and sigmoid colon. The large bowel is responsible for absorbing the remaining water from the indigestible contents, to assist in maintaining the body's fluid level, and for transporting the contents through the remainder of the colon and rectum and finally to the anus to be expelled. Simultaneously, bacteria in the colon are acting on the remaining contents, which break down into a final solid waste called *feces*.

Occasionally, the vermiform appendix, a small appendage of the cecum, becomes full and inflamed by the indigestible material. This is commonly known as *appendicitis* and in many cases is demonstrable with ultrasound.

URINARY SYSTEM

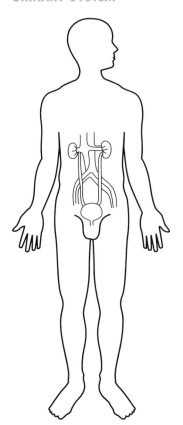

The urinary system is composed of paired kidneys (one on each side of the body), paired ureters (one on each side of the body), the urinary bladder, and the urethra. The *kidneys* are bean-shaped organs about the size of an adult man's fist. Each kidney has its own artery, vein, and ureter that pass through the renal hilum. The renal pelvis is a funnel-shaped reservoir that collects urine from all parts of the kidney and then empties it into the *ureter*, which transports the urine to the bladder. The *bladder* temporarily stores the urine, eventually expelling it from the body via the *urethra*.

The main functions of the urinary system include:
- Regulating blood volume and composition
- Regulating blood pressure
- Producing red blood cells

The urinary system regulates blood volume and composition by filtering waste from the blood that passes through the kidneys, which forms urine (for release from the body). **Urine** is composed of waste products such as urea, ammonia, bilirubin, drugs, and toxins. Important substances such as water, salt, glucose, and amino acids that the body requires are reabsorbed.

Blood pressure is regulated by the urinary system by controlling blood volume, adjusting the flow of blood into and out of the kidneys, and secreting **renin**, an enzyme that helps control blood pressure. Further, the kidneys uniquely possess an additional capillary bed that affords them the ability of maintaining a state of blood pressure equilibrium even when the systemic pressure changes as a result of problems in the cardiovascular system (see Table 5-1).

The kidneys release **erythropoietin**, a hormone notifying the bone marrow to increase production of red blood cells when inadequate oxygen levels are detected in the blood.

Anatomy

Kidneys are retroperitoneal organs situated on either side of the spine, directly anterior to the deep muscles of the back, inferior to and behind the liver and spleen. Each kidney lies at a slight angle, with the superior portion closest to the spine. An adrenal gland is closely related to the superomedial surface.

As urine collects in the renal pelvis of each kidney, it travels with the flow of gravity down the ureters, which are 8- to 10-inch-long narrow tubes that run between the renal pelvis (to which they are attached) and the urinary bladder (to which they are attached). The ureters enter the bladder posterolaterally.

The urinary bladder is normally located in the midline of the pelvic cavity, in front of (or anterior to) most of the pelvic organs. It opens into the urethra inferiorly. It is a hollow, muscular organ shaped like a balloon. The walls of the bladder stretch and become thinner as it fills with urine. The bladder can hold up to 2 cups (or 16 ounces) of urine comfortably for 2 to 5 hours. At the level where the bladder opens into the urethra, there are circular sphincter muscles that close tightly around the opening in order to prevent leakage. Sensory receptors in the bladder send a message to the brain when the bladder is full, and the urge to empty intensifies. Voluntary skeletal muscles can temporarily postpone the bladder from emptying. However, at some point, the brain signals the sphincter muscles to relax, and the smooth muscle in the bladder walls tightens to induce urination, also known as **micturition**. The bladder expels the urine through the urethra, where it is discharged from the body. A lack of voluntary control over the process is known as *incontinence*.

Filtration

Each kidney contains about a million *nephrons*, or filtering units. Each nephron has a *glomerulus*, a cluster or ball of capillaries derived from an arteriole. The glomerulus is contained within a capsule called *Bowman's capsule*. Bowman's capsule opens into a long, twisting tubule. The glomerulus releases water and dissolved waste from the blood into the capsule and then through to the tubule. Inside the tubule, glucose, salts, amino acids, and any other substances that the body might require are absorbed back into the bloodstream. What remains in the tube becomes urine. The urine flows through a series of collecting tubes, the renal pelvis that connects to the ureter, and on into the bladder.

RESPIRATORY SYSTEM

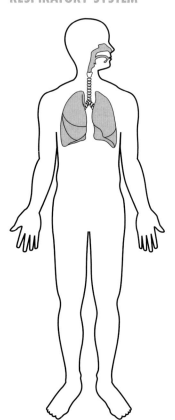

The respiratory system is composed of a long unobstructed airway, beginning in the pharynx and nasal cavity and followed by the larynx, trachea, bronchus, and lungs. The primary function of these structures is to sustain life by:

- Providing the means to supply oxygen to the blood while eliminating carbon dioxide, a natural by-product of cellular activity. This is achieved when inhalation occurs. The **diaphragm** contracts, air enters the body via the nose and/or mouth, travels through the pharynx, and rushes past the larynx, down the trachea, and into the lungs. Within the lungs, air from the trachea passes into the main bronchi, which is subdivided into smaller bronchi, and bronchioles that pass the air into the alveoli, where the exchange of gases (oxygen and carbon dioxide) takes place. Each alveolus is inflated by the air and forms a small sac lined with very thin tissue to facilitate the exchange of gases with adjacent blood capillaries. The muscular diaphragm relaxes, exhalation occurs, the diaphragm contracts, and the cycle of respiration continually repeats.

Anatomy

Air inhaled through the nose is warmed, filtered, and moistened as it goes through the nasal passages and into the pharynx.

The *pharynx* is commonly known as the throat. It is situated posterior to the nasal cavity and superior to the larynx and trachea. Both air and food travel through the pharynx on their way to the trachea and esophagus, respectively. Food in the pharynx is prevented from entering the trachea by the epiglottis, a flap of connective tissue.

The *larynx* lies between the pharynx (superiorly) and trachea (inferiorly). It is commonly referred to as the voice box, a cartilaginous "box" with two pairs of membranes stretched across the inside; these are the vocal cords. When air passes the larynx, it vibrates the vocal cords, thus enabling us to make sound.

The *trachea* is commonly known as the windpipe, or main airway. It is 12 cm long and 2.5 cm wide and is held open by rings of cartilage within its walls. The trachea descends in front of the esophagus and bifurcates into two main bronchi that enter each lung.

The *bronchi* formed by the division of the trachea are also held open by cartilaginous rings within their walls. They enter the lungs and branch out into smaller bronchial tubes, which divide and subdivide into tiny bronchioles. As the branches divide, they narrow and their walls become thinner with less and less cartilage.

The tiny bronchioles end at air chambers that resemble a bunch of grapes. Each chamber contains multiple alveoli, cup-shaped cavities that inflate with the inhaled air and exchange it for carbon dioxide from adjacent blood capillaries. Exhalation causes the alveoli to deflate, and reverse airflow expels the carbon dioxide waste from the body.

Contained within the thoracic cavity, the paired *lungs* enclose the branching bronchial tree and alveoli. It is estimated that each lung consists of 300 million alveoli. The lungs, in turn, are enclosed by a double-walled sac called the **pleura** (visceral and parietal pleura). These two sacs, with pleural fluid between them, enable the lungs to expand and contract without adhering to the chest walls.

Each lung is somewhat triangular in shape, with its apex superior and base inferior. They are separated from the abdominal cavity by the muscular diaphragm located at the margin of their base. For descriptive purposes, the lungs are divided into lobes, with the right lung having three lobes and the left having two.

CHAPTER 6

Anatomy Layering and Sectional Anatomy

BETTY BATES TEMPKIN AND ALEXANDER LANE

OBJECTIVES

Define the layering concept.

Describe structure orientation and its significance in cross-sections of anatomy.

Define how body structure relationships apply to sonography.

Explain the importance of using two different scanning planes.

KEY WORDS

Abdominal Cavity — Division of the ventral cavity and peritoneal cavity that extends inferiorly from the diaphragm and is continuous with the pelvic cavity through the pelvic inlet.

Diaphragm — Large muscle that assists inspiration and divides the ventral cavity into upper thoracic and lower peritoneal cavities.

Dorsal Cavity — One of two main body cavities. Situated on the posterior (dorsal) side of the body. Contains the cranial cavity and spinal cavity.

False Pelvis — Descriptive term given to the area superior to the pelvic inlet (linea terminalis) and inferior to the iliac crests. Also called greater pelvis or pelvis major.

Greater Sac — Peritoneal compartment of the abdominal cavity that extends from the diaphragm to the pelvis and covers the width of the abdomen.

Intraperitoneal — Refers to certain body structures enclosed within the parietal peritoneal sac and covered by peritoneum. They are connected to the cavity wall by mesentery, double folds of peritoneum.

Lesser Sac — Peritoneal compartment posterior to the stomach that is a diverticulum of the greater sac. Also known as the omental bursa.

Linea Terminalis — Imaginary line drawn from the symphysis pubis around to the sacral promontory, marking the dividing plane between the true and false pelves. The circumference of this plane is termed the *pelvic inlet*.

Mesentery — Double folds of peritoneum that connect intraperitoneal body structures to the cavity wall.

Omentum — A double layer of peritoneum that extends from the stomach to adjacent abdominal organs. Classified as two parts: the greater omentum and the lesser omentum.

Parietal Peritoneum — Portion of peritoneal lining that forms a closed sac (except in females, in whom a portion of the fallopian tubes opens into it).

Pelvic Cavity — Division of the ventral cavity and peritoneal cavity that extends superiorly from the iliac crests to the pelvic diaphragm inferiorly. Continuous with the abdominal cavity.

Pelvic Inlet — Describes the circumference of the linea terminalis.

Peritoneal Cavity — Division of the ventral cavity. Largest body cavity, encompassing the abdomen and pelvis. Also known as abdominopelvic cavity.

Peritoneum or Peritoneal Membrane — Thin, membranous sheet of tissue that secretes serous fluid. Serves as a lubricant and facilitates free movement between organs.

Retroperitoneal — Refers to certain body structures that lie behind or posterior to the parietal peritoneal sac. Only their anterior surface is in contact with the peritoneal lining.

Thoracic Cavity — Division of the ventral cavity. An enclosed area that basically corresponds to the rib cage. Separated from the abdominal cavity by the diaphragm. Contains the bronchi and lungs.

True Pelvis — Descriptive term given to the region deep to the pelvic inlet (linea terminalis). Also called lesser pelvis or pelvis minor.

Ventral Cavity — One of two main body cavities. Situated on the anterior (ventral) side of the body. Divided by the diaphragm into the abdominopelvic (or peritoneal) cavity and thoracic cavity.

Visceral Peritoneum — Portion of peritoneal lining that completely covers various organs and body structures.

This chapter relates to the methodology for learning sectional anatomy. Advances and expansions in the field of radiologic diagnostic medicine demanded an update in the teaching of human anatomy. Therefore a new methodology guided by computer imaging modalities was formulated. Each computer imaging modality, including ultrasound, depicts the body in sections in various views, layer by layer. Thus an analysis of body sections is essential to the interpretive process.

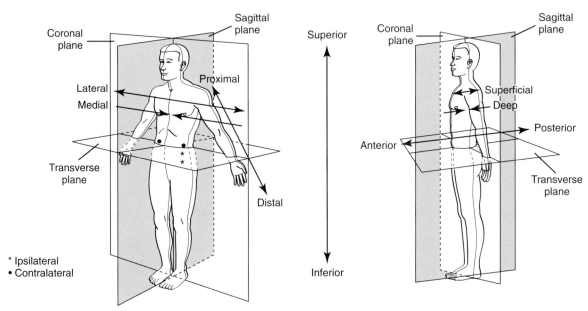

FIGURE 6-1   Body Planes and Directional Terms.

The guidelines for the sonographic study of sectional anatomy can be standardized and use a systematic search pattern for the accurate identification and description of layered anatomy, sectional anatomy, cadaver sections, and clinical images. These eight orientation guidelines for sectional anatomy are outlined as follows:

1. DIRECTIONAL TERMINOLOGY
Understanding the directional terminology that sonographers use is key to accurate descriptions and communication (Figure 6-1). This terminology is discussed in detail in Chapter 7, First Scanning Experience.

2. BODY DIVISIONS
Sonographers must be able to differentiate the natural cavities and spaces of the body, not only because of the bulk of structures they contain, but also because of the potential abnormalities that can invade them. As seen in Figure 6-2, the human body consists of two main cavities, the *dorsal cavity* and the *ventral cavity*:

Dorsal Cavity
Situated on the posterior (dorsal) side of the body, the **dorsal cavity** consists of the cranial cavity and spinal cavity.

Ventral Cavity
Situated on the anterior (ventral) side of the body, the **ventral cavity** is divided into *thoracic* and *peritoneal cavities* by the **diaphragm**, a muscular partition that assists with inspiration.

- The **thoracic cavity** is the enclosed area that corresponds to the rib cage, encompassing the chest.
- The **peritoneal cavity**, also referred to as the abdominopelvic cavity, is the largest body cavity, encompassing the abdomen and pelvis. It is lined by the **peritoneal membrane** or **peritoneum**, a thin sheet of tissue that secretes serous fluid, which serves as a lubricant and facilitates free movement between organs. The peritoneum is classified as *visceral* and *parietal*:
  ○ **Visceral peritoneum** is the portion of peritoneum covering the organs.
  ○ **Parietal peritoneum** is the portion of peritoneum lining the cavity that forms a closed sac, except in females, in whom a portion of the fallopian tubes opens into it. The enclosed structures are termed **intraperitoneal**, and the structures located posterior to the sac and covered anteriorly with peritoneum are termed **retroperitoneal**.
    - Intraperitoneal structures include the following, which are attached to the cavity wall by **mesentery** (double folds of peritoneum): stomach, ovaries, gallbladder, intestines (majority of), spleen (except hilum), and liver (except a bare area posterior to dome).
    - Retroperitoneal applies to the following structures: kidneys, ureters, urinary bladder, pancreas, aorta, inferior vena cava, adrenal glands, uterus, prostate gland, ascending colon, descending colon, somatic nerves, duodenum (majority of), and lymph nodes (abdominal).
  ○ The **omentum** is a double layer of peritoneum that extends from the stomach to adjacent abdominal

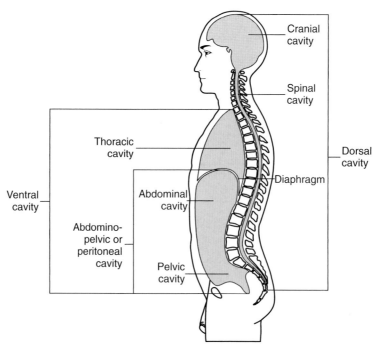

FIGURE 6-2 **Body Cavities.** Ventral cavity includes the thoracic and abdominopelvic cavities. The thoracic cavity is an enclosed area that basically corresponds to the rib cage. It is separated from the abdominal cavity by the diaphragm. The abdominopelvic cavity extends from the diaphragm (superiorly) to the pubic bone (inferiorly). Dorsal cavity includes the cranial and spinal cavities. The cranial cavity ("calvarium") contains the brain; the spinal cavity contains the spinal cord.

organs. It is classified as the *greater omentum* and the *lesser omentum*. In some instances, there are folds of peritoneum running from one organ to another, called ligaments. The names of the ligaments are directly related to the organs to which they are attached.

- The *greater omentum* attaches to the anterior surface of the transverse colon.
- The *lesser omentum* attaches the lesser curvature of the stomach and first part of the duodenum to the porta hepatis (liver portion where the hepatic artery and main portal vein enter the liver and the biliary ducts exit—also known as the liver hilum).

○ The peritoneal cavity is divided into two spaces or compartments: the *greater sac* and the *lesser sac*. The neck, or area of communication between the sacs, is termed *epiploic foramen* or foramen of Winslow.

- The **greater sac** extends from the diaphragm to the pelvis, covering the width of the abdomen.
- The **lesser sac**, also known as the omental bursa, is located posterior to the stomach. It is a diverticulum of the greater sac.

○ Table 6-1 summarizes additional peritoneal cavity spaces created by the complex arrangement of the peritoneum. These spaces are particularly

appreciated sonographically when filled with free fluid.

○ The **abdominal cavity** or abdominal portion of the peritoneal cavity is bordered:
- Superiorly by the diaphragm
- Anteriorly by the abdominal wall muscles
- Posteriorly by the vertebral column, ribs, and iliac fossa

It is continuous with the pelvic cavity inferiorly through the pelvic inlet. Contents of the abdominal cavity include the liver, gallbladder and biliary tract, pancreas, adrenal glands, kidneys, ureters, spleen, stomach, intestines, and lymph nodes. Also included are the abdominal aorta and its branches, which supply blood to these structures, and the inferior vena cava and the main portal vein, which receive and remove blood from them. The left and right crura of the diaphragm (muscular bands that arise from the lumbar vertebrae and insert into the diaphragm) are also within the abdominal cavity.

○ The **pelvic cavity** or pelvic portion of the peritoneal cavity is bordered:
- Anteriorly and laterally by the hipbones
- Posteriorly by the sacrum and coccyx

■ ■ ■ **Table 6-1** Peritoneal Cavity Spaces

Space	Location
Supracolic compartment (supramesocolic space)	The area above the transverse colon constitutes the supracolic compartment, which includes the right subhepatic space, left subhepatic space, right subphrenic space, and left subphrenic space.
Subhepatic spaces	Classified as right and left because they are located posterior to the right and left lobes of the liver, respectively. The right subhepatic space includes Morison's pouch, which lies between the superior pole of the right kidney and the posterior aspect of the right lobe of the liver. The left subhepatic space includes the lesser sac.
Subphrenic spaces	Classified as right and left because they are located on each side of the falciform ligament, respectively. The spaces lie between the diaphragm and the anterior portion of the right and left lobes of the liver.
Infracolic compartment (inframesocolic space)	The area inferior to the transverse colon constitutes the infracolic compartment, which includes the right paracolic gutter, left paracolic gutter, the gutter to the right of the mesentery, and the gutter to the left of the mesentery.
Paracolic gutters	The right paracolic gutter is located between the right lateral abdominal wall and the ascending colon. The left paracolic gutter is between the left lateral abdominal wall and the descending colon. The gutter to the right of the mesentery is a space between the mesentery and the ascending colon. The gutter to the left of the mesentery is a space between the mesentery and the descending colon.
Perirenal space	An area located around the kidney, adrenal gland, and fat, surrounded by fascia (Gerota's fascia).
Pararenal space	Classified as anterior and posterior. The anterior pararenal space is located between the anterior surface of the renal fascia (Gerota's fascia) and the posterior portion of the peritoneum. The posterior pararenal space is located between the posterior surface of the renal fascia and the transversalis fascia.
Posterior cul-de-sac (*pouch of Douglas* or *rectouterine pouch*)	The most posterior and dependent portion of the peritoneal sac. A space located between the urinary bladder and rectum in the male and the rectouterine pouch in the female.
Anterior cul-de-sac (*vesicouterine pouch*)	A shallow space located between the anterior wall of the uterus and the urinary bladder. This space all but disappears as the urinary bladder fills with urine. This space does not exist in the male.

It extends superiorly from the iliac crests to the pelvic diaphragm inferiorly. Contents of the pelvic cavity include the distal portion of the ureters, urinary bladder, urethra, distal portion of the ileum, cecum, appendix, sigmoid colon, rectum, lymph nodes, and iliac vessels. Additionally, the female pelvis includes the uterus, fallopian tubes, and ovaries, and the male pelvis contains the prostate gland and seminal vesicles.

The pelvic cavity is descriptively divided into the *true* and *false pelves*, which are based on an oblique plane in the pelvis defined by the **linea terminalis**, an imaginary line drawn from the symphysis pubis around to the sacral promontory and marking the dividing plane. The circumference of this plane is described as the **pelvic inlet**.

- **True pelvis**: the region deep to the pelvic inlet. Also called the lesser pelvis or pelvis minor.

- **False pelvis**: the area superior to the pelvic inlet and inferior to the iliac crests. Also called the greater pelvis or pelvis major.

3. TISSUE LAYERS
Tissue layers (anatomic layers) are classified into four categories, based on location: *somatic, extravisceral (visceral), intravisceral luminal*, and *intravisceral nonluminal*.

Somatic Layers
- These include the multilayers found on each body region from skin to cavity.
- Located in a region where no cavity exists, the somatic layers encompass the entire region from peripheral to deep.

Extravisceral Layers (Visceral Layers)
- These layers indicate the serial sequence of viscera (internal organs), blood vessels, and spaces between each organ within each cavity.

- The extravisceral layers of the abdomen and pelvis are outlined and discussed, going from deep to superficial. Each organ layer, including muscles and blood vessels from posterior to anterior, is named and discussed. This layering approach is the best method for clarifying the intricate relationships of adjacent body structures and reinforces the concept that familiarity with how anatomy is layered leads to easier recognition of the same anatomy in cross-sections. Layers of the abdomen and pelvis are illustrated in Figures 6-14 through 6-29 at the end of this chapter.

Intravisceral Luminal Layers
- These are found within the walls of organs with a lumen, such as the stomach or urinary bladder.

Intravisceral Nonluminal Layers
- These layers involve organs without a prominent lumen. The adrenal glands are an excellent example of intravisceral nonluminal organs.

4. STRUCTURE CLASSIFICATION

Classification of the structures in cadaver and ultrasound sections into four anatomic units follows mastery of the anatomic layers. The four units are the *musculoskeletal, vascular, visceral,* and *enclosing units.* See Figures 6-14 through 6-29 for assistance in classifying structures.

Musculoskeletal Unit
- Skeletal muscles in the body wall are specified.

Vascular Unit
- Origin and distribution of the vessels are noted.

Visceral Unit
- Organ location and course are discussed.

Enclosing Unit
- This unit includes membranes, fossae, spaces, depressions, and recesses.

5. STRUCTURE ORIENTATION

Structure orientation refers to the way body components are typically situated inside the body. The orientation, or lie, is determined by the length or long axis of a structure. Internal components lie or are situated in one of the following:

Vertical Orientation
- Examples include the aorta, superior mesenteric artery, inferior vena cava, common carotid artery, internal jugular vein, and uterus.

Vertical Oblique Orientation
- Examples include the kidneys, common hepatic duct, common bile duct, portal vein, gastroduodenal artery, proper hepatic artery, superior and inferior mesenteric veins, common iliac arteries, uterus, quadratus lumborum, and psoas major muscles.

Horizontal Orientation
- Examples include renal arteries and veins, splenic vein, and thyroid isthmus.

Horizontal Oblique Orientation
- Examples include the pancreas and liver.

Variable Orientation
- Examples include the gallbladder and ovaries.

• • •

Figure 6-3 illustrates these examples. Knowledge of structure orientation makes identification more recognizable on cadaver and ultrasound sections.

Examples of how to describe structure orientation in ultrasound imaging are seen in Figure 6-4, *A* to *E.*

6. SECTIONAL PLANES

Classic body planes are *transverse, sagittal,* and *coronal* (see Figure 6-1). Scanning planes used in sonography are the same as anatomic body planes; however, their interpretations depend on the location of the transducer and sound wave approach. (This will be discussed in greater detail in Chapter 7; see Figures 7-3, 7-4, and 7-5).

Transverse Plane
- Divides the body into unequal superior and inferior sections perpendicular to the long axis of the body.

Sagittal Plane
- Divides the body into equal right and left sections parallel to the long axis of the body from a midsagittal plane.
- Divides the body into unequal right and left sections parallel to the long axis of the body from parasagittal planes.

Coronal Plane
- Divides the body into equal anterior and posterior sections perpendicular to the sagittal planes and parallel to the long axis of the body from the midaxillary line or midcoronal plane.
- Divides the body into unequal anterior and posterior sections perpendicular to the sagittal planes and parallel to the long axis of the body from paracoronal planes.

Text continued on p. 56

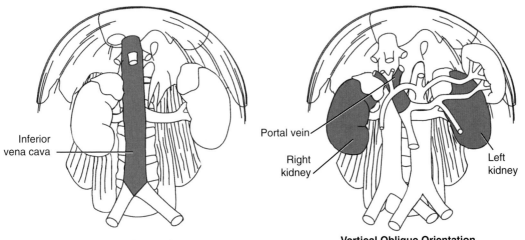

Inferior vena cava

Vertical Orientation

Portal vein

Right kidney

Left kidney

Vertical Oblique Orientation
(the superior pole of the kidneys is medial to the inferior pole—
the portal vein's inferior portion is medial to its superior portion)

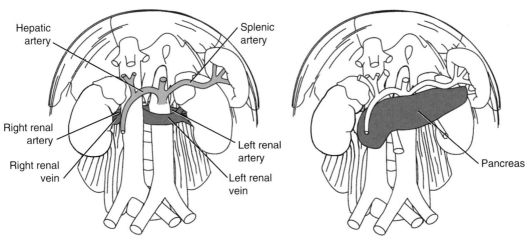

Hepatic artery

Splenic artery

Right renal artery

Left renal artery

Right renal vein

Left renal vein

Horizontal Orientation

Pancreas

Horizontal Oblique Orientation
(the lateral end of the pancreas is slightly more
superior than the medial end)

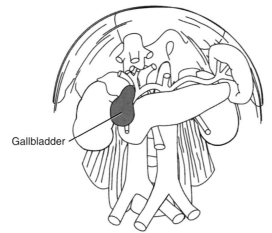

Gallbladder

Variable Orientation
(the variable position of the gallbladder is dependent on the amount of bile
it contains and/or the length of its mesenteric attachment)

FIGURE 6-3 Structural Orientation.

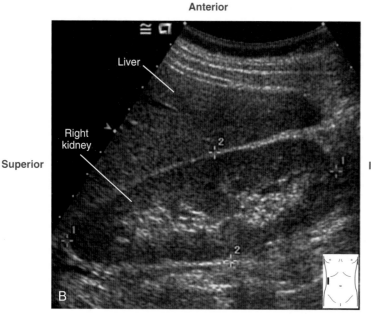

Anterior

Right

Left

Posterior

Transverse scanning plane image showing:
A longitudinal section of the
- Right renal artery (RRA)
- Right renal vein (RRV)

An axial section of the
- Midportion of the right kidney
- Inferior vena cava (IVC)
- Gallbladder (GB) fundus
- Liver

FIGURE 6-4   **A,** Describing structure orientation.

Anterior

Superior

Inferior

Posterior

Sagittal scanning plane image showing:
A longitudinal section of the
- Liver

A long axis section of the
- Right kidney

FIGURE 6-4   **B,** Describing structure orientation.

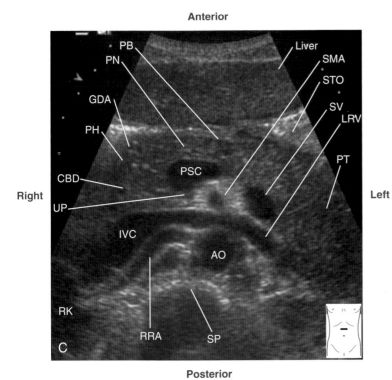

Anterior

PB
PN
GDA
PH
CBD
UP
IVC
RK
RRA
SP
AO
PSC
Liver
SMA
STO
SV
LRV
PT

Right   **Left**

C

Posterior

FIGURE 6-4   **C,** Describing structure orientation.

Transverse scanning plane image showing:
A longitudinal section of the
- Right renal artery (RRA)
- Left renal vein (LRV)
- Splenic vein (SV)
- Stomach (STO)
- Portal splenic confluence (PSC)

A long axis section of the
- Pancreas: uncinate process (UP), head (PH), neck (PN), body (PB), tail (PT)

An axial section of the
- Anterior vertebral surface spine (SP)
- Aorta (AO)
- Inferior vena cava (IVC)
- Superior mesenteric artery (SMA)
- Superior pole, right kidney (RK)
- Common bile duct (CBD)
- Gastroduodenal artery (GDA)
- Liver

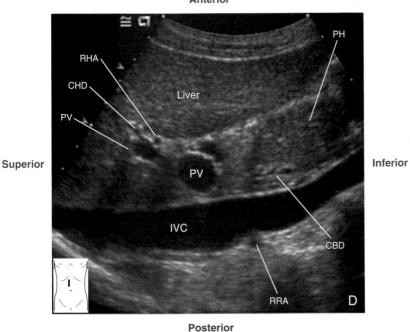

Anterior

RHA
CHD
PV
Liver
PH
PV
IVC
CBD
RRA
D

Superior   **Inferior**

Posterior

FIGURE 6-4   **D,** Describing structure orientation.

Sagittal scanning plane image showing:
A longitudinal section of the
- Inferior vena cava (IVC)
- Common bile duct (CBD)
- Common hepatic duct (CHD)
- Liver

An axial section of the
- Right renal artery (RRA)
- Portal vein (PV)
- Right hepatic artery (RHA)
- Pancreas head (PH)

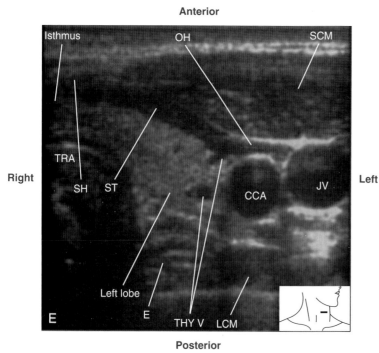

Anterior

Isthmus   OH   SCM

TRA

Right   SH   ST   CCA   JV   **Left**

Left lobe

E   E   THY V   LCM

Posterior

Transverse scanning plane image showing:
A longitudinal section of the
- Isthmus

An axial section of the
- Trachea (TRA)
- Thyroid (Left lobe)
- Esophagus (E)
- Common carotid artery (CCA)
- Internal jugular vein (JV)
- Inferior thyroid vessels (THY V)
- Strap muscles: omohyoid (OH), sternothyroid (ST), sternohyoid (SH), sternocleidomastoid (SCM)
- Longus colli muscle (LCM)

FIGURE 6-4   **E,** Describing structure orientation.

7. BODY STRUCTURE RELATIONSHIPS

Describing the relationship of adjacent body structures helps identify anatomy in ultrasound image sections. Documented ultrasound images include the specific area of the body being imaged, patient position, and the scanning plane. Together, image documentation and determination of the relationship of adjacent structures classify or identify the anatomy in an ultrasound image section. As noted in Chapter 7, this is particularly significant when disease processes are present that affect the typical location(s) and appearance(s) of internal body structures. It is important to note that the standard sonographic appearance of body structures does not depend on the scanning plane from which they are imaged.

In a *sagittal scanning plane* image, the target organ or area of interest is always related to a structure immediately:
- Anterior to it
- Posterior to it
- Superior to it
  and
- Inferior to it

For example, in the following transabdominal sagittal scanning plane image (Figure 6-5) taken just to the left of the midline of the body, if the body of the pancreas is the area of interest, you can see that the:
- Liver is anterior to it
- Splenic vein, superior mesenteric artery, and aorta are posterior to it
- Splenic artery is superior to it
- Stomach is inferior to it

Even if you did not know that was the body of the pancreas, you could take the adjacent relationships and apply them to anatomic layers or even look them up

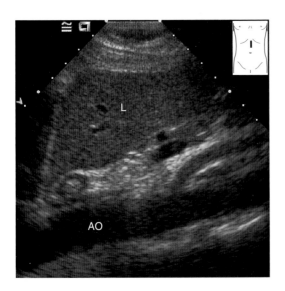

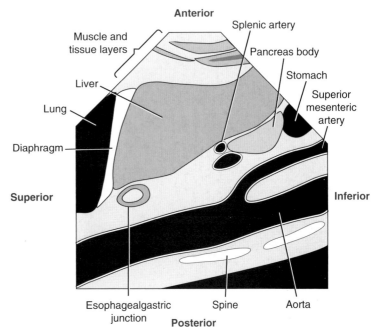

FIGURE 6-5

in an anatomy book to find the answer. If you were only able to conclude that the area of interest (body of the pancreas) has the echo texture of an organ and you could only identify the liver and the aorta in the image, a deduction could still be made by determining how many organs lie directly between the liver and the aorta. When the origin of pathology cannot be identified, it is treated in the same respect.

The same principle can be applied to every structure in Figure 6-5. For example, if the esophageal gastric junction is the area of interest, then the:

- Liver is anterior to it
- Aorta is posterior to it
- Diaphragm is superior to it
- Splenic artery, splenic vein, pancreas body, stomach, and superior mesenteric artery are inferior to it

If the midaorta is the area of interest, the:

- Superior mesenteric artery, splenic vein, pancreas body, splenic artery, and liver are anterior to it
- Spine is posterior to it
- Proximal aorta is superior to it
- Distal aorta is inferior to it

In a *coronal scanning plane image*, the target organ or area of interest is always related to a structure immediately:

- Right or left lateral to it
- Medial to it
- Superior to it
  and
- Inferior to it

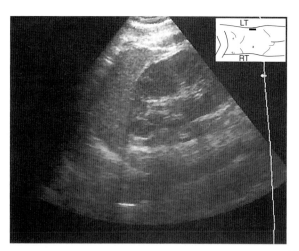
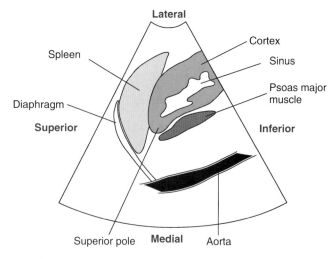

FIGURE 6-6

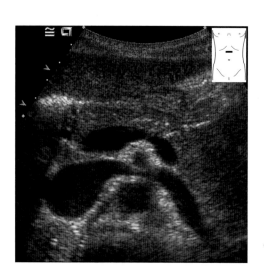
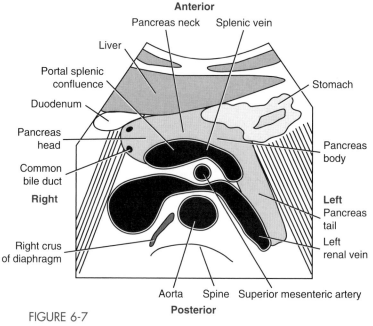

FIGURE 6-7

For example, in the above coronal scanning plane image (Figure 6-6) taken from a left lateral approach, using the superior pole of the left kidney, you can see that the:
- Spleen is left lateral to it
- Psoas major muscle and aorta are medial to it
- Spleen is superior to it
- Lower pole is inferior to it

In a *transverse scanning plane* image from an anterior or posterior approach, the target organ or area of interest is always related to a structure immediately:
- Anterior to it
- Posterior to it
- Right lateral to it
  and
- Left lateral to it

For example, in the above transabdominal transverse scanning plane image (Figure 6-7), if the neck of the pancreas is the area of interest, you can see that the:
- Liver is anterior to it
- Portal splenic confluence and inferior vena cava are posterior to it

- Portion of the pancreas head, gastroduodenal artery, common bile duct, and duodenum are right lateral to it
- Pancreas body and the stomach are left lateral to it

In a *transverse scanning plane* image from either a right or left lateral approach, the target organ or area of interest is always related to a structure immediately:

- Right or left lateral to it
- Medial to it
- Anterior to it

    and

- Posterior to it

Multiple scanning planes are utilized in ultrasound imaging because single-plane views do not provide enough confirmation to make definitive judgments. Multiple scanning planes provide multiple dimensions, which generate not only volume measurements, but also an overall complete assessment. If something visualized in one scanning plane can be verified in the perpendicular scanning plane, then the findings are considered confirmed and reliable.

It is good practice to compare the anatomic relationships recognized sonographically to gross anatomy. For example, Figure 6-8 is a transabdominal sagittal scanning plane image taken just to the right of the midline of the body (represented by the solid line on the layering illustrations). By twisting the

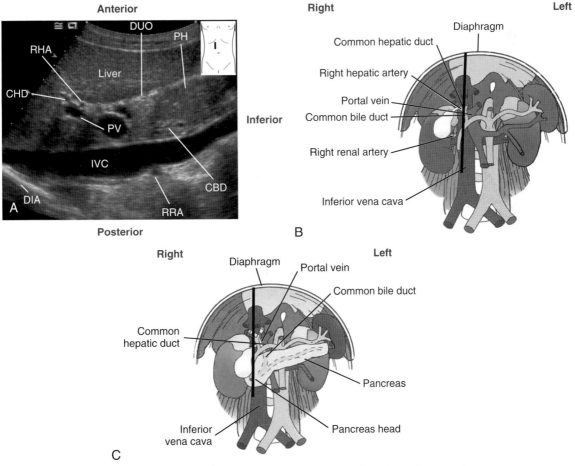

FIGURE 6-8 **Comparing Ultrasound Image Section to Corresponding Gross Anatomy Layers.** **A,** Transabdominal sagittal scanning plane image just to the right of the midline of the body demonstrating an axial section of the head of the pancreas and adjacent structures. DIA (diaphragm), RRA (right renal artery), IVC (inferior vena cava), PV (portal vein), CBD (common bile duct), PH (pancreas head), CHD (common hepatic duct), RHA (right hepatic artery), DUO (duodenum). **B,** Corresponding gross anatomy represented in an illustrated layer of the abdomen (solid line represents the sagittal scanning plane position). **C,** Corresponding gross anatomy represented in an illustrated layer of the abdomen anterior to the layer in **B**.

transducer 90 degrees (usually to the right for correct orientation) into the perpendicular plane—in this case the transverse scanning plane (represented by the dotted line on the layering illustrations, Figure 6-9)—the anatomy can not only be confirmed but also examined in another dimension, thereby affording a broader perspective.

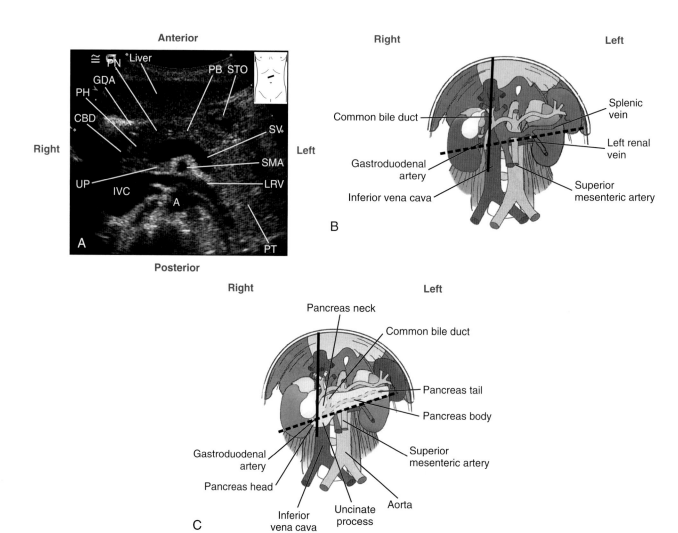

FIGURE 6-9 **Comparing Ultrasound Image Section to Corresponding Gross Anatomy Layers.** **A,** Transabdominal transverse scanning plane image of the mid to lower epigastrium, demonstrating the long axis of the pancreas and adjacent structures. A (aorta), IVC (inferior vena cava), LRV (left renal vein), SMA (superior mesenteric artery), UP (uncinate process of the pancreas), PT (pancreas tail), SV (splenic vein), SMA (superior mesenteric artery), PH (pancreas head), CBD (common bile duct), PN (pancreas neck), GDA (gastroduodenal artery), PB (pancreas body), STO (stomach). **B,** Corresponding gross anatomy represented in an illustrated layer of the abdomen (dotted line represents the transverse scanning plane position, solid line represents sagittal scanning plane position). **C,** Corresponding gross anatomy represented in an illustrated layer of the abdomen anterior to the layer in **B.**

8. COMPARISON OF CADAVER SECTIONS AND ULTRASOUND IMAGE SECTIONS

It is immediately apparent that the size, shape, and relationship of adjacent structures, positional orientation, and location of body structures do not change in regard to cadaver sections and ultrasound images.

In the following comparison of cadaver section and ultrasound image at the level of the tenth thoracic vertebra (Figure 6-10), it is clear that the size, shape, and positional orientation of the caudate lobe of the liver, ligamentum venosum, inferior vena cava, and stomach are the same.

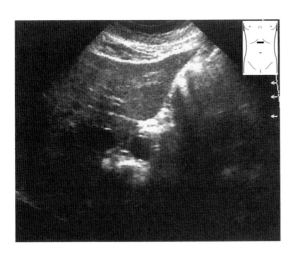
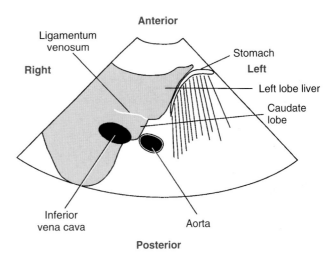

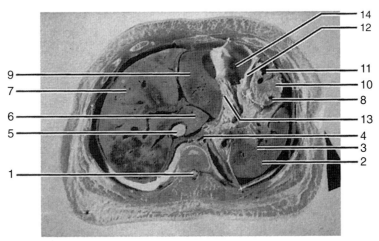

1. Spinal cord
2. Spleen
3. Hilum of spleen
4. Descending abdominal aorta
5. Inferior vena cava
6. Caudate lobe
7. Right lobe of the liver
8. Descending colon
9. Left lobe of the liver
10. Splenic flexure (left colic flexure)
11. Transverse colon
12. Greater curvature of stomach
13. Lesser curvature of stomach
14. Lumen of stomach

FIGURE 6-10   **Comparing Image and Cadaver Sections.** (From Bowden RL et al: *Basic atlas of modern section anatomy*, Philadelphia, 2006, Saunders.)

When comparing this cadaver section and ultrasound image at the level of the twelfth thoracic vertebra (Figure 6-11), it is apparent that the size, shape, positional orientation, and location of the pancreas and adjacent structures are the same. Note that the head of the pancreas rests against the duodenum and sits directly anterior to the inferior vena cava. Also observe the locations and adjacent relationships of the aorta, tail of the pancreas, and left kidney.

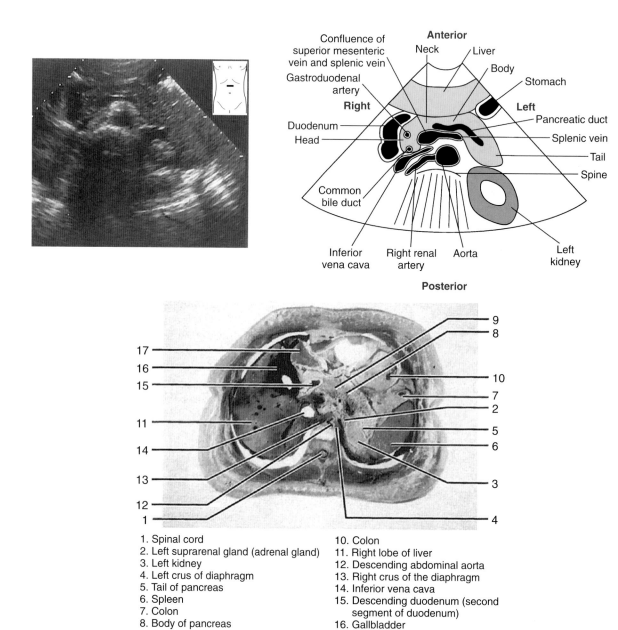

FIGURE 6-11 **Comparing Image and Cadaver Sections.** (From Bowden RL et al: *Basic atlas of modern section anatomy*, Philadelphia, 2006, Saunders.)

1. Spinal cord
2. Left suprarenal gland (adrenal gland)
3. Left kidney
4. Left crus of diaphragm
5. Tail of pancreas
6. Spleen
7. Colon
8. Body of pancreas
9. Head of pancreas
10. Colon
11. Right lobe of liver
12. Descending abdominal aorta
13. Right crus of the diaphragm
14. Inferior vena cava
15. Descending duodenum (second segment of duodenum)
16. Gallbladder
17. Stomach

This cadaver and ultrasound section (Figure 6-12) is at the level of the second lumbar vertebra. Compare the identical size, location, and positional orientation of the superior mesenteric artery, aorta, right renal artery, and inferior vena cava. Note the location of the kidneys.

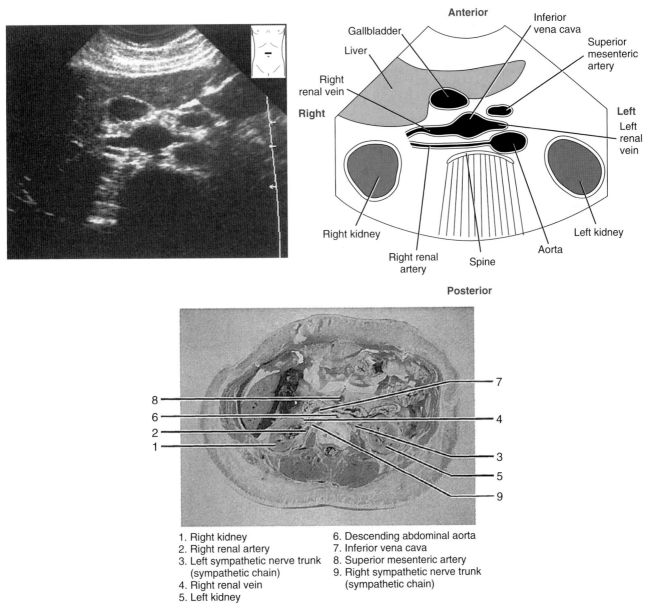

1. Right kidney
2. Right renal artery
3. Left sympathetic nerve trunk (sympathetic chain)
4. Right renal vein
5. Left kidney
6. Descending abdominal aorta
7. Inferior vena cava
8. Superior mesenteric artery
9. Right sympathetic nerve trunk (sympathetic chain)

FIGURE 6-12   **Comparing Image and Cadaver Sections.** (From Bowden RL et al: *Basic atlas of modern section anatomy*, Philadelphia, 2006, Saunders.)

In the comparison of cadaver section and ultrasound image at the level of the fifth vertebra of the sacrum shown in Figure 6-13, it is obvious that the size, shape, and positional orientation of the uterus are the same on both sections. Observe the comparable locations of the urinary bladder. Also, notice the location and adjacent relationships of the rectum, rectouterine pouch (posterior cul-de-sac), and ovary, as indicated on the cadaver section.

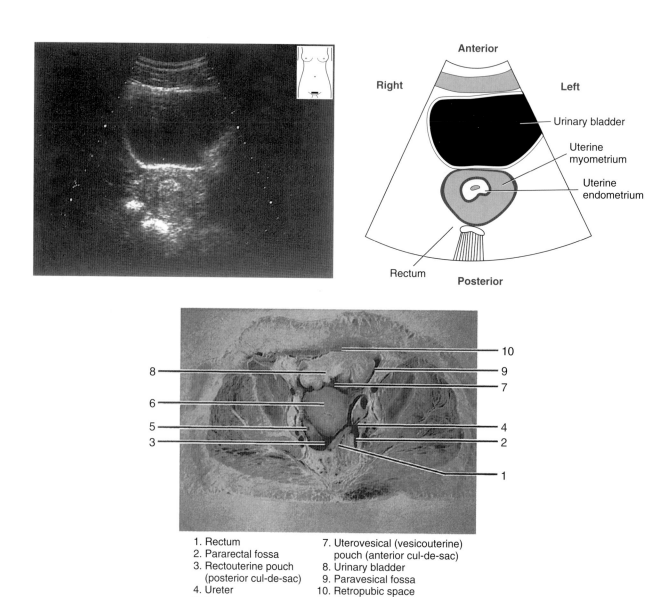

1. Rectum
2. Pararectal fossa
3. Rectouterine pouch (posterior cul-de-sac)
4. Ureter
5. Ovary
6. Uterus (womb)
7. Uterovesical (vesicouterine) pouch (anterior cul-de-sac)
8. Urinary bladder
9. Paravesical fossa
10. Retropubic space

FIGURE 6-13 **Comparing Image and Cadaver Sections.** (From Bowden RL et al: *Basic atlas of modern section anatomy*, Philadelphia, 2006, Saunders.)

ABDOMINAL LAYERS

A valuable exercise is to use Play-Doh to duplicate abdominal layers (Figures 6-14 through 6-23). Choose one color of Play-Doh for the muscles, another for the arteries, still another for the veins, and so on. This exercise helps differentiate the intricate relationships of internal body structures, and it reinforces the concept that familiarity with how anatomy is layered leads to easier recognition of the same anatomy in cross-sections.

Muscle Layer

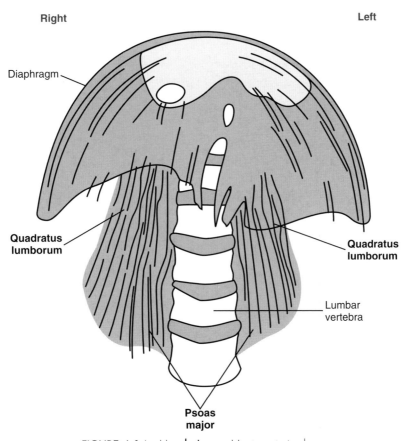

FIGURE 6-14 **Muscle Layer.** Most posterior layer.

Quadratus Lumborum Muscle
- Bilateral
- Extends from the iliolumbar ligament, adjacent portion of the iliac crest, and the transverse processes of the lower lumbar vertebrae. Courses upward, lateral to the psoas major muscle, until it terminates at the twelfth rib.

Psoas Major Muscle
- Bilateral
- Somewhat triangular
- Originates from the lower thoracic and lumbar vertebrae. Courses slightly anterior and lateral as it descends through the lower abdomen just lateral to the spine. Near the fifth lumbar vertebra it courses more laterally, away from the spine, on its descent to the iliac crests, where it terminates.
- The iliac vessels run through the space left between the spine and psoas when it courses laterally.

Kidneys and Adrenal Glands

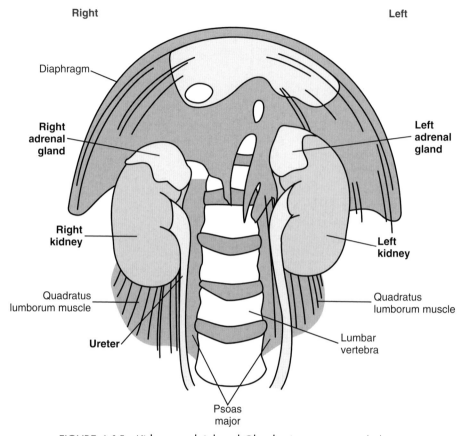

Right   Left

Diaphragm

Right adrenal gland

Left adrenal gland

Right kidney

Left kidney

Quadratus lumborum muscle

Quadratus lumborum muscle

Ureter

Lumbar vertebra

Psoas major

FIGURE 6-15 **Kidneys and Adrenal Glands.** Anterior to muscle layer.

Kidneys
- Bilateral; vertical oblique orientation
- Retroperitoneal, between the twelfth thoracic and fourth lumbar vertebrae. Directly anterior to the quadratus lumborum and psoas major muscles.

Adrenal Glands
- Bilateral; vertical oblique orientation
- Retroperitoneal. Just superoanterior and slightly medial to each kidney. Directly anterior to the quadratus lumborum and psoas major muscles.

Inferior Vena Cava (IVC)

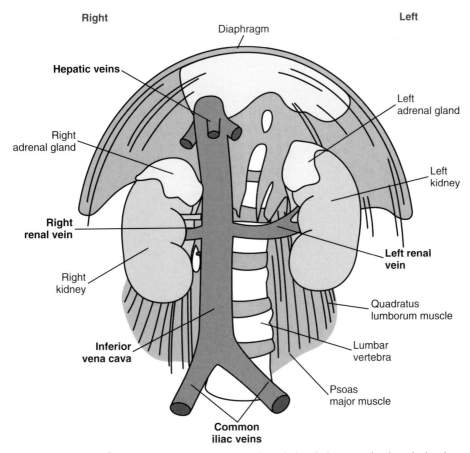

FIGURE 6-16   **Inferior Vena Cava.** Anterior and medial to kidneys and adrenal glands.

Inferior Vena Cava (IVC)
- Vertical orientation. Originates at the junction of the common iliac veins, just anterior to the fifth lumbar vertebra.
- Ascends the retroperitoneum anterior to the spine and psoas major muscle.
- Pierces the diaphragm to enter the right atrium of the heart.

IVC Tributaries
- **Left and right renal veins.** Enter the IVC bilaterally. Horizontal orientations.
- **Left, right, and middle hepatic veins.** Enter the IVC anteriorly. Vertical orientations.

Abdominal Aorta

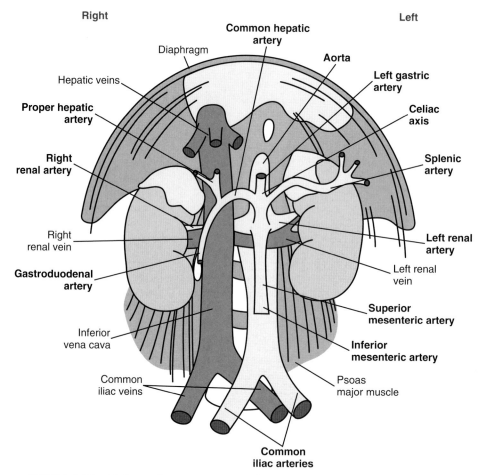

FIGURE 6-17 **Abdominal Aorta.** Anterior and medial to kidneys and adrenal glands.

Abdominal Aorta

- Vertical orientation. Originates at the left ventricle of the heart, then descends through the chest (thoracic aorta) to pierce the diaphragm and enter the abdominal cavity.
- Descends the retroperitoneum anterior to the spine and psoas major muscle.
- Bifurcates into the common iliac arteries near the level of the fourth lumbar vertebra.

Aorta Branches

- **Celiac artery/axis.** Arises anteriorly from the aorta. Vertical orientation. Has 3 branches:
  1. **Splenic artery.** Horizontal orientation, courses left lateral to the spleen, anterior to the left kidney and left adrenal gland. Typically tortuous.
  2. **Common hepatic artery.** Horizontal orientation on its right lateral course to the liver. Has two branches:
     a. **Proper hepatic artery.** Vertical oblique orientation, runs superiorly and slightly right lateral to the liver hilum.
     b. **Gastroduodenal artery.** Vertical orientation, runs inferiorly to the pylorus of the stomach and the duodenum.
  3. **Left gastric artery.** Vertical then horizontal orientation (tortuous). Travels to the stomach and esophagus.

- **Superior mesenteric artery.** Arises anteriorly from the aorta. Vertical orientation. Runs inferiorly, parallel to the aorta on its course to the small bowel and pancreas. Is anterior to the horizontally orientated left renal vein.
- **Left and right renal arteries.** Arise bilaterally from the aorta. Horizontal orientations. Posterior to the right and left renal veins. Right renal artery runs directly posterior to the vertically oriented inferior vena cava.
- **Inferior mesenteric artery.** Arises anteriorly from the aorta. Vertical orientation. Runs inferiorly to the large bowel and rectum.

Portal Venous System

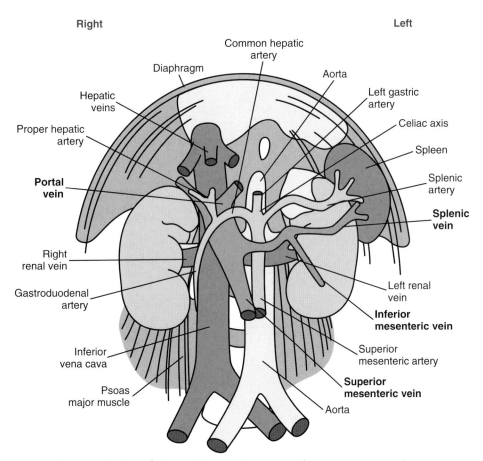

FIGURE 6-18 **Portal Venous System.** Anterior to inferior vena cava and aorta.

Portal Venous System
- Encompasses the superior mesenteric vein, inferior mesenteric vein, and splenic vein, which unite to form the portal vein. This portal splenic confluence occurs directly posterior to the pancreas neck.
- **Superior mesenteric vein.** Vertical oblique orientation. Ascends from the small bowel, anterior to the uncinate process of the pancreas, and terminates posterior to the pancreas neck, where it joins the splenic vein to from the portal vein. Runs just right lateral to the superior mesenteric artery. Runs parallel and right lateral to the inferior mesenteric vein.
- **Inferior mesenteric vein.** Vertical oblique orientation. Ascends from the large bowel and terminates when it enters the splenic vein.
- **Splenic vein.** Horizontal orientation. Inferoposterior to the splenic artery. Travels medially from the spleen and terminates posterior to the pancreas neck, where it unites with the superior mesenteric vein to form the portal vein. On its course,

it runs along the posterior aspect of the pancreas tail, body, and neck. It passes directly anterior to the left kidney and the superior mesenteric artery.

- **Portal vein.** Horizontal then vertical oblique orientation. Formed by the union of the superior mesenteric and splenic veins directly posterior to the neck of the pancreas. Ascends to the liver hilum, directly posterior to the common and proper hepatic arteries. Divides into right and left branches inside the liver.

Gallbladder and Biliary Tract

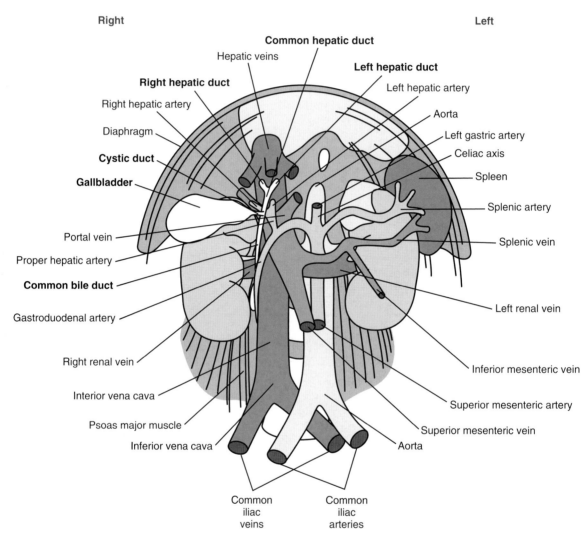

FIGURE 6-19 **Gallbladder and Biliary Tract.** Anterior to portal vein, inferior vena cava, and right kidney.

Biliary Tract
- Intraperitoneal
- Composed of *right* and *left hepatic ducts, common duct,* and *cystic duct*
  - ○ **Right and left hepatic ducts.** Vertical oblique orientation. Bile-filled intrahepatic ducts that unite at the liver hilum to form the common duct.
  - ○ **Common duct.** Vertical oblique orientation. Descriptively divided into a proximal portion, the common hepatic duct, and a distal portion, the common bile duct.
    - • **Common hepatic duct.** From the liver hilum, it runs a short distance inferiorly, passing anterior to the right hepatic artery on its course to meet the

cystic duct, which is connected to the gallbladder. From this level, the common hepatic duct continues as the common bile duct.
- **Common bile duct**. Courses inferomedially, running behind a portion of the first part of the duodenum on its way to the head of the pancreas, where it meets the pancreatic duct. Either together or separately, the common bile duct and pancreatic duct terminate after they enter the duodenum.
    - ○ **Cystic duct**. Vertical oblique orientation. A short duct that joins the gallbladder with the common duct. Typically located adjacent to the cystic artery.

Gallbladder
- Intraperitoneal. Orientation is variable, only the gallbladder neck is fixed in its position.
- Descriptive divisions are the *neck, body,* and *fundus.*
    - ○ **Neck.** Is the "S"-shaped curve situated above the body of the gallbladder that connects to the cystic duct.
    - ○ **Body.** Portion of the gallbladder lying between the neck and fundus.
    - ○ **Fundus.** Lower free, expanded end of the gallbladder. Often located anterior to the superior pole of the right kidney.

Pancreas

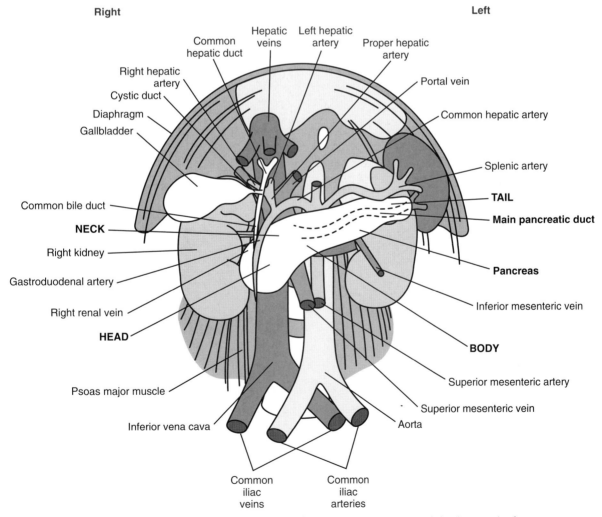

FIGURE 6-20 Pancreas. Anterior to the portal venous system, common bile duct, and inferior vena cava.

Pancreas

- Retroperitoneal. Horizontal oblique orientation. Extends from the hilum of the spleen to the duodenum.
- Descriptively composed of a *head, uncinate process, neck, body,* and *tail.*
  - **Pancreas head.** Sits directly anterior to the inferior vena cava between the duodenum on the right and the superior mesenteric vein on the left. Lies at a level slightly inferior to the level of the neck, body, and tail. Is posterior and medial to the gastroduodenal artery. Is anterior and medial to the distal common duct (common bile duct).
  - **Uncinate process.** Medial projection of the pancreas head that varies in size, but typically is situated directly anterior to the inferior vena cava and posterior to the superior mesenteric vein and pancreas neck. It can extend as far to the left to lie between the superior mesenteric artery anteriorly and aorta posteriorly.
  - **Pancreas neck.** Just medial to the pancreas head, directly anterior to the superior mesenteric vein (inferiorly) and portal splenic confluence (superiorly). Inferior to common and proper hepatic arteries. Separated from the uncinate process by the superior mesenteric vein.
  - **Pancreas body.** Just medial to the pancreas neck. Anterior to, in order of occurrence, the splenic vein, superior mesenteric artery, left renal vein, and aorta. Inferior to common hepatic and splenic arteries. Extends left laterally to the tail.
  - **Pancreas tail.** Extends left lateral from the pancreas body to the hilum of the spleen. Anterior to the splenic vein and superior pole of the left kidney. Typically inferior to the splenic artery.

Gastrointestinal Tract

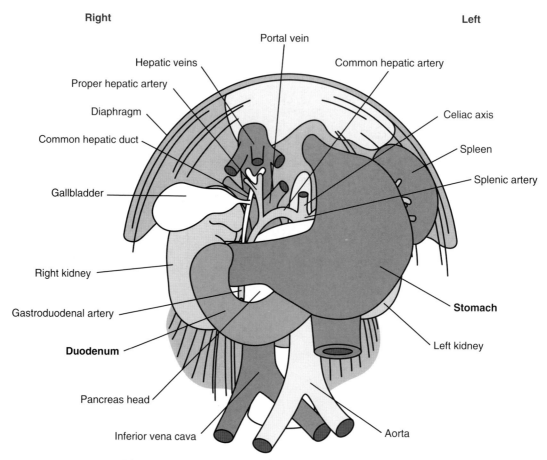

FIGURE 6-21 **Gastrointestinal Tract.** Anterior to the pancreas.

Stomach

- Vertical then horizontal orientation
- Anterior to the diaphragm, spleen, left adrenal gland, superior pole of the left kidney, anterior aspect of the pancreas body and tail, and splenic flexure of the colon

Duodenum

- Presents an unusual orientation—it is in the shape of an imperfect circle so that its termination is not far removed from its starting point.
- Begins at the pylorus of the stomach and runs horizontally to the neck of the gallbladder. Typically posterior to the gallbladder and anterior to the gastroduodenal artery, pancreas head, common bile duct, common hepatic artery, and portal vein.
- Takes a sharp curve and descends along the right margin of the pancreas head for a variable distance, usually to the level of the superior edge of the fourth lumbar vertebra.
- Curves again, passing horizontally, right to left with a slight inclination upward, anterior to the inferior vena cava, aorta, and vertebral column.
- Ends opposite the second lumbar vertebra at the jejunum.

Liver

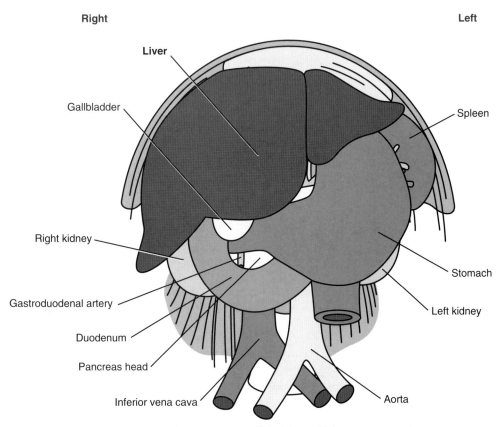

FIGURE 6-22 Liver. Anterior to the pancreas, gallbladder and biliary tract, portal venous system, aorta, inferior vena cava, and kidneys.

Liver

- Horizontal oblique orientation. Occupies the right upper quadrant and often extends across the midline of the body into the left upper quadrant.
- Intraperitoneal except for a bare area that is posterior to its dome.
- Most anterior organ of the peritoneal cavity.
- Descriptively divided into *right* and *left lobes*.
  - **Right lobe.** Immediately anterior to the gallbladder, right kidney (primarily the superior pole), right adrenal gland, and head of the pancreas.
  - **Left lobe.** Immediately anterior to the stomach and body of the pancreas.
- Superior and lateral surfaces border the diaphragm.

Muscle Layer

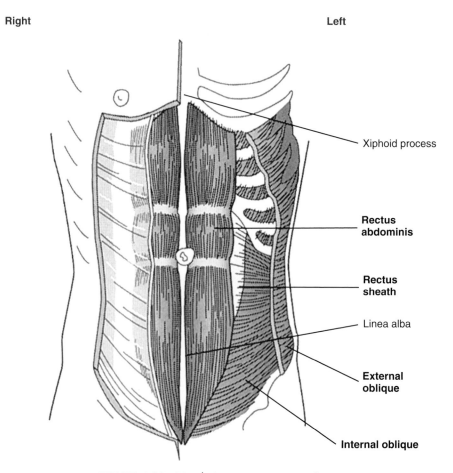

FIGURE 6-23 **Muscle Layer.** Most anterior layer.

Anterior Muscles

- Abdominal wall is the most anterior abdominal layer.
- Extends from the xiphoid process of the sternum to the pelvic bones.
- Consists of *subcutaneous tissue* and *muscles*.
  - **Subcutaneous tissue.** Contains fat, fibrous tissue, fascia, small vessels, and nerves.
  - **Muscles.** Rectus abdominis is bilateral to the linea alba, a white line of connective tissue in the midline of the peritoneal cavity. Vertical orientation. Originates at the pubis, then ascends to insert at the xiphoid process and costal cartilages of the fifth, sixth, and seventh ribs. Enclosed by the rectus sheath, layers of the oblique and transversus muscles.

PELVIC LAYERS

A valuable exercise is to use Play-Doh to duplicate the pelvic layers (Figures 6-24 through 6-29). Choose one color of Play-Doh for the muscles, another for the arteries, still another for the veins, and so on. This exercise helps differentiate the intricate relationships of internal body structures and reinforces the concept that familiarity with how anatomy is layered leads to easier recognition of the same anatomy in cross-sections.

True Pelvis Muscle Layer

Right   Left

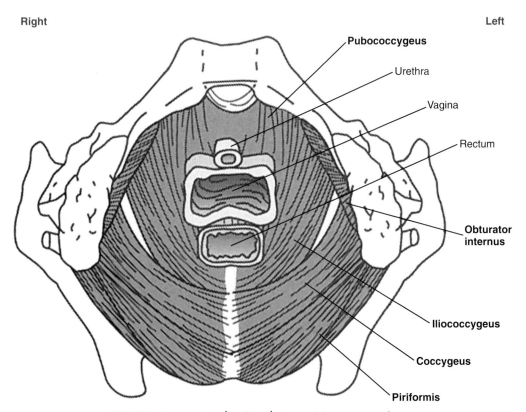

FIGURE 6-24 True Pelvis Muscle Layer. Most posterior layer.

True Pelvis Muscles
- The true pelvis muscle layer is the deepest layer of the pelvis.
- Muscles of this layer include the *obturator internus, piriformis, coccygeus, iliococcygeus,* and *pubococcygeus.*
  - **Obturator internus muscle.** Triangular, bilateral muscle tissue that originates at the pelvic brim. Courses parallel and adjacent to the lateral pelvic wall, narrowing inferiorly to pass through the lesser sciatic foramen to the greater trochanter of the femur. Lateral to the pelvic viscera.
  - **Piriformis muscle.** Triangular, bilateral muscle that originates from the sacrum. Extends laterally, narrowing to pass through the greater sciatic foramen to the greater trochanter of the femur.
  - **Pubococcygeus, iliococcygeus, and coccygeus muscles.** Referred to as the pelvic diaphragm. Line the floor of the true pelvis.
  - **Pubococcygeus, puborectalis, and iliococcygeus muscles.** Referred to as the levator ani muscles, a hammock-like portion of the pelvic floor. The pubococcygeus muscles course from the pubic bone to the coccyx. A separation in a section of the muscle, termed the *genital hiatus,* allows the passage of the urethra, vagina, and rectum (as demonstrated here). In males, the levator

prostate, a section of the puborectalis muscle, embraces the sides of the prostate. This portion is called the pubovaginalis in women.

○ **Pubococcygeus muscle pair.** The most medial and anterior muscles of the pelvic diaphragm.

○ **Iliococcygeus muscles.** Extend from the ischial spine to the coccyx. Lie just lateral to the pubococcygeus muscles.

○ **Coccygeus muscles.** Course from the ischial spine to the coccyx. They are the most posterior muscle pair of the pelvic diaphragm.

False Pelvis Muscles

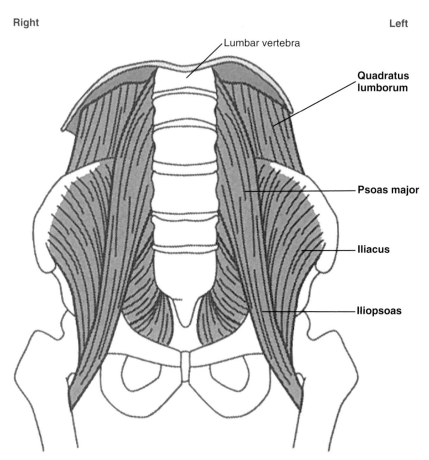

Right   Left

Lumbar vertebra

Quadratus
lumborum

Psoas major

Iliacus

Iliopsoas

FIGURE 6-25   **False Pelvis Muscle Layer.** Anterior to true pelvis muscles.

False Pelvis Muscles

• Muscles of the posterior body wall and false pelvis include the *quadratus lumborum, psoas major, iliacus,* and *iliopsoas.*

○ **Quadratus lumborum muscle.** A bilateral muscle tissue. Vertical orientation. Extends from the iliolumbar ligament to the adjacent portion of the iliac crest, and the transverse processes of the lower lumbar vertebrae. Courses upward, lateral to the psoas major muscle, until it reaches the twelfth rib.

○ **Psoas major muscle.** Somewhat triangular, bilateral muscle that originates from the lower thoracic and lumbar vertebrae. Vertical oblique orientation. Courses slightly anterolaterally as it descends through the lower abdomen right next to the spine. Near the fifth lumbar vertebra, the psoas major separates from the spine and runs laterally on its descent to the iliac crests. This separation creates a space between the vertebral column and the psoas major,

through which the iliac vessels travel. At the level of the iliac crests, the psoas major muscles join the iliacus muscles to form the iliopsoas muscles.
- ○ **Iliacus muscles.** Originate from the iliac fossa and the base of the sacrum. Extend to meet the psoas major muscle.
- ○ **Iliopsoas muscles.** Descend laterally passing over the pelvic inlet to insert into the lesser trochanter of the femur.

Rectum/Colon

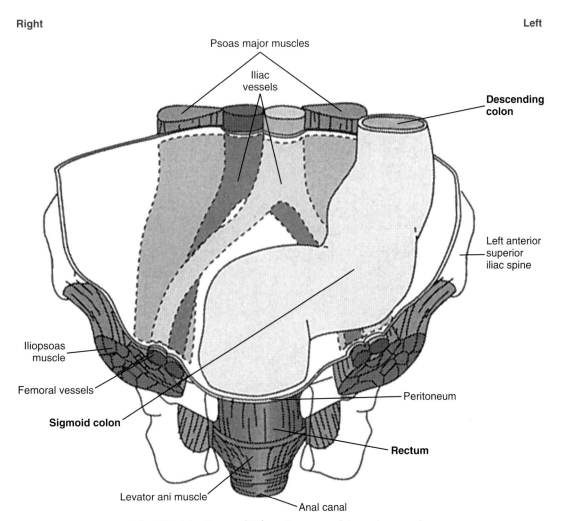

FIGURE 6-26   Rectum/Colon. Anterior to false pelvis muscles.

Rectum/Colon
- This layer includes the *rectum* and portions of the *colon.*
  - ○ **Descending colon.** Passes downward through the peritoneal cavity along the lateral border of the left kidney. Curves medially at the inferior pole of the kidney toward the lateral border of the psoas major muscle. Descends in the angle between the psoas major and quadratus lumborum muscle to the iliac crest. Distal portion (iliac colon) begins at the iliac crest and runs just anterior to the psoas major and iliacus muscle to the sigmoid portion of the colon.
  - ○ **Sigmoid colon.** Continuous with the descending colon. Passes horizontally, anterior to the sacrum to the right side of the pelvis. Curves toward the left to reach the midline of the pelvis, where it bends downward and ends at the rectum. Anterior to the external iliac vessels and the left piriformis muscle.

○ **Rectum.** Continuous with the sigmoid colon. Ends in the anal canal below. Courses inferiorly, anterior to the coccyx, where it bends back sharply into the anal canal. This inferior portion lies directly anterior to the sacrum, coccyx, and levator ani muscle.

Uterus/Bladder

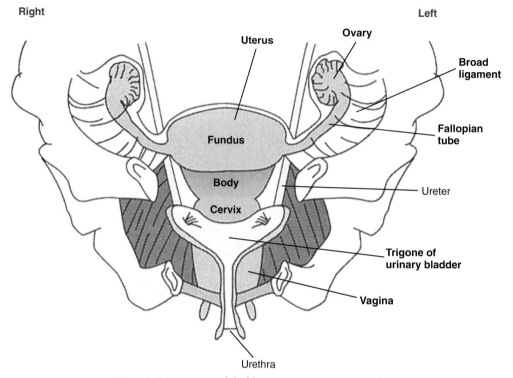

FIGURE 6-27   Uterus/Bladder. Anterior to rectum/colon.

> **NOTE:** A large portion of the bladder has not been drawn to facilitate the location of the organs immediately adjacent to it.

Uterus/Urinary Bladder
• **Uterus.** An organ of the female pelvis. The nonpregnant uterus is located in the true pelvis, anterior to the rectum and posterior to the bladder. Typically oriented vertically. There are spaces (not demonstrated here) posterior and anterior to the uterus that are referred to as the posterior cul-de-sac (pouch of Douglas or rectouterine pouch) and anterior cul-de-sac, formed by the peritoneum. Descriptively divided into the *fundus, body,* and *cervix.*
  ○ **Fundus.** The superior, anteriorly tilted part of the uterus.
  ○ **Body.** The vertical, oblique portion between the fundus and the cervix.
  ○ **Cervix.** Inferior to the body of the uterus and continuous with the vagina.
• Other organs of the female pelvis include the *vagina, fallopian (uterine) tubes,* and *ovaries.*
  ○ **Vagina.** A vertically oriented, elongated structure located just anterior to the rectum and posterior to the bladder (trigone) and urethra. Note that the distal portion of the ureters is lateral to the vagina.

○ **Fallopian tubes.** Lie in the superior part of the broad ligament and extend laterally toward the ovaries. The broad ligament is actually a double fold of peritoneum covering the anterior surface of all of the pelvic viscera except for the ovaries.

○ **Ovaries.** Located on the posterior portion of the broad ligament and entirely inside the peritoneal sac. The ovaries are not demonstrated here because, although "attached" laterally to the uterus by the fallopian tubes and broad ligament, they are posterior to both structures. The ovary is also immediately anterior to a portion of the ureter and internal iliac vessels.

• **Urinary bladder.** Situated in a vertical oblique orientation in the anterior pelvis. The superior portion is anterior to the inferior portion.

Prostate Gland/Bladder

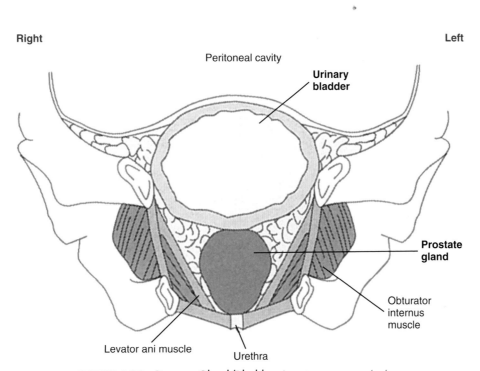

FIGURE 6-28 **Prostate Gland/Bladder.** Anterior to rectum/colon.

Prostate Gland/Urinary Bladder

• The organs of the male pelvis appreciated at this layer are the *prostate gland* and *urinary bladder*.

○ **Prostate gland.** Retroperitoneal. Anterior to the rectum and inferior to the bladder. Lateral surfaces are in close proximity to the levator prostate muscles, which are separated from the gland by a plexus of veins. Not demonstrated here, but important to note, is the fact that the prostate is perforated by the urethra and ejaculatory duct, and the seminal vesicles lie superior to the prostate gland and posterior to the bladder.

○ **Urinary bladder.** Vertical oblique orientation in the anterior pelvis. The superior portion is anterior to the inferior portion. Directly anterior to the rectum.

Muscle Layer

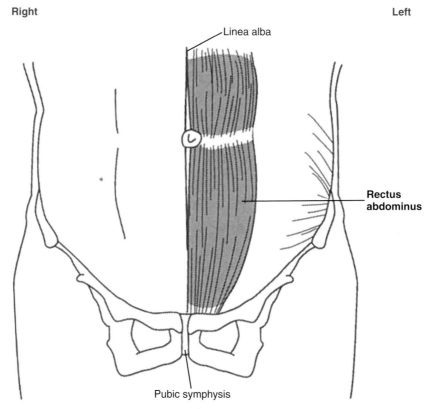

FIGURE 6-29 **Muscle Layer.** Most anterior layer.

Rectus Abdominus Muscle
- Most anterior muscle of the pelvis
- Bilateral muscle tissue immediately lateral to the linea alba (a white line of connective tissue in the median of the abdomen)
- Originates at the pubis and then ascends to insert at the xiphoid process of the sternum and costal cartilages of the fifth, sixth, and seventh ribs

CHAPTER 7

First Scanning Experience

BETTY BATES TEMPKIN AND KATHRYN A. GILL

OBJECTIVES

Become familiar with ultrasound terminology.
Describe the criteria for interpreting ultrasound scanning planes.
Describe clinical and professional standards.
Describe the significance of using an ultrasound scanning protocol.
Learn how to scan the abdominal aorta.
Describe the criteria for case presentations.

Identify standards that determine whether images in an ultrasound study meet the criteria for diagnostic purposes.
Describe the difference between diffuse and localized disease.
Describe the possible compositions of a mass and the characteristics of each.
Identify ways to describe the sonographic appearance of abnormal ultrasound findings within the scope of a sonographer's legal parameters.

Sonographers are medical professionals with specialized education and the ability to acquire, view, modify, analyze, and communicate diagnostic information obtained with ultrasound. They are required to have an in-depth understanding of cross-sectional anatomy, physiology, ultrasound physics, and clinical and communication skills, as well as highly developed psychomotor skills that are specific to the profession.

Sonographers work with complex, high-tech imaging machinery and instrumentation, which includes a handheld transducer that transmits nonionizing sound waves (in a rectangular or cone-shaped beam) and collects the reflected echoes to form an image of internal anatomy that may be photographed, videotaped, recorded on disc, or transmitted to an interpreting physician for diagnosis.

During an ultrasound scan, sonographers evaluate the images, looking for visual clues that draw a distinction between normal and abnormal echo patterns. They determine whether the images meet the criteria for diagnostic purposes, and then select which ones best represent the study. Sonographers also prepare an oral or written technical observation of the ultrasound findings—including any measurements, calculations, and analysis of the results—to accompany the images when the case is presented to the physician.

Because of the high degree of decisional latitude and technical analysis, sonographers play an integral role in patient evaluation, which carries a high level of responsibility in the diagnostic process.

As described in Chapter 1, sonographers have multiple duties that define their role in allied health and medicine. Among these duties is obtaining the required ultrasound images that are representative of study findings for physician interpretation. Image quality is directly proportional to the technical proficiency and scanning expertise of the sonographer.

SURFACE LANDMARKS

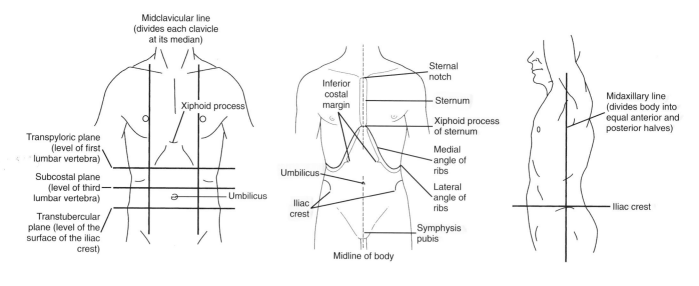

REGIONAL DIVISIONS OF THE ABDOMEN

QUADRANT DIVISIONS OF THE ABDOMEN

FIGURE 7-1 How to Describe the Location of Abdominopelvic Cavity Structures. Descriptive divisions and surface landmarks of the abdominopelvic cavity.

Accomplished scanning techniques are a result of practice and knowledge of the following:

- **Location of anatomy.** Body structures are accurately identified on ultrasound images by their location—*not* by their sonographic appearance, since it may be altered by pathology or other factors (Figure 7-1).
- **Sonographic appearance of normal body structures** (Table 7-1 on page 87) **and the terms used to describe their appearance** (Table 7-2 on page 89). An understanding of the normal sonographic appearance provides the baseline against which to recognize abnormalities.
- **Body planes, directional terms, and how to interpret ultrasound scanning planes** (Figures 7-2 and 7-3, *A* to *C*).
- **Imaging criteria** as described previously.
- **Sonographic characterization of ultrasound findings and the terms used to describe them.**

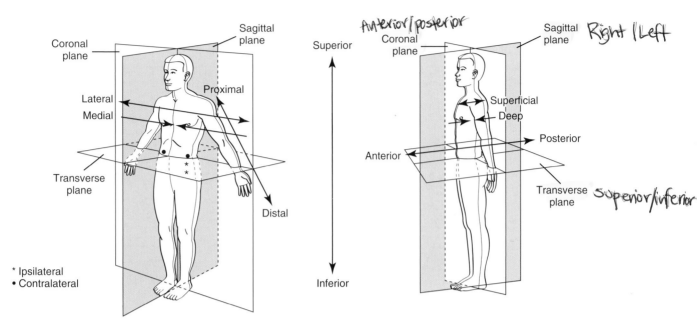

FIGURE 7-2 **Body Planes and Directional Terms.** View of the body in the anatomic position: standing erect, arms at the sides, face and palms directed forward. Body planes are sagittal, coronal, and transverse. Directional terms are superior to inferior; anterior to posterior; medial to lateral; superficial to deep; proximal to distal; and ipsilateral to contralateral.

BODY PLANES

The classic anatomic body planes are *transverse, sagittal,* and *coronal planes* (see Figure 7-2).

Transverse plane:
- Divides the body into unequal superior and inferior sections.
- Perpendicular to the long axis of the body.

Sagittal plane:
- Midsagittal plane divides the body into equal right and left halves.
- Parasagittal planes divide the body into unequal right and left sections.
- Parallel to the long axis of the body.

Coronal plane:
- Midcoronal plane runs along the midaxillary line and divides the body into equal anterior and posterior halves.
- All other coronal plane sections divide the body into unequal anterior and posterior sections.
- Perpendicular to sagittal planes and parallel to the long axis of the body.

ULTRASOUND SCANNING PLANES

The scanning planes used in sonography are the same as anatomic body planes (see Figures 7-2 and 7-3, A to C), but their interpretations depend on the *location of the transducer* and the *sound wave approach* (where the sound waves enter the body).

Figure 7-3, A to C demonstrates standard ultrasound scanning plane interpretations. Endocavital scanning plane interpretations are shown in Figure 7-4 on page 86. Figure 7-5 on page 86 demonstrates how to interpret neurosonography (neonatal brain) scanning planes.

Positional orientation of the transducer verifies the scanning plane. In most cases the manufacturer of the transducer sets the positional orientation. Sagittal scanning plane orientation, for example, is usually indicated by a notch or raised portion on the top surface of the transducer. Once the transducer orientation is established, the scanning plane can be changed by turning the transducer 90 degrees.

Text continued on p. 94

Saggital Scanning Plane
2 Approaches: Anterior or Posterior

1. Anterior Approach

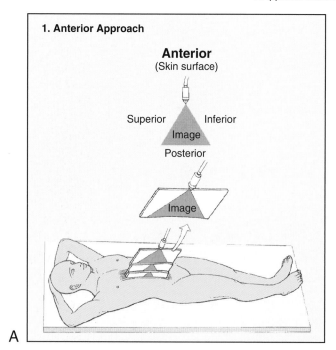

2. Posterior Approach

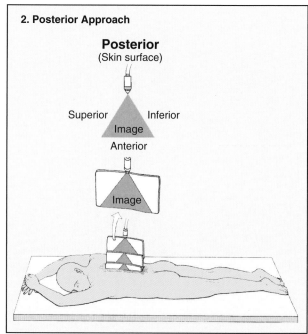

FIGURE 7-3   **A,** How to Interpret Sagittal Scanning Planes.

Coronal Scanning Plane
2 Approaches: Left Lateral or Right Lateral

1. Left Lateral Approach

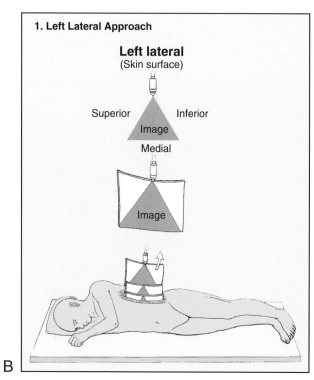

2. Right Lateral Approach

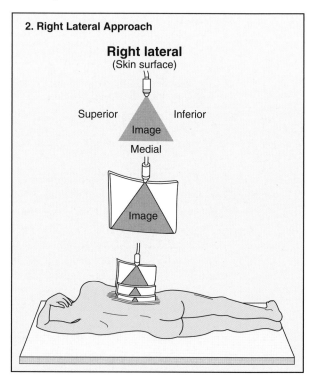

FIGURE 7-3, cont'd   **B,** How to Interpret Coronal Scanning Planes.

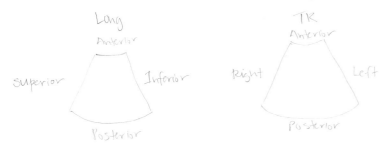

Transverse Scanning Plane
4 Approaches: Anterior or Posterior or Left Lateral or Right Lateral

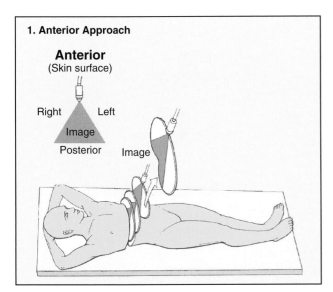

1. Anterior Approach

Anterior
(Skin surface)

Right   Left
Image
Posterior   Image

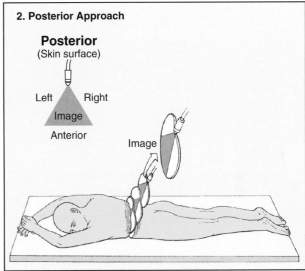

2. Posterior Approach

Posterior
(Skin surface)

Left   Right
Image
Anterior

Image

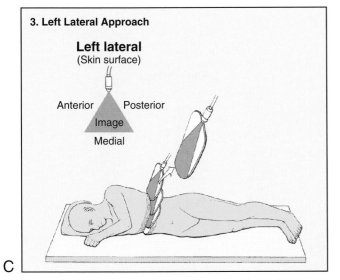

3. Left Lateral Approach

Left lateral
(Skin surface)

Anterior   Posterior
Image
Medial

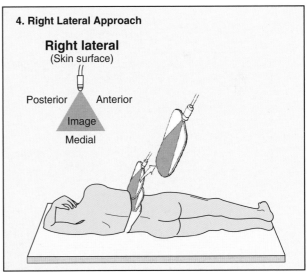

4. Right Lateral Approach

Right lateral
(Skin surface)

Posterior   Anterior
Image
Medial

C

FIGURE 7-3, cont'd   **C,** How to Interpret Transverse Scanning Planes.

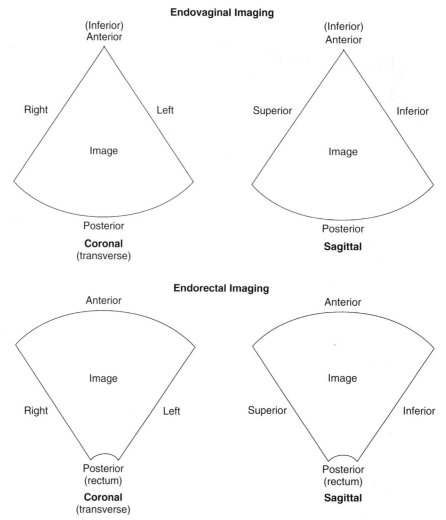

FIGURE 7-4 **Endocavital Scanning Plane Interpretations.** Endovaginal imaging and endorectal imaging are obtained from an inferior transcavital approach, which is technically organ oriented. Image orientation still varies among institutions, authors, and textbooks. These examples represent the majority.

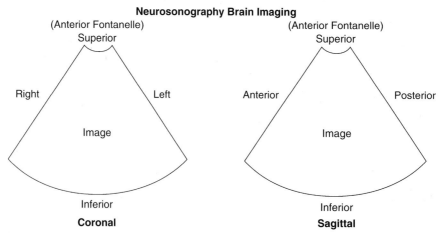

FIGURE 7-5 **Neurosonography/Neonatal Brain Scanning Plane Interpretations.** The anterior fontanelle is used as the primary acoustic window or approach when imaging the neonatal brain. In some instances the posterior fontanelle and mastoid fontanelles are utilized (see Chapter 26).

Table 7-1 How to Describe the Sonographic Appearance of Normal Body Structures

Body Structures	Image	Normal Sonographic Appearance
Organ parenchyma	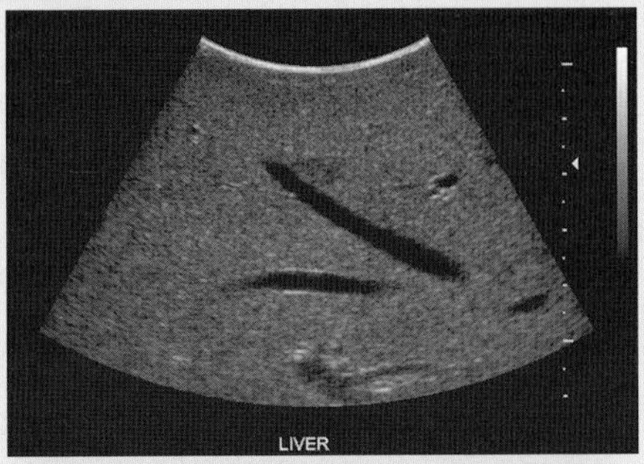 LIVER	■ Homogeneous or uniform echo texture with ranges in echogenicity. ■ Liver parenchyma, for example, could be described as homogeneous and moderately echogenic.
Muscle	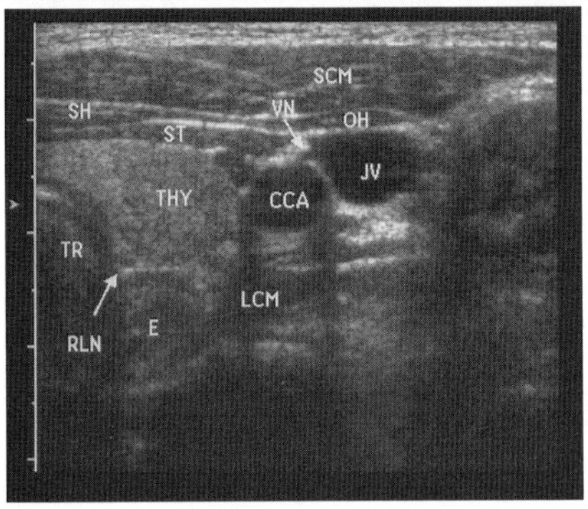 SCM (sternocleidomastoid muscle), OH (omohyoid muscle), ST (sternothyroid muscle), SH (sternohyoid muscle), LCM (longus colli muscle), THY (thyroid), CCA (common carotid artery), JV (jugular vein), E (esophagus), TR (trachea), RLN (recurrent laryngeal nerve), VN (vagus nerve)	■ Homogeneous or uniform echo texture with low echogenicity. ■ Muscles typically appear hypoechoic or less echogenic relative to the organ(s) or body structure(s) they are adjacent to. ■ Skeletal muscle bundles are distinctly separated by bright symmetric bands of fibroadipose septate that appear hyperechoic or more echogenic compared with the low gray appearance of the muscle.
Placenta	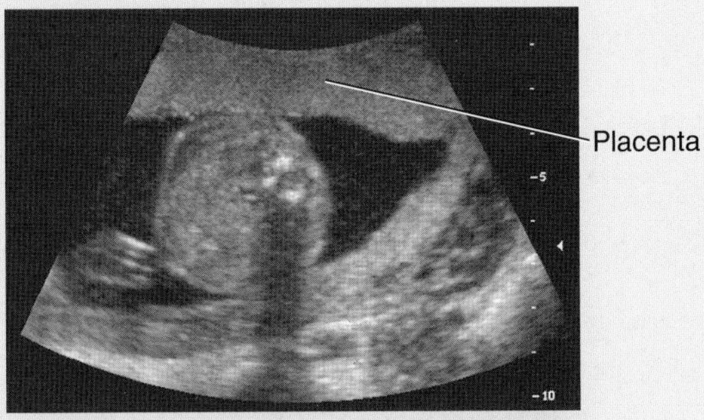	■ Echo texture changes throughout a pregnancy, from homogeneous or uniform with moderate to high echogenicity to heterogeneous or mixed echo pattern, when interrupted by multiple vascular components. ■ Normally hyperechoic or brighter appearance relative to uterine myometrium.
Tissue	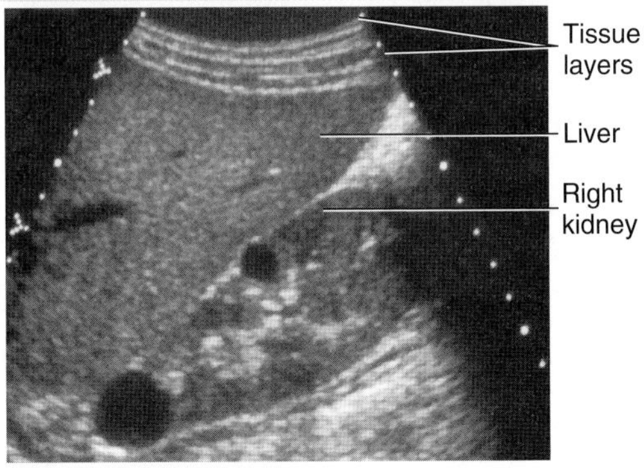	■ Echo texture is homogeneous or uniform and moderately echogenic. ■ Margins appear very bright or hyperechoic compared with adjacent structures.

Continued

■ ■ ■ **Table 7-1**   How to Describe the Sonographic Appearance of Normal Body Structures—cont'd

Body Structures	Image	Normal Sonographic Appearance
Fluid-filled structures: Blood vessels Ducts Umbilical cord Amniotic sac Brain ventricles Ovarian follicles Renal calyces Urine-filled urinary bladder Bile-filled gallbladder Bursa	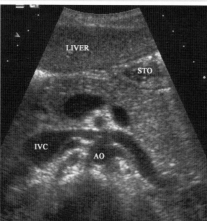 Common hepatic duct · Hepatic artery · Gallbladder · Portal vein · Inferior vena cava · Through transmission · Through transmission	■ Lumens appear anechoic (black; echo-free). ■ Walls appear bright; highly echogenic or hyperechoic compared with adjacent structures. ■ May exhibit bright posterior through transmission, making them easy to distinguish sonographically. *enhancement*
Gastrointestinal (GI) tract *Digestive tract*	LIVER · STO · IVC · AO STO (stomach), AO (aorta), IVC (inferior vena cava)	■ Walls are thin and generally appear hypoechoic or less echogenic compared with adjacent structures; however, they can appear very bright if they are surrounded by an extensive amount of fat. ■ The appearance of the GI tract lumen varies depending on its contents. ■ A fluid-filled lumen appears anechoic. ■ A gas- or air-filled lumen will appear bright, highly echogenic, and generally hyperechoic relative to adjacent structures. ■ The lumen can also have a complex or mixed appearance, displaying anechoic portions from fluid, along with echogenic portions that vary in brightness depending on their composition (partially digested food, indigestible material, gas, air). ■ All or individual sections of the GI tract may cast a posterior shadow where air or gas is present in the lumen. ■ Empty, collapsed bowel has a distinctive "bull's eye" appearance due to the contrast between the very bright, collapsed lumen and hypoechoic walls.
Bones, fat, air, fissures, ligaments, tendons, and the diaphragm	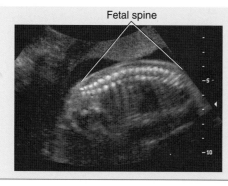 Fetal spine	■ Appear echogenic and vary in brightness depending on the density of the structure, its distance from the sound beam, and the angle at which the beam strikes the structure. ■ Because these structures either reflect or attenuate the sound beam, they appear hyperechoic or brighter compared with adjacent structures; they may cast a posterior shadow.

Table 7-1 How to Describe the Sonographic Appearance of Normal Body Structures—cont'd

Body Structures	Image	Normal Sonographic Appearance
Nerves	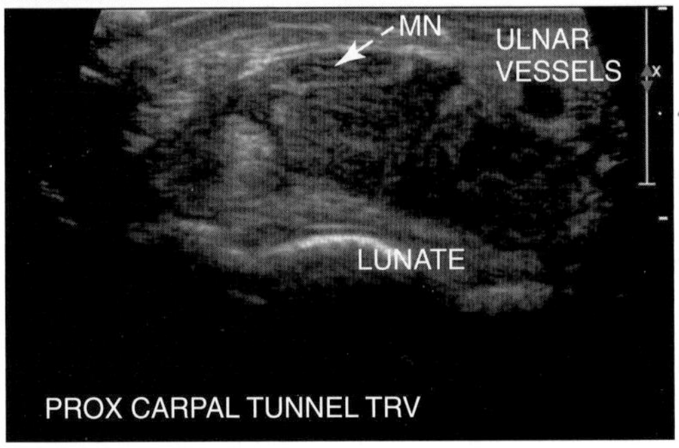 MN ULNAR VESSELS LUNATE PROX CARPAL TUNNEL TRV *to mucs* *to tendon* MN (median nerve)	■ Appearance is generally described in comparison with adjacent structures: hyperechoic or brighter when compared with the appearance of muscle; hypoechoic or less echogenic when compared with the appearance of tendons. ■ Peripheral nerve fibers present as very low gray or echo-poor with a distinctive internal echo pattern that appears stippled in axial sections and honey-combed in longitudinal sections.

Table 7-2 Common Ultrasound Terms

Term	Definition	Example
Acoustic enhancement	"Increased echo amplitude" or "posterior through transmission" visualized posterior to a structure that does not attenuate (decrease, stop, impede, or absorb) the sound beam. Considered a type of sonographic artifact. *low attenuating structure*	Bright posterior through transmission can be visualized posterior to the urinary bladder.
Acoustic impedance	The resistance a material provides to the passage of sound waves.	Bone portrays more acoustic impedance than tissue.
Acoustic shadows	"Reduced echo amplitude" or echo "drop off" posterior to a structure that attenuates (decreases, stops, impedes, or absorbs) the sound beam. Margins of the shadow are generally sharp and well defined. Considered a type of sonographic artifact. *high attenuating struc*	Black posterior shadowing can be visualized posterior to the fetal femur.
ALARA (as low as reasonably achievable)	The prudent use of diagnostic sonography; dictates that the output level and exposure time to ultrasound is minimized while obtaining diagnostic data.	Always consider ALARA when scanning. The thermal index (TI) and mechanical index (MI) are components of ultrasound bioeffects that should be monitored while scanning. The TI and MI values are usually located in the upper right side of the display screen.
Anechoic	Term used to describe an echo-free appearance on a sonographic image.	A true cyst appears anechoic.
Anterior (ventral)	Situated at or directed toward the front. A structure in front of another structure.	The liver is situated anteriorly in the body. The body of the pancreas is anterior to portions of the: splenic vein; superior mesenteric artery; left renal vein; abdominal aorta; spine. The head of the pancreas is anterior to the inferior vena cava.
Artifact	Image artifacts are echo features or structures observed on ultrasound images that are unassociated with the object being imaged.	Acoustic shadows are one type of sonographic artifact.
Ascites	Accumulation of serous fluid anywhere in the abdominopelvic cavity.	Ascites may be visualized in the posterior cul-de-sac of the abdominopelvic cavity.
Attenuation	Decrease in the intensity of the sound beam as it passes through a structure, caused by absorption, scatter, or beam divergence.	The density, composition, and angle of the sound beam when it strikes an object determine how much of the sound beam is attenuated.

Continued

■ ■ ■   **Table 7-2**   Common Ultrasound Terms—cont'd

Term	Definition	Example
Axial (short axis) (view or section)	At right angles to longitudinal sections. Term used to describe the section of a structure portrayed within a scanning plane image.	Axial views of the aorta may be seen in transverse scanning plane images. Axial sections of the pancreas can be visualized in sagittal scanning plane images of the midhypogastrium.
Beam divergence	Widening of the sound beam as it travels.	The pyramid appearance of an ultrasound image typifies beam divergence.
Calculi/"stones"	Concentration of mineral salts that may accompany some disease processes. *most common in Galbladder.*	Calculi are often visualized within the gallbladder as bright, movable structures that vary in size and cast posterior shadows.
Calipers (electronic)	Two or more measurement cursors that can be manipulated to calibrate the distance between echoes of interest on the imaging screen.	Measurement calipers are used to obtain length, width, and anteroposterior measurements to provide the dimensions or total volume of a structure of interest.
Color flow Doppler	Doppler shift information in a two-dimensional presentation superimposed on a real-time gray-scale anatomic cross-sectional image.	Flow directions are presented as different colors on the ultrasound display screen.
Complex mass	Abnormal mass within the body that is composed of both tissue and fluid.	A complex mass is classified as an abnormal tissue and fluid collection within the body that disrupts the otherwise normal echo pattern of body structures on an ultrasound image.
Contralateral	Situated on or affecting the opposite side.	The ovaries are contralateral organs.
Contrast	A comparison to show differences.	An ultrasound image produces a preponderance of dark and light comparative gray-scale tones.
Coronal scanning planes	Any plane parallel to the long axis of the body and perpendicular to sagittal scanning planes.	A coronal scanning plane image demonstrates the anatomy visualized in a lateral to medial dimension and superior to inferior dimension.
Coupling agent	Substance used to reduce air between the ultrasound transducer and surface of the skin.	Gel is a typical coupling agent used in sonography.
Crura of diaphragm	Right and left crus or fibromuscular bands arising from the lumbar vertebrae that insert into the central tendon of the diaphragm.	The crura of the diaphragm are often visualized on ultrasound images as curvilinear structures immediately adjacent to the spine. Their sonographic appearance varies from bright to hypoechoic relative to adjacent structures.
Cystic	Describes the sonographic appearance of a fluid collection within the body that does not meet the criteria to be considered a true cyst.	Ascites is said to be cystic in nature.
Deep	Internal. Situated away from the surface.	The kidneys are deep structures within the body.
Depth of penetration	Maximum distance the sound beam travels from the transducer through a medium.	The greater the intensity of the ultrasound beam, the greater the distance the beam will travel through a medium. The greater the attenuation of a medium, the less the distance of travel.
Diffuse disease	Infiltrative disease throughout an organ that disrupts the otherwise normal sonographic appearance of organ parenchyma.	Infiltrative disease alters the normal echo pattern throughout an organ.
Distal	Situated farthest from the point of origin.	The abdominal aorta is distal to the thoracic aorta.
Doppler (effect)	Change in observed sound frequency caused by relative motion between the source of the sound or reflector and the observer.	Doppler is used to detect blood flow through vessels. It detects not only the presence of flow but also the direction of flow by measuring the difference in the frequency of the reflected sound compared with the transmitted sound.
Echogenic	Describes a structure that is able to produce echoes or echo patterns on sonograms.	Body structures are echogenic or capable of producing echoes.

■ ■ **Table 7-2** Common Ultrasound Terms—cont'd

Term	Definition	Example
Echopenic	Few echoes/ No Echoes	The bile-filled gallbladder may appear echopenic.
Echo texture	Describes the sonographic appearance of soft tissue structures within the body.	Normal organ parenchyma (soft tissue) is characterized sonographically as homogeneous or uniform in echo texture. If disrupted or changed by disease, the parenchyma typically assumes an irregular or heterogeneous echo texture or pattern. The nature of this change may be diffuse disease (infiltrative; focal) or localized disease (a mass or multiple masses circumscribed to a specific area).
Extraorgan pathology	Abnormal disease process that originates outside of an organ.	An extraorgan mass may be visualized originating outside of an organ, causing abnormalities such as displacement of other organs and structures, obstruction of other organs or structures from view, internal invagination of organ capsules, and discontinuity of organ capsules.
Focal/multifocal change	Disease process confined to isolated area(s) of an organ.	A focal area of altered echo pattern may be visualized in only a part of an organ.
Focal zone	The point at which the sound beam is the narrowest and the resolution is the best.	Different transducers have different depths where their focus or focal zone is optimal. Therefore, the depth of a structure (of interest) within the body determines which transducer should be used.
Gray scale	Scale of achromatic colors having multiple graduations from white to black. *w/o color*	Sonographic display format where echo amplitude (intensity) is recorded and presented as variations in brightness of shades of gray.
Heterogeneous	Describes an irregular or mixed echo pattern on a sonographic image.	An organ can appear heterogenous when pathology disrupts its otherwise normal, uniform sonographic appearance.
Homogeneous	Describes uniform or similar echo patterns on a sonographic image.	Most normal organ parenchyma appears homogeneous on ultrasound images.
Hyperechoic	Comparative term used to describe an area in a sonographic image where the echoes are brighter or more intense compared to surrounding structures.	The pancreas typically appears hyperechoic relative to the liver.
Hypoechoic	Comparative term used to describe an area in a sonographic image where the echoes are not as bright compared to surrounding structures.	The kidney typically appears hypoechoic relative to the liver.
Inferior (caudal)	Toward the feet. Situated below or directed downward. A structure lower than another structure.	The uterus is situated inferiorly in the body. The superior mesenteric artery is inferior to the celiac axis. The body of the pancreas is inferior to the esophageal gastric junction. The bifurcation of the aorta is inferior to the level of the renal arteries.
Infiltrative disease *everywhere*	Diffuse disease process that spreads throughout an entire organ.	The echo pattern of an organ is altered throughout due to infiltrative disease.
Interface	The boundary between two materials or structures.	Use the bright sonographic appearance of fat interfaces to differentiate body structures from each other.
Intraorgan pathology	Abnormal disease process that originates within an organ.	An intraorgan mass may be visualized originating within an organ and causing abnormalities such as disruption of the normal internal architecture, external bulging of the organ's capsule, and displacement or shifting of adjacent body structures.

Continued

■ ■ ■ **Table 7-2** Common Ultrasound Terms—cont'd

Term	Definition	Example
Intraperitoneal	Abdominopelvic structures enclosed in the sac formed by the parietal peritoneum.	The liver (except for the bare area posterior to the dome), gallbladder, spleen (except for the hilum), stomach, the majority of the intestines, and the ovaries are considered intraperitoneal.
Ipsilateral	Situated on or affecting the same side.	The spleen and left kidney are ipsilateral.
Isogenic/isosonic *Isoechoic*	Comparative term used to describe an area in a sonographic image where the echo patterns are equal in echogenicity.	The spleen may appear isogenic relative to the liver.
Lateral	Pertaining to the right or left of the middle or midline of the body. Describes a structure situated at, on, or toward the side.	The spleen is situated left laterally in the body. The carotid arteries are lateral to the thyroid gland. The pancreas head, neck, and tail are lateral to the pancreas body. The kidneys are lateral to the spine.
Localized disease *Same as focal*	Represents a circumscribed mass or multiple masses.	Masses may be classified as solid, cystic, or complex.
Long axis (view or section)	Represents the longest length of a structure.	It is standard practice in sonography to measure the long axis section of most structures.
Longitudinal (view or section)	Pertains to length; running lengthwise.	Longitudinal views of the aorta may be seen in coronal or sagittal scanning plane images. A longitudinal section of the splenic vein can be visualized in transverse scanning plane images of the mid hypogastrium.
Mass	Circumscribed disease process. *Circular*	A mass is defined according to its composition: solid, cystic, or complex.
Medial	Situated at, on, or toward the middle or midline of the body.	The spine is situated medially within the body. The pancreas neck is medial to the head of the pancreas; the pancreas body is medial to the head, neck, and tail of the pancreas.
Medium	Any material through which sound waves travel.	Most fluid collections are nonattenuating mediums, whereas bone is an attenuating medium.
Mesentery	A double fold of peritoneum that connects intraperitoneal organs to the abdominal cavity wall.	Gallbladder position is variable due to its long mesentery.
Midsagittal and parasagittal scanning planes	Any plane parallel to the long axis of the body and perpendicular to coronal scanning planes.	A sagittal scanning plane image demonstrates the anatomy visualized in an anterior-to-posterior (or posterior-to-anterior) dimension and superior-to-inferior dimension.
Mirror image artifact (non-Doppler)	The sonographic image of a structure is duplicated in an atypical position and appears as a mirror image of the original.	Mirror images usually occur when scanning structures that share a distinctly curved interface, such as the interface between the diaphragm and liver and diaphragm and spleen.
Necrotic	Degeneration or "death" of tissue.	Many complex masses are described as necrotic.
Neoplasm	New, abnormal growth of existing tissues; either benign or malignant.	A neoplasm is characterized as a tumor or mass.
Orthogonal	At right angles; perpendicular.	Coronal planes are orthogonal to sagittal planes.
Parenchyma	Tissue composing an organ.	Normal organ parenchyma appears homogeneous on an ultrasound image.
Peritoneum	Thin sheet of tissue that lines the peritoneal cavity and secretes serous fluid, which serves as a lubricant and facilitates free movement between organs. Classified as *parietal* (portion of lining that forms a closed sac) and *visceral* (portion of lining that directly covers organs and various body structures). Characterized as *intraperitoneal* (inside the sac) and *retroperitoneal* (posterior or behind the sac).	Structures enclosed and generally covered by peritoneum include the liver, gallbladder, spleen, stomach, majority of the intestines, and ovaries. Structures behind and only anterior surfaces are covered by peritoneum include the pancreas, inferior vena cava, abdominal aorta, urinary system, colon, and uterus.

■ ■ ■ **Table 7-2** Common Ultrasound Terms—cont'd

Term	Definition	Example
Pleural effusion	A collection of fluid inside the lung.	A pleural effusion appears anechoic and hypoechoic relative to the bright appearance of adjacent ribs.
Posterior (dorsal)	Situated at or directed toward the back. A structure behind another structure.	The kidneys are situated posteriorly in the body. The inferior vena cava is directly posterior to the head of the pancreas. The splenic vein is directly posterior to the pancreas tail and body. The right renal artery runs posterior to the inferior vena cava along its course to the right kidney.
Proximal	Situated closest to the point of origin or attachment.	The common hepatic duct is proximal to the common bile duct.
Retroperitoneum	Area of the abdominopelvic cavity located behind or posterior to the peritoneum.	Structures posterior to the peritoneum include the pancreas, inferior vena cava, abdominal aorta, urinary system, adrenal glands, colon, and uterus. Only their anterior surfaces are in contact with the parietal peritoneal lining.
Reverberation	Ultrasound image artifact caused when sound waves pass through and beyond a structure whose acoustic impedance is noticeably different from an adjacent structure, causing a huge amount of reflection back to the transducer.	Reverberation is a common artifact seen on ultrasound images when scanning intercostally. Generally, an image of a structure (in this case a rib) is repeated, with the repeated images taken at an equal distance from the others.
Septations	Thin, membranous inclusion(s) within a mass. _Seperates a mass_	Single or multiple septations may be visualized in cystic or complex masses.
Solid mass	Abnormal mass within the body composed of one thing, tissue.	A solid mass is classified as an abnormal tissue collection within the body that disrupts the otherwise normal echo pattern of body structures on an ultrasound image.
Sonogram	Pictorial record with ultrasound.	Image records representative of the findings during an ultrasound examination.
Sonographer	Highly skilled allied-health professional qualified by technological education to perform ultrasound examinations of patients and document the results under the supervision of a physician.	Sonographers are responsible for gathering pertinent data during an ultrasound examination and documenting the necessary representative images of the study for physician interpretation or diagnosis.
Sonologist	The physician who interprets a sonogram.	During an ultrasound examination, a sonologist may scan and take images or use images provided by a sonographer to ultimately make a diagnosis based on the ultrasound findings.
Superficial	External. Situated on or toward the surface.	The testicles are superficial structures. The thyroid is a superficial gland.
Superior (cranial) _cephalad_	Toward the head. Situated above or directed upward. A structure higher than another structure.	The lungs are situated superiorly in the body. The diaphragm is the superior margin of the abdominopelvic cavity.
Systemic	Pertains to the body as a whole.	Systemic circulation transports blood from the heart to all parts of the body (except for the lungs) and back again.
TGC (time-gain compensation)	Increase in receiver gain with time to compensate for loss in echo amplitude, usually due to attenuation, with depth.	Most ultrasound machines include a group of sliding potentiometers to control the amplification of received echoes. Most ultrasound displays include a TGC curve, which is a graphic display of the settings of the receiver's gain controls.
Through transmission	"Increased echo amplitude" or "acoustic enhancement" visualized posterior to a structure that does not attenuate (decrease, stop, impede, or absorb) the sound beam. Considered a type of sonographic artifact.	A true cyst must exhibit posterior through transmission.

Continued

■ ■ ■ **Table 7-2** Common Ultrasound Terms—cont'd

Term	Definition	Example
Transducer (ultrasound)	A device capable of converting electrical energy to mechanical energy, and vice versa.	Ultrasound transducers include linear sequential array and curved linear array. Annular array, sector-phased array, and single element. Transesophageal, intraoperative, and endocavital.
Transmission	Term implying passage of energy through a material.	A sonographic image is the result of configured transmissions.
Transverse scanning planes	Any plane perpendicular to the long axis of the body.	A transverse scanning plane image demonstrates the anatomy visualized in an anterior-to-posterior (or posterior-to-anterior) dimension and right-to-left dimension or a lateral-to-medial dimension and anterior-to-posterior dimension.
True cyst (simple cyst)	Abnormal mass within the body composed of fluid.	To be classified as a true or simple cyst, the mass must meet three specific sonographic appearance criteria: (1) anechoic, (2) well-defined and thin, smooth walls, and (3) exhibits posteriorly through transmission. If not, the mass is characterized as cystic in nature. Either way, a true cyst or cystic mass disrupts the otherwise normal echo pattern of organ parenchyma.
Ultrasound	Sound at frequencies above 20 kilohertz or above the range of human hearing.	Used to obtain a sonogram, which is any image produced with ultrasound.

(handwritten annotations: "if all 3", "if 1-2 of 3 = cystic mass", "enhancement→")

CLINICAL CRITERIA

Whether you are in a classroom or clinical setting, certain professional and clinical standards should be followed:

- Wear appropriate attire.
- Wear a personal identification badge.
- Introduce yourself to patients; put them at ease and make them as comfortable as possible.
- Practice courteous and respectful interactions with patients and staff.
- Conversations with patients should be proper and professional. Never discuss the sonographic findings or offer your opinion of the study results. **Only physicians can legally render a diagnosis.**
- Check every patient's identification bracelet (or patient number) against the patient's chart; make very sure you have the correct patient.
- Briefly explain the examination process to the patient.
- Inquire about the patient's symptoms and history of illness or surgeries.
- Instruct the patient in a slow, clear, and appropriate manner.
- When required, help the patient to dress in an examination gown.
- Assist patients with any medical equipment that may be attached to them, such as an oxygen tank.
- Before helping the patient onto the examination table or stretcher, check that the brakes are set to ensure that the table or stretcher cannot move. Have a handled step stool available to assist shorter patients onto the table.
- Drape patients properly and explain to them why it is necessary to do so.
- Be familiar with your institution's isolation policies.
- Be familiar with sterile techniques.
- Be familiar with procedures to assist physicians with special studies.
- Most transabdominal pelvic studies require the patient to have a full urinary bladder. Because this can cause the patient discomfort, scan prudently to complete the examination in a timely manner.
- Most institutions require patients to sign a consent form prior to endocavital studies. Further, it is recommended that the examination should be witnessed by

another sonographer or appropriate health care professional. The sonographer's and a witness's initials should be part of the permanent record.

- Know how to handle all ultrasound equipment. Practice attaching and detaching transducers from the machine.
- Be comfortable operating the image documenting system.

IMAGING CRITERIA

- Begin with a transducer best suited to the structure(s) of interest. Use real-time transabdominal or endocavital scanners with sector or curved linear transducers.
- Use a coupling agent such as gel to remove the air between the transducer and the surface of the patient's skin.
- Patient comfort and the amount of transducer pressure exerted on the patient are important considerations. Experiment by using different amounts of transducer pressure on your own skin surface.
- Perform comprehensive scanning surveys. A survey is a detailed assessment and inclusive observation. All ultrasound examinations should begin with a longitudinal and axial survey of either all abdominal structures or the area of interest and immediate adjacent structures.
- No images are taken during a survey. This is a time to fine-tune technique, establish the optimal patient position(s) and breathing technique(s), thoroughly and methodically investigate the area(s) of interest, and rule out normal variants or abnormalities.
- Adjust field size to best view the area of interest.
- Focus near and far gain settings to enhance visualization of the area of interest.
- Adjust contrast to help differentiate structures from one another.
- Adjust gain settings so that the margins of structures are well defined.
- Power settings should be low. Compensate with adjusted TGC (time-gain compensation) slope (see Table 7-2).
- Avoid areas of fade-out on an image whenever possible. Try increasing or adjusting the TGC slope, or switch to a more powerful transducer.
- Follow a scanning protocol—this ensures standardization and is essential for comparing studies.

SCANNING

Your first scan will be of the abdominal aorta. Review the location, gross anatomy, and sonographic appearance of the aorta detailed in Chapter 10. A valuable exercise is to use Play-Doh to duplicate the abdominal layers that include the aorta. Use the layering illustrations from Chapter 6 as a guide. Choose one color of Play-Doh for arteries, another for veins, and so on. This exercise helps differentiate the intricate relationship the abdominal aorta has with surrounding structures, and it reinforces the concept that familiarity with how anatomy is layered leads to easier recognition of the same anatomy in cross-sections. The following is a suggested protocol for sonographic evaluation of the abdominal aorta.

A. Patient Preparation

- The patient should fast for at least 8 hours before the study. This should help reduce the amount of gas in the overlying bowel, which can obscure visualization of portions of the abdominal aorta.
- In the instance that a patient has recently eaten, still attempt the study on the chance that you may be able to visualize the aorta.

B. Patient Position

- The best patient position is determined by what will produce optimal views of areas of interest.
- For instructional purposes, a supine position will be used as the best position for evaluating the abdominal aorta.

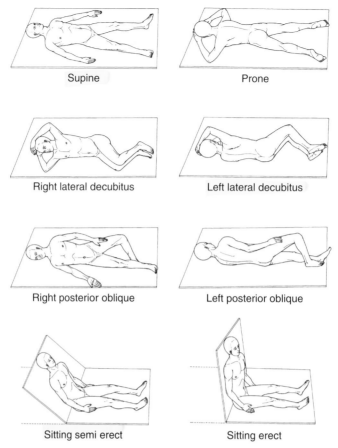

Supine   Prone

Right lateral decubitus   Left lateral decubitus

Right posterior oblique   Left posterior oblique

Sitting semi erect   Sitting erect

FIGURE 7-6 Standard Patient Positions.

- Alternative patient positions for viewing the abdominal aorta include right or left lateral decubitus, right or left posterior oblique, or sitting semierect to erect (Figure 7-6). This should alert you to the fact and advantage that multiple options are available for solving imaging challenges. Simply put, if it does not work in one patient position, try another position.

C. How to Choose and Use a Transducer
Choosing a Transducer
- As you learned in Chapter 2, the higher-number megahertz (MHz) transducers are best for imaging superficial structures, and the lower-number megahertz transducers are best for evaluating deep structures.
- Because the abdominal aorta is retroperitoneal and one of the deepest structures of the body, the transducer of choice is usually a 3.0 or 3.5 MHz. If the patient is very thin, a 5.0 MHz transducer may be the best choice.
- If you are not achieving the desired results with one transducer, switch to another.

Using a Transducer
- Holding the transducer like you would a pencil puts the least amount of strain on the wrist and affords ease of movement. See ergonomic specifics in Chapter 4.
- Scanning should be very fluid, not rigid.
- The transducer is easily manipulated into different positions, which provides you with multiple options for obtaining the best views and images of structures of interest (Figure 7-7).
- Slightly twisting/rotating the transducer first one way and then the other obliques or angles the scanning plane so that the largest margins of structures can be resolved and examined in their entirety.

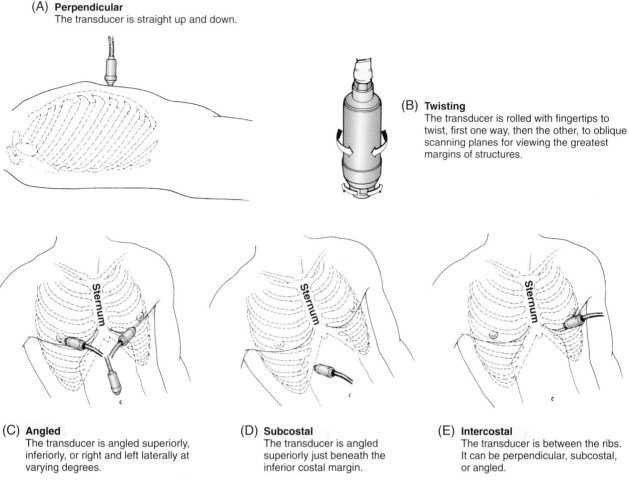

(A) Perpendicular
The transducer is straight up and down.

(B) Twisting
The transducer is rolled with fingertips to twist, first one way, then the other, to oblique scanning planes for viewing the greatest margins of structures.

(C) Angled
The transducer is angled superiorly, inferiorly, or right and left laterally at varying degrees.

(D) Subcostal
The transducer is angled superiorly just beneath the inferior costal margin.

(E) Intercostal
The transducer is between the ribs. It can be perpendicular, subcostal, or angled.

FIGURE 7-7 **Transducer Positions and Motions.** Different transducer positions and motions are routinely used to achieve the optimal image. They include the following: (**A**) Perpendicular, (**B**) Twisting/Rotating, (**C**) Angled, (**D**) Subcostal, (**E**) Intercostal.

- The amount of pressure exerted on the skin surface by the transducer can be varied to improve imaging results. Always check with patients to make sure the pressure from the transducer is not too much and that they are comfortable. Encourage patients to let you know if they feel any discomfort from the transducer.

D. Breathing Technique

- Respiration moves internal body structures. Deep inspiration forces the diaphragm and everything below it in the abdomen to move down. Deep exhalation does the opposite—everything moves upward.
- The suggested breathing technique when imaging the abdominal aorta is normal respiration.
- If you find that a patient's normal respiration causes too much movement to adequately visualize the aorta, have the patient momentarily stop breathing without inhaling or exhaling.

E. The Survey

- The survey of the aorta usually begins longitudinally from an anterior (transabdominal) approach in the sagittal scanning plane. Alternatively, the aorta may also be examined from a left lateral approach in the coronal scanning plane.

ABDOMINAL AORTA • LONGITUDINAL SURVEY
Sagittal Plane • Transabdominal Anterior Approach

1. Begin scanning with the transducer perpendicular, at the midline of the body, just inferior to the xiphoid process of the sternum (see Figures 7-1 and 7-7, and below). Always use a scanning couplant, such as gel, to reduce air between the transducer and surface of the skin.

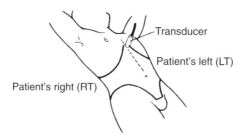

2. To distinguish the abdominal aorta from the inferior vena cava (IVC), slightly move or angle the transducer from the midline position to the patient's right. A long, tubular, anechoic structure with bright walls should come into view posterior to the liver; passing through the diaphragm. This is the distal portion of the IVC.

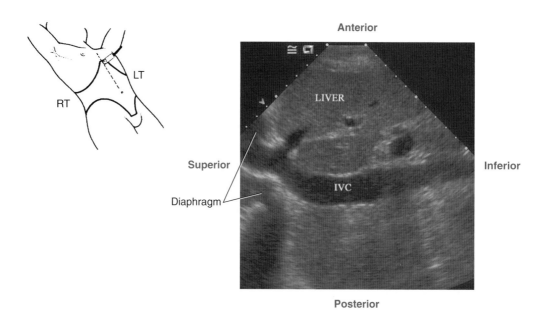

3. Return to the midline and slightly move or angle the transducer to the patient's left (as seen in the drawing below). The long, anechoic, tubular structure with bright walls in the posterior portion of the image is the proximal abdominal aorta (AO). It should come into view posterior to the liver (L) and the diaphragm (appears as the thick, bright, vertical line in the superior portion of the image below, separating the lung from the liver).

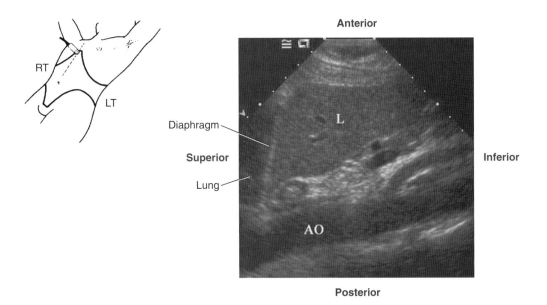

Next, find the longest axis (greatest length) of the aorta by either sliding the transducer a little to the right or left or slightly twisting/rotating the transducer, or both.

If the celiac artery and superior mesenteric artery (anterior branches of the aorta) are not visualized, try barely twisting the transducer first one way, then the other. This should oblique or angle the scanning plane enough to help resolve the small, anechoic, long sections of the vessels.

4. Once the long axis and anterior branches have been resolved, very slightly rock the transducer right and left enough to scan through the aorta. Continue rocking and slowly slide the transducer inferiorly, following along the length of the aorta, as illustrated below. Keep your eyes on the monitor screen; use the image as a guide to evaluate the appearance of the aorta until you scan completely through the mid and distal portions to the bifurcation (usually seen at or near the level of the umbilicus) and right and left common iliac arteries.

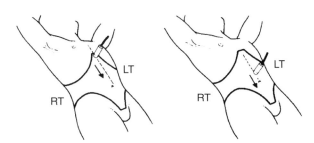

5. In some cases the bifurcation site and common iliac arteries can be better visualized with the transducer angled from the lateral aspects of the most distal portion of the aorta. Move the transducer slightly toward the patient's left, then angle the transducer at varying degrees, aiming the sound beam back toward the aorta until you relocate the most distal viewable portion. Keeping this angle, slowly slide the transducer inferiorly until the bifurcation site and long sections of the common iliac arteries come into view, as shown below. If the bifurcation is unresolved from the left lateral aspect, follow the same steps from the right lateral aspect.

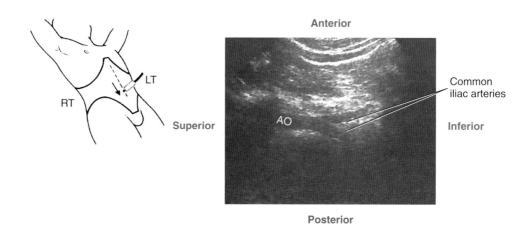

■ ■ ■ ■ BIFURCATION ALTERNATIVE

If the longitudinal bifurcation is still unresolved, it may be easier to visualize from a coronal plane, as seen in the illustration below.
* Patient positioned in right lateral decubitus. Left lateral approach.
* Begin with the transducer perpendicular, mid-coronal plane, just superior to the iliac crest.
* Look for the inferior pole of the left kidney as a landmark. It is usually easy to identify at this level or by sliding the transducer superiorly until it comes into view.
* When the inferior pole of the left kidney is located, the distal aorta, bifurcation site, and common iliac arteries should be seen in the medial and inferior portions of the image. It may be necessary to slightly twist the transducer varying degrees to resolve the long axis.

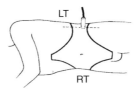

The next step is the axial survey of the aorta. In most cases this is performed from an anterior approach in the transverse scanning plane. Alternatively, like the longitudinal views of the aorta, the axial views may also be obtained from a left lateral approach in the transverse scanning plane.

ABDOMINAL AORTA • AXIAL SURVEY
Transverse Plane • Transabdominal Anterior Approach

1. As shown below, begin scanning with the transducer perpendicular, at the midline of the body, just inferior to the xiphoid process of the sternum.

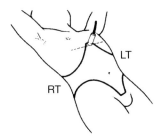

2. Now angle the transducer superiorly until the heart is identified by its pulsations, as seen below. Keeping your eyes on the screen, very slowly return the transducer to a perpendicular position while looking for the aorta in the posterior portion of the image, anterior and just to the left of the bright reflective spine. The axial sections of the aorta will appear as relatively large, round, anechoic structures with bright walls.

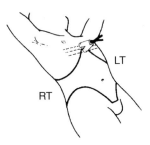

NOTE: *Axial sections of the proximal aorta may also be located by starting with a longitudinal section of the proximal aorta in the sagittal scanning plane. Keeping your eye on the long section of the aorta, simply turn the transducer 90 degrees into the transverse scanning plane, visualizing the aorta the entire time.*

3. Continue by very slightly rocking the transducer right and left, just enough to scan through the aorta. Continue rocking as you slowly slide the transducer inferiorly. Keep your eyes on the monitor screen; use the image as a guide. Move slowly and try to avoid losing sight of the aorta, which can be challenging if it is tortuous. As you scan through the proximal aorta (AO), note the celiac artery/ axis (CA), an anterior branch. It may also be possible to distinguish the longitudinal sections of the splenic artery (SA) and hepatic artery (HA) branches of the celiac axis, as seen in the image below (IVC, inferior vena cava; PV, portal vein). In some cases, a small section of the tortuous gastric artery branch of the celiac can also be visualized.

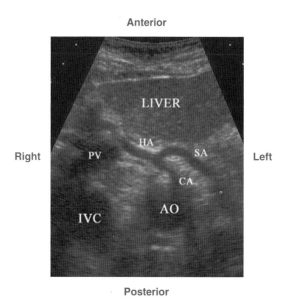

Just inferior to this level, the superior mesenteric artery (SMA) appears anterior to the aorta (AO) as a distinctive, relatively small, and anechoic round structure with bright walls, shown in the image below. Also at this level, notice how the left renal vein passes through the space between the AO and SMA.

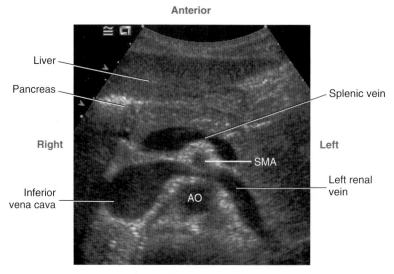

4. As seen in the illustration and image below, keep rocking and very slowly sliding the transducer inferiorly beyond the proximal aorta and through the mid aorta (A) where longitudinal sections of the aorta's lateral branches, the right renal artery (RRA) and left renal artery (LRA), can be identified. Very slight twisting of the transducer can help resolve the renal arteries if they are not immediately visualized.

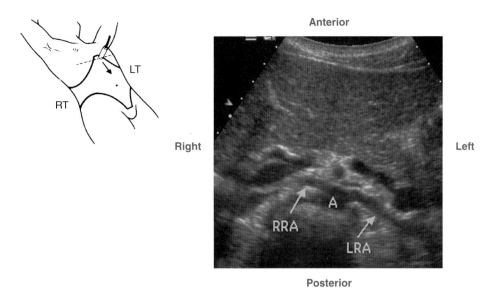

5. Continue to slowly rock and slide beyond the mid aorta and then through the distal aorta to the bifurcation, as shown below. At the level of the bifurcation, the image will change from the single, axial section of the aorta to two small, round, axial sections of the right common iliac artery (RIA) and left common iliac artery (LIA). Continue to scan inferiorly through the iliacs until you lose sight of them.

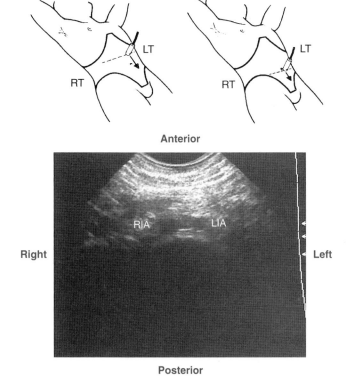

F. Image Documentation Criteria

- Labeling should be confined to the margins surrounding the images. Labels should not cover any part of an image being submitted for diagnostic interpretation because it could potentially cover information pertinent to the diagnosis. If labeling or measurement calipers are used on an image, it is standard practice to document that same image with the labels or calipers removed.
- For legal purposes and standardization, the following information **must** be included on image documentation:
  - ✓ Patient name and identification number
  - ✓ Date and time
  - ✓ Scanning site (name of hospital, private office, etc.)
  - ✓ Name or initials of person performing the study
  - ✓ Name or initials of endocavital studies witness
  - ✓ Transducer megahertz
  - ✓ Patient position
  - ✓ Scanning plane
  - ✓ Area of interest: general (i.e., aorta) and specific (i.e., proximal, mid, or distal)
- Use up-to-date, calibrated ultrasound machinery.
- Documented areas of interest or required images must be represented in at least two scanning planes that are perpendicular to each other to give a more dimensional and therefore more accurate representation. Single plane representation of a structure is not enough confirmation.
- Required images must be documented in a logical sequence. Follow a scanning protocol.
- In most institutions, abnormal ultrasound findings are documented after a scanning protocol's sequence of required images. Otherwise, the documentation becomes confusing for the interpreting physician.
- Abnormal ultrasound findings are also documented in at least two scanning planes that are perpendicular to each other to give a more dimensional and accurate representation and to calculate volume measurements.

G. Required Images

■ ■ □   CLINICAL CORRELATION

The images you take should be the best representation of the ultrasound findings; they should provide data necessary for a physician to render a diagnosis.

- In this case, keep in mind that you survey the abdominal aorta in its entirety—from its proximal portion, through mid and distal sections, to its bifurcation—but you take only one representative longitudinal and axial image of each major section. Therefore those images have to embody the overall condition of the aorta.
- It is standard practice to use a scanning protocol to document specific views of body structures that give the physician the most information possible. In some institutions additional views may be required for physician personal preference. Although slight variations may exist in the scanning protocol according to the interpreting physician, the basic comprehensive images should always be the same.
- Typically, the scanning planes used during the survey should be the same scanning planes used to document the images.

- To accurately measure structures, begin by scanning as perpendicular to the structure as possible for the truest representation of its size. If the sound beam is not perpendicular to the structure, the size of the structure will be distorted on the image even though it might not appear to be. The degree of distortion is proportional to the angle of the sound beam—the greater the angle, the greater the distortion.
- The following section lists the routine longitudinal and axial required images of the abdominal aorta and how they should be labeled.

ABDOMINAL AORTA • LONGITUDINAL IMAGES

Sagittal Plane • Transabdominal Anterior Approach

1. Longitudinal image of the **PROXIMAL AORTA** (inferior to the diaphragm and superior to the celiac trunk).

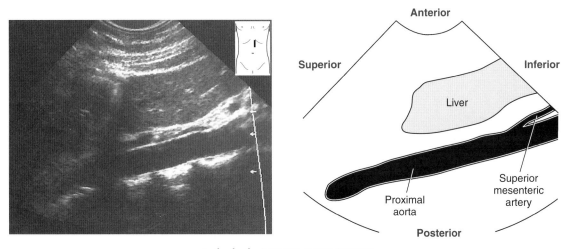

Labeled: **AORTA SAG PROX**

2. Longitudinal image of the **MID AORTA** (inferior to the celiac trunk; along the length of the superior mesenteric artery).

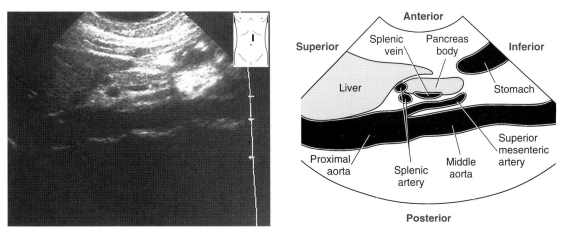

Labeled: **AORTA SAG MID**

3. Longitudinal image of the **DISTAL AORTA** (inferior to the superior mesenteric artery; superior to the bifurcation).

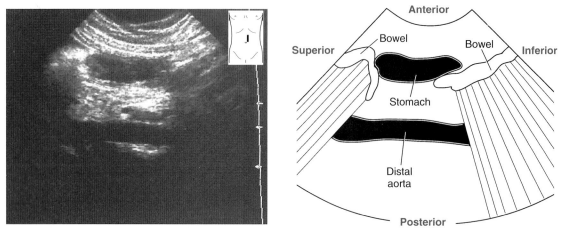

Labeled: **AORTA SAG DISTAL**

4. Longitudinal image of the **AORTA BIFURCATION/COMMON ILIAC ARTERIES.**

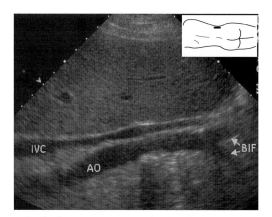

Labeled: **AORTA RT COR BIF** *or*
AORTA LT COR BIF *or*
AORTA SAG BIF RT or LT

ABDOMINAL AORTA • AXIAL IMAGES
Transverse Plane • Transabdominal Anterior Approach

5. Axial image of the **PROXIMAL AORTA** (inferior to the diaphragm and superior to the celiac trunk) with anteroposterior measurement (calipers placed outside wall to outside wall).

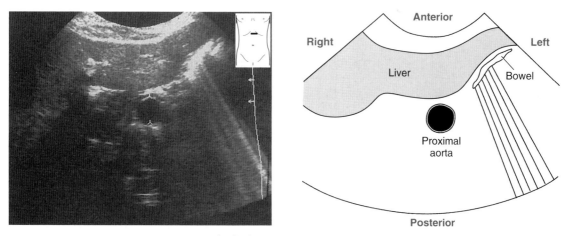

Labeled: **AORTA TRV PROX**

> **NOTE:** *Some studies suggest that a good method to decrease observer variation when measuring the aorta is to take the anteroposterior measurements in longitudinal sections. To ensure consistent results, follow your institution's preference and always be diligent in the technique used to measure the aorta.*

6. Same image as in no. 5 without measurement calipers.

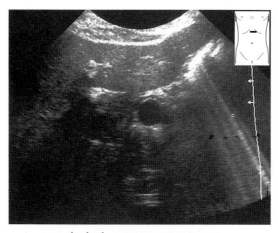

Labeled: **AORTA TRV PROX**

7. Axial image of the **MID AORTA** (inferior to the celiac trunk, at the level of the renal arteries, and along the length of the superior mesenteric artery) with anteroposterior measurement (calipers placed outside wall to outside wall).

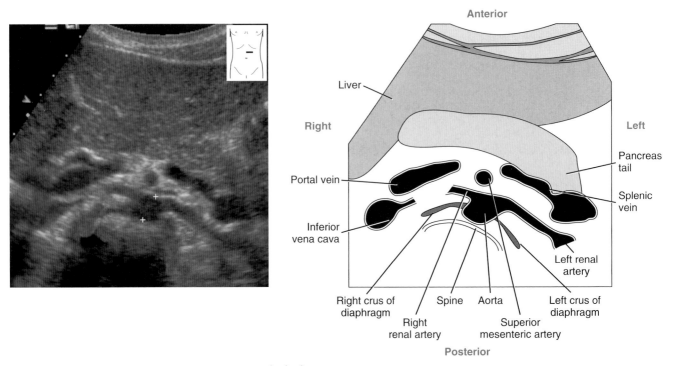

Labeled: **AORTA TRV MID**

8. Same image as in no. 7 without measurement calipers.

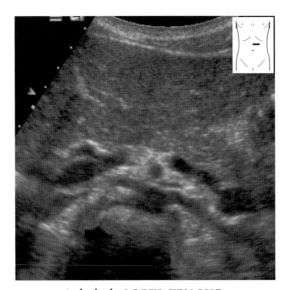

Labeled: **AORTA TRV MID**

NOTE: *If the renal arteries are not represented on the previous image, an additional image(s) that includes the right and left renal arteries must be taken here and labeled accordingly.*

9. Axial image of the **DISTAL AORTA** (inferior to the superior mesenteric artery and superior to the bifurcation) with anteroposterior measurement (calipers placed outside wall to outside wall).

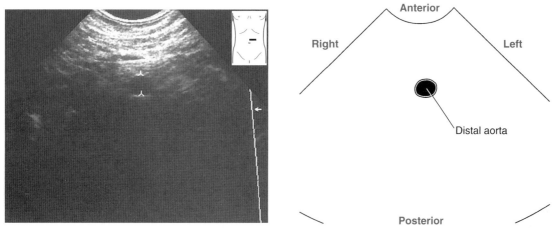

Labeled: **AORTA TRV DISTAL**

10. Same image as in no. 9, without measurement calipers.

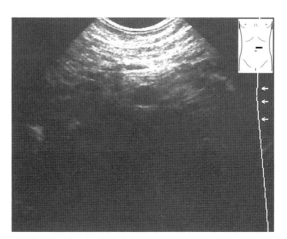

Labeled: **AORTA TRV DISTAL**

11. Axial image of the AORTA BIFURCATION (common iliac arteries).

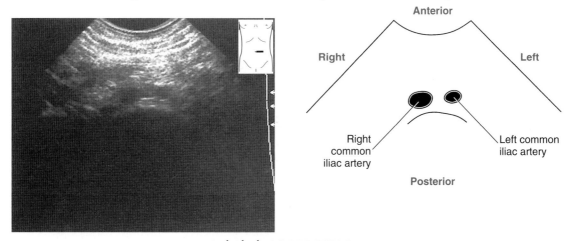

Labeled: **AORTA TRV BIF**

H. Abnormal Findings

Keep in mind that if you observe something abnormal during the survey, you must be prepared to document it. Basically, all abnormalities or pathology can be evaluated and documented the same way:

- First, during the survey determine the *number*—how many? Then the *origin* of the abnormality—which organ(s) or structure(s) is (are) primarily involved? Which of the adjacent structures, if any, are involved?
- Second, determine the *composition* of the abnormality. Is it solid, cystic, complex (solid and cystic), or septated? (Discussed in greater detail later in this chapter.)
- Third, pathology images are documented following the standard protocol images and include the *size* of the abnormality(ies) with volume measurement(s) (greatest dimensions in at least two scanning planes) and *high and low gain images* (gain range helps to resolve composition) in at least two scanning planes.

I. Case Presentation

Case presentation is the method of presenting the images and related details of an ultrasound study to the interpreting physician.

- State the type of examination and reason for it.
- Present patient history.
- Relate patient's lab data and any other known correlative information such as reports and films from other imaging modality studies.
- Present documentation in the sequence it was taken.
- Be capable of justifying your technique and procedures.
- Be able to describe the ultrasound findings using appropriate sonographic terminology (see How To Describe Ultrasound Findings, below).

■ ■ ■　CLINICAL CORRELATION

- Sonographers hold a unique position among other allied health professionals specializing in imaging modalities because sonography is operator dependent. The images are only as good as the sonographer taking them.
- Scanning competency is not certified by registry or licensing, so it takes personal initiative and discipline to judge proficiency and master scanning skills. Match the quality of your images with established protocol images and use feedback from your instructors and/or physicians to help monitor your personal progress.

HOW TO DESCRIBE ULTRASOUND FINDINGS

The purpose of this section is to give sonographers the knowledge base to accurately and appropriately describe the sonographic appearance of ultrasound findings within the scope of a sonographer's legal parameters. As discussed in Chapter 1, this specific need arises with the understanding that physicians exclusively render diagnoses. Sonographers *acquire, assess, modify, analyze, document,* and *describe* the ultrasound findings using ultrasound terminology in an oral or written technical observation (Table 7-3; also see Table 7-2).

It is important to note that although a sonographer's written technical observation may act as a reference for the interpreting physician, it is the documented images provided by the sonographer that the physician ultimately utilizes to

■ ▓ ▒ Table 7-3 Describing Echogenicity on Ultrasound Images

Term	Definition
Homogeneous	Uniform or similar echo patterns
Heterogeneous	Irregular or mixed echo patterns
Anechoic	Echo free
Isogenic/isosonic/isoechoic	Same echogenicity
Hypoechoic	Decreased echogenicity compared to an adjacent structure(s)
Hyperechoic	Increased echogenicity compared to an adjacent structure(s)

determine a diagnosis. If a sonographer, for example, fails to make an accurate description in the technical observation but demonstrates the findings on the images, he or she has performed within the legal guidelines of the scope of practice for diagnostic medical sonographers.

Therefore, as mentioned in Chapter 1, it is not essential to be familiar with all of the various pathologies detectable with ultrasound to be able to accurately describe their sonographic appearance or to take the correct images for physician interpretation. That is not to say that sonographers would not benefit from having knowledge of diseases and their sonographic presentation; however, it is not essential to the ultrasound imaging process.

Once a sonographer becomes practiced at recognizing the echo patterns of normal anatomy, it stands to reason that any change in that normal appearance would suggest that an abnormality is present. Even if a sonographer does not know what is causing the change or deviation in the normal echo pattern, *recognizing it as a deviation is what is most important*. Remember that:
- **differentiating** abnormal echo patterns from normal echo patterns,
- **documenting** any differences in echo pattern appearance, and
- **describing** any difference in echo pattern appearance using sonographic terminology

afford the interpreting physician with the comprehensive sonographic details of a study on which the diagnosis is based.

Every internal body structure visualized with ultrasound has a typical normal appearance of its *shape, size, contour,* and *position within the body,* and—for soft tissue structures—the *parenchymal texture* as well. This appearance is highly consistent among persons, with only small variations seen. All pathology visualized with ultrasound disrupts, in some way, the normal sonographic appearance of the structure involved. It does this by changing one, some, or all of the characteristics of the structure's typical normal appearance.

As mentioned, ultrasound terms are used to describe the sonographic appearance or echogenicity of body structures—*homogeneous, heterogeneous, isosonic, anechoic, hyperechoic,* and *hypoechoic.* These terms refer to texture (uniform or irregular) and quantity (ranging from an abundance of echoes to an absence of echoes) (see Tables 7-2 and 7-3).

Normal organ parenchyma (soft tissue) is described sonographically as **homogeneous,** or uniform in texture. If disrupted or changed by disease, the parenchyma typically assumes an irregular, or **heterogeneous,** echo pattern. The nature of this change may be *diffuse disease* (infiltrative) or *localized disease* (a mass or multiple masses circumscribed to a specific area).

Describing Diffuse Disease

Infiltrative diffuse disease spreads throughout an entire organ. Sonographically, the parenchymal texture is altered and often appears heterogeneous with varying degrees of echogenicity, depending on the extent of the disease. In some cases an infiltrative change in parenchyma may be described as simply as:

> "The liver appears enlarged and hyperechoic compared to the pancreas."

As the disease advances, organ parenchyma can become more coarse or patchy looking with necrotic (degenerating), blood-filled spaces. Sonographic appearance of progressive diffuse disease could be characterized by a sonographer as:

> "Liver shape appears altered with coarse, scattered increases in echogenicity and multiple fluid-filled, anechoic spaces 1 to 5 mm in diameter throughout."

Changes in the size, shape, and position of an organ affected by infiltrative diffuse disease may be subtle and unrecognizable, or they may be immediately obvious. When diffuse disease causes enlargement of an organ, the sonographer must determine the extent of increase and describe whether any adjacent structures have been compromised. All or just a portion of an organ may extend far beyond its normal boundaries, possibly displacing other organs and structures from their normal positions or blocking them entirely from view. A description of the diffuse enlargement, shown in Figure 7-8 below, can be described as:

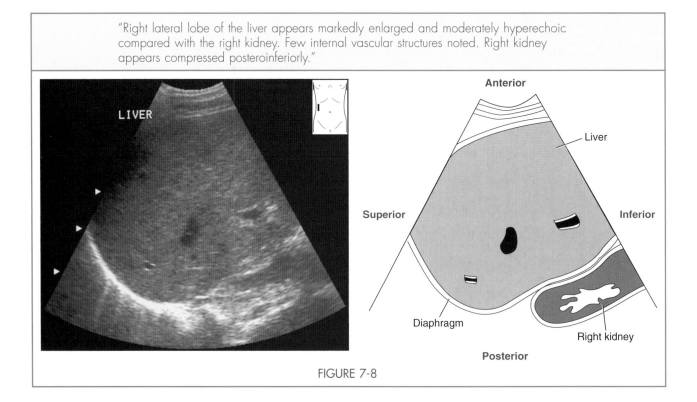

"Right lateral lobe of the liver appears markedly enlarged and moderately hyperechoic compared with the right kidney. Few internal vascular structures noted. Right kidney appears compressed posteroinferiorly."

FIGURE 7-8

Diffuse infiltrative disease of the spleen can displace adjacent structures, particularly the left kidney. A description might be:

> "Spleen appears enlarged and hyperechoic relative to the left kidney, which is displaced inferomedially. Superior pole of kidney appears flattened by the lumpy contour of the spleen."

Another example of diffuse disease that can affect neighboring structures is enlargement of the pancreas head, which can cause biliary duct obstruction, dilate the common bile duct (CBD), and compress the anterior surface of the inferior vena cava (IVC). Some of these cases present with duodenal obstruction as well. A proper description would be:

> "Pancreas appears heterogeneous and markedly hyperechoic relative to the liver. Small shadowing calcifications throughout, and irregular outline are noted. Head appears focally enlarged: 6 cm anteroposteriorly. There is posterior displacement (or anterior compression) of the IVC. CBD appears dilated: 12 mm. The duodenum is not seen."

Describing Localized Disease

A localized change in the normal appearance of parenchyma represents a mass or multiple masses, which are circumscribed to a specific area. Mass descriptions should include *origin (or location), size, composition, number,* and *any associated complications with adjacent structures.*

Origin

When describing the origin of pathology, it is routine to classify localized disease as *intraorgan* (originates within an organ) or *extraorgan* (originates outside an organ).

Intraorgan features include:
- Disruption of the normal internal architecture
- External bulging of organ capsules
- Displacement or shift of adjacent body structures

Figures 7-9 and 7-10 show intraorgan pathology that illustrates these features. The findings in Figure 7-9 below can be characterized as:

"Transvaginal image showing an intraorgan uterine mass pushing on the posterior margin of the endometrium; displacing it anteriorly. Mass appears solid and hypoechoic relative to the myometrium. Contour appears smooth and even. 3 cm anteroposterior, 2.5 cm long."

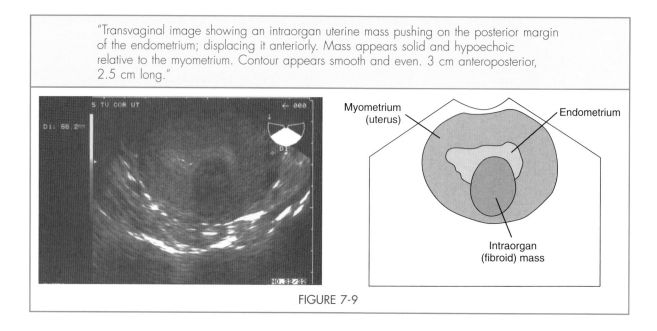

FIGURE 7-9

Figure 7-10 demonstrates another intraorgan mass. A proper description of the abnormal findings would be:

"Primarily solid, heterogeneous, 10 x 10 cm complex, intrahepatic mass. Central portion has irregular borders and appears hypoechoic relative to mass periphery. Interrupted anteroposteriorly by an anechoic area, anteroposterior long axis 4.2 cm, 1.5 cm long, walls grossly irregular. Periphery appears hyperechoic relative to the center, has slightly irregular borders. There is a slight bulge of the liver capsule posterosuperiorly. Inferior vena cava is not visualized."

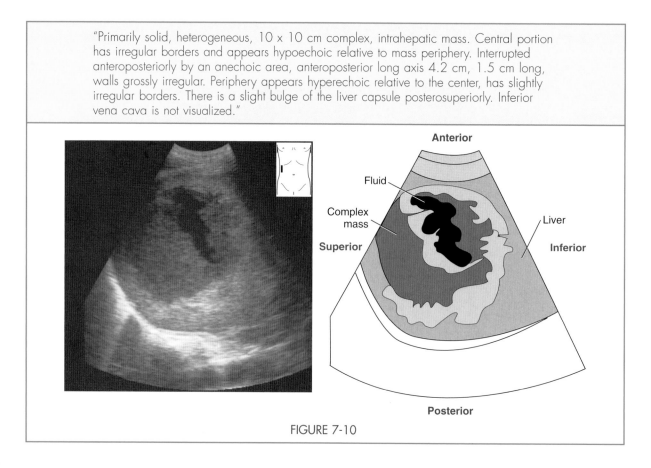

FIGURE 7-10

Extraorgan features include:
- Displacement of other organs and structures
- Obstruction of other organs or structures from view
- Internal invagination of organ capsules
- Discontinuity of organ capsules

It may be impossible to determine the origin of a mass from any single ultrasound image; however, for the sake of description, review of Figure 7-11 below demonstrates some conclusive determinations. It is highly probable that the mass is adrenal in origin and is obstructing the view of the small gland. The findings could be related to the interpreting physician as:

"Right upper quadrant, solid, homogeneous mass. Appears hypoechoic compared to the liver and right kidney. Borders appear uniform. Anteroposterior long axis measures 6.2 cm, width 5 cm. Mass appears extrahepatic. Evidence of discontinuity of liver capsule is visualized. Right adrenal gland is not visualized. Right kidney is seen anteromedially; separate from the mass."

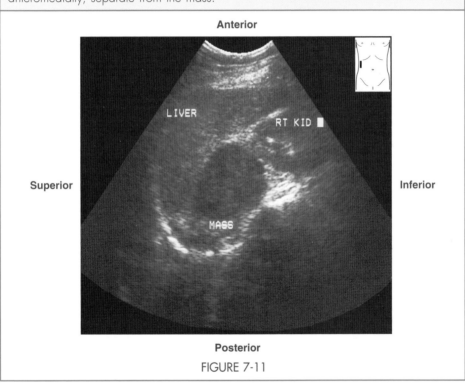

FIGURE 7-11

Masses are generally distinctive in appearance and, unless very small, readily identified with ultrasound. In some cases the organ that a mass arises from is obvious. In other cases, the origin of a mass may be difficult to determine, depending on the extent of the pathologic process. Large masses, such as the one in Figure 7-12 below, can present the greatest challenge in trying to determine their primary site, especially if their size obstructs the organ of origin and complicates adjacent structures as well. The findings could be related to the interpreting physician as:

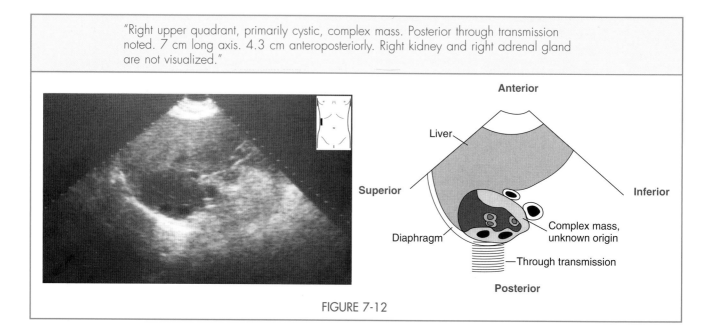

"Right upper quadrant, primarily cystic, complex mass. Posterior through transmission noted. 7 cm long axis. 4.3 cm anteroposteriorly. Right kidney and right adrenal gland are not visualized."

FIGURE 7-12

Size

It is standard practice to measure the long axis, greatest width, and greatest depth of a mass in order to calculate a volume measurement:

$$(L \times W \times AP) = V$$

The size and number of localized tumors are variable. In some cases a mass or multiple masses can affect the overall size of an organ. In these cases, if the individual tumors can be distinguished from each other and from organ parenchyma, they should be measured individually.

Composition

A mass may be described as *solid, cystic,* or *complex* according to its composition.

Solid Masses

Although there are numerous varieties of solid masses or neoplasms (abnormal growth of existing tissues, either benign or malignant), they are all one thing, tissue. Therefore, on an ultrasound image, a solid mass appears as echogenic shades of gray representing its tissue composition on an ultrasound image. The level of echogenicity and appearance of tissue texture depend on:

- What type of localized disease is present
- The degree of its density
- Its effect on internal architecture

Solid tissue masses are characterized sonographically in the same manner as soft tissue organs, with the terms: *homogeneous, heterogeneous, isosonic, hyperechoic,* and *hypoechoic* (see Tables 7-2 and 7-3).

Figure 7-13 shows an intrahepatic, single fluid collection and multiple solid masses that appear brighter than the surrounding liver parenchyma. These findings can be characterized sonographically as:

"Right lobe of the liver appears heterogeneous. 1- to 2-cm multiple, solid, intrahepatic masses appear coarse and hyperechoic relative to liver parenchyma. Anechoic fluid collection located in the medial portion of the right lobe measures 5 cm. Walls are well defined and smooth. Posterior enhancement is noted."

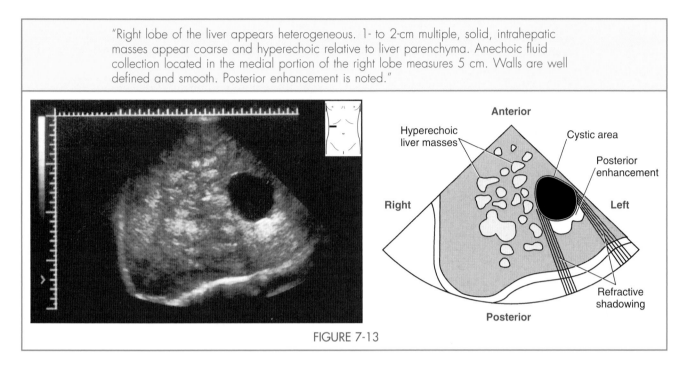

FIGURE 7-13

Figure 7-14 shows a solid mass that appears darker than the parenchyma surrounding it. This could be related as:

"A solid, homogeneous breast mass that appears hypoechoic compared with surrounding structures. Long axis measures 10 cm. Measures 6 cm anteroposteriorly."

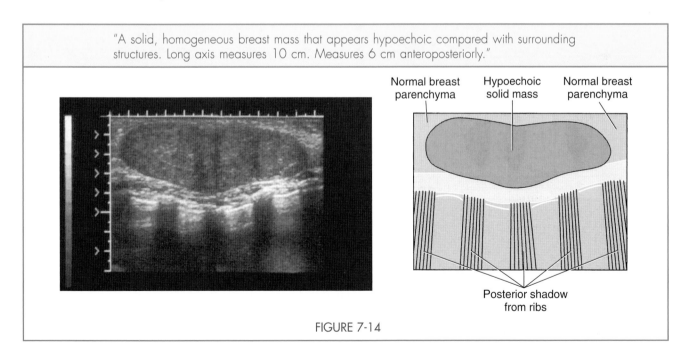

FIGURE 7-14

When a solid mass appears isosonic to the organ parenchyma it is part of, the mass is only distinguishable by its walls. This border differentiation may be the only clue to the presence of an isosonic mass or masses.

Cystic Masses

To be considered a simple or true cyst, the mass in question must meet 3 sonographic criteria:

1. Mass must appear *anechoic* with no internal echoes.
2. Mass *walls* must be *well defined, thin,* and *smooth.*
3. Mass must *exhibit posterior through transmission* or increased echo amplitude visualized posterior to a structure that does not attenuate (decrease, stop, or absorb) the sound beam. There are 2 situations in which the posterior through transmission criterion may be difficult to meet: (1) A cyst located deep in the body beyond the focal zone of the transducer, which means not enough sound waves are being generated to pass through the fluid to create the enhancement effect; and (2) A cyst located directly anterior to a bony structure, which absorbs the sound waves, preventing through transmission.

A fourth "soft" simple cyst criterion is the refractive edge shadows that emanate from the edge margins of rounded structures. Simple cysts are generally round and therefore may also exhibit refractive shadowing (see Figure 7-13).

If one of the three simple cyst criteria is not met, the mass is not a true cyst. A mass that meets only one or two of these criteria is said to be *cystic* in nature.

The image in Figure 7-15 below demonstrates two simple cysts. The findings can be described as:

"Right kidney presents with a 2-cm diameter anechoic mass, superior pole and 1-cm diameter anechoic mass anterosuperior margin of midportion. Both masses have smooth, well-defined, thin walls. Posterior through transmission is noted."

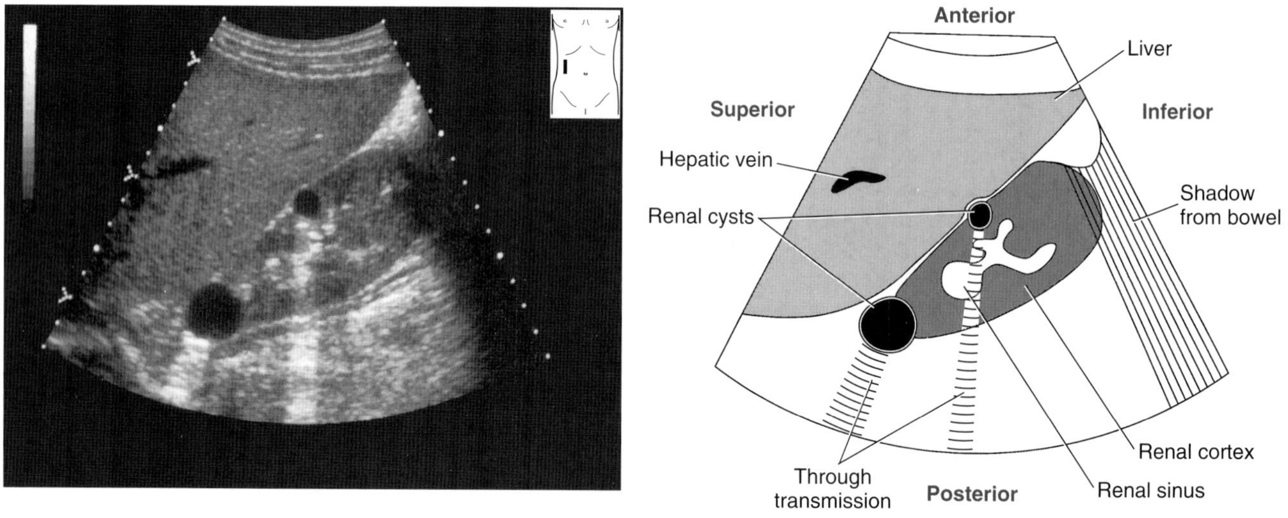

FIGURE 7-15

In some cases it is normal to observe "cystic noise" or anterior reverberation within a simple cyst; that is, low-level echoes may be located near the anterior wall. Echoes rarely occur in the posterior portion of a true cyst.

Septations are thin, membranous inclusions found in some cystic masses. Whether single or multiple, they are generally easy to visualize because of their bright sonographic appearance. A multilocular renal cyst could be described as:

"Renal mass with multiple, 1- to 3-cm, fluid-filled areas separated by highly echogenic, thin, linear, inclusions."

Complex Masses

A mass containing both fluid *and* tissue components is said to be complex. Complex masses may be primarily cystic or primarily solid. The combination of both appearances within the same structure gives rise to the term *complex*. The sonographic appearance of the walls of complex masses varies from well defined and smooth to poorly defined and irregular.

The appearance of the internal composition of any mass may vary with time. This is especially true of vascular masses, which may appear anechoic when the blood is fresh, but become complex and even solid as the blood thickens and eventually forms clots.

Some solid masses, such as uterine fibroids, may degenerate over time. These benign tumors may remain very stable for years and then, as a result of various hormonal changes, begin to change internally. This type of degenerative process, often referred to as necrosis, usually means that a solid mass has begun to liquefy and thereby assume a more complex sonographic appearance. A sonographer could describe these findings, as seen in Figure 7-16, as:

"Uterine mass that appears complex and primarily cystic. Posterior enhancement is noted. Mass measures 10 cm wide and 7 cm anteroposteriorly. The anterior and lateral walls appear smooth and thin. Posteriorly, the wall thickens and appears to give rise to a solid component that measures 5 × 5 cm. Solid component appears heterogeneous with small anechoic portions and irregular borders; partially fills the posterior half of the mass."

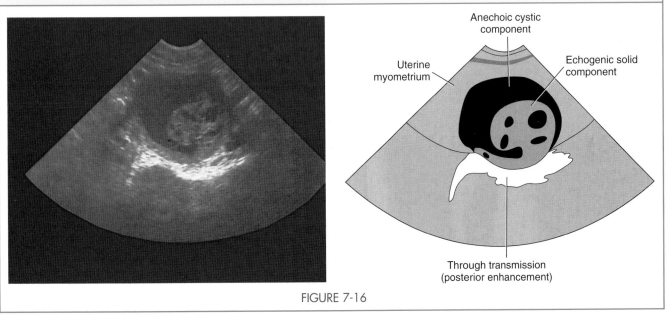

FIGURE 7-16

Figures 7-17 and 7-18 demonstrate complex breast masses that could be described as:

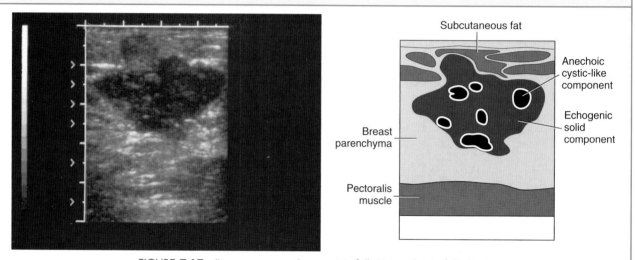

"A single, primarily solid, complex breast mass. Appears heterogeneous and hypoechoic compared to adjacent breast tissue, with slightly thick, irregular borders. 6 cm long axis measurement, 4 cm anteroposteriorly. 1.5- to 2-cm multiple anechoic structures noted throughout."

Subcutaneous fat

Anechoic cystic-like component

Echogenic solid component

Breast parenchyma

Pectoralis muscle

FIGURE 7-17 (Image courtesy Sentara Norfolk General, Norfolk, Va.)

"A single, primarily solid, heterogeneous, complex breast mass. Border is thick and relatively smooth. Long axis measurement 2.2 cm, anteroposterior measurement 1.9 cm. Central, 1.3-cm anechoic area with smooth, thin walls."

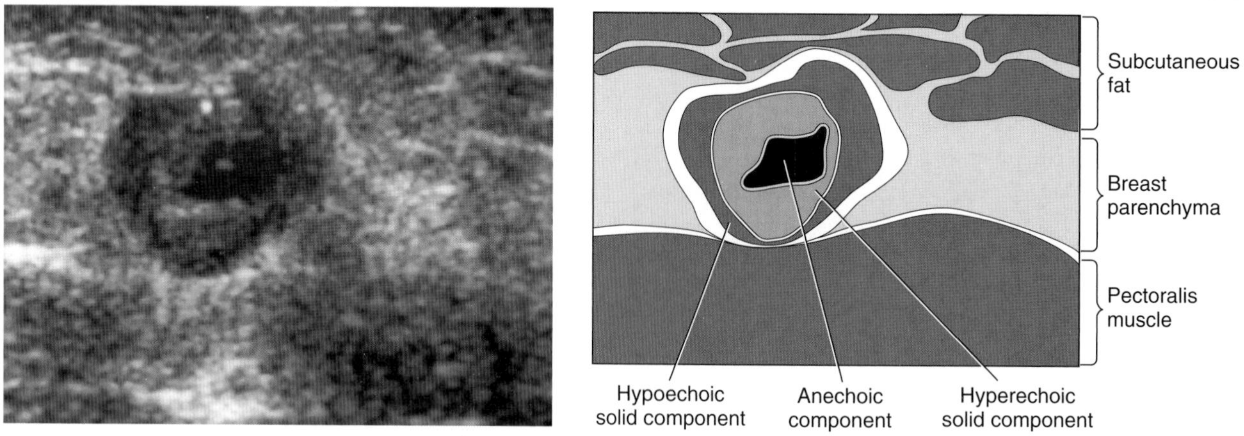

Subcutaneous fat

Breast parenchyma

Pectoralis muscle

Hypoechoic solid component

Anechoic component

Hyperechoic solid component

FIGURE 7-18 (Image courtesy Acuson Corp., Mountain View, Calif.)

A complex intrahepatic mass is seen in Figure 7-19 below. Notice the description of the sonographic appearance of the walls and borders of the mass. It is very important to convey the appearance of mass borders to the interpreting physician. As previously noted, this means describing the borders as *smooth* or *irregular*, *thin* or *thick*, and including whether they appear *uniform* or *uneven* throughout. The findings in Figure 7-19 could be described as:

"Primarily solid, heterogeneous, 10 × 10-cm complex, intrahepatic mass. Central portion has irregular borders and appears hypoechoic compared to mass periphery and adjacent liver. Anechoic component measures 4.2 cm anteroposteriorly, and is approximately 1.5 cm deep; walls are markedly irregular. Mass periphery appears hyperechoic relative to the central portion and adjacent liver; borders are slightly irregular. There is a slight bulge of the liver capsule posterosuperiorly."

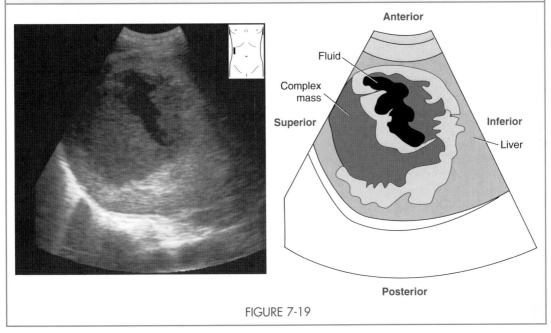

FIGURE 7-19

Notice how the walls of the mass in the color flow Doppler image below are characterized in the description of Figure 7-20:

"Single, interior bladder mass appears solid, heterogeneous, and hyperechoic compared to adjacent structures. 7.5 cm long axis, 5 cm anteroposterior measurement. Superior, inferior, and anterior borders are markedly irregular. Most anterior margin meets the anterior bladder wall. Posterior margin is slightly irregular and adjacent to the posterior bladder wall. Borders appear thick posteriorly and inferiorly; slightly thinner anteriorly and superiorly. Anechoic fluid (urine) is noted superior and inferior to the mass."

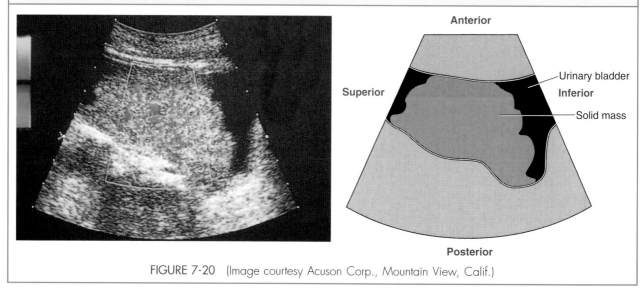

FIGURE 7-20   (Image courtesy Acuson Corp., Mountain View, Calif.)

The right upper quadrant complex mass seen in Figure 7-21 below could be described as:

"A primarily solid, complex, intrahepatic mass. Anteroposterior measurement 9.5 cm, width measures 7 cm. Appears heterogeneous, coarse, and primarily hyperechoic compared to the liver. Mass borders are extremely irregular and thin except for a portion of the superior and inferior borders, which appear slightly thicker. Posterior portion is composed of an area with markedly irregular walls that is hypoechoic bordering on anechoic when compared to the rest of the mass and adjacent liver; it measures 5 cm wide and 4 cm anteroposteriorly. Additional small, scattered anechoic areas are noted throughout the mass."

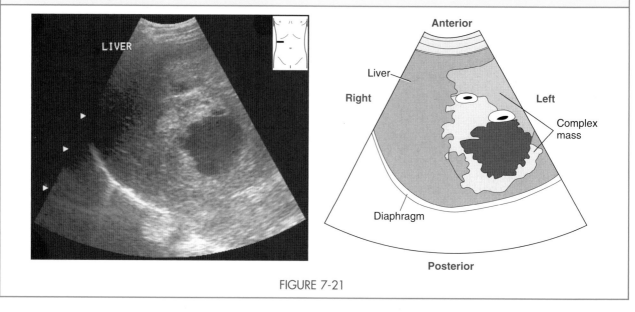

FIGURE 7-21

Other Considerations

Some disease processes are accompanied by the formation of calculi, or "stones," which further interrupt the normal appearance of an organ or body structure. Calculi are distinguished sonographically by the fact that they reflect and impede or stop sound waves. As a result, their surface appears highly echogenic and bright, and posteriorly, they cast shadows. This distinctive sonographic appearance makes calculi easy to identify and distinguish from normal echo patterns. Further, the posterior shadows generally present with sharp, well-defined edges. Figure 7-22 (below) demonstrates calculi within the bile-filled gallbladder. A sonographer could characterize this ultrasound finding as:

"Multiple echogenic foci are visualized within the gallbladder. Posterior shadowing is present."

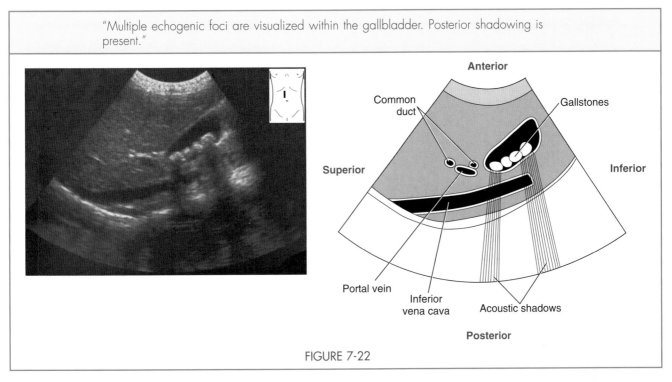

FIGURE 7-22

The next ultrasound image, Figure 7-23, shows another example of calculi and can be described as:

"Intraluminal gallbladder density with well-defined posterior shadowing."

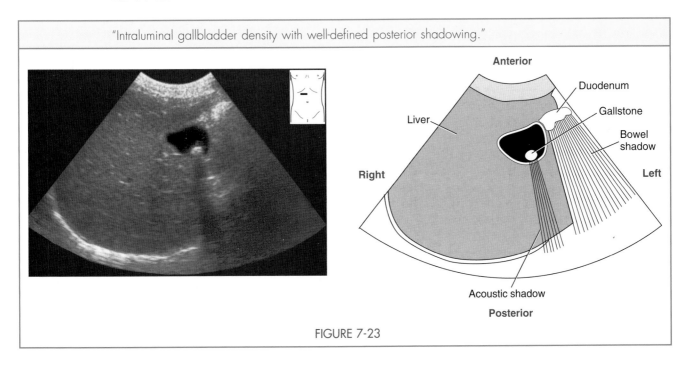

FIGURE 7-23

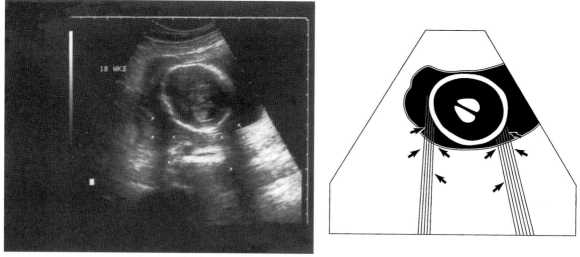

FIGURE 7-24   **Refractive Shadowing. A,** Fetal skull with refractive shadowing *(arrows).* (Image courtesy the Group for Women, Norfolk, Va.)

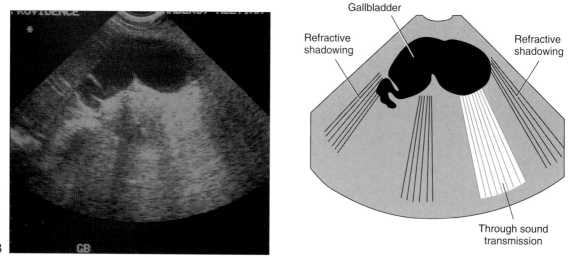

FIGURE 7-24, cont'd   **B,** Longitudinal section of the gallbladder with refractive shadows seen at the curved edges.

It is important to note that not all distal shadows visualized with sonography are representative of pathology. As previously mentioned, refraction shadows can occur at edge margins, especially on round structures. Refraction is a change in direction of sound as it passes through a boundary. Images of the fetal skull are a good example (Figure 7-24, *A*). Refractive shadows can also be visualized at the edges of the gallbladder neck and fundus when they are imaged longitudinally. Even though the longitudinal sections of the gallbladder do not appear round, the rounded edges of the curvaceous neck and bulb-shaped fundus still refract the sound beam (Figure 7-24, *B*).

CHAPTER 8

Embryology*

AVIAN L. TISDALE, REVA ARNEZ CURRY, AND BETTY BATES TEMPKIN

OBJECTIVES

Describe the three layers of the embryo and the organs formed from each layer.

List the embryologic age at initial organ formation.

Compare and contrast the development of the gastrointestinal (GI) tract and accessory GI organs.

Compare and contrast the development of the heart, aorta, and inferior venous cava.

Compare and contrast the function of the umbilical arteries and the umbilical vein.

Describe the differences between an embryo and fetus.

Explain the difference between gestational age, postovulatory age, and the Carnegie staging system.

KEY WORDS

Accessory Gastrointestinal (GI) Organs — Liver, pancreas, and biliary system, which assist gastrointestinal tract function.

Cardinal Venous System — Portion of embryo that, along with the embryonic vitelline vein, eventually develops into the inferior vena cava and tributaries.

Carnegie Stages — System used by embryologists to assess embryo development using a numbering system that is based on morphologic features and age.

Cytogenesis — Cell development.

Diencephalon — Composed of the thalamus and hypothalamus. Located in the center of the brain just above the brain stem.

Ductus Venosus — Shunts oxygenated blood past the liver directly into the inferior vena cava.

Ectoderm — Outermost layer of an embryo that develops into the epidermis, nervous tissue (brain, spinal cord, spine, spinal nerves), and sense organs.

Embryo — Developmental stage of human offspring from implantation to completion of the 8th post-conception week.

Embryogenesis — Formation and growth of an embryo.

Embryology — Study of embryos and their development, from the beginning of

gestation to the end of the second month (8 weeks' gestation).

Embryonic Stage — Stage of development from conception or uterine implantation to 8 weeks.

Endoderm — Innermost layer of an embryo, which develops into the respiratory and digestive tract linings and the urinary bladder.

Fetal Stage — Stage of development from 8 weeks to birth.

Fetus — Unborn fetus following the eighth week of development; gestation from the third to ninth months (9 to 40 weeks).

Foregut — Develops from the primitive gut and gives rise to portions of the mouth, pharynx, esophagus, stomach, and proximal duodenum.

Genital Tubercle — Elevated area between coccyx and umbilical cord in both male and female embryos; in males, tubercle elongates to become the penis.

Gestational Age — Estimate of embryonic/fetal age, which begins 2 weeks from the first day of the last menstrual period.

Hemopoiesis — Production of red blood cells.

Hindgut — Develops from the primitive gut and gives rise to the distal portion of the colon.

Histogenesis — Development of tissues.

Ligamentum Teres — Postnatal degeneration of the umbilical vein.

Ligamentum Venosum — Postnatal ductus venosus.

Mammary Ridges — Tissue along each side of the developing embryo from which breast tissue will develop.

Meconium — Discharge of fetal bowel, composed of cells, mucus, and bile.

Mesoderm — Middle layer of the embryo from which the heart, early circulatory system, bones, muscles, kidneys, and reproductive system develop.

Mesonephros — Second of three stages of renal development.

Metanephros — Third and last stage of renal development.

Midgut — Develops from the primitive gut and gives rise to the latter portion of the duodenum, small bowel, and proximal colon.

Müllerian Ducts — Paramesonephric ducts that develop alongside the mesonephros (second stage of kidney development) into the female genital tract.

Myelination — Lipoprotein covering of nerve fibers.

Neural Tube — Arises from the neurologic plate to form the early brain.

Continued

---

*This embryologic chapter is a compilation of the prenatal explanations given at the beginning of each chapter in the first and second editions, along with additional material from numerous references. The information has been moved into one chapter for those who want a brief review of embryology before proceeding to the body organs and structures chapters.

Organogenesis — Development of organs.

Peristalsis — Movement of intestines that propels internal contents forward.

Phagocytosis — Engulfment of harmful substances by lymphocytes.

Postovulatory Age — Length of time since last ovulation before pregnancy; used to assess embryonic age.

Pronephros — First of three stages of renal development.

Prosencephalon — Forebrain from which the paired olfactory bulbs and optic tracts, as well as the unpaired pineal and pituitary glands, are formed.

Proximal Vitelline Veins — Veins in the early embryo that contribute to development of the hepatic portion of the inferior vena cava.

Reticuloendothelial — Network of cells and connective tissue.

Septum Transversum — Embryonic structure that becomes connective tissue framework for the liver.

Subcardinal Veins — Veins in the early embryo that contribute to the development of prerenal and renal portions of the inferior vena cava, carrying venous blood from the renal and urogenital tracts.

Supracardinal Veins — Veins in the early embryo that contribute to the development of prerenal and renal portions of the inferior vena cava, carrying blood from the body wall of the embryo.

Tailgut — Part of the primitive gut that reabsorbs during the embryonic stage.

Telencephalon — End brain from which the cerebral hemispheres, basal ganglia, and lateral ventricles are formed.

Umbilical Arteries — Arteries that branch off inferior aspect of anterior aorta and return deoxygenated blood to the placenta.

Umbilical Veins — Veins that carry blood from the embryonic portion of the placenta to the embryonic heart. Some of these veins degenerate, and the remaining left umbilical vein carries all the blood from the placenta to the fetus.

Vitelline Artery Complex — Developing arteries that branch anteriorly from aorta and branch into the yolk sac.

Vitelline Veins — Veins that carry blood from the yolk sac to the developing embryo.

Wolffian Ducts — Paramesonephric ducts that develop alongside the mesonephros (second stage of kidney development) into the male genital tract.

■ ■ ■   NORMAL MEASUREMENTS

Gestational Age (weeks)	CRL (cm)	CRL (inches)
6.1	0.4 cm	0.2 in
7.2	1.0 cm	0.4 in
8.0	1.6 cm	0.6 in
9.2	2.5 cm	1.0 in
9.9	3.0 cm	1.2 in
10.9	4.0 cm	1.6 in
12.1	5.5 cm	2.2 in
13.2	7.0 cm	2.8 in
14.0	8.0 cm	3.1 in

■ ■ ■   CLINICAL CORRELATION

Many gross anatomic abnormalities result from interrupted or deranged cytogenesis. This is largely due to genetic abnormalities.

Understanding human **embryology** will guide the reader's recognition of sonographic findings during prenatal and postnatal development of anatomic structures, as well as help the reader to comprehend the medical terminology associated with those structures.

Organ development in the **embryo** occurs in three specific stages:

1. **Cytogenesis**, the development of cells
2. **Histogenesis**, the formation of cells into tissues
3. **Organogenesis**, the formation of tissues into organs (Table 8-1)

The **embryonic stage** of development is from conception or uterine implantation to 8 weeks. The **fetal stage** of development is from 8 weeks to birth.

■ ■ ■   Table 8-1   Organogenesis

Embryologic Weeks	Organogenesis
3	Aorta and tributaries form as two dorsal vessels that fuse into one
3	First and second pharyngeal pouches
3–4	Neural tube emerges
4	Liver, gallbladder, biliary ducts, and pancreas emerge from ventral diverticulum into primitive gut
4	GI—foregut, midgut, hindgut, tailgut
4–5	Urinary system—pronephros to mesonephros to metanephros
5	Spleen—from left mesogastrium
5–6	Neural tube begins brain formation
6	Breasts form from mammary ridges
6–8	IVC and tributaries develop from vitelline veins
8	Portal vein emerges from vitelline veins
8	Sex differentiation seen on embryo from genital tubercle

Fertilization takes place shortly after ovulation, approximately 2 weeks after the end of the last menstrual period. A zygote is formed from the union of the sperm and ova (egg cell), comprising 23 chromosomes from the female and 23 from the male. The zygote is diploid—that is, it contains two sets of chromosomes (46 versus 23). Three weeks after the last menstrual period, the zygote has traveled through the fallopian tube, grown rapidly to approximately 500 cells, and has implanted in the uterus as a blastocyst. In the fourth week after the last menstrual period, the embryonic period begins.

The embryo consists of three layers:
1. The outer layer is the **ectoderm**, from which the brain, spinal cord, spine, and spinal nerves will develop.
2. The middle layer is the **mesoderm**, from which the heart, early circulatory system, bones, muscles, kidneys, and reproductive system develop.
3. The inner layer is the **endoderm**, from which the lungs, intestines, and urinary bladder will develop.

These layers are illustrated in Figure 8-1. There are different ways to assess embryonic growth. **Gestational age** is considered to be 2 weeks from the first day of the last menstrual period. Some clinicians prefer to use the term **postovulatory age**, which is the length of time from the last ovulation to when pregnancy occurred. In many cases this offers a better estimation of the time fertilization took place and a more accurate embryonic age. Another method of assessing embryonic age is the Carnegie staging system. **Carnegie stages** are used by embryologists to describe the maturity of embryos based on physical characteristics, using a numbering system from 1 to 23, with 23 being the most advanced development.

EMBRYOLOGIC DEVELOPMENT
Heart and Abdominal Aorta Development
The cardiovascular system is the first system to become functional in the embryo. This is necessary to provide an adequate supply of nutrients and oxygen to the other body systems as they develop. The embryonic heart is formed at the same time as the aorta and begins beating at approximately 22 days of actual embryonic age. Several studies show the variance of heart rate in the embryo. One study took embryonic heart rate measurements between 45 days and 15 weeks after the first day of the last menstrual period. It showed a gradual increase from 123 bpm (beats per minute) at 45 days' gestational age to 177 bpm at 9 weeks, then an average decrease to 147 bpm by 15 weeks. Another study resulted in different findings. It examined 319 embryos between 6 and 14 weeks' gestational age and found the maximum heart rate at 8 weeks, then a gradual decrease to 161 bpm by 14 weeks' gestational age. Embryologic heart rates can vary widely, as shown by a third study, which found a mean difference of 0 to 8 bpm in serial embryo heart

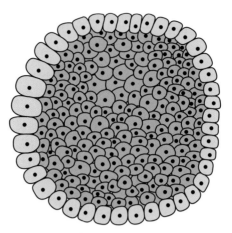
Blastocyst cross section

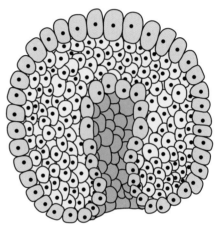
Gastrulation (involution)

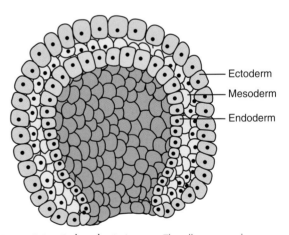

FIGURE 8-1 **Embryologic Layers.** This illustration demonstrates how the three embryologic layers are definitively formed, but ultimately involute. These structures are dynamic, rapidly dividing into new cells that will form more sophisticated tissues.

rate measurements taken 4 minutes apart in gestational ages of 6 to 10 weeks, compared with a wider variability at a higher embryologic age: 0 to 18 bpm in serial heart rate measurements taken 4 minutes apart in embryos between 10 and 13 weeks' gestational age.

The vascular portion of the cardiovascular system develops from mesodermal cells, called the angioblasts, during the third week. At this time, all vessels are composed of endothelium; thus the location of vessels in relation to the heart determines which vessels are arteries and which vessels are veins. During the third week, there are two dorsal aortas, which are extensions of the two endocardial heart tubes (Figure 8-2). The aortas quickly fuse into a single vessel after this period.

The single aorta has several branches. Numerous intersegmental arteries branch posteriorly and feed the embryo. Eventually, many of these arteries become the lumbar arteries (see Figure 8-2). In addition, the common iliac arteries and the median sacral artery develop from intersegmental arteries. The **vitelline artery complex** branches anteriorly from the aorta and extends into the yolk sac. The celiac artery (CA), superior mesenteric artery (SMA), and inferior mesenteric artery (IMA) develop from this complex. The two **umbilical arteries** branch off the inferior aspect of the anterior aorta and return the deoxygenated blood to the placenta. The umbilical arteries eventually give rise to the internal iliac arteries and superior vesical artery. The majority of the remaining vessels develop from the primitive vascular network by forming channels connecting the organ systems to existing capillaries and vessels. Umbilical arteries in the embryo and fetus, and the pulmonary artery postnatally, are the only arteries in the body that carry deoxygenated blood.

Inferior Vena Cava Development

The development of the inferior vena cava (IVC) is complex, which predisposes it to multiple anatomic variations. The IVC and its tributaries are formed from a portion of the **vitelline vein** and portions of the **cardinal venous system** within the embryo (Figures 8-3

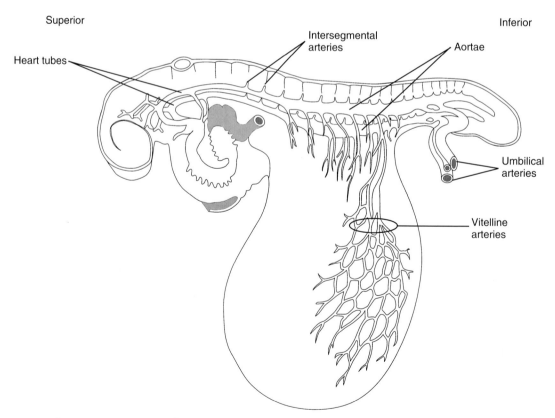

FIGURE 8-2 **Aortic Development.** Representation of aortic development of approximately the third embryologic week.

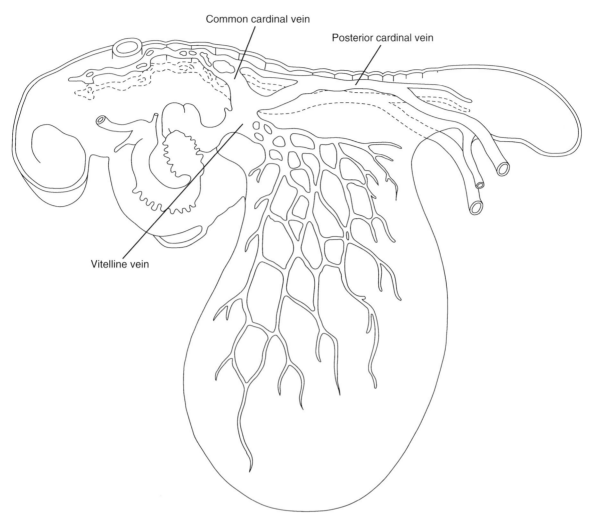

Common cardinal vein

Posterior cardinal vein

Vitelline vein

FIGURE 8-3 **Inferior Vena Cava Development.** Origin of the IVC and associated tributaries in the embryo.

and 8-4). The posterior cardinal veins (PCVs), subcardinal veins, and supracardinal veins are formed during the sixth, seventh, and eighth weeks of embryonic development, respectively. The PCVs regress during this period and do not evolve into a portion of the IVC; however, they do serve as a base for the development of the subcardinal and supracardinal veins. Enormous anastomoses and regressions of these veins give rise to the IVC and its tributaries. **Subcardinal veins** carry venous blood from the renal and urogenital tracts, whereas **supracardinal veins** carry blood from the body wall of the embryo.

Venous blood reaches the embryonic heart in three ways: (1) the vitelline veins carry blood from the yolk sac, (2) the umbilical veins carry oxygenated blood from the placenta, and (3) the left umbilical vein passes through the liver on its way to the heart.

The IVC has four sections (see Chapter 11, Figure 11-1). Beginning superiorly, the first area encountered is the hepatic section, located directly posterior to the liver, where the hepatic veins empty into the IVC. The hepatic section of the IVC and hepatic veins develop from the **proximal vitelline vein** (Table 8-2). The next section is termed the *prerenal* section. It extends from just inferior to the hepatic veins to slightly superior to the renal veins and is derived from a subcardinal vein. The renal section is the next most inferiorly located area of the IVC. The renal veins and multiple tributaries are located within this section, which terminates almost immediately after branching off from the renal veins. The subcardinal and supracardinal veins undergo multiple anastomoses to form this level. The final section is the postrenal section, which is formed from a supracardinal vein. The postrenal section of the IVC extends

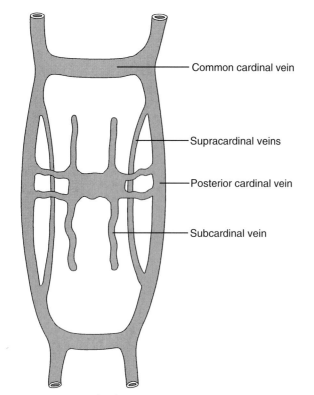

FIGURE 8-4 **Cardinal Venous System.** Anterior view of the cardinal venous system.

- Common cardinal vein
- Supracardinal veins
- Posterior cardinal vein
- Subcardinal vein

from just inferior to the renal veins until the common iliac veins converge into the IVC.

Portal Venous Development

The portal vein develops approximately during the eighth embryologic week. The vitelline veins undergo several anastomoses, forming a vascular network that gives rise to the main portal vein (Figure 8-5). The venous tributaries are also formed from the primitive vascular network), and they join the main portal vein at its inferior aspect.

Biliary System Development

Accessory gastrointestinal (GI) organs are non-GI tract structures that assist in digestion. The liver, pancreas,

■ ■ ■ **Table 8-2** Inferior Vena Cava (IVC) Sections at 6 to 8 Embryologic Weeks

Section of IVC	Originates From ...
Hepatic section of IVC and hepatic veins	Proximal vitelline vein
Prerenal section of IVC	Subcardinal vein
Renal section of IVC	Subcardinal and supracardinal veins
Postrenal section of IVC	Supracardinal vein

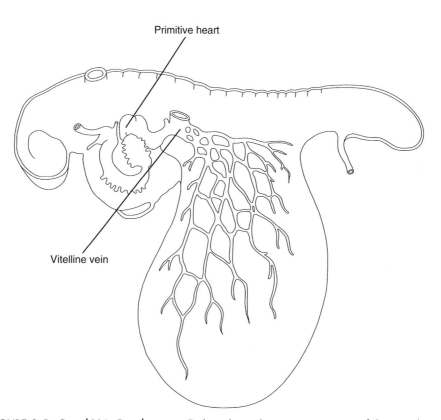

Primitive heart

Vitelline vein

FIGURE 8-5 **Portal Vein Development.** Early embryo demonstrating origin of the portal vein.

gallbladder, tongue, teeth, salivary, gastric, and intestinal glands are categorized as accessory organs. The oral cavity, pharynx, esophagus, stomach, and the small and large intestines are part of the gut, or gastrointestinal tract.

The liver, gallbladder, bile ducts, and part of the pancreas are formed by a ventral diverticulum, or sac, which turns into the septum transversum. The septum transversum is a mesodermal structure that becomes the connective tissue framework of the liver. This process begins at approximately 4 weeks, or when the embryo is approximately 2.5 mm in length. The gallbladder is present in the fetus and is often noted on sonography. It is nonfunctional until birth.

Liver Development
The primitive gut is formed during the fourth week of embryonic life and is composed of three parts: a foregut, a midgut, and a hindgut. A fourth part, the tailgut, is reabsorbed. The liver develops from the foregut (Figure 8-6).

The distal or caudal foregut outpouches between the layers of the ventral mesentery. The head of the outpouch demonstrates a superior diverticulum (a circumscribed sac), also known as the extrahepatic biliary ducts. The diverticulum tissue moves into the septum transversum and divides to form the right and left hepatic lobes.

■ ■ ■ **CLINICAL CORRELATION**

Sonographic visualization of the gallbladder is key. Sometimes the gallbladder is incompletely formed. In cases where it is not present at all (a condition known as biliary atresia), immediate medical attention after birth is required.

The endodermal cells of the diverticulum give rise to the liver parenchymal cells, the hepatocytes. These cells become arranged in a series of branching and anastomosing plates. Hepatic cells are corded within and join the blood sinuses of the umbilical and vitelline veins to complete the formation of hepatic parenchyma.

The umbilical veins bring oxygenated blood from the embryonic portion of the placenta to the embryonic tubular heart, whereas the vitelline veins return blood from the yolk sac to the heart. The liver tissue sequentially moves into the vitelline veins and then the umbilical veins. As the liver tissue moves into the vitelline

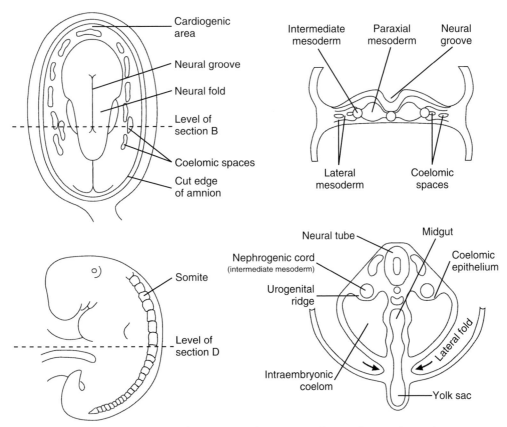

FIGURE 8-6 Primitive Gut Development. Median section of an embryo outlining the primitive gut.

veins, their midsection becomes capillarized, whereas their caudal ends become the primitive portal veins and their cranial ends become the early hepatic veins.

The right umbilical vein and part of the left umbilical vein degenerate. The remaining left umbilical vein portion carries oxygenated blood from the placenta to the fetus. The **ductus venosus** concurrently develops as a large shunt that passes through the liver to connect the umbilical vein to the inferior vena cava, thus allowing some blood to flow directly from the placenta to the heart. Postnatally, the umbilical vein becomes the **ligamentum teres**, and the ductus venosus becomes the **ligamentum venosum**.

The hepatic parenchyma is composed of hepatocytes interspersed with Kupffer cells and organized into lobules approximately 1 × 2 mm in size. Typically, approximately 1 million lobules are found in the liver. Peripherally around each lobule are several portal triads, each containing portal venules, bile ductules, and hepatic arterioles.

The Kupffer cells and the fibrous and hematopoietic tissue are derived from the splanchnic mesenchyme of the septum transversum.

The liver grows rapidly and bulges into the midportion of the abdominal cavity. **Hemopoiesis**—the formation and development of blood cells—begins during the sixth week of embryonic life and is primarily responsible for the liver's large size.

The inferior portion of the hepatic diverticulum enlarges to form the gallbladder. The common bile duct is derived from the stalk, which connects the hepatic and cystic ducts to the duodenum.

Anomalies of the liver include the left-sided liver (situs inversus), congenital cysts, congenital hemangioma, and intrahepatic biliary duct atresia or stenosis.

Pancreas Development

The pancreas gland is formed from ventral and dorsal diverticula of the primitive foregut. The diverticula rotate and fuse, with the ventral portion forming most of the head of the pancreas and the dorsal portion forming the entire body and tail. The ductal system drains into the dorsal duct, the duct of Wirsung, which empties into the duodenum, or common bile duct. The ventral duct, the duct of Santorini, is an accessory duct that is small and sometimes absent. It enters the duodenum separately from Wirsung's duct.

Urinary System Development

The kidneys pass embryonically through three developmental stages. The **pronephros** and **mesonephros** appear in the fourth to fifth week of gestation and are precursors to the **metanephros** (Figure 8-7). The embryonic kidneys are drained by the mesonephric (**wolffian**) ducts. The paramesonephric ducts are located alongside

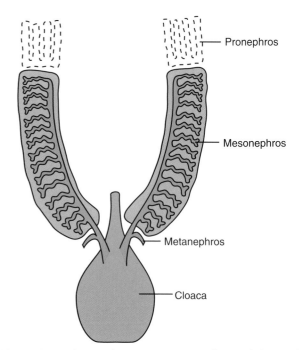

FIGURE 8-7 The renal pre-structures are illustrated here. The pronephros is shown in dash form because it serves as precursor tissue to the metanephros. The mesonephros is a collection of ducts that will coalesce and form the metanephros. These represent permanent kidney tissue comprising functional units called nephrons.

the mesonephric ducts. The reproductive organs will develop from this site. The permanent kidney—the metanephros—appears toward the end of the fifth week of gestation. It is derived from the mesodermal tissue of the embryo and is not functional until the end of the eighth week. The kidneys initially lie in the pelvic cavity. As the embryo grows, the kidneys move up into the abdomen.

Congenital defects in renal development include ectopic kidney (located away from the normal position), renal agenesis (unilateral or bilateral absence of the kidney[s]), and horseshoe kidney (both kidneys are joined together at their superior or inferior poles). Variants in the renal vasculature and ureters may also occur. For example, multiple renal arteries occur in 25% of the U.S. population. Variations of the ureter occur much less frequently, in only 2% of that population. Seventy-five percent of these variations consist of partial bifurcation of the ureter, with the remaining 25%, total duplication of the ureter along its entire length.

Spleen Development

Development of the spleen begins at about the fifth week of gestation and arises from mesodermal cells. It begins as a thickening in the mesenchyme on the left side of the mesogastrium, or the omentum bursa. These mesenchymal cells differentiate into two types of cells—reticular cells and primitive free cells, which resemble adult lymphocytes. The spleen is separated from the stomach by the gastrolienal ligament and from the left kidney by the lienorenal ligament. The fetal spleen is normally quite lobulated (Figure 8-8).

During embryonic life, the spleen is important in producing red and white blood cells. It begins to perform this hematopoietic, or blood cell–producing, function by approximately the eleventh week of gestation. This activity is a result of tissue-myeloid functions. These functions generally end shortly after birth but may reactivate in certain pathologic conditions. In adult life the spleen will continue to produce lymphocytes and monocytes.

By the fifth or sixth month of gestation, the spleen begins to assume its smooth, ovoid adult shape and its adult functions. Its white pulp, which contains Malpighian corpuscles, performs the lymphocytic functions. This distinct portion of the spleen begins to form late in fetal development.

The spleen's red pulp carries out various functions. The splenic cords house reticular cells responsible for the **reticuloendothelial** functions of the spleen, which includes **phagocytosis**. This portion does not develop until after birth, when primary fetal blood cell formation ceases, and the purpose of the red pulp in the spleen after birth is to destroy the degenerating red blood cells.

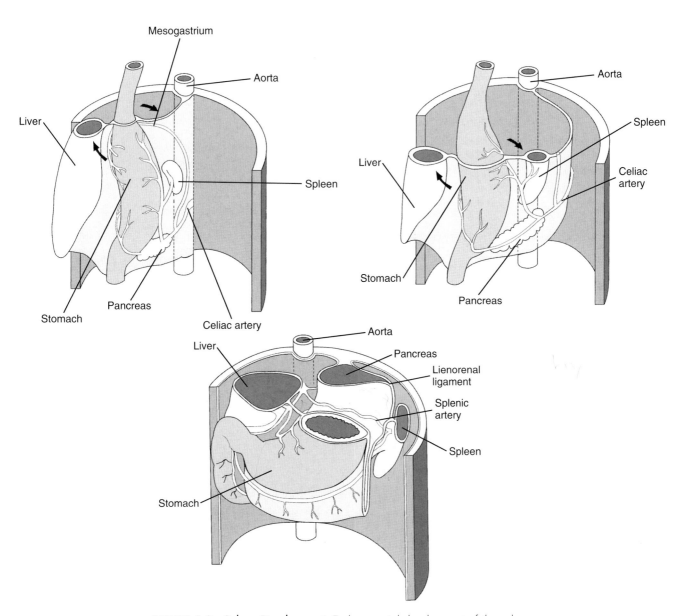

FIGURE 8-8 **Spleen Development.** Early prenatal development of the spleen.

Gastrointestinal Tract Development

The primitive gut develops from the posterior portion of the yolk sac during the fourth week of embryonic development. It is divided into four parts: the foregut, the midgut, the hindgut, and the tailgut (Table 8-3).

A portion of the mouth and all of the pharynx, esophagus, stomach, and proximal duodenum originate from the foregut and are supplied with blood from the celiac axis artery. The remainder of the duodenum, the small bowel, and the colon as far as the middle and left thirds of the transverse colon originate from the midgut. Blood supply to the midgut is from the superior mesenteric artery. The hindgut gives rise to the remainder of the colon, supplied with blood from the inferior mesenteric artery (see Table 8-3). In the adult, these regions retain the same blood supply. As previously mentioned, the tailgut is resorbed.

The mouth and pharynx develop from the cranial part of the foregut. The tracheoesophageal septum divides the cranial portion of the foregut into the laryngotracheal tube and the esophagus.

The stomach originates as a fusiform dilatation of the caudal portion of the foregut. It is suspended from the dorsal wall of the abdominal cavity by the dorsal mesentery and attaches (along with the duodenum) to the developing liver and the ventral abdominal wall by the ventral mesentery. As it grows into the ventral

mesentery, the liver divides it into the falciform ligament and the lesser (gastrohepatic) omentum. The dorsal mesentery bulges ventrally as the greater omentum; the spleen appears in its craniolateral portion.

The final position of the stomach is the result of two rotations. The first rotation is 90 degrees around a vertical axis, moving the dorsal mesogastrium to the left and creating the omental bursa (lesser peritoneal cavity). The second rotation is around an anteroposterior axis, moving the pylorus to the right and superiorly and the proximal portion of the stomach to the left, resulting in the gastric cavity running from superior left to inferior right.

During **embryogenesis** the midgut herniates out of, and then back into, the abdominal cavity (Figure 8-9). While outside the cavity, the midgut rotates 270 degrees counterclockwise and then returns to the abdomen. Thus the root of the mesentery becomes fixed, with one end at the ligament of Treitz and the other in the right iliac fossa. The colon returns next—distal bowel first and cecum last. The colon wraps around the central small bowel and becomes fixed around the edge of the abdomen. This creates a "picture frame" for the small bowel (Figure 8-10).

■ ■ □ Table 8-3 Primitive Gut

Primitive Gut Section	Gives rise to ...
Foregut	Part of mouth; all of pharynx, esophagus, stomach, and proximal duodenum
Midgut	Distal duodenum, proximal colon
Hindgut	Remainder of colon
Tailgut	Resorbed

> **■ ■ □ CLINICAL CORRELATION**
>
> In some this process does not take place (a condition known as situs inversus) resulting in abnormally placed abdominal organs.

> **■ ■ □ CLINICAL CORRELATION**
>
> If this process does not take place, the fetus is born with a condition known as omphalocele in which the bowel is covered in a membrane and remains outside the abdomen.

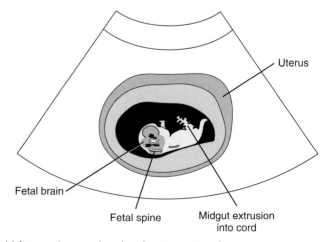

FIGURE 8-9 **Midgut Development.** A 10-week-old fetus with normal midgut herniation into the cord.

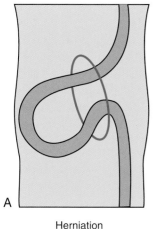
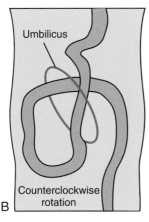
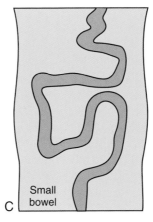
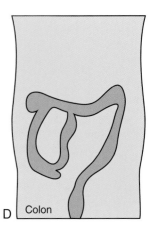

Herniation   Affixed framework

FIGURE 8-10 Herniation and placement of intestinal tissue along with the remainder of the gastrointestinal tract is complex. **A,** The intestines herniate through the umbilicus. **B,** It completes a 270-degree, counterclockwise rotation before returning to the abdomen and becoming fixed. It is important that the small bowel returns first and the colon returns last. **C,** In normal anatomy the small bowel extends from the stomach, performing the first steps in digestion. **D,** The colon extends from the small bowel leading to the rectum. Primary functions of the colon include water reabsorption and storage of stool.

The duodenum develops from both the caudal portion of the foregut and the cranial portion of the midgut, forming a C-shaped loop that projects ventrally. The lumen of the duodenum becomes reduced and may be obliterated by epithelial cells. Normally, the duodenum recanalizes and the lumen is restored.

The embryonic duodenum is the site of origin of the liver and pancreas; thus the excretory ducts of these two organs discharge into the developed structure.

The intestines project into the umbilical cord during the fifth week of embryonic development and return to the abdomen, coiling, during the tenth week, when the abdominal cavity has enlarged. **Peristalsis** occurs by the eleventh week, and swallowing begins at week 12; the intestines begin to fill with **meconium**, which is discharged in the fetal bowel and consists of sloughed off cells, mucus, and bile. By the twentieth week the GI tract has reached its normal configuration and relative size.

The anal canal opens during week 7, when a membrane that separates the rectum from the exterior ruptures.

Male Pelvis Development

Gender is initially determined by the presence (male) or absence (female) of the Y chromosome during conception. Until the seventh or eighth week of gestation, male and female embryos appear identical.

The testicles arise in the fetal upper abdomen near the developing kidneys. In the fourth month the testes descend to the level of the urinary bladder, where they remain until approximately the seventh month of gestation. The testes descend through the inguinal canal and into the scrotum after the seventh month. This descent is hormonally controlled and usually happens during the last month of gestation, but it occasionally does not occur until the first weeks of neonatal life.

The external genitals of both male and female embryos remain undifferentiated until the eighth week of gestation. Before the eighth week, all embryos have a region called the **genital tubercle**. The genital tubercle is an elevated area between the coccyx and the umbilical cord, where the mesonephric and paramesonephric ducts empty. In males, the genital tubercle elongates and develops into the penis (Figure 8-11).

Female Pelvis Development

The reproductive organs develop with the urinary system from two urogenital folds in the early embryo. Each urogenital fold consists of a gonad and a mesonephros.

Differentiation of the gonads into ovaries or testes depends on the genetic makeup of the embryo. The gonads are initially located in the cephalad position and descend into the true pelvis during fetal development.

The mesonephros is the precursor of the metanephros, the urogenital sinus, the wolffian (mesonephric) ducts, and the müllerian (paramesonephric) ducts. The metanephros and the urogenital sinus form the urinary system. The wolffian and **müllerian ducts** form the male and female genital tracts, respectively. The müllerian ducts of the female embryo fuse midline to form the vagina, uterus, and fallopian tubes. The wolffian ducts degenerate in the female embryo, leaving only remnants along the broad ligaments and vaginal walls.

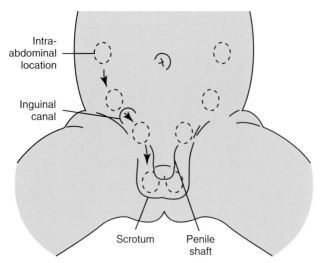

FIGURE 8-11 *Visualize a tissue sheath extending (in the embryo) from the abdomen to the scrotum. Within this sheath the male testicles descend to their final anatomic location. The delayed descent (usually within the inguinal canal) results in testicles retained within the abdominal cavity.*

Congenital uterine malformations result in anatomic variations of the uterus, cervix, and vagina, resulting from the incomplete fusion or agenesis of the müllerian ducts (Figure 8-12). The bicornuate uterus is the most common of the congenital malformations of the female genital tract. It is recognized sonographically by the presence of two endometrial canals that usually communicate at the level of the cervix. Bicornuate uterus is best appreciated in short axis sections, as seen in Figure 8-13. Note the gestational sac in the right horn of the uterus and myometrial tissue separating the two endometrial canals.

Congenital ovarian malformations include unilateral müllerian duct anomaly; gonadal dysgenesis; and accessory, lobulated, and supernumerary ovaries. The unilateral müllerian duct anomaly results in a uterus-like periovarian mass characterized by a central cavity lined by endometrial tissue surrounded by a thick, smooth muscle wall. Gonadal dysgenesis is the absence of both ovaries. It is usually hereditary in nature and associated with an abnormal chromosomal karyotype. In rare cases, unilateral ovarian agenesis may occur. Accessory, lobulated, and supernumerary ovaries are among the rarest of gynecologic malformations.

Breast Development

The mammary glands develop along two strips of ectoderm, the **mammary ridges**, which run along each side of the developing embryo. These are visible by 6 weeks' gestational development. The ridge-like appearance adds texture and dimension to these structures, which

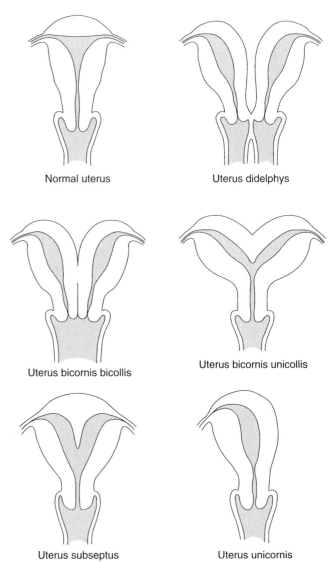

FIGURE 8-12 Congenital Uterine Malformations. This figure illustrates some congenital uterine malformations with anatomic variations of the uterus, cervix, and vagina, resulting from the incomplete fusion or agenesis of the müllerian ducts. Complete duplication of the vagina, cervix, and uterine horns is seen in *uterus didelphys*. The bicornuate uterus has two uterine horns that are fused at one cervix *(uterus bicornis unicollis)* or at two cervices *(uterus bicornis bicollis)*. *Uterus subseptus* is a milder anomaly marked by a midline myometrial septum within the endometrial canal. In some cases only one müllerian duct develops, forming a single uterine horn and a uterine tube continuous with one cervix and vagina *(uterus unicornis)*.

will later undergo more complex development to form breast tissue (Figure 8-14).

By 8 weeks' gestation a bud has developed in the ectoderm, along the mammary ridges, and extends into the underlying connective tissue. This bud will continue to develop, and by the fourth month of gestation it will begin to extend outward into secondary buds. These will further develop into the lactiferous ducts during puberty. More complex development will occur during pregnancy due to hormonal stimulation (Figure 8-15).

In the fetus the externally located nipple site of the mammary gland is slightly recessed, forming what is known as the mammary pit. By birth, it will be slightly raised on the skin surface. Further development of breast tissue will not continue until puberty.

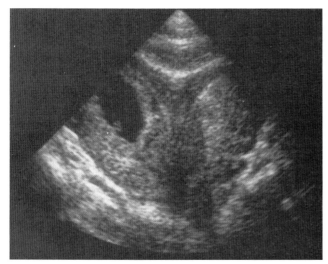

FIGURE 8-13 Congenital Uterine Malformation. This transverse scanning plane, transabdominal image of the pelvis demonstrates a bicornuate uterus containing a gestational sac within the right endometrial cavity. The gestational sac is anechoic and is surrounded by the hyperechoic decidual reaction of the endometrial lining. Myometrial tissue separates the endometrial canals of the left and right uterine horns.

Thyroid and Parathyroid Development

The thyroid gland arises from a median, saclike entodermal diverticulum (the thyroid sac), which begins to thicken during the third week of embryologic development. It arises at the level of the first and second pharyngeal pouches (epithelial entodermal-lined cavities that give rise to a number of vital organs within the embryo) of the ventral wall of the pharynx. The stalk between the thyroid and the tongue is called the thyroglossal duct. It opens in the embryo at the foramen cecum, located at the base of the tongue. The thyroglossal duct atrophies by the sixth week of embryonic development, and thyroid follicles begin to form by the eighth week. They acquire colloid by the third month of development. The thyroglossal duct normally closes after birth. If it persists, a cyst, fistula, or accessory pyramidal lobe may develop.

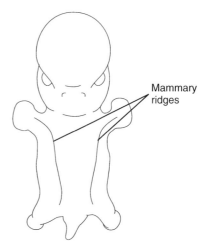

FIGURE 8-14 Breast Development. Mammary ridges seen during prenatal development of fetus.

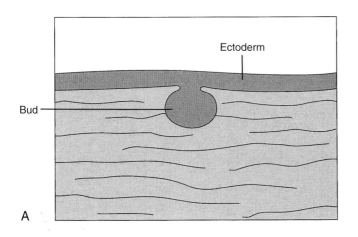

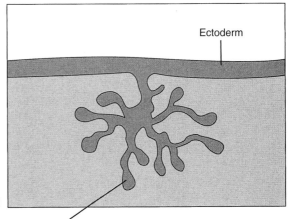

FIGURE 8-15 Breast Development. A, Connective tissue bud seen at approximately 10 weeks' gestational age. **B,** Outward extensions into lactiferous ducts seen at approximately 4 months' gestational age.

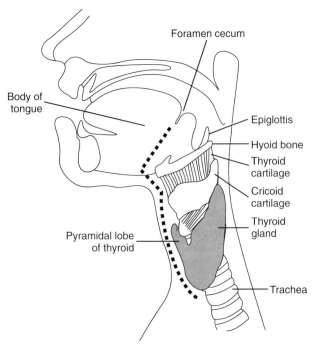

FIGURE 8-16 **Thyroid Development.** Embryonic migration of the thyroid gland. Broken line indicates migration.

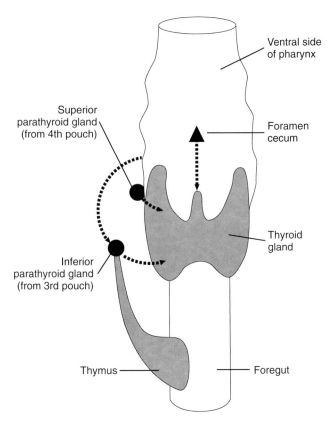

FIGURE 8-17 **Parathyroid Development.** Migration of the thymus and parathyroid glands.

Aberrant thyroid tissue may be found anywhere along the path of the thyroid gland (Figure 8-16). The lingual type accounts for 90% of ectopic thyroids.

The parathyroid glands develop from the third and fourth pharyngeal pouches. They are epithelial entodermal-lined cavities that give rise to a number of vital organs. Parathyroid-3 tissue descends and rests on the dorsal surface of the thyroid gland and forms the inferior parathyroid gland. It originates from the third pouch in conjunction with the thymic primordium in the fifth embryonic week. These primordia lose their connection with the pharyngeal wall and migrate together caudally to lie in a lower position in the neck. Parathyroid-4 loses its contact with the wall of the pharynx and attaches to the caudally migrating thyroid. It eventually rests on the dorsal surface of the upper thyroid gland and forms the superior parathyroid gland (Figure 8-17). The thymus descends to the thorax and lies behind the sternum anterior to the pericardium and great vessels (Figure 8-18).

Neonatal Brain Development

Organogenesis can be divided into several specific developmental events. The first major event, **neural tube** formation, has a peak occurrence at 3 to 4 weeks' gestation. The evolving neural plate involutes and closes dorsally to form the embryonic neural tube, which gives rise to the early brain and spinal cord. By the end of this period, three primary brain vesicles are apparent: the forebrain (prosencephalon), the midbrain (mesencephalon), and the hindbrain (rhombencephalon) (Figure 8-19).

At 5 to 6 weeks' gestation the most anterior brain vesicle, the **prosencephalon**, diverticulates (folds) to form the separate telencephalon (end brain) and the **diencephalon** (in-between brain) (Figure 8-20). The **telencephalon** gives rise to the large cerebral hemispheres, basal ganglia, and lateral ventricles. The diencephalon forms the thalamus and hypothalamus (Table 8-4). The paired olfactory bulbs, optic tracts, and unpaired pineal and pituitary glands also arise from the diverticulation of the forebrain (prosencephalon). Figure 8-21 shows the prosencephalon, diencephalon, and telencephalon. The prosencephalon (forebrain) forms the olfactory bulbs and optic tracts, which are located anteriorly in the neurologic tract. The diencephalon (mid or in-between brain) forms the thalamus and hypothalamus. Note that in the fully developed brain, this important gland is located deep within the cerebral hemispheres. The telencephalon (end brain) gives rise to the cerebral hemispheres and lateral ventricles.

Another major event involves the proliferation of the developing brain's neurons (nerve cells). This occurs between 2 and 4 months of gestation. All the neurons

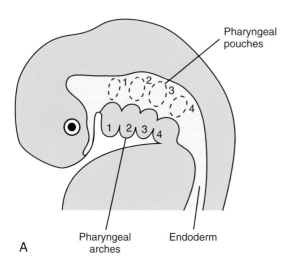

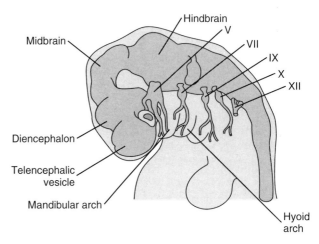

FIGURE 8-20 **Brain Development.** Developing brain at 5½ weeks.

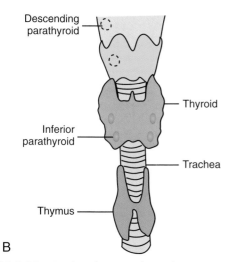

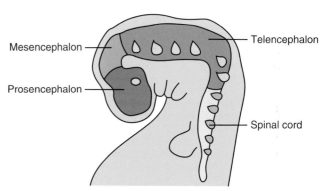

FIGURE 8-18 **A,** The pharyngeal pouches are responsible for the development of a wide range of tissues including glandular, respiratory, and gastrointestinal. **B,** The parathyroid glands migrate to their location on the anterior thyroid gland. There are 4 parathyroid glands in normal anatomy.

FIGURE 8-21 The prosencephalon, diencephalon, and telencephalon are labeled in this figure. The prosencephalon (forebrain) forms the olfactory bulbs and optic tracts, located anteriorly in the neurologic tract. The diencephalon (mid or in-between brain) forms the thalamus and hypothalamus. Note that in the fully developed brain, this important gland is located deep within the cerebral hemispheres. The telencephalon (end brain) gives rise to the cerebral hemispheres and lateral ventricles.

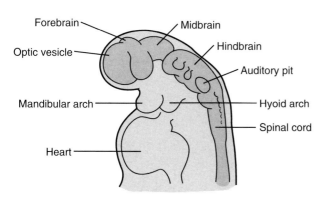

FIGURE 8-19 **Brain Development.** First stage of early development of the brain at 3½ weeks.

Table 8-4 Brain Area Formation: 3 to 4 Embryologic Weeks

Brain Portion	Forms ...
Prosencephalon: forebrain	Paired olfactory bulbs and optic tracts, unpaired pineal and pituitary glands
Diencephalon: in-between brain	Thalamus and hypothalamus
Telencephalon: hindbrain	Cerebral hemispheres, basal ganglia, and lateral ventricles

are located in the subependymal region and thereby proliferate from both ventricular and subventricular areas. Unfortunately, very little is known about the quantitative aspects of this event. Disorders of neuronal proliferation can result in either microencephaly or macroencephaly.

Neuronal migration primarily occurs during between 3 and 5 months of gestation. During this time, a remarkable series of occurrences take place. Millions of neurons in their original ventricular and subventricular sites migrate to new locations within the central nervous system, where they will reside permanently. Again, disorders in this major event result in severe neurologic disturbances.

From approximately the sixth month of gestation to several years after birth, major organizational events occur. These events settle the elaborate circuitry that distinguishes the human brain. One example of an organizational event is the proper alignment, orientation, and layering of the neurons of the cerebral cortex.

Finally, myelination, the laying down of a highly specialized myelin membrane, takes place. This event takes a very long time, continuing from the second trimester of pregnancy into adult life.

REFERENCE CHARTS

■ ■ ■ ASSOCIATED PHYSICIANS

- **Embryologist:** Physician specializing in embryology, a branch of medicine involving early development and growth of embryos.
- **Obstetrician:** Physician specializing in the branch of medicine that addresses care of women during pregnancy, childbirth, and recovery.
- **Sonologist/Radiologist:** Physician specializing in performing and/or interpreting sonograms (ultrasound examinations).

■ ■ ■ COMMON DIAGNOSTIC TESTS

Category of Tests (multiple tests represented by each category)	When Performed
Genetic tests	Before pregnancy or first trimester
Testing RE: maternal health conditions	Before pregnancy through first trimester
Pregnancy assessment	Throughout pregnancy
Fetal anomalies detection	First or second trimester
Fetal maturity	Second or third trimester, as indicated by symptoms

■ ■ ■ LABORATORY VALUES

Test	Change Between Nonpregnant and Pregnant Levels
Hemoglobin	Slight decrease
Hematocrit	Slight decrease
Kidney-serum creatinine	Slight decrease
Kidney-BUN	Slight increase
Kidney-urine glucose	Increase
Liver-ALT, AST	Unchanged
Liver-alkaline phosphatase	Increase (up to 2 to 4 times nonpregnant level)
Liver-LDH	Slight increase

■ ■ ■ AFFECTING CHEMICALS

Product labels now warn of the dangers alcohol and tobacco pose to an unborn child.

CHAPTER 9

Introduction to Laboratory Values

TIANA V. CURRY-McCOY AND REVA ARNEZ CURRY

OBJECTIVES

Explain the role of laboratory tests and normal range of values.

Contrast patient's values to normal, high, and low lab values.

List methods used to obtain lab samples.

Describe the importance of quality control in laboratory testing.

Discuss the purpose of Westgard rules.

KEY WORDS

Alanine Aminotransferase (ALT) — Previously referred to as serum glutamic pyruvic transaminase (SGPT). ALT is normally present in large concentrations in the liver.

Amylase — Carbohydrates are digested by amylase, which is produced in the salivary glands and the pancreas.

Aspartate Aminotransferase (AST) — Previously referred to as serum glutamic oxaloacetic transaminase (SGOT). AST is present in the brain, kidneys, muscle, heart, and liver.

Bilirubin — Results from the degradation of heme by reticuloendothelial liver cells, causing a reddish bile pigment.

Blood Urea Nitrogen (BUN) — Formed when protein breaks down.

Cholesterol — A soft, waxy substance found in all body parts and needed for proper bodily function.

Creatine Phosphokinase (CPK) — An enzyme found in muscle tissues (heart, brain, and skeletal).

Creatinine — An end product of creatine breakdown in muscle. Creatinine is found in urine, muscle, and blood.

Glucose — The main metabolite consumed by the body for energy; excreted through urine.

Hematocrit — This value shows the ratio of the packed red blood cell volume.

Human Chorionic Gonadotropin (hCG) — Used to confirm pregnancy and can be determined by blood or urine test; levels detected as early as 10 days after a missed period in a menstrual cycle.

Lactate Dehydrogenase (LD) — When cells are damaged or destroyed they release LD into the blood. LD is an indicator of tissue damage and certain diseases.

Lipase — An enzyme that helps absorb body fat and is released from the pancreas to the small intestine.

Prostate Specific Antigen (PSA) — A protein produced by prostate cells; can be used to detect prostate cancer in men.

Prothrombin — The clotting factor prothrombin is a precursor to thrombin, which is needed for the formation of normal blood clots.

Quadruple Screen Test (Quad Screen) — A blood test performed during 15 to 22 weeks of pregnancy to screen for certain birth defects.

Quality Control (QC) — The process by which standards are employed to determine if lab assays are working properly and are within equipment and value control standards.

Thyroid Stimulating Hormone (TSH) — Produced by the pituitary gland. TSH directs the thyroid to produce and release triiodothyronine (T_3) and thyroxine (T_4).

Westgard Rules — Universal computational rules designed to determine if analytical runs are within control limits; helps to determine if samples are viable in their current conditions (samples may need to be diluted, re-obtained, etc).

AGENCY OVERSIGHT OF LABORATORY TESTING

There are many health care agencies, personnel, and facilities in the United States that work together to ensure proper oversight of acquisition, evaluation, and quality control of laboratory values. It is the duty of the Health Care Financing Administration to ensure that medical laboratory testing in the United States is regulated to ensure quality control. **Quality control (QC)** in clinical laboratories is composed of extensive equipment maintenance and testing to ensure that laboratory results are correct and equipment is working properly within parameter limits. Clinical Laboratory Improvement Amendments (CLIA), overseeing laboratory quality control, are enforced by the Center for Clinical Standards and Quality to approximately 244,000 laboratories in the United States. Laboratory methods, techniques, and equipment are standardized with QC methods to ensure patient safety in diagnosis.

The major agencies used to assist laboratories in maintaining CLIA are the Commissions of Office Laboratory

Accreditation, The Joint Commission (TJC), and the College of American Pathologists Laboratory Accreditation Program (CAP-LAP). CLIA standards are a part of the International Organization of Standardization (ISO). Accreditation and monitoring of these agencies are maintained through various techniques, such as self-studies, regular quality control sampling, reports, and inspections. This regulation allows medical personnel and patients to be secure in the results output by laboratories, research results to be compared, and medical records and testing to be universally translated and trusted. Refer to Table 9-1 for a definition of the agencies and an explanation of how they work together to ensure quality control and standardization.

QUALITY CONTROL OF LABORATORY VALUES

Westgard rules are mathematical calculations to establish control limits. A Levey-Jennings chart (Figure 9-1) is a common quality control tool that determines if standards are within set control limits over a period of time. If standards are out of control limits, accuracy and imprecision errors can be detected. A full explanation of control limits and Westgard rules can be found at www.westgard.com. Analytical variations can be detected by quality control. Westgard rules establish statistical limits of variation for all analytic methods, evaluate quality controls, and allow for correction of errors by taking corrective steps and then reanalyzing controls and patient samples.

Laboratories have standards for how long they monitor new equipment or new control lots to verify that readings maintain acceptable ranges. Agencies such as CLIA and CAP-LAP also require laboratories to participate in external proficiency testing in addition to daily QC. Proficiency testing allows these agencies to compare laboratories all over the country. During the proficiency testing, unknown samples are received from the agency and tested in the same manner as patient samples, and results are reported back to the agency. All participating laboratory results are compiled by the agency, and performance reports are sent back to the participating laboratories. Laboratories using the same methods are graded by the samples-defined performance criteria.

Laboratories have many rules, regulations, and standards in place to provide the best possible patient care. The values detected in patient samples, in conjunction with sonographic images obtained by sonographers, assist the physician in diagnosis and application of treatment. The following are some of the major methods used in obtaining patient samples and the value ranges that are important to the body systems reviewed in this

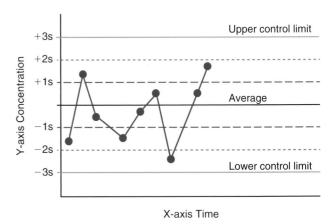

FIGURE 9-1 Levey-Jennings chart.

■ ■ ■ Table 9-1 Organizations Related to Laboratory Value Acquisition and Quality Control

Center for Clinical Standards and Quality (CCSQ)	Office within the CMS responsible for implementation of CLIA; policies; quality, clinical, and medical science issues; and survey and certification of their programs.
Centers for Medicare and Medicaid Services (CMS)	Federal agency housed in the U.S. Department of Health and Human Services; responsible for CLIA.
Clinical Laboratory Improvement Amendments (CLIA)	Used to regulate human laboratory testing in the United States through quality laboratory testing; governs approximately 244,000 laboratories.
College of American Pathologists Laboratory Accreditation Program (CAP-LAP)	Voluntary accreditation program used to ensure labs meet or exceed laboratory quality requirements; governs approximately 7,000 laboratories.
Commissions of Office Laboratory Accreditation (COLA)	Independent organization that accredits approximately 8,000 laboratories and assists them in meeting and complying with CLIA standards.
Health Care Financing Administration (HCFA)	Governing body that uses CLIA to regulate all medical laboratory testing in the United States.
International Organization for Standardization (ISO)	Constructed of 163 member countries, this voluntary agency is nongovernmental and serves to ensure products, services, and systems have international safety, quality, and efficiency.
The Joint Commission (TJC)	Independently inspects laboratories, hospitals, and health organizations; certifies and accredits over 20,500 health care programs, organizations, and facilities.

book. Please note the ranges here may vary slightly from the ranges listed in other chapters, because laboratory values may vary among different laboratories and institutions. The information provided in this chapter is meant to be an extended review of the main clinical laboratory values listed in other chapters of this book.

LABORATORY VALUES

Laboratory values are like captions that give details about symptoms a patient may or may not be able to verbalize. Sonographic images add more detail to the captions by providing images and details to help sonologists and clinicians arrive at differential diagnoses and optimal treatment plans. Laboratory values, primary organs associated with the value, value ranges, and implications for low or high values are shown on the following charts.

Laboratory Value: Bilirubin
Primary Organs: Liver, Gallbladder
Bilirubin results from the degradation of heme by reticuloendothelial liver cells, causing a reddish bile pigment. Bilirubin can be tested in two ways. The first method is blood test by venipuncture. To prepare for this test the patient should not eat or drink for a minimum of 4 hours before the test. Health care providers will instruct patients on medications that may interfere with the test results. The second method is urine test by collection bag. Instructions about interfering medication also apply for this method of testing. Both tests may be used to diagnose liver or gallbladder disease.

■ ■ □ **Table 9-2** Bilirubin Reference Values

Sample	Normal Values	Implications of High Values
Urine	None (not normally found in urine)	Liver or gallbladder tumors Biliary tract gallstones Biliary tract disease Liver disease Hepatitis Cirrhosis Hemolytic anemia
Blood (newborn)	340 μmol/L	Jaundice Neurologic defects Seizures Abnormal eye movements and reflexes
Blood (adult)		
Direct (conjugated) Total	0–0.3 mg/dL 0.3–1.9 mg/dL	Jaundice Hemolytic anemia Transfusion reaction Erythroblastosis fetalis Gilbert's syndrome Rotor syndrome Liver disease Hepatitis Cirrhosis Medical drug interference (pharmaceutical or chemo) Gallstones Cancer of pancreas or gallbladder Biliary stricture Crigler-Najjar syndrome Dubin-Johnson syndrome Choledocholithiasis

Laboratory Value: Alanine Aminotransferase (ALT) and Aspartate Aminotransferase (AST)
Primary Organs: Liver, Pancreas

Alanine aminotransferase (ALT) was previously referred to as serum glutamic pyruvic transaminase (SGPT). Aspartate aminotransferase (AST) was previously referred to as serum glutamic oxaloacetic transaminase (SGOT). However, most laboratories will show results as ALT and AST. AST is present in the brain, kidneys, muscle, pancreas, heart, and liver. Whereas ALT is normally present in large concentrations in the liver, when ALT levels rise in the blood it serves as an indicator of specific liver damage. These levels are often run in a panel and compared to total protein, bilirubin, and alkaline phosphatase (ALP). Total protein is a measurement of albumin and globulin in the fluid portion of blood. ALP is found in all body tissues; however, high levels are seen in liver, bone, and bile ducts. AST can be directly compared to ALT, giving an AST/ALT calculated ratio. All of the aforementioned tests can be collected by venipuncture and can be used to indicate liver damage. Normal ranges of these proteins can vary with age, pregnancy, and gender. High levels of these proteins may indicate the patient is alcoholic and may be the cause of liver damage.

■ ■ ■ **Table 9-3** ALT, AST, ALP, Total Protein Levels

Blood Sample	Normal Value	Implications of Low Values	Implications of High Values
ALT	10–40 International Units/liter (IU/L)		Hepatitis Cirrhosis Liver necrosis Hemochromatosis Liver tumor/cancer Liver ischemia Mononucleosis Pancreatitis Liver toxic medications Viral hepatitis A
AST	10–34 IU/L		Heart attack Muscle trauma/disease Hepatitis Cirrhosis Liver necrosis Hemochromatosis Liver tumor/cancer Liver ischemia Mononucleosis Pancreatitis Liver toxic medications Viral hepatitis A
ALP	44–147 IU/L	Protein deficiency Malnutrition Wilson's disease Hypophosphatemia	Rickets Sarcoidosis Leukemia Lymphoma Paget's disease Hepatitis Osteoblastic tumor Osteomalacia Biliary obstruction Hyperparathyroidism Blood type O or B consuming high fatty meals Pancreatitis Renal cancer Gallstones

■ ■ ■ **Table 9-3** ALT, AST, ALP, Total Protein Levels—cont'd

Blood Sample	Normal Value	Implications of Low Values	Implications of High Values
Total protein	6–8.3 g/dL	Hemorrhage Extensive burns Agammaglobulinemia Glomerulonephritis Liver disease Malabsorption Malnutrition Protein losing enteropathy Nephrotic syndrome	Pregnancy Chronic inflammation HIV Hepatitis B Hepatitis C Waldenström's disease Multiple myeloma

Laboratory Value: Cholesterol and Triglycerides
Primary Organs: Liver, Heart

Cholesterol is found in all body parts, and this soft, waxy substance is needed for proper bodily function. There are 3 major types of cholesterol: low-density lipoprotein (LDL; bad), high-density lipoprotein (HDL; good), and very low-density lipoprotein (VLDL; bad). Cholesterol carries lipids (triglycerides and other fats) through the blood to the liver. Blood tests can be done to measure cholesterol and triglyceride levels.

■ ■ ■ **Table 9-4** Cholesterol and Triglyceride Levels

Measurement	Value (mg/dL)	Level	Notes
Total cholesterol	<200 200–239 240 and above	Good Moderately high High	
LDL	<100 100–129 130–159 160–189 190 and above	Good for history of heart disease Good Moderately high High Extremely high	High levels linked to cardiovascular disease
HDL			Carry lipids to liver
Men Women Men Women	<40 <50 40–49 50–59 60 and above	Not good Not good Good Good Extremely good	
VLDL	5–40	Normal	Helps build cholesterol on artery walls
Triglycerides	<150 150–199 200–499 500 and above	Good Moderately high High Extremely high	High levels linked to coronary artery disease

Laboratory Value: Blood Urea Nitrogen (BUN)
Primary Organs: Liver, Kidney

The **blood urea nitrogen (BUN)** test measures urea nitrogen in the blood. When protein breaks down, urea nitrogen is formed. Urea nitrogen can be measured in the blood by venipuncture. Many medicines can interfere with this test, and a physician should be consulted before the test is performed.

■ ■ ■ **Table 9-5** Blood Urea Nitrogen Levels

Sample	Normal Value	Implications of Low Values	Implications of High Values
Blood	6–20 mg/dL	Liver failure Low dietary protein Hyperhydration Malnutrition	Gastrointestinal bleeding Kidney failure or disease Shock Urinary tract obstruction Hypovolemia Excessive gastrointestinal tract protein levels Heart attack Congestive heart failure

Laboratory Value: Creatinine

Primary Organ: Kidney

When creatine in muscles is broken down, a byproduct is creatinine. Creatinine can be measured by 24-hour urine collection or blood drawn by venipuncture. A physician should be consulted about interfering medications.

■ ■ ■ **Table 9-6** Creatinine Levels

Sample	Normal Value	Implications of Low Values	Implications of High Values
Blood	**mg/dL**		
Men	0.7–1.3	Muscular dystrophy	Kidney damage, failure, or infection
Women	0.6–1.1	Myasthenia gravis	Dehydration Urinary tract blockage Eclampsia/pre-eclampsia Rhabdomyolysis
Urine	**mg/kg of body mass/day**		
Men	14–26	Myasthenia gravis	Kidney damage, failure, or infection
Women	11–20		Low blood flow to kidneys Urinary tract blockage High-meat diet Rhabdomyolysis

Laboratory Value: Amylase, Lipase

Primary Organ: Pancreas

Carbohydrates are digested by amylase, which is produced in the salivary glands and the pancreas. Pancreatic disease can cause a release of amylase into the blood. Irregular levels of amylase can be detected by venipuncture or urine test. The urine test may be performed by 24-hour catch or clean catch.

Lipase is an enzyme that helps absorb body fat and is released from the pancreas to the small intestine. Measurements of lipase can be performed by blood draw from the vein. A patient normally fasts for 8 hours before this test, and a doctor must be consulted about medications.

■ ■ ■ **Table 9-7** Amylase Levels and Lipase Levels

Sample	Normal Value	Implications of Low Values	Implications of High Values
Amylase Levels			
Blood	23–85 U/L	Pancreatic cancer or damage Kidney disease Toxemia in pregnancy	Ovarian, lung, or pancreatic cancer Acute pancreatitis Intestinal obstruction Mumps Salivary gland obstruction Cholecystitis Perforated ulcer Macroamylasemia Severe gastroenteritis Gallbladder disease Bile duct or pancreas obstruction Ruptured tubal pregnancy
Urine	2.6–21.2 IU/hr		Ovarian, lung, or pancreatic cancer Acute pancreatitis Intestinal obstruction Mumps Salivary gland obstruction Cholecystitis Perforated ulcer Alcohol consumption Ectopic or ruptured tubal pregnancy Pelvic inflammatory disease Pancreatic duct blockage Gallbladder disease
Lipase Levels			
Blood	0–160 U/L	Permanent damage to pancreatic lipase producing cells Cystic fibrosis	Celiac disease Pancreatic cancer Duodenal ulcer Bowel obstruction Pancreatic infection or swelling Kidney disease Gallbladder inflammation Acute pancreatitis

Laboratory Value: Glucose

Primary Organs: Pancreas, Liver, Thyroid

A glucose test measures the amount of glucose (sugar) in a patient sample. A glucose test can be performed by venipuncture or urine collection. A blood glucose test can be performed in two ways: random (anytime during the day) and fasting (at least 8 hours of not eating). Glucose is not normally found in the urine. A urine glucose test can be performed by direct urine sample, which is tested with a dipstick, or by 24-hour home collection of urine. Urine glucose tests are performed often during pregnancy as an indicator of gestational diabetes. Glucose tests are indicators of diabetes; however, a fasting glucose test and a glucose tolerance test (GTT) are better indicators. There are two types of GTT. The first, the IV glucose tolerance test (IGTT), is rarely used and is never used to diagnose diabetes. In IGTT, glucose blood measurements are made before and 1 minute and 3 minutes after an injection of glucose directly into the patient's vein. The oral glucose tolerance test (OGTT) consists of the patient ingesting approximately 75 grams of a glucose liquid drink. Blood levels are taken before (sometimes) and every 30 to 60 minutes after consumption for up to 3 hours, depending on the doctor's request. Some patients feel nauseated after OGTT consumption; if a patient vomits the liquid he or she will have to retake the test. Health care providers must be notified of all medications before the glucose test.

■ ■ **Table 9–8** Glucose Levels

Sample	Value (mg/dL)	Implications of Low Values	Implications of High Values
Blood			
Random normal	≤125	Hypoglycemia	Diabetes
Fasting normal	70–99	Adrenal insufficiency	Insulinoma
Fasting pre-diabetic	100–125	Severe liver disease	High insulin or
Fasting diabetic	126 and above	Insulin overdose	diabetes medication
		Excessive alcohol intake	Cushing syndrome
		Hypopituitarism	Pancreatitis
		Hypothyroidism	Pancreatic cancer
		Insulinoma	Chronic kidney failure
		Starvation	Acromegaly
		Underactive thyroid gland	Overactive thyroid
		Low food intake	
		Renal disease	
Urine			
Normal	0–15	Normal	Diabetes
			Renal glycosuria
			Gestational diabetes
OGTT			
Fasting normal	60–100		Pre-diabetes
Non-fasting			Gestational diabetes
1 hour normal	<200		Diabetes
2 hour normal	<140		Cushing syndrome
2 hour pre-diabetes	140–200		Pancreatic damage
2 hour diabetes	200 and above		Kidney failure

Laboratory Value: Lactate Dehydrogenase (LD)
Primary Organ: Heart
When cells are damaged or destroyed they release lactate dehydrogenase (LD) into the blood. LD is an indicator of tissue damage and certain diseases. LD levels from a blood test can help determine anemia, acute or chronic tissue damage, determine or monitor cancers, and detect severe infections. Body fluid (cerebrospinal or pleural) LD can distinguish meningitis and help determine injury or inflammation, or imbalance from blood pressure or protein in the blood. LD levels range with age, and reference values may vary on different machinery. Samples are drawn from either a vein (normally in the arm) or from body fluid, such as a spinal tap.

■ ■ ■ **Table 9–9** Lactate Dehydrogenase Levels

Sample	Values (Units/L)	Implications of High Values
Serum		
Child 1–3	160–370	Myocardial infarction
Child 4–17	105–370	Pulmonary infarction or embolism
Adult	122–222	Leukemia
		Hypoxia
		Liver or renal disease
		Severe shock
		Hodgkin's disease
Blood		
Newborn	160–450	Sepsis
Infant	100–250	Acute kidney or liver disease
Child	60–170	Acute muscle injury
Adult	100–190	Pancreatitis
		Bone fractures
		Cancer
		Anemia
		Infections (HIV, meningitis, encephalitis)
Cerebrospinal Fluid		
Newborn	≤70	Jakob-Creutzfeldt disease
Adults	≤40	Bacterial meningitis
		Neurosyphilis
		Tumors

Laboratory Value: Creatine Phosphokinase (CPK)

Primary Organs: Heart, Brain, Skeletal

Creatine phosphokinase (CPK) is an enzyme found in muscle tissues (heart, brain, and skeletal). Levels can be measured by blood sample obtained by venipuncture. CPK has three isoforms (BB brain type, MM muscle type, and MB muscle/brain type), which can help distinguish body injury. The physician should be consulted about medications or treatments that may interfere with measurements.

■ ■ ■ **Table 9-10** Creatine Phosphokinase Levels

Isoforms	Value (mcg/L)	Location	Implications of High Values
CPK-1 or CPK-BB (brain type)		Brain Lung	Cancer Stroke Brain bleeding Seizure Pulmonary infarction Electroconvulsive therapy
CPK-2 or CPK-MB (muscle/brain type)		Heart	Myocarditis Heart defibrillation Electrical injury Heart injury or surgery
CPK-3 or CPK-MM (muscle type)		Skeletal muscle	Myositis Crush injuries Rhabdomyolysis Seizures Surgery Strenuous exercise Electromyography
Total CPK	10–120		

Laboratory Value: Prostate Specific Antigen (PSA)
Primary Organ: Prostate
Prostate cells produce a protein called prostate specific antigen (PSA). PSA can be used to detect prostate cancer in men. Blood samples can be obtained through venipuncture to examine PSA levels. PSA screening normally occurs between the ages of 50 and 75 in men with no risk factors for prostate cancer. For men with a family history or of African-American ethnicity, PSA screening starts between the ages of 40 and 45. PSA levels can differ in age and alter slightly after a prostate examination.

■ ■ ■ **Table 9-11** Prostate Specific Antigen Levels

Age	Blood Sample Values	Implications of High Values
Normal	4 ng/mL	Prostatitis
50 or younger	2.5 ng/mL	Enlarged prostate
		Prostate cancer
		Urinary tract infection
		Recent cystoscopy or prostate biopsy
		Recent bladder catheter tube

Laboratory Value: Estrogen
Primary Organ: Female and Male
There are three components of estrogen that may be measured in an estrogen test: E1 (estrone), E2 (estradiol), and E3 (estriol). Each measurement can be used for a different diagnosis. E1 and E2 levels can be detected in males as well as females. E2 levels may vary during menstrual cycles. Unconjugated or free E3 (uE3) may be used as a marker in pregnancy for abnormalities. Levels of estrogen vary for sex and age. This test is performed by blood draw.

■ ■ ■ **Table 9-12** Estrogen Levels

Type, Sex	Values (pg/mL)	Implications of Low Values	Implications of High Values
E1			
Adult male	10–60		Delayed puberty
			Testicular or adrenal gland cancer
			Gynecomastia
			Cirrhosis
			Hyperthyroidism
Female premenopausal	17–200	Turner syndrome	Early puberty
Female postmenopausal	7–40	Polycystic ovarian syndrome	Ovarian or adrenal tumors
		Anorexia	Cirrhosis
		Hypopituitarism	Hyperthyroidism
		Hypogonadism	
		Extreme exercise endurance	
		Stein-Levanthal syndrome	
E2			
Adult male	10–50		Gynecomastia
			Klinefelter syndrome
Female premenopausal	30–400	Turner syndrome	Early puberty
Female postmenopausal	0–30	Menopause	Amenorrhea
		Polycystic ovarian syndrome	Ovarian hypofunction
		Anorexia	Rapid weight loss
		Hypopituitarism	Low body fat
		Hypogonadism	
		Extreme exercise endurance	
		Stein-Levanthal syndrome	

Table 9-12 Estrogen Levels—cont'd

Type, Sex	Values (pg/mL)	Implications of Low Values	Implications of High Values
E3			
Pregnant female	10–100 nM	Eclampsia Offspring Down syndrome Failing pregnancy	
Nonpregnant female	<7 nM		
uE3			
Males	<0.07 ng/mL		
Females	<0.08 ng/mL		

During pregnancy		<0.3 multiples of
		  gestational age median
		Fetal termination
		Aromatase deficiency
		1 or 2 fetal adrenal
		  insufficiency
		Smith-Lemli-Opitz
		  syndrome
		X-linked ichthyosis
			>2.1 ng/mL
			Fetal congenital
			  adrenal
			  hyperplasia
			Pending labor

Laboratory Value: Human Chorionic Gonadotropin (hCG)

Primary Focus: Pregnancy

Human chorionic gonadotropin (hCG) is used to detect pregnancy and can be determined by blood or urine test as early as 10 days after conception. A urine test can be performed by direct collection in a container. A blood test performed by venipuncture can be measured qualitatively (presence of hCG used to determine pregnancy) or quantitatively (how much hCG determination of fetal age, and diagnosis of abnormal pregnancy). HCG levels rapidly rise in the first trimester of pregnancy and then slowly decline. HCG levels should double every 48 hours early in the pregnancy. HCG levels can also be used to diagnose gestational trophoblastic disease of the testes or ovaries.

Table 9-13 Human Chorionic Gonadotropin Levels

Value	Implications of Abnormally Rising and/or Low Values	Implications of High Values

<25–50 mIU/mL will
  result in a negative
  pregnancy test result
	Miscarriage
	Tubal pregnancy
	Fetal death
	Ectopic pregnancy
	Partial miscarriage
		Pregnancy
		More than one fetus
		Uterine or ovarian cancer
		Uterine hydatidiform mole
		Testicular cancer
		Gestational trophoblastic disease

Laboratory Value: Alpha Fetoprotein (AFP)

Primary Focus: Pregnancy

Alpha fetoprotein (AFP) is produced in the fetal yolk sac and liver of a developing fetus. AFP is used in a **quadruple screen test (quad screen)** for fetal birth defects. AFP levels are drawn by venipuncture. Quad screening is a blood test that includes AFP, hCG, uE3, and inhibin A (placenta-released hormone) administered between 15 and 22 weeks of pregnancy. AFP levels can also be used to diagnose liver, ovarian, testicular, stomach, colon, lung, breast, and lymphoma cancers. Increased levels can also be observed in cases of cirrhosis and hepatitis.

■ ■ ▫ **Table 9-14** Alpha Fetoprotein Levels

Patient	Values	Implications of Low Values	Implications of High Values
Males and nonpregnant females	<40 mcg/L		
Pregnant females 0–32 weeks	0.2–250 ng/mL	Down syndrome Edward syndrome	More than one fetus Anencephaly Miscarriage Spina bifida Turner syndrome Tetralogy of Fallot Duodenal atresia Hepatitis and cirrhosis for nonpregnant females and males

Laboratory Value: Thyroid Stimulating Hormone, T₃, T₄

Primary Organs: Thyroid and Parathyroid Glands

Thyroid stimulating hormone (TSH) is produced by the pituitary gland. TSH directs the thyroid to produce and release triiodothyronine (T_3) and thyroxine (T_4). TSH, T_3, and T_4 can be measured at the same time by venipuncture. A physician should be consulted about medications that may interfere with this test. Normal ranges may vary during pregnancy.

■ ■ ▫ **Table 9-15** Thyroid Hormone Levels

Hormone	Normal Values	Implications of Low Values	Implications of High Values
THS	0.4–4 mIU/L	Graves' disease High iodine levels Toxic nodular goiter	Hypothyroidism
T_3	100–200 ng/dL	Thyroiditis Starvation Underactive thyroid gland Short- or long-term illness	Graves' disease Liver disease Toxic nodular goiter Thyrotoxicosis Medications or supplements Pregnancy Birth control pill Estrogen
T_4	4.5–11.2 mcg/dL	Malnutrition Fasting Illness Medications Hypothyroidism	Graves' disease Trophoblastic disease Toxic multinodular goiter Germ cell tumors Iodine-induced hyperthyroidism Subacute thyroiditis High-thyroid hormone medication Pregnancy Birth control pills Estrogen Liver disease Inherited condition

Laboratory Values: Hematocrit and Prothrombin

Primary Focus: Blood and Vital Organs

A **hematocrit** value is the ratio of the packed red blood cell volume in a centrifuged blood sample, which is expressed as a percentage. The patient blood sample is collected and measured either by automated machine (a calculation based on the amount of hemoglobin and average volume of red blood cells) or manually by centrifugation of the blood sample (plasma is separated from red blood cells that are packed at the bottom). Hematocrit levels change with age and differ for gender in adults. Reference values may differ slightly based on the laboratory testing the samples.

■ ■ ■ **Table 9-16** Hematocrit Levels

Age Range, Sex	Normal Values (%)	Implications of Low Values	Implications of High Values
Newborn	45–68	Anemia or sickle sell	Chronic smoking
Infant	30–49	Loss of blood	Living at high altitudes
Adult male	41–54	Nutritional deficiencies	Erythrocytosis
Adult female	36–46	Colon cancer/leukemia	Hypoxia
		Kidney failure	Polycythemia
		Overhydration	Dehydration
			Polycythemia vera
			Tumors
			Pulmonary fibrosis
			Erythropoietin abuse

The clotting factor **prothrombin** is a precursor to thrombin, which is needed for the formation of normal blood clots. The measurement of the time taken for plasma to clot is called prothrombin time (PT). The prothrombin test can also be called INR, which means international normalized ratio, which is how protrombin tests are standardized. This test is performed by venipuncture and addition of chemicals to the blood sample to measure clotting time. PT is commonly measured to monitor clotting levels when patients are taking blood-thinning medication, determine liver function, and detect abnormal bleeding. A similar test, partial thromboplastin time (PTT), performed in the same manner is used to measure the ability of clotting proteins or factors and is normally performed in conjunction with PT. The health care provider should be aware of medications taken by the patient, especially warfarin, and will advise on preparation for the test.

■ ■ ■ **Table 9-17** Prothrombin Levels

Assay	Normal Values (seconds or INR)	INR above 1.1 without Warfarin	High or Low With Warfarin
PT	11–13.5 sec or 0.8–1.1 INR Warfarin medication 2–3 INR	Low levels of vitamin K Liver disease Bleeding disorders Disseminated intravascular coagulation	Alcohol consumption Wrong medication dose Over-the-counter medication interference Food complications
PTT	Normal values 25–35 sec Blood-thinning medication 2.5 × normal value range	Abnormal values (too long) Hemophilia A or B Factor XII or factor XI deficiency Liver disease Lupus anticoagulants Hypofibrinogenemia Malabsorption Vitamin K deficiency Disseminated intravascular coagulation Von Willebrand's disease	

Laboratory Value: Blood Cell Count and Sediment Rate

Primary Focus: Blood

There are several types of blood counts that can be performed on a patient: complete blood count (CBC), red blood count (RBC), and white blood count (WBC). CBC measures total hemoglobin, hematocrit, platelet, WBC, and RBC, also provides average red blood size (MCV), hemoglobin per red blood cell (MCH), and hemoglobin concentration per red blood cell (MCHC). CBC is used to diagnose infections and allergies, detect blood and clotting disorders, and evaluate production/destruction of red blood cells. RBC measures the amount of red blood cells a person has and is used to diagnose anemia, scarring of bone marrow, white blood cell cancer, kidney disease that is damaging blood vessels, and premature breakdown of red blood cells. WBC is used to detect infection or allergies and is a total measurement of basophils, eosinophils, lymphocytes, monocytes, and neutrophils. All of these counts are measured by venipuncture.

■ ■ ▢ **Table 9-18** Blood Cell Counts

Assay	Normal Values	Implications of Low Values	Implications of High Values

CBC	RBC: see below
	WBC: see below
	Hematocrit
	    Male 40%–50%
	    Female 36%–44%
	Hemoglobin
	    Male 13.8–17.2 g/dL
	    Female 12–15 g/dL
	MCV 80–95 femtoliter
	MCH 27–31 pg/cell
	MCHC 32–36 g/dL
		RBC: see below
		WBC: see below
		Hemoglobin-anemia
		Blood loss
			RBC: see below
			WBC: see below

RBC	Female 4.2–5.4 cells/μL Male 4.7–6.1 million cells/μL	Bleeding Anemia Leukemia Malnutrition Multiple myeloma Overhydration Pregnancy RBC hemolysis Bone marrow failure Specific drugs Nutrition deficiencies Erythropoietin deficiency	Cigarette smoking Congenital heart disease Cor pulmonale Dehydration Hypoxia Pulmonary fibrosis Polycythemia vera Kidney tumor Specific drugs

WBC	4500–10,000 cells/μL	Leukopenia, WBC <4500,
		    neutrophils <1700
		Failure, deficiency, or
		    cancer of bone
		    marrow
		Liver or spleen disease
		Autoimmune disorders
		Bacterial infection
		Viral illnesses
		Cancer drugs or radiation
			Tissue damage
			Leukemia
			Mental or physical stress
			Cigarette smoking
			Allergy
			Inflammatory disease
			Specific drugs or
			    medications
			Splenectomy

Erythrocyte sedimentation rate (ESR) is a measurement of bodily inflammation. This test is performed by venipuncture when a patient presents with unexplained fevers, muscle symptoms, specific arthritis, and other vague symptoms. The test can also be used to monitor cancers, bone infections, autoimmune disorders, tissue death, specific arthritis, and inflammatory diseases.

■ ■ ■ **Table 9-19** Erythrocyte Sedimentation Rate

Age, Sex	Normal Values (mL/hr)	Implications of Low Values	Implications of High Values
Newborn	0–2	Hypofibrinogenemia	Kidney disease
Child	3–13	Leukemia	Pregnancy
Woman <50 yr	<20	Polycythemia	Anemia
Woman >50 yr	<30	Sickle cell anemia	Cancer
Man <50 yr	<15	Liver or kidney disease	Thyroid disease
Man >50 yr	<20	causing low plasma	Autoimmune disorders
		protein	Systemic infection
		Congestive heart failure	Rheumatic fever
		Hyperviscosity	Tuberculosis
			Bone infections
			Skin infections
			Heart or heart valve infection
			Necrotizing vasculitis
			Macroglobulinemia
			Hyperfibrinogenemia
			Allergic vasculitis
			Giant cell arteritis
			Polymyalgia

■ ■ ■ **Table 9-20** Review Table

Organ	Laboratory Test
Abdominal aorta Neonatal brain	Hematocrit
Liver	Bilirubin
Liver Pancreas	ALT AST ALP Total protein levels
Liver Heart	LDL HDL VLDL Total proteins
Liver Kidney	BUN Creatinine
Pancreas	Amylase Lipase Glucose
Heart	LD CPK
Male pelvis	PSA
Female pelvis Obstetrics	Estrogen (E1, E2, E3) hCG AFP
Thyroid gland Parathyroid gland	THS T_3 T_4

SUMMARY

This chapter highlighted the quality control measures in the laboratory and reviewed some of the laboratory values that are significant to sonography. Table 9-20 provides a reference for the laboratory tests associated with each organ. The values reviewed here are only part of the overall package presented to a physician for diagnosis. While high or low values may be indicative of a problem, the sonographic image may show the exact location and severity of an abnormal condition. Values and images working in conjunction with each other can lead to diagnosis and treatment, possibly eliminating invasive measures.

Imagine every patient is a book. Patients come with narrators for their story (themselves, family, or referring physicians). However, some patients may not have effective narration, increasing the likelihood of the physician missing important details. Laboratory values are like captions that help provide effective narration by giving details about symptoms a patient may or may not be able to verbalize. With knowledge of the appropriate laboratory values and whether they are within normal or abnormal range, the sonographer is guided on what area(s) to focus on to produce the most effective images most likely to aid in differential diagnoses.

CHAPTER 10

The Abdominal Aorta

MYKA BUSSEY-CAMPBELL AND REVA ARNEZ CURRY

OBJECTIVES

Describe the normal location, course, and size of the aorta.

Describe the layers (gross anatomy) of an artery.

Describe the location of the aortic branches and the organs supplied by those branches.

Discuss the function of the aorta.

Describe the sonographic appearance of the aorta and its branches.

Describe the associated laboratory values and diagnostic tests.

KEY WORDS

Angiotensin II — A hormone released in the event of bleeding to initiate vasoconstriction and help maintain blood pressure.

Aorta — A retroperitoneal, tubular structure coursing inferiorly from the heart, just to the left side of the spine, through the chest and abdomen until it bifurcates into the common iliac arteries. Along its course, the aorta gives off multiple branches that supply body structures with oxygen-rich blood.

Celiac Artery (CA) — Abdominal aorta anterior branch. Superior to and within centimeters of the superior mesenteric artery. Also known as the celiac trunk and celiac axis. Branches into the left gastric artery (LGA), splenic artery (SPA), and common hepatic artery (CHA).

Common Hepatic Artery (CHA) — Celiac artery branch. Courses horizontally to the right and branches into the gastroduodenal artery (GDA) and proper hepatic artery (PHA).

Common Iliac Arteries — Abdominal aorta division into right and left common iliac arteries. Supply the pelvis and lower extremities.

Gastroduodenal Artery (GDA) — Common hepatic artery branch. Courses inferiorly. Supplies the right side of the greater curvature of the stomach via the right gastroepiploic artery and the pancreatic duodenal area via the superior-anterior and superior-posterior pancreatic duodenal arteries.

Gonadal Arteries — Abdominal aorta anterior branches inferior to the renal arteries. Course inferiorly. Supply their respective organs.

Inferior Mesenteric Artery (IMA) — Abdominal aorta anterior branch. Inferior to the superior mesenteric and renal arteries. Courses anteroinferiorly, dividing into several other smaller arteries supplying the transverse colon, descending colon, and rectum.

Left Gastric Artery (LGA) — Celiac artery branch. Courses superior and left lateral. Supplies the left side of the lesser curvature of the stomach and eventually anastomoses with the right gastric artery.

Proper Hepatic Artery (PHA) — Common hepatic artery branch. Courses right lateral and superiorly. Supplies the liver via the right, middle, and left hepatic arteries.

Renal Arteries — Abdominal aorta bilateral branches located a few centimeters within the origin of the SMA. Course horizontally to each kidney.

Renin — Released from the kidneys in the event of bleeding. Acts on angiotensin II, which initiates vasoconstriction; thus blood pressure is maintained.

Splenic Artery (SPA) — Celiac artery branch. Courses horizontally to the left with a slight inferior-to-superior angulation. Supplies the spleen, pancreas, and left side of the greater curvature of the stomach.

Superior Mesenteric Artery (SMA) — Abdominal aorta anterior branch. Inferior to and within centimeters of the celiac artery. Courses anteroinferiorly. Divides into several arteries that supply the largest portion of the small intestine and the ascending colon and part of the transverse colon. The inferior-anterior pancreatic duodenal artery and the inferior-posterior pancreatic duodenal artery originate from the SMA and feed the pancreatic head and duodenal area.

Suprarenal Arteries — Abdominal aorta bilateral branches. Also known as the adrenal arteries. Course horizontally to each adrenal gland at a level between the CA and SMA.

■ ■ ■ **NORMAL MEASUREMENTS**

Anatomy	Measurement
Proximal abdominal aorta	2 cm
Distal abdominal aorta	1.5 cm
Common iliac arteries	0.8 and 1.0 cm

Although all body vessels are important, the aorta is especially vital because the blood flowing to the abdominal organs and lower extremities must pass through at least some part of this vessel to reach its destination. Because of the large volume of blood that it transports, the aorta is considered one of the two great vessels of the abdomen, the other being the inferior vena cava.

The arterial vascular system is complex. The sonographer should be well acquainted with its anatomy, physiology, sonographic appearance, and associated tests to ensure that the patient receives the highest quality of care.

LOCATION

The **aorta** is a retroperitoneal structure coursing in a superior-to-inferior direction along the left side of the spine (Table 10-1). This tubular structure originates from the heart at the left ventricular outflow tract and follows a candy cane–shaped loop down into the thoracic cavity. This portion, considered the thoracic aorta, is not visualized when an abdominal sonogram is performed. After the aorta passes posteriorly to the diaphragm at the aortic hiatus on the posterosuperior portion of the diaphragm, it is termed the *abdominal aorta* (AO). It continues to course inferiorly, giving off several branches, many of which can be visualized by sonography. The AO bifurcates into the common iliac arteries slightly left lateral to the spine, at the level of the umbilicus (Figure 10-1). It is posterior to the left lobe of the liver, body of the pancreas, pylorus of the stomach, splenic artery, splenic vein, and left renal vein. It is anterior to the psoas major muscle of the back.

The AO has many branches (Figures 10-2 and 10-3). There is considerable variation in the origin and course *Second Branch* of these vessels; therefore only the most common configurations will be discussed.

Directly after the aorta passes posteriorly to the diaphragm, the inferior phrenic arteries branch off the anterior-lateral aspect of the aorta and course superiorly to supply the underside of the diaphragm. At approximately the same level, the celiac trunk—also known as *First Branch of Aorta* the **celiac artery (CA)** and celiac axis—branches anteriorly from the aorta. The CA, often measuring less than 1 cm, further branches into the left gastric artery (LGA), *Third Branch* splenic artery (SPA), and common hepatic artery (CHA).

The CA and its branches are of extreme importance in supplying the majority of the abdominal organs, the stomach, and the duodenum.

- The **left gastric artery (LGA)** courses superiorly and to the left. It doubles back to supply the left side of the lesser curvature of the stomach and eventually anastomoses with the right gastric artery.
- The **splenic artery (SPA)** supplies the spleen, pancreas, and left side of the greater curvature of the stomach as it courses horizontally to the left with a slight inferior-to-superior angulation. The pancreas is supplied primarily via the main, dorsal, caudal, and great pancreatic arteries, which branch from the SPA. The left side of the greater curvature of the stomach is supplied by the left gastroepiploic artery, which branches from the distal end of the SPA.
- The **common hepatic artery (CHA)** pursues a horizontal course to the right and branches into the gastroduodenal artery (GDA) and proper hepatic artery (PHA).
  - The **gastroduodenal artery (GDA)** courses inferiorly, supplying the right side of the greater curvature of the stomach via the right gastroepiploic artery and the pancreatic duodenal area via the superior-anterior and superior-posterior pancreatic duodenal arteries.
  - The **proper hepatic artery (PHA)** courses right lateral and superiorly, supplying the liver via the right, middle, and left hepatic arteries. The cystic artery feeds the gallbladder after it branches from the right hepatic artery. The right gastric artery, which supplies the right side of the lesser curvature of the stomach, commonly originates from the PHA, GDA, or CHA.

The origin of the next most inferiorly located branch of the aorta varies. The **suprarenal arteries**, also termed the *adrenal arteries*, originate bilaterally from the lateral aspect of the aorta and course horizontally to the adrenal glands. These arteries commonly originate between the level of the CA and the level of the superior mesenteric artery (SMA), which is located a few centimeters inferior to the CA.

Moving inferiorly, the **superior mesenteric artery (SMA)** branches from the anterior aspect of the aorta within centimeters of the CA. The SMA continues an anterior-inferior course and divides into several arteries that supply the largest portion of the small intestine and the ascending colon and part of the transverse colon. In addition, the inferior-anterior pancreatic duodenal artery and the inferior-posterior pancreatic duodenal artery originate from the SMA and feed the pancreatic head and duodenal area.

Within a few centimeters of the origin of the SMA, the right and left **renal arteries** branch from the lateral aspect of the aorta. Both arteries course horizontally and

■ ■ ■ Table 10-1 Location of Abdominal Aorta and Branches Routinely Visualized With Ultrasound

	Aorta (can be tortuous)	Celiac Artery	Left Gastric Artery (very tortuous)	Splenic Artery (tortuous)
Anterior to	Spine, psoas major muscle	Aorta	Celiac artery, splenic artery, CHA	Celiac artery, pancreas tail, superior pole of lt kidney
Posterior to	Lt renal vein, SMA, splenic vein, pancreas body/tail, celiac artery, splenic artery, CHA, lt gastric artery, inferior duodenum, stomach, peritoneum, liver, diaphragm (proximal abdominal aorta)	Lt gastric artery, peritoneum, liver	Liver, peritoneum	Liver, lt gastric artery, stomach, peritoneum
Superior to		SMA, pancreas body, splenic vein	Celiac artery, splenic artery, SMA	Pancreas body, splenic vein, SMA
Inferior to	Diaphragm	Diaphragm, EGJ	Diaphragm, celiac artery, splenic artery, CHA	Diaphragm
Medial to	Splenic artery, lt renal artery, lt kidney, lt ureter, lt adrenal gland, pancreas tail, ascending duodenum, lt crus of diaphragm	Splenic artery, cardiac end of stomach		Spleen
Lt lateral to	Spine, IVC, rt renal artery, rt kidney, rt adrenal gland, rt crus of diaphragm, CHA, PHA, GDA	Liver caudate lobe, CHA	Celiac artery	Celiac artery, lt gastric artery, CHA, aorta
Rt lateral to			Celiac artery	

	Common Hepatic Artery	Proper Hepatic Artery	Gastroduodenal Artery	Superior Mesenteric Artery
Anterior to	Celiac artery, IVC	Portal vein	IVC, CBD, pancreas neck/head	Aorta, lt renal vein
Posterior to	Liver, lt gastric artery, peritoneum	Common duct, peritoneum	Liver, peritoneum	Splenic vein, pancreas body, liver, SMV, peritoneum
Superior to	Pancreas neck/head, SMA	GDA		Renal arteries, renal veins, common iliac arteries, common iliac veins
Inferior to		Rt & lt hepatic arteries, porta hepatis	PHA	Diaphragm, celiac, artery, splenic artery, lt gastric artery
Medial to	PHA, common duct, portal vein	Common duct, rt and lt hepatic arteries, porta hepatis, cystic duct	Duodenum	Splenic vein, pancreas tail, lt ureter
Lt lateral to				SMV, IMV, PSC, IVC
Rt lateral to	Celiac artery, splenic artery	CHA	CHA, SMA, SMV, splenic vein	

Continued

■ ■ ■ **Table 10-1** Location of Abdominal Aorta and Branches Routinely Visualized With Ultrasound—cont'd

	Rt Renal Artery	**Lt Renal Artery**	**Rt Common Iliac Artery**	**Lt Common Iliac Artery**
Anterior to	Rt crus of diaphragm	Lt crus of diaphragm	Rt common iliac vein, proximal IVC, spine	Lt common iliac vein, spine
Posterior to	IVC, rt renal vein, peritoneum, PSC, pancreas head/uncinate	Lt renal vein, peritoneum, pancreas tail, splenic vein	Peritoneum, small intestine, rt ureter	Peritoneum, small intestines, lt ureter
Superior to	Common iliac arteries, common iliac veins, rt ureter	Common iliac arteries, common iliac veins, lt ureter		
Inferior to	SMA, celiac artery, rt adrenal gland	SMA, celiac artery, lt adrenal gland, splenic artery	SMA, renal arteries and veins	SMA, renal arteries and veins
Medial to	Rt kidney	Lt kidney	Rt common iliac vein, proximal IVC, psoas major muscle	Psoas major muscle
Lt lateral to		Aorta, SMA		Lt common iliac vein, rt common iliac artery, rt common iliac vein
Rt lateral to	Aorta, SMA		Lt common iliac vein, lt common iliac artery	

CBD, common bile duct; **CHA,** common hepatic artery; **EGJ,** esophageal gastric junction; **GDA,** gastroduodenal artery; **IMV,** inferior mesenteric vein; **IVC,** inferior vena cava; **PHA,** proper hepatic artery; **PSC,** portal splenic confluence; **SMA,** superior mesenteric artery; **SMV,** superior mesenteric vein.

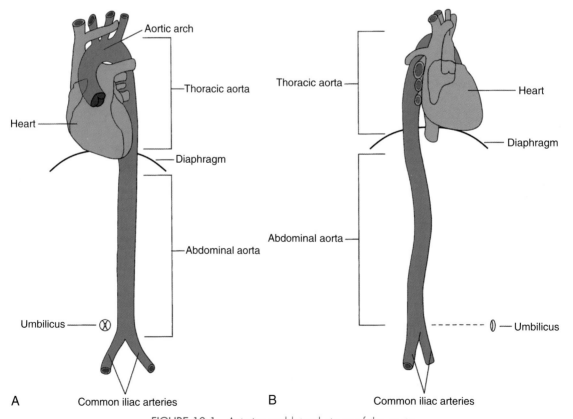

FIGURE 10-1 Anterior and lateral views of the aorta.

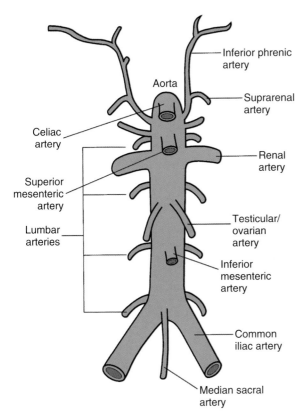

Celiac artery
Aorta
Inferior phrenic artery
Suprarenal artery
Renal artery
Superior mesenteric artery
Lumbar arteries
Testicular/ ovarian artery
Inferior mesenteric artery
Common iliac artery
Median sacral artery

FIGURE 10-2 Initial branches of the abdominal aorta.

supply the kidneys; however, the right renal artery (RRA) has a longer course than the left renal artery (LRA) because the aorta sits on the left side of the spine, which forces the RRA to travel a greater distance to reach the right kidney. In addition, it should be noted that the RRA normally courses posterior to the inferior vena cava (IVC) and anterior to the spine on its course to reach the right kidney.

Fourth branches Inferior to the SMA and renal arteries, the **gonadal arteries** originate from the anterior aspect of the aorta and course inferiorly to their respective organs. The left artery often originates slightly superiorly to the right artery. The male gonadal arteries are termed the *testicular arteries,* and the female gonadal arteries are termed the *ovarian arteries.*

The **inferior mesenteric artery (IMA)** is the next major artery that branches from the aorta. It originates from the anterior aspect of the aorta and pursues an antero-inferior course dividing into several other smaller arteries supplying the transverse colon, descending colon, and rectum.

The median sacral artery supplies the sacrum and is the most inferior branch of the aorta, followed by the aorta's bifurcation into the **common iliac arteries**, which along with their branches supply the pelvis and lower extremities. Also note that the lumbar arteries originate

bilaterally from the lateral aspect of the aorta throughout the entire length of the aorta (see Figure 10-2).

SIZE

Although the size of the normal abdominal aorta varies depending on body habitus, it is accepted that the average anteroposterior diameter is 2 cm at the most superior portion of the adult abdomen. Coursing inferiorly, it decreases in size with an average measurement of 1.5 cm at its bifurcation into the common iliac arteries. The abdominal portion of the aorta is approximately 14 cm long, beginning at the aortic hiatus (an opening in the diaphragm at approximately the twelfth thoracic vertebra), and extending inferiorly to the fourth lumbar vertebra. The aorta then bifurcates into the common iliac arteries, which vary in diameter between 0.8 cm and 1.0 cm.

The abdominal aorta should not exceed 3 cm at any level. It has been suggested that the best method to decrease observer variation when measuring the aorta is to take the anteroposterior measurement in a longitudinal section, as opposed to an axial section. To ensure consistent results, always be diligent in the technique used to measure this vessel.

GROSS ANATOMY

The aorta, like other vessels, has three layers: *tunica intima, tunica media,* and *tunica adventitia.* Their thickness varies, as seen in Figure 10-4. Arteries often have a thicker tunica media to allow for greater elasticity.

PHYSIOLOGY

The primary function of the aorta and its branches is to channel blood to organs and tissues to ensure oxygenation and metabolism. Although other functions such as blood pressure maintenance and assisting in the control of bleeding are primarily the responsibility of the arteriole-capillary system, the aorta does participate in these functions as well. The venous system is capable of maintaining blood pressure through its valves; however, valves are not present in the arterial system. Thus the aorta and large arteries use a different mechanism to maintain blood flow during diastole. As the ventricles contract during systole, blood is quickly sent into the aorta, forcing the expansion of the vessel wall. As a result, potential energy is stored in the vessel wall. When the aortic valve in the heart closes and diastole ensues, the arterial wall recoils to release the stored potential energy. The wall recoil forces blood to continue its forward movement; thus the blood pressure is maintained.

In addition, multiple nerve and chemical receptors are present throughout the arterial system that responds to various stimuli. The many local and systemic chemical and neurologic events can cause vasoconstriction or

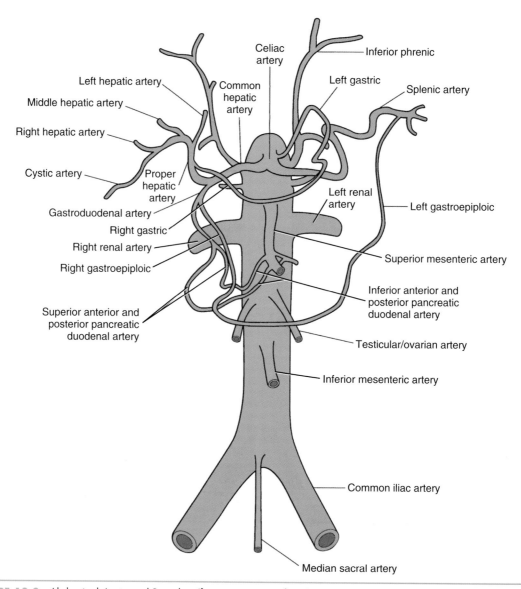

■ ■ ■ **FIGURE 10-3** Abdominal Aorta and Branches (from superior to inferior)

Vessel	Location
Abdominal aorta (AO)	Left lateral to the spinal column Posterior to the left lobe of the liver, body of the pancreas, pylorus of the stomach, splenic artery, splenic vein, and left renal vein
Celiac artery (CA)	Arises anteriorly from the aorta approximately at the same level of the inferior phrenic arteries Branches into LGA, SPA, and CHA
Left gastric artery (LGA)	Branch of the CA Courses superiorly to the left and then back toward the right to eventually anastomose with the right gastric artery Supplies the left side of the lesser curvature of the stomach
Splenic artery (SPA)	Branch of the CA Courses to the left to supply the spleen Branches into the left gastroepiploic artery to supply the greater curvature of the stomach
Common hepatic artery (CHA)	Branch of the CA Pursues a horizontal course to the right and branches into the proper hepatic artery and gastroduodenal artery
Proper hepatic artery (PHA)	Branch of the CHA Courses right lateral and superiorly, supplying the liver via the right, middle, and left hepatic arteries

Vessel	Location
Superior mesenteric artery (SMA)	Branches from the anterior aspect of the aorta and continues an anteroinferior course
	Branches into inferior-anterior and posterior pancreatic duodenal artery, which anastomose with the superior-anterior and posterior pancreatic duodenal artery
Suprarenal arteries	Originate bilaterally from the lateral aspect of the aorta
	Course horizontally to the adrenal glands
Renal arteries (RA)	Originate bilaterally from the lateral aspect of the aorta
	Course horizontally to the kidneys
	Right renal artery runs posterior to the inferior vena cava
Gonadal arteries	Arise inferior to the superior mesenteric artery and renal arteries
	Originate from the anterior aspect of the aorta and course inferiorly to their respective organs (testes or ovaries)
	Left gonadal artery originates slightly superior to the right gonadal artery
	Also called *testicular arteries* or *ovarian arteries*
Inferior mesenteric artery (IMA)	Arises inferiorly on the anterior aspect of the abdominal aorta
	Supplies the transverse colon, descending colon, and rectum
Median sacral artery	The most inferior branch of the aorta
	Supplies the sacrum
	Marks the level of the bifurcation of the aorta into right and left common iliac arteries
Common iliac arteries	Formed by the division of the distal portion of the aorta
	Supply the lower extremities

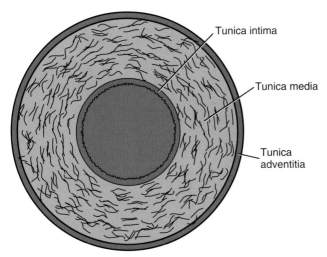

Tunica intima

Tunica media

Tunica adventitia

FIGURE 10-4 Cross-section of the arterial wall.

vasodilatation. For instance, **renin** is released from the kidney in the event of bleeding. Renin acts on **angiotensin II**, which initiates vasoconstriction; thus blood pressure is maintained through vasoconstriction. Further, chemical-humoral reactions allow for vasoconstriction of certain arterial segments, which can result in increased organ perfusion or heat dissipation. As is evident, the aorta and its branches play a critical role in homeostasis.

SONOGRAPHIC APPEARANCE

Arterial vasculature should normally display an anechoic lumen with bright, echogenic walls that clearly delineate it from adjacent structures. Larger vessels will often display significant pulsatility, which will assist in proper identification. In the sagittal or coronal scanning plane the aorta is seen as a longitudinal, tubular, highly pulsatile structure, slightly anterior and to the left of the spine. The proximal portion of the abdominal aorta often appears curvilinear as it courses posteroanteriorly after passing behind the diaphragm into the retroperitoneum. The aorta continues to run anteriorly until it bifurcates; however, this slight degree of posterior-to-anterior angulation results in the mid and distal portions displaying more of a linear configuration than the proximal portion (Figures 10-5 and 10-6). Note that the aorta is often tortuous; thus identification of a significant longitudinal portion can be difficult.

Although it is not always possible, one should attempt to identify the layers of the abdominal aorta to assist in excluding pathology. The tunica intima often appears as a bright echogenic line on the innermost portion of the vessel wall. The tunica media is believed to be represented by the echo-free area between the bright tunica intima and tunica adventitia. The tunica adventitia is the fibrous outermost section of the vessel that appears

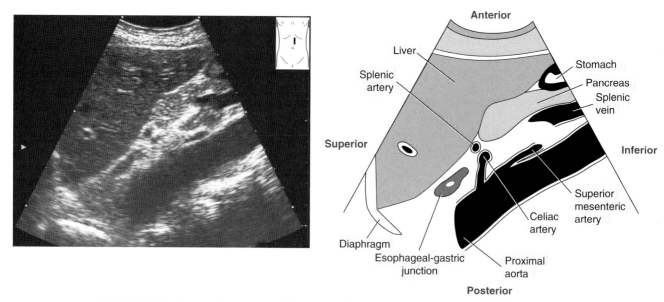

FIGURE 10-5   Longitudinal section of the proximal portion of the abdominal aorta in a sagittal scanning plane.

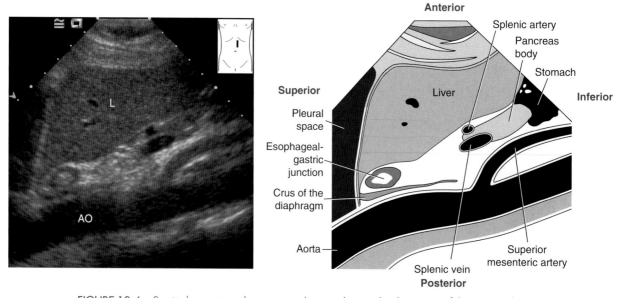

FIGURE 10-6   Sagittal scanning plane image showing longitudinal sections of the proximal aorta and superior mesenteric artery. Note the left lobe of the liver anteriorly. Also notice the body of the pancreas posterior to the left lobe and anterior to the superior mesenteric artery.

as a moderately bright line differentiating the vessel from other structures.

Even though the aorta has many branches, the branches demonstrated with reasonable consistency on ultrasound are the CA, SMA, renal arteries, and common iliac arteries. The CA is easily visualized at a level slightly superior to the body of the pancreas. In the transverse scanning plane the CA and its branches are recognizable by displaying the characteristic shape of a seagull (Figure 10-7). The longitudinal sections of the SPA and the CHA

represent the wings of the bird, and the short tubular section of the CA represents the body.

The SMA is also easy to identify. Longitudinally, the superior mesenteric artery appears as a linear structure branching anteriorly from the aorta slightly inferior to the CA (Figure 10-8). It runs inferiorly and parallel to the aorta. In axial sections the SMA is seen as a small, round, anechoic structure surrounded by bright, echogenic parapancreatic fat directly posterior to the splenic vein (Figures 10-9 and 10-10).

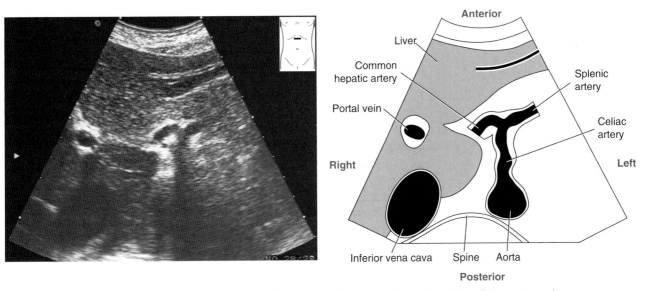

FIGURE 10-7 Transverse scanning plane image showing a short axis section of the aorta and longitudinal sections of the celiac artery, common hepatic artery, and splenic artery.

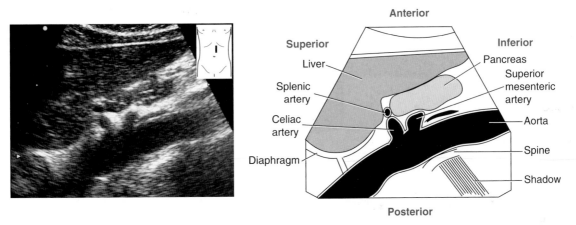

FIGURE 10-8 Sagittal scanning plane image of a longitudinal section of the mid aorta and its anterior branches, the celiac artery and superior mesenteric artery.

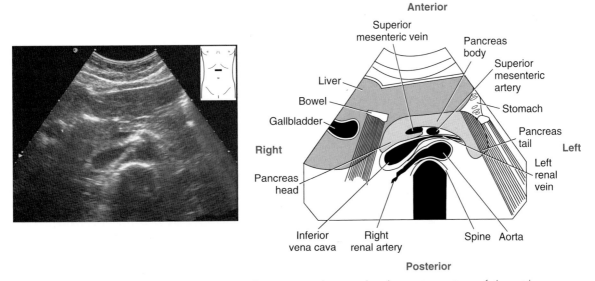

FIGURE 10-9 Transverse scanning plane image showing the short axis sections of the mid abdominal aorta and its superior mesenteric artery branch.

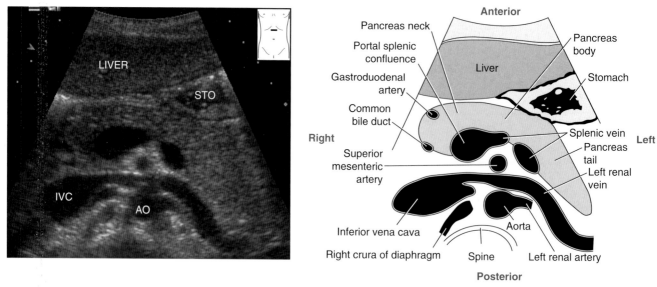

FIGURE 10-10 This transverse scanning plane image shows another axial section of the abdominal aorta (AO), as well as the superior mesenteric artery. Note how the superior mesenteric artery is anterior to the aorta and longitudinal section of the left renal vein. Directly anterior to the superior mesenteric artery, portions of the splenic vein can be seen forming a posterior border of the tail and body of the pancreas. The portal-splenic confluence can be seen anterior and slightly right lateral to the superior mesenteric artery.

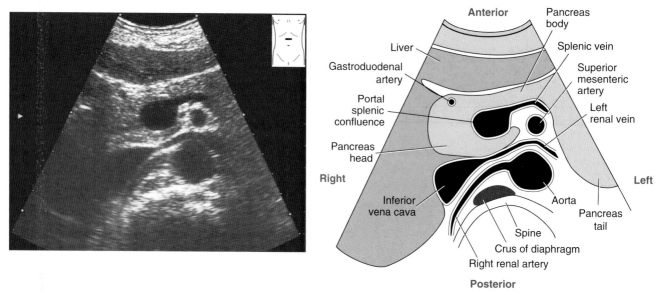

FIGURE 10-11 Transverse scanning plane image displaying short axis section of the mid aorta and longitudinal, curvilinear section of the right renal artery.

The renal arteries are usually most easily seen in the transverse scanning plane as small-diameter, curvilinear, longitudinal structures branching right and left laterally from the aorta and then running toward their respective kidney (Figure 10-11). Although the axial sections of the LRA can be challenging to identify, the axial RRA can usually be seen directly posterior to a longitudinal section of the IVC (Figure 10-12). The IMA is the next most inferiorly located vessel; however, it is not consistently demonstrated.

As was previously discussed, the aorta bifurcates into the common iliac arteries at about the level of the umbilicus or fourth lumbar vertebrae. Just before the bifurcation, the distal portion of the aorta narrows slightly (Figure 10-13).

The bifurcation is most easily demonstrated in the transverse scanning plane. One will see the single, axial, distal portion of the aorta divided into two separate axial vessels as the transducer is angled or moved inferiorly (Figures 10-14 and 10-15).

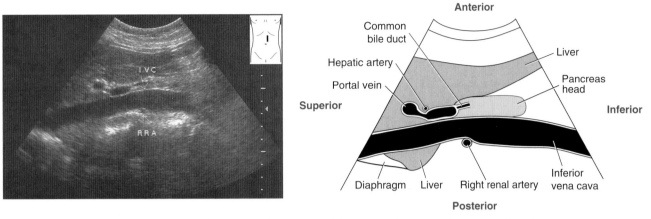

FIGURE 10-12 Sagittal scanning plane image delineating a longitudinal section of the inferior vena cava and short axis section of the right renal artery.

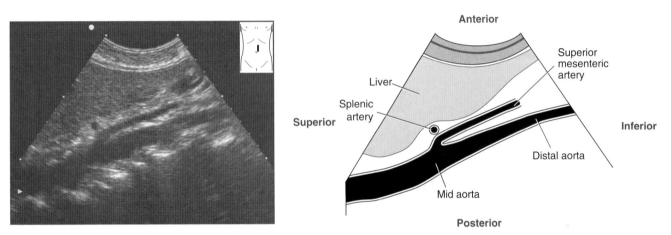

FIGURE 10-13 Longitudinal section of the distal aorta *(arrows)*. Note decrease in aortic diameter.

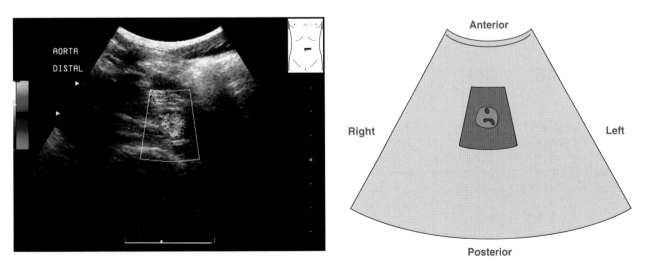

FIGURE 10-14 Color Doppler transverse scanning plane image showing an axial section of the distal aorta just before bifurcation into the common iliac arteries.

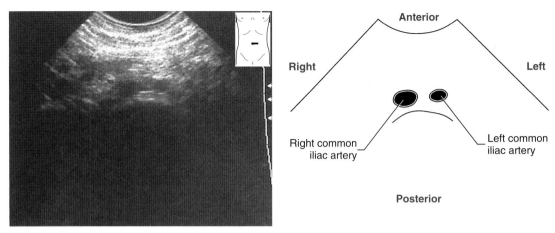

FIGURE 10-15 Transverse scanning plane image showing axial sections of the common iliac arteries just distal to the aortic bifurcation.

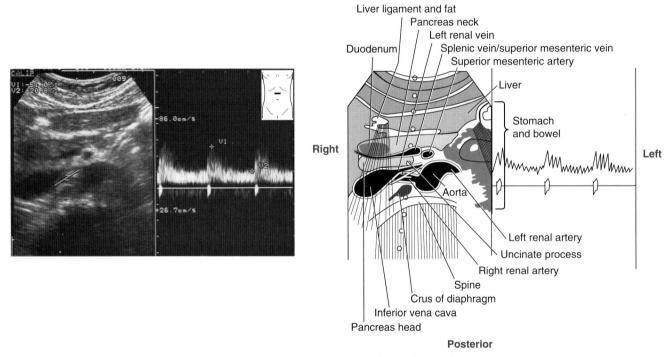

FIGURE 10-16 Normal right renal artery Doppler waveform. This is a low-resistance waveform (the diastolic flow is approximately one third of the peak systolic flow, indicating a low-resistance vascular bed).

Doppler assessment of the abdominal aorta and its branches is extremely useful in understanding systolic and diastolic flow. Normal waveforms are explained in the Common Diagnostic Tests chart at the end of this chapter (Figures 10-16 through 10-21).

SONOGRAPHIC APPLICATIONS
The aorta and its branches are primarily evaluated to detect aneurysms and stenosis; however, arterial grafts are routinely evaluated as well.

- Fusiform, saccular, and dissecting aneurysms can be readily identified.
- Stenosis of the CA, SMA, renal artery, and common iliac arteries can also be identified with the aid of Doppler sonography. Stenosis is often the causative factor in other disease states, such as bowel ischemia resulting from SMA stenosis or renovascular hypertension caused by renal artery stenosis.
- Grafts can be evaluated for patency and complications using Doppler sonography.

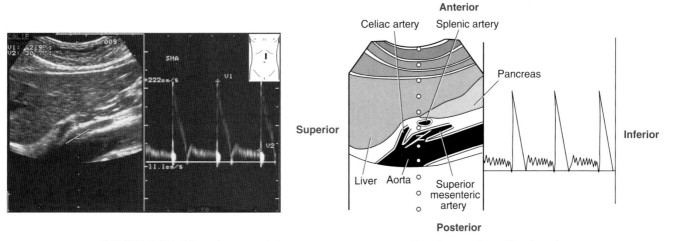

FIGURE 10-17 Normal preprandial superior mesenteric artery Doppler waveform. The diastolic flow, as compared with the low-resistance renal artery waveform, is much less in relation to the peak systolic flow. The preprandial superior mesenteric artery waveform is considered a high-resistance waveform.

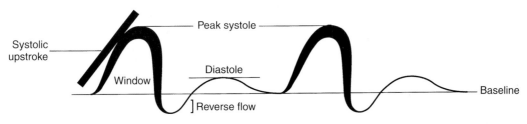

FIGURE 10-18 Doppler waveform throughout two cardiac cycles.

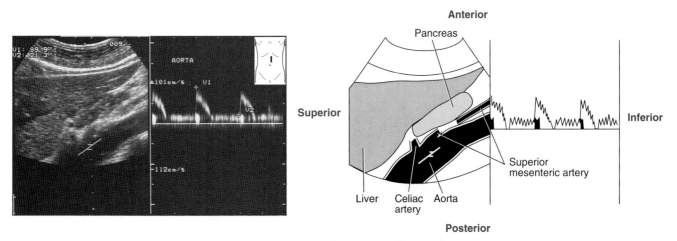

FIGURE 10-19 Normal aortic Doppler waveform.

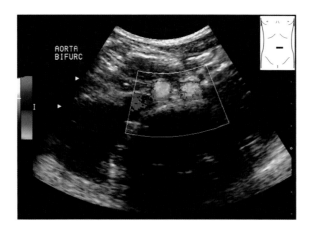
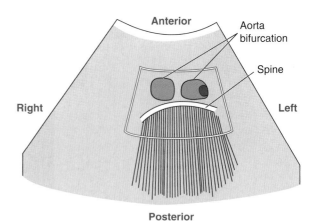

FIGURE 10-20   Color Doppler, transverse scanning plane sonogram demonstrating axial sections of the common iliac arteries.

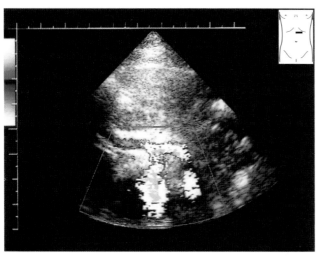
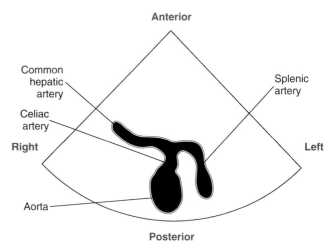

FIGURE 10-21   Color Doppler, transverse scanning plane sonogram demonstrating flow within the aorta, celiac artery, splenic artery, and common hepatic artery.

REFERENCE CHARTS

■ ■ ■   ASSOCIATED PHYSICIANS

Many physicians may be involved in care of the patient with a disorder of the aorta or its branches, depending on the organ(s) affected.

- **Interventional radiologist:** Specializes in identification, diagnosis, and endovascular treatment of vascular disorders.
- **Vascular surgeon:** Specializes in the surgical and endovascular treatment of vascular disorders.

■ ■ ■   COMMON DIAGNOSTIC TESTS

Diagnostic tests to evaluate the arterial system include duplex Doppler sonography, color-flow Doppler, plethysmography, segmental blood pressures, arteriography, computed tomography, and magnetic resonance imaging.

- **Duplex Doppler sonography:** Can indicate flow patterns within the vasculature; abnormalities indicate certain disease states such as stenosis and aneurysms. (This chapter includes only a limited discussion of Doppler sonography as an aid in evaluating the aorta and its branches.) The normal Doppler waveform may be a low-resistance waveform, a high-resistance waveform, or a combination waveform. A low-resistance waveform occurs when there is no reverse flow, and significant diastolic flow is present throughout the cardiac cycle. This is generally seen when the diastolic flow is approximately one third of the normal peak systolic flow. A low-resistance waveform should be present in arteries that feed low-resistance beds such as the brain, kidneys, and abdominal organs (see Figure 10-16). A normally high-resistance waveform will exhibit a sharp systolic upstroke along with reduced diastolic flow, and it may display reverse flow. High-resistance waveforms will be seen in the external carotid artery, extremities, and the preprandial SMA (see Figure 10-17). A combination waveform will show attributes of both low- and high-resistance waveforms. This type of waveform is seen in the common carotid artery and abdominal aorta (see Figure 10-19). In addition, most waveforms should not exhibit spectral broadening. Spectral broadening can be detected as excessive echoes within the window of the waveform. Various abnormalities within these waveforms such as increased peak systolic velocities, increased diastolic velocities, significant spectral broadening, flow reversal, and other findings assist in ascertaining the presence of pathology in the vessel or the organ supplied by the vessel. (It should be noted that this discussion does not explain Doppler sonography sufficiently to allow one to interpret Doppler waveforms.) A sonographer or vascular technologist performs this examination. A physician, usually a radiologist or vascular surgeon, interprets the study.

- **Color-flow Doppler (color imaging):** Often gives results similar to those of duplex sonography; however, its main use is to facilitate location of vessels for duplex sonography or to ascertain the presence and location of flow in a structure (see Figure 10-21). Recent improvements in equipment may soon allow for color imaging to be used much like duplex sonography. A sonographer or vascular technologist performs this examination. A physician, usually a radiologist or vascular surgeon, interprets the study.
- **Plethysmography and segmental blood pressure:** Although primarily used to evaluate vascular disease of the extremities, these tests can assist in determining the presence and extent of occlusive aortic disease. There are several types of plethysmographs; the function of each is to measure volume changes within an area. Thus one can ascertain the volume of blood and extent of arterial disease within that particular area. In addition, segmental blood pressures can be used in conjunction with plethysmography or separately to ascertain blood flow to an area. When compared with normal values, the pressure information can also indicate the presence or severity of disease. A sonographer or vascular technologist performs this examination. A vascular surgeon usually interprets the examination.
- **Arteriography:** Most often considered the gold standard when evaluating the aorta and its branches. In the arteriogram, dye is injected into the vessel supplying the target area and several radiographs are then taken. An interventional radiologist performs this examination, assisted by a radiologic technologist. The radiologist interprets the study.
- **Computed axial tomography (CT) scan:** Often used to evaluate the aorta, this examination consists of a series of sequential radiographs taken over the target area. The images are computer reconstructed in two or three dimensions, enabling excellent identification and differentiation of structures. Structures can be evaluated with or without the aid of contrast material. A radiologic technologist performs this examination, and a radiologist interprets it. CT and ultrasound measurements of the aorta and common iliac arteries in normal patients and those with aneurysms have been performed. One study showed that both CT and ultrasound introduce some variability when measuring diameters, with ultrasound

slightly underestimating the diameter in normal aortas and slightly overestimating the diameter in patients with aortic aneurysm. This can be addressed by comparing normal CT and ultrasound measurements against surgery and pathology findings and by reducing operator variability through established scanning protocols.
- **Spiral computed axial tomography (spiral CT):** An innovation of the traditional CT technique, spiral CT uses continuous radiation and continuous table movement for up to 100 seconds to produce a large volume of data resembling a spiral or helix instead of individual slices. These data can be obtained with a single breath hold, which is an advantage over traditional CT. The large volume of data that can be reconstructed to better depict lesions and abnormalities is another advantage of spiral CT. Spiral CT has provided improved imaging on aortic and common iliac artery aneurysms.
- **Magnetic resonance imaging (MRI):** MRI applications are rapidly increasing and now include the vascular area. MRI images are similar in format to those of CT scans. The resolution is often superior to CT. Another advantage is that the images are created using a magnetic field, not with ionizing radiation, as used in CT scanning. An MRI technologist or radiologic technologist performs this procedure, and a radiologist interprets the examination.

■ ■ ■ LABORATORY VALUES

Many laboratory values are based on the arterial system, most of which indicate the functioning of other organs.
- **Hematocrit** (the percentage of red blood cells to whole blood) is used to measure possible bleeding from the arterial system; measurement of red blood cells aids in this determination. An abnormal decrease in red blood cells may also point to bleeding. Levels of cholesterol and lipids may indicate the potential for pathology or suggest the current arterial disease state; however, they cannot directly measure either.

■ ■ ■ VASCULATURE

Abdominal aorta → inferior phrenic → celiac → superior mesenteric → renals → inferior mesenteric → gonadals → common iliacs
Celiac artery → left gastric → splenic → common hepatic
Common hepatic → proper hepatic → gastroduodenal
Proper hepatic → right hepatic → middle hepatic → left hepatic
Gastroduodenal → right gastroepiploic → superior-anterior and posterior pancreatic duodenal → inferior-anterior and posterior pancreatic duodenal

■ ■ ■ AFFECTING CHEMICALS

Nonapplicable

CHAPTER 11

The Inferior Vena Cava

MYKA BUSSEY-CAMPBELL AND REVA ARNEZ CURRY

OBJECTIVES

Discuss the normal location and course of the inferior vena cava (IVC).

Discuss the major tributaries that feed into the IVC, along with the organs that are emptied by the tributaries.

Discuss the function of the IVC.

Describe the sonographic appearance of the IVC and commonly visualized tributaries.

Describe associated diagnostic tests related to the IVC.

KEY WORDS

Common Iliac Veins (Right and Left) — Bilateral veins that empty the lower extremities and pelvis and converge at approximately the level of the umbilicus to form the inferior vena cava.

Gonadal Veins (Right and Left) — Bilateral veins that empty either the testes or ovaries. Superior to the lumbar veins, the right gonadal vein courses parallel to the IVC and empties into its anterolateral aspect of the IVC; the left gonadal vein courses parallel and lateral to the IVC and empties into the left renal vein.

Hepatic Veins (Right, Middle, Left) — Normally, three hepatic veins meet at the superior aspect of the liver and empty into the anterior aspect of the IVC. Generally, the right hepatic vein empties the right lobe of the liver, the middle hepatic vein empties the caudate lobe, and the left hepatic vein empties the left lobe of the liver.

Inferior Phrenic Veins — Veins that bilaterally drain the diaphragm and empty into the lateral aspect of the IVC; they course in a superior-to-inferior direction.

Inferior Vena Cava (IVC) — A retroperitoneal, tubular structure coursing superiorly from the convergence of the common iliac veins in the lower abdomen, just to the right of the spine, through the abdomen and chest until it reaches the right atrium of the heart. Along its course, it receives multiple tributaries filled with deoxygenated blood from body structures.

IVC Sections (Hepatic, Prerenal, Renal, Postrenal) — The hepatic section is located directly posterior to the liver, where the hepatic veins empty into the IVC. The prerenal section extends from just inferior to the hepatic veins to slightly superior to the renal veins. The renal section includes the renal veins and multiple tributaries. This section terminates almost immediately after the branching of the renal veins. The postrenal section extends from just inferior to the renal veins to the convergence of the common iliac veins.

Lumbar Veins — Veins that bilaterally empty the posterior abdominal wall into the lateral aspect of the IVC, just superior to the convergence of the common iliac veins. There can be multiple pairs up to the level of the renal veins.

Renal Veins (Right and Left) — Veins that bilaterally empty the kidneys into the lateral aspect of the IVC. The right renal vein generally empties only the right kidney but sometimes assists the right adrenal gland via the right suprarenal vein. The left renal vein empties the left kidney and is subject to more tributaries than the right renal vein, such as the left gonadal vein, left suprarenal vein, and many smaller tributaries.

Suprarenal Veins (Right and Left) — Veins that bilaterally empty the adrenal glands. The left suprarenal vein follows a course similar to that of the left renal vein, into which it eventually empties. When the right suprarenal vein does not empty into the right renal vein, it empties directly into the IVC at a level slightly superior to the right renal vein.

■ ■ ■ NORMAL MEASUREMENTS	
Anatomy	**Measurement**
Common iliac veins	1.6 to 1.8 cm diameter
Right common iliac vein	5.5 cm long
Left common iliac vein	7.5 cm long
Inferior vena cava	2.5 cm diameter

The inferior vena cava (IVC) is one of the two great abdominal vessels; the other being the aorta. The abdominal organs all have tributaries that empty deoxygenated blood into the IVC; thus a sonographer must have a full understanding of this vasculature to adequately evaluate the abdomen during a sonographic examination and ensure that each patient receives the best possible care.

LOCATION

Joining

The IVC is formed by the convergence of the common iliac veins, which empty the lower extremities and pelvis (Table 11-1). The IVC continues to course superiorly through the retroperitoneum along the anterior, right lateral aspect of the spine and to the right of the aorta. It then travels through the diaphragm and empties into the right atrium of the heart. It is important to note that the IVC can have many possible congenital variations, including double IVC, IVC located on the left, absence of certain portions of the IVC, or a combination of these. These variations are possible because of the complex embryologic development of the IVC, as discussed in Chapter 8.

Many tributaries, including the lumbar veins, right gonadal vein, renal veins, and hepatic veins, will empty into the IVC as it continues its superior course and pierces the diaphragm at the caval hiatus to enter the right atrium of the heart. The IVC is located posterior to the intestines and the body of the liver. It is medial to the right kidney. The IVC is located more posteriorly as it courses superiorly.

The IVC is considered to have four sections (Figure 11-1). Beginning superiorly, the **hepatic section** is located directly posterior to the liver, where the hepatic veins empty into the IVC. The next section is termed the **prerenal section**. It extends from just inferior to the hepatic veins to slightly superior to the renal veins. The **renal section** is the next most inferiorly located area of the IVC. The renal veins and multiple tributaries are located within this section, which terminates almost immediately after the branching of the renal veins. The final section is the **postrenal section**, which extends from just inferior to the renal veins until the common iliac veins converge into the IVC.

The IVC has many tributaries; however, several contain multiple configurations that are not suitable for sonographic evaluation. Thus only major tributaries will be discussed here (Figure 11-2). As previously mentioned, the IVC is formed from the convergence of the **right and left common iliac vein** tributaries, which empty the lower extremities and pelvis at approximately the level of the umbilicus. The **lumbar veins**, which empty into the lateral aspect of the IVC, are the next most

■ ■ ■   **Table 11-1**   Location of Inferior Vena Cava and Tributaries Routinely Visualized With Ultrasound

	Inferior Vena Cava	Hepatic Veins	Rt Renal Vein	Lt Renal Vein	Rt Common Iliac Vein	Lt Common Iliac Vein
Anterior to	Spine, rt crus of diaphragm, rt psoas major muscle, rt renal artery, rt adrenal gland	IVC	Quadratus lumborum muscle, rt renal artery	Aorta, lt renal artery	Psoas major muscle	Psoas major muscle
Posterior to	Pancreas head/uncinate process, transverse duodenum, portal vein, CBD, posterior surface of liver, hepatic veins		Pancreas head	Pancreas body/tail	Rt common iliac artery	Lt common iliac artery
Superior to		Renal veins	Common iliac veins	Common iliac veins		
Inferior to	Diaphragm	Diaphragm	SMA, rt adrenal gland	SMA, lt adrenal gland	Renal veins	Renal veins
Medial to	Rt renal vein, rt kidney, rt ureter, rt adrenal gland		Rt kidney	Lt kidney		Lt common iliac artery
Lt lateral to				IVC		Rt common iliac vein and artery
Rt lateral to	Lt renal vein, aorta, caudate lobe of liver		IVC		Lt common iliac vein and artery, rt common iliac artery	

IVC, Inferior vena cava; **SMA,** superior mesenteric artery.

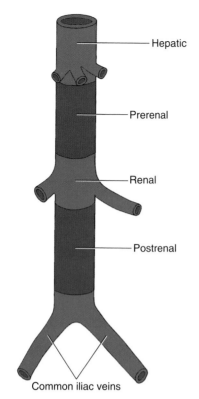

FIGURE 11-1 Sections of the inferior vena cava.

inferior tributaries. These horizontally coursing veins empty the posterior abdominal wall and are located bilaterally. In addition, there is usually more than one pair that continues emptying into the IVC up to the level of the renal veins.

Moving superiorly, the **right gonadal vein**, which courses parallel to the IVC, empties into the anterior lateral aspect of the IVC. Within a few centimeters superiorly, the renal veins also empty into the IVC. Although the **right renal vein** generally empties only the right kidney, it sometimes assists the right adrenal gland via the right suprarenal vein. The **left renal vein** is normally much longer than the right renal vein as it runs from the left kidney to the IVC. It courses posteriorly to a portion of the splenic vein and pancreas tail and between the aorta and SMA, making it subject to more tributaries than the shorter right renal vein. The **left gonadal vein** follows a course parallel and lateral to the IVC and empties into the left renal vein. In addition, the **left suprarenal vein** follows a course similar to that of the left renal vein, into which it eventually empties. Many smaller tributaries may also drain into the left renal vein. When the **right suprarenal vein** does not empty into the right renal vein, it empties directly into the IVC at a level slightly superior to the right renal vein.

The next major IVC tributaries are the hepatic veins. There are most commonly three hepatic veins, which course from the inferior aspect, deep within the liver, to the superior aspect of the liver, where they empty into the IVC. Generally, the **right hepatic vein** empties the right lobe of the liver, the **middle hepatic vein** empties the caudate lobe, and the **left hepatic vein** empties the left lobe of the liver.

The most superior tributaries of the IVC are the **inferior phrenic veins**, which course in a superior-to-inferior direction, draining the diaphragm and emptying into the lateral aspect of the IVC. One should note that several vein locations are parallel to the locations of their sister arteries.

SIZE

The IVC is formed by the union of the left and right common iliac veins, which measure 1.6 to 1.8 cm in diameter. The common iliac veins join to the right of the spine, which means that the left common iliac vein will be slightly longer than the right common iliac vein, at 7.5 cm and 5.5 cm, respectively. The diameter of the IVC is approximately 2.5 cm. The diameter will increase during a Valsalva maneuver or inspiration and commonly decrease during expiration. Asking the patient to "sniff" will cause the IVC to momentarily collapse. Although it will vary with respiration, the IVC should not exceed 3.7 cm.

GROSS ANATOMY

In general, venous walls are thinner because their tunica media is thin compared with that of the arterial system. A highly tensile vessel is not needed because the venous network is a low-pressure system.

PHYSIOLOGY

The IVC and its associated tributaries have the primary function of returning deoxygenated blood to the heart. Because the pressure on the venous side of the circulatory system is low compared with the arterial side, venous circulation contains valves, which prevent backflow of blood during diastole.

The momentum of the blood during systole forces the valves open. Once the momentum decreases and the blood is not pushed forward, the valve closes and prevents retrograde flow. In various diseases, the valves may not function, and this will cause retrograde blood flow. Blood is also moved forward by a decrease in thoracic pressure, which pulls the blood into the right atrium. In this case the IVC simply acts as a transportation vehicle.

SONOGRAPHIC APPEARANCE

Venous vasculature should normally display an anechoic lumen with thin, bright, echogenic walls. During real-time examination, the sonographer will note that the IVC displays significant variation in diameter compared with arterial vasculature. Additionally, small moving echoes are often noticed within the lumen of the IVC.

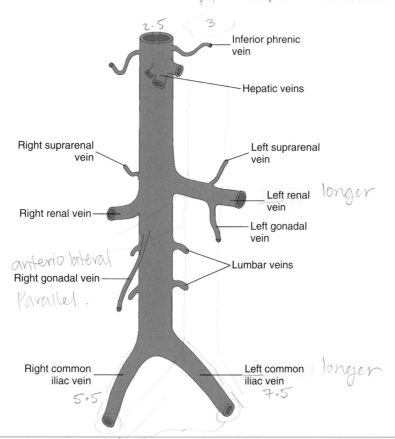

Handwritten annotations: AO · 2.5 · 3 · longer · anterio lateral · Parallel · 5.5 · 7.5 · longer · 1.6 – 1.8

■ ■ ■ **FIGURE 11-2** IVC and Major Tributaries

Vein(s)	Location
Common iliac veins	• Iliac veins drain the lower extremities and pelvis at the approximate level of the umbilicus.
Inferior vena cava	• The IVC is formed by the convergence of the common iliac veins. • It continues to course superiorly through the retroperitoneum along the anterolateral aspect of the spine and to the right of the aorta. Vessels that drain into the IVC are listed in order below, from inferior to superior.
Lumbar veins	• Lumbar veins drain into the IVC along most of its course. • Both right and left lumbar veins empty into the lateral aspect of the IVC. • Both right and left veins course horizontally and empty the posterior abdominal wall.
Gonadal veins (right and left)	• The right gonadal vein follows a course parallel to the IVC and empties into the lateral aspect of the IVC. • The left gonadal vein courses parallel and laterally to the IVC and empties into the left renal vein.
Renal veins	• The left renal vein passes anteriorly to the aorta and posteriorly to the superior mesenteric artery as it courses from the left kidney.
Suprarenal veins (right and left)	• The right suprarenal vein often empties into the IVC slightly superior to the right renal vein. • The left suprarenal vein follows a course similar to the left renal vein, into which it eventually empties.
Hepatic veins (right, middle, and left)	• All branches course from the inferior aspect, deep within the liver, to the superior aspect of the liver where they empty into the IVC. • The right hepatic vein empties the right lobe of the liver. • The middle hepatic vein empties the caudate lobe. • The left hepatic vein empties the left lobe of the liver.

The reason for these echoes has been debated; however, it is agreed that they are related to the flow of blood within the vessel.

In a sagittal scanning plane in the epigastric area, the hepatic section of the IVC can be seen as a longitudinal, tubular, elastic structure located directly posterior to the liver (Figure 11-3).

In some instances the IVC may appear to be coursing through the liver parenchyma, especially in the most superior section of the liver. The hepatic veins can often be seen at this level as anechoic, linear structures, with nondescript walls, originating in the liver and emptying into the IVC (Figures 11-4 to 11-6).

As seen in Figure 11-7, *A*, hepatic veins increase in diameter as they approach the IVC. In this transverse scanning plane image the hepatic veins appear as anechoic linear structures, whose walls are not obvious, emptying into the IVC. One often notices a characteristic "bunny ear" or "reindeer sign" pattern, also seen in this image. Figure 11-7, *B*, shows a color Doppler image of the hepatic veins emptying into the IVC.

Moving inferiorly, the renal veins are the next IVC tributaries consistently recognized with ultrasound. In a transverse scanning plane image the left renal vein is seen longitudinally as a curvilinear structure emptying into the medial aspect of the IVC as it follows a course

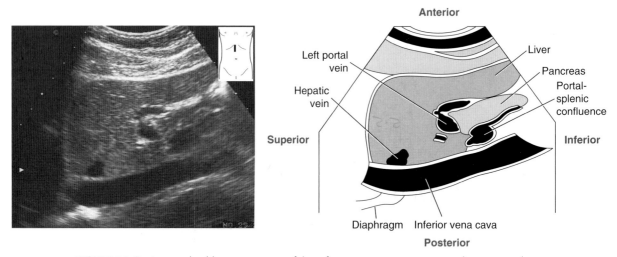

FIGURE 11-3 Longitudinal hepatic section of the inferior vena cava in a sagittal scanning plane image.

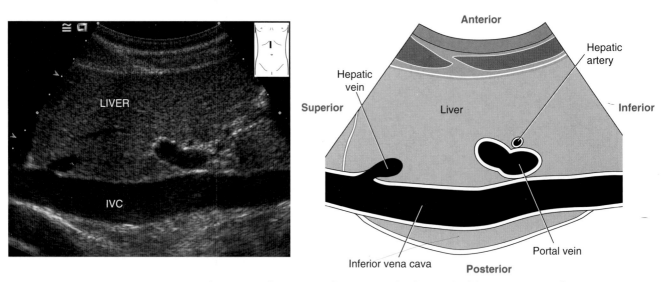

FIGURE 11-4 Sagittal scanning plane image showing another longitudinal hepatic section of the IVC coursing posteriorly to the liver.

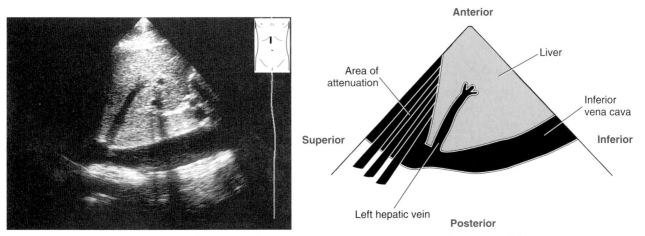

FIGURE 11-5   Sagittal scanning plane image demonstrating a longitudinal section of left hepatic vein emptying into the IVC.

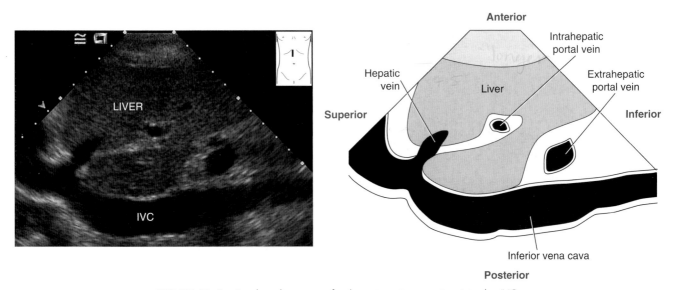

FIGURE 11-6   Another depiction of a hepatic vein emptying into the IVC.

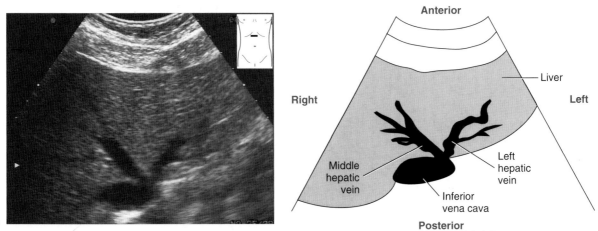

FIGURE 11-7   **A,** Axial section of the liver showing the middle hepatic vein and left hepatic vein emptying into the IVC.   *Continued*

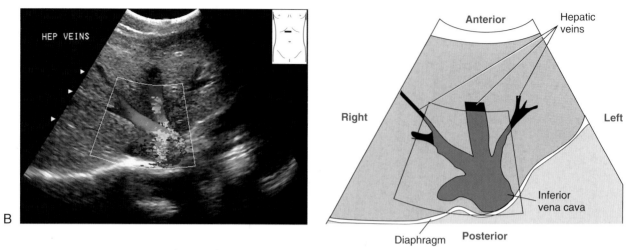

FIGURE 11-7, cont'd **B,** Color image demonstrating the hepatic veins emptying into the IVC.

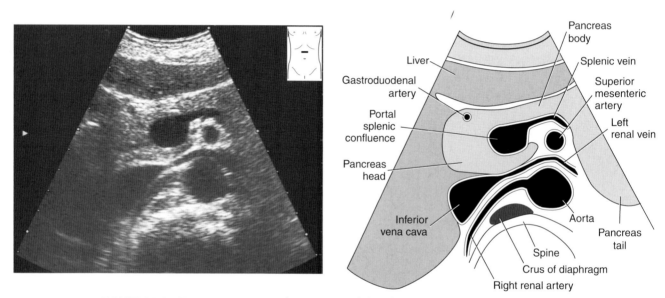

FIGURE 11-8 Transverse scanning plane section of the abdominal vasculature demonstrating axial sections of the IVC, aorta, and superior mesenteric artery, along with the longitudinal, curvilinear section of the left renal vein following a coursing posterior to the superior mesenteric artery and anterior to the aorta. Note the longitudinal section of the right renal artery.

anterior to the aorta and posterior to the superior mesenteric artery from its origin in the left kidney (Figure 11-8).

The right renal vein can also be seen as a longitudinal, curvilinear structure emptying into the lateral aspect of the IVC at this level (Figure 11-9). The gonadal vein and lumbar veins are not consistently imaged. However, the common iliac veins are most easily visualized in the transverse scanning plane at approximately the level of the umbilicus immediately before they converge to form the IVC.

SONOGRAPHIC APPLICATIONS

The IVC and its visible branches are primarily evaluated sonographically to detect intraluminal thrombosis and tumor invasion. The venous system can be evaluated by various diagnostic modalities. However, sonography is continually increasing in diagnostic accuracy and acceptance by medical professionals as the study of choice.

- Thrombosis may be the result of numerous causes.
- Tumor invasion most commonly occurs in the renal veins and often extends into the IVC.

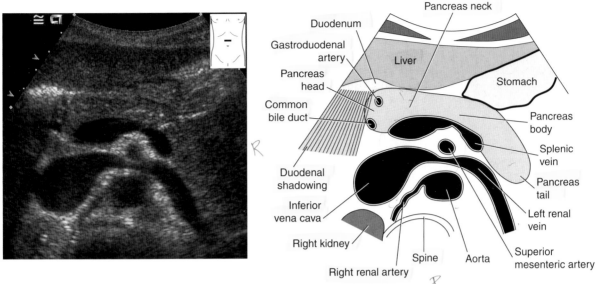

FIGURE 11-9 An axial section of the IVC is clearly shown in this transverse scanning plane image. Note the longitudinal section of the left renal vein entering the medial aspect of the IVC. Anterior and medial to the IVC is an axial section of the SMA. Anterior to the SMA is a longitudinal section of the splenic vein. The most posterior vessel in this image is an axial section of the aorta, from which the longitudinal, curvilinear section of the right renal artery can be seen coursing its way to the right kidney.

NORMAL VARIANTS

Because of its complex formation, the IVC can have many variations, such as the following:
- Double IVC
- Left-positioned IVC
- Absence of a portion of the IVC (rare)

REFERENCE CHARTS

■ ■ ■ ASSOCIATED PHYSICIANS

Generally, vascular surgeons treat the patient whose disorder involves the venous system. However, other physicians are often involved depending on the other organs or organ systems involved. In addition, internists—internal medicine practitioners—often render care to patients who do not require surgery.
- **Interventional radiologist:** Specializes in identification, diagnosis, and endovascular treatment of vascular disorders.
- **Vascular surgeon:** Specializes in the surgical and endovascular treatment of vascular disorders.

■ ■ ■ COMMON DIAGNOSTIC TESTS

The following diagnostic tests are commonly used to evaluate the venous system: duplex Doppler sonography, color Doppler, continuous-wave Doppler sonography, impedance flow plethysmography, venography, computed tomography, and magnetic resonance imaging.

- **Duplex Doppler sonography:** Although veins of the extremities can be evaluated with B-mode imaging and compression, one also needs to assess the flow dynamics of the area. Thus duplex Doppler is necessary to ensure an adequate examination. A normal venous flow pattern should be spontaneous and phasic (changes with respiration). Proximal compression and distal augmentation are also used to assess venous flow. Abnormalities often suggest disease. The abdominal venous system displays characteristic Doppler waveforms (Figure 11-10). A sonographer or vascular technologist performs this examination. A physician, usually a radiologist or a vascular surgeon, interprets the findings.
- **Color-flow Doppler:** Color Doppler can often assist in determining flow characteristics in the abdomen and extremities by quickly identifying flow and turbulence. Continuous-wave Doppler is also helpful in determining the status of extremity veins. The Doppler signal is amplified by a loudspeaker, which allows the examiner to hear an audible signal. Abnormalities in this signal indicate disease. A sonographer or vascular technologist performs this examination. A physician, usually a radiologist or a vascular surgeon, interprets the findings.
- **Impedance flow plethysmography:** Impedance flow plethysmography is the technique of measuring the blood volume change of an area. Strain gauge plethysmography is generally used when evaluating veins. Bilateral inflatable cuffs are placed on the proximal portion of the extremities, along with gauges that measure change in extremity size. As the cuffs are inflated, the flow of blood toward the heart is stopped

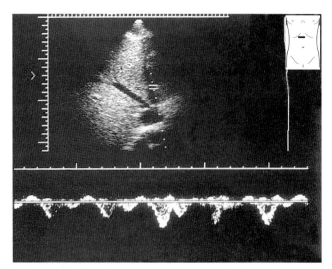

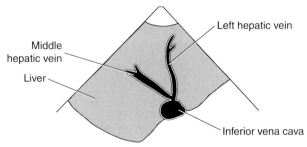

FIGURE 11-10 Axial section of the liver demonstrating a normal spontaneous and phasic Doppler pattern from the left hepatic vein.

and blood accumulates distal to the cuff, causing the extremity to increase in size. Next, the cuffs are deflated, allowing the blood to rush from the extremity back toward the heart. The strain gauge presents a readout of this rate of volume change. The results between extremities are compared as well to established normals. If the flow of blood toward the heart is abnormally slow, some type of blockage should be considered; this test should be done in conjunction with B-mode imaging, continuous-wave sonography, and/or duplex sonography to ensure accuracy. A sonographer or vascular technologist performs this examination. A physician, usually a radiologist or a vascular surgeon, interprets the findings.

- **Venography:** Venography is considered by many the gold standard when detecting venous disease. Dye (contrast material) is injected into the target vein, and serial radiographs are taken. Defects in filling indicate the presence of disease. This is a highly invasive test, and reactions to the injected dye are of great concern. This procedure is performed by a radiologist, assisted by a radiologic technologist. The radiologist interprets this examination.
- **Computed axial tomography (CT) scan:** CT is sometimes done to evaluate the abdominal venous system; however, it is rarely used to determine the disease state of extremities. This examination consists of a series of sequential radiographs, which are computer-reconstructed to identify various structures. A radiologic technologist performs this examination, and a radiologist interprets the findings.
- **Magnetic resonance imaging (MRI):** MRI is infrequently called on to evaluate the venous system. Furthermore, it

is not used to assess the extremity veins. The images are similar in format to those of CT; however, the images are generated using a strong magnetic field instead of radiation, as in CT. An MRI technologist or radiologic technologist performs this examination and a radiologist interprets the examination.

■ ■ ■ LABORATORY VALUES

Almost all blood laboratory values are taken from the venous system; however, the majority of examinations indicate the status of other organs or body systems. As with the arterial system, the percentage of red blood cells to whole blood (hematocrit) indicates possible bleeding from the venous system.

■ ■ ■ VASCULATURE

INFERIOR TO SUPERIOR
Iliac veins → IVC
Lumbar veins → IVC
Gonadal veins → IVC
Renal veins → IVC
Hepatic veins → IVC
Inferior phrenic veins → IVC

■ ■ ■ AFFECTING CHEMICALS

Nonapplicable

CHAPTER 12
The Portal Venous System

MYKA BUSSEY-CAMPBELL, REVA ARNEZ CURRY, AND BETTY BATES TEMPKIN

OBJECTIVES

Discuss the normal location, course, and size of the portal vein.

Discuss the normal location of the portal vein tributaries.

Describe the function of the portal venous system.

Describe the sonographic appearance of the portal vein and its tributaries.

Discuss associated diagnostic tests.

KEY WORDS

Hilum — Indentation, depression, or pit on an organ forming a doorway or area of entrance and exit for vessels, ducts, and nerves; also called *hilus.*

Intrahepatic — Completely enclosed by liver tissue.

Left Portal Vein — The left branch of the main portal vein. Courses to the left and branches into medial and lateral subdivisions that give off multiple subdivisions.

Main Portal Vein — Formed by the union of the splenic vein and superior mesenteric vein posterior to the neck of the pancreas. Along with its tributaries, it delivers blood from the spleen and gastrointestinal tract

(esophagus, stomach, and small and large intestines) to the liver for metabolism and detoxification. Divides into the right and left branches.

Portal Triad — Composed of hepatic arteries and bile ducts that run alongside portal veins in triads surrounded by a sheath of connective tissue. The triads radiate throughout the liver.

Right Portal Vein — The right branch of the main portal vein. Courses to the right and branches into anterior and posterior subdivisions that give off multiple subdivisions.

Splenic Vein — Drains the spleen and courses from lateral to medial directly posterior to the tail, body, and neck of the pancreas, where it unites with the superior mesenteric vein to form the portal vein.

Superior Mesenteric Vein — Courses from inferior to superior and drains the small intestine and portions of the large intestine via several smaller branches. Unites with the splenic vein posterior to the neck of the pancreas to form the portal vein.

■■■ NORMAL MEASUREMENTS

Anatomy	Measurement
Portal vein	5 to 6 cm long/mean length 8.3 cm
	13-mm diameter/mean diameter 11.6 cm
	1.45-mm mean diameter/preprandial
	1.48-mm mean diameter/postprandial

The portal system is unique because it carries blood and nutrients from the bowel and abdominal organs to the liver for metabolism and detoxification. This system includes all veins that drain blood from the spleen, pancreas, gallbladder, and gastrointestinal tract, with the exception of the lower rectum. The blood is then delivered to the liver by the portal vein. Disruption to the flow can cause multiple adverse effects.

Abnormalities that affect other organs are often the reason for portal vein pathology. Therefore it is imperative that the sonographer understand the many factors associated with the portal system and have a good awareness of its interdependence with other body systems to ensure that the patient receives the highest quality sonographic examination possible.

LOCATION

The **main portal vein** is formed by the confluence or junction of the splenic vein and the superior mesenteric vein at the level of the second lumbar vertebra, directly posterior to the neck of the pancreas and anterior to the inferior vena cava (Table 12-1 and Figure 12-1). From here, the portal vein runs approximately 5 to 6 cm

■ ■ ■ **Table 12-1** Location of the Portal Venous System Routinely Visualized With Ultrasound

	Portal Vein	Splenic Vein	Superior Mesenteric Vein	Inferior Mesenteric Vein
Anterior to	IVC, pancreas uncinate process	Lt kidney, lt renal vein, lt renal artery, SMA, rt renal artery	Pancreas/inferior head/ uncinate process, IVC, rt ureter, inferior duodenum	Lt common iliac vessels, lt psoas major muscle
Posterior to	Pancreas neck, superior duodenum, CHA, PHA, common duct, peritoneum	Pancreas neck/body/ tail, peritoneum	Pancreas neck, peritoneum	Pancreas body, peritoneum
Superior to	Pancreas head, SMV, IMV, splenic vein	SMV, IMV		
Inferior to	Porta hepatis, rt portal vein branch, lt portal vein branch	Splenic artery, portal vein	Splenic vein, portal vein	Splenic vein, portal vein
Medial to	Cystic duct	Spleen, portal vein	Pancreas head, duodenum	SMV, portal vein, pancreas head
Lt lateral to		IVC, pancreas head		Splenic vein
Rt lateral to	SMV, IMV, splenic vein, pancreas head, aorta, celiac artery	SMA, aorta	IMV, splenic vein, SMA	

CHA, Common hepatic artery; IVC, inferior vena cava; PHA, proper hepatic artery; SMV, superior mesenteric vein.

superoposteriorly to the second portion of the duodenum and then ascends to the liver hilum (area of entrance and exit for the vessels, ducts, and nerves of the liver), where it divides into right and left branches that run alongside corresponding hepatic artery branches into the liver. Along this course to the liver, the portal vein runs posteriorly and between the common bile duct and hepatic artery, with the artery lying medial to the duct.

The left branch, the left portal vein, is longer and smaller than the right branch. It runs horizontally to the left and branches into medial and lateral subdivisions that send branches into the caudate lobe and then the left lobe of the liver. Along its course, it is posterior to the ligamentum teres (obliterated umbilical vein). The right branch of the main portal vein, the right portal vein, enters the right lobe of the liver and branches into anterior and posterior subdivisions that give off multiple subdivisions throughout the right lobe.

Portal vein tributaries include splenic, superior mesenteric, cystic, and pyloric. Other portal vein tributaries—the left and right gastric, pancreaticoduodenal, gastroepiploic, and inferior mesenteric—vary significantly in terms of where they enter the portal vein system. The splenic vein drains the spleen and courses from lateral to medial directly posterior to the pancreas. The superior mesenteric vein courses from inferior to superior and drains the small intestine and portions of the large intestine via several smaller branches. The inferior mesenteric vein also courses from inferior to superior as it drains the large intestine via several smaller branches. This vessel most often empties blood into the splenic vein; however, there is considerable variance regarding where the inferior mesenteric vein joins the portal system.

SIZE

The main portal vein is an intraabdominal structure normally measuring up to 13 mm in diameter, with a length of approximately 5 to 6 cm before it divides into right and left portal vein branches. One research study on 40 adult cadavers showed a mean vein length of 8.3 cm and a mean vein diameter of 11.6 mm. Another study in 48 adults showed a preprandial (before a meal) mean portal vein diameter of 1.45 cm (14.6 mm), which increased slightly to 1.48 cm postprandial (following a meal). A subset of this study group, adults 31–40 years of age, showed a mean vein diameter of 1.30 cm (13 mm).

GROSS ANATOMY

Refer to Location.

PHYSIOLOGY

As mentioned, the function of the portal vein and its tributaries is to drain blood from the abdominal organs and bowel and deliver it to the liver for metabolism and detoxification. This system is much different from that of the arterial supply to the liver or the systemic venous supply, which drains the liver.

Portal veins terminate in the liver in sinusoids or capillary-like vessels that deliver the blood to the hepatic veins and, in turn, to the inferior vena cava, which transports the blood to the heart. Consequently, portal venous blood is filtered twice—first, through the capillaries of the pancreas, spleen, gallbladder, and

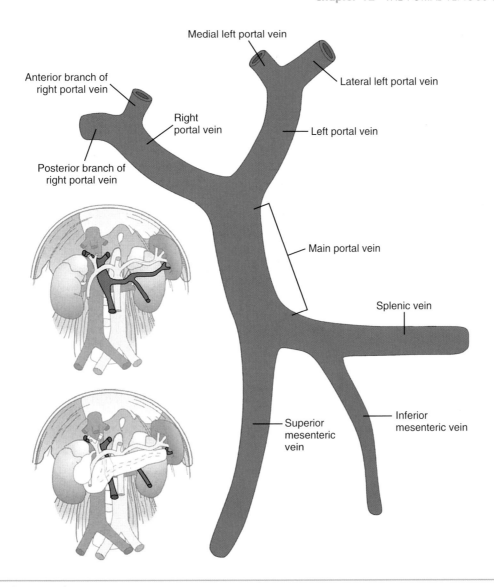

FIGURE 12-1   Portal Venous System

Vessel	Course
Superior mesenteric vein	• Courses from inferior to superior as it drains the large intestine via several smaller branches. • Joins splenic vein to form main portal vein.
Splenic vein	• Courses laterally from the spleen and then medially, directly posterior to the pancreas neck. • Joins superior mesenteric vein to form main portal vein.
Inferior mesenteric vein	• Courses from inferior to superior. • Drains the large intestine via several smaller branches. • Usually joins the splenic vein, but can vary widely as to where it actually joins the portal venous system.
Main portal vein	• Formed by the union of splenic vein and superior mesenteric vein posterior to the neck of the pancreas. • Courses superiorly approximately 5 to 6 cm and then divides into intrahepatic right and left branches. • Smaller veins also empty into the main portal vein with considerable variation as to where they join the portal venous system, including the left and right gastric veins, pancreaticoduodenal veins, and gastroepiploic veins.
Right portal vein	• Courses right from the main portal vein and branches into anterior and posterior divisions.
Left portal vein	• Courses left, horizontally, from the main portal vein and branches into medial and lateral divisions.

gastrointestinal tract; then by the sinusoids in the liver. As noted, this is a vital and unique function.

SONOGRAPHIC APPEARANCE

Intrahepatic (completely enclosed by liver tissue) arteries and bile ducts accompany portal veins in triads that are enclosed by a sheath of connective tissue. The **portal triads** spread throughout liver lobes and segments. Sonographically, the surrounding connective tissue, combined with the high-collagen content in the walls of the portal veins, makes their walls appear very bright in contrast to their anechoic lumens and thus makes it easy to differentiate them from other structures in the liver, especially the hepatic veins (Figure 12-2).

In a transverse scanning plane, at the mid-epigastrium, the origin of the portal vein or portal splenic confluence appears as an oval or round structure where the splenic vein and superior mesenteric vein unite, directly posterior to the neck of the pancreas (Figure 12-3). At a level just superior to this, in an oblique transverse scanning plane, a longitudinal section of the portal vein can be seen coursing right laterally into the liver (Figure 12-4). Moving slightly right lateral and superiorly should reveal the main portal vein as it branches into right and

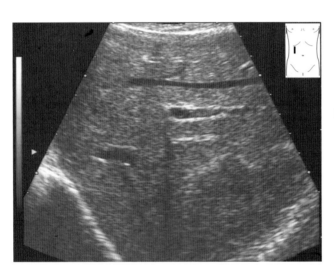
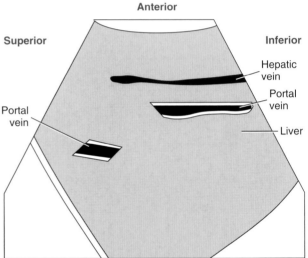

FIGURE 12-2 **Portal Vein Walls.** Sagittal scanning plane image of the right lobe of the liver showing the difference between the sonographic appearance of portal vein walls and hepatic vein walls. Portal vein walls appear distinctively *brighter* because of their high-collagen content and sheath covering.

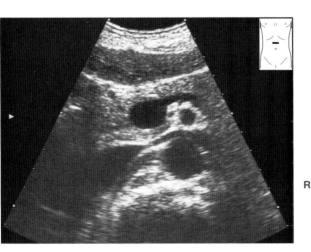
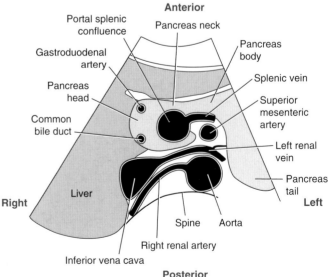

FIGURE 12-3 **Portal Splenic Confluence.** Transverse scanning plane image of the mid-epigastrium demonstrating the origin of the portal vein.

left portal veins (Figure 12-5). The left portal vein can often be followed farther to the left and can be seen branching into its medial and lateral subdivisions (Figure 12-6). The left lateral branch is more commonly visualized than the medial branch. The right portal vein can be followed farther to the right and seen branching into its anterior and posterior divisions (Figure 12-7).

In a sagittal oblique scanning plane just to the right of the midline of the body, at the level of the neck of the pancreas, an anechoic, longitudinal section of the superior mesenteric vein can be identified passing between axial sections of the pancreas neck and uncinate process to become the portal vein, which continues to course superiorly toward the liver (Figure 12-8). Moving laterally, a small, round, anechoic axial section of the right portal vein can be imaged. The bile ducts are generally imaged as small, linear, anechoic structures located anterior to the axial right portal vein (Figure 12-9). In the left lobe of the liver, it is often more difficult to image the left portal vein unless it is abnormally enlarged. However, in a sagittal scanning plane, it normally appears as a small, round, anechoic axial structure with bright walls (Figure 12-10).

Evaluating the portal vein with color Doppler and duplex Doppler produces far superior diagnoses than does B-mode imaging. Figure 12-11 shows a normal pulsed-wave Doppler of the portal vein. Figure 12-12 shows color flow into the liver toward the transducer and therefore is red in color.

SONOGRAPHIC APPLICATIONS

- Portal vein hypertension (the most common reason for examination of the portal vein; however, this pathology involves structures in addition to the portal vein, including the abdominal cavity, spleen, and liver)
- Detect tumor invasion
- Detect thrombosis

NORMAL VARIANTS

Nonapplicable

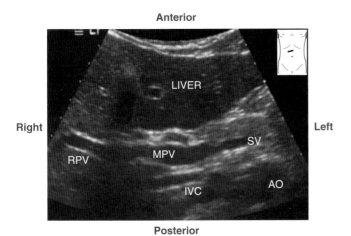

FIGURE 12-4 Relationship of Splenic Vein and Main Portal Vein. Transverse oblique scanning plane image of the mid-epigastrium showing a longitudinal section of a portion of the splenic vein becoming the main portal vein.

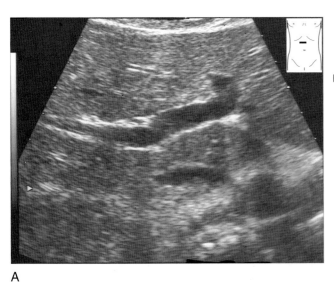

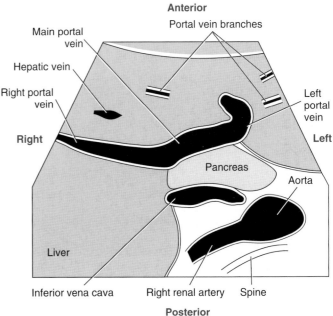

FIGURE 12-5 Main Portal Vein Branches. A, Transverse scanning plane image of a longitudinal section of the main portal vein and its right and left branches. *Continued*

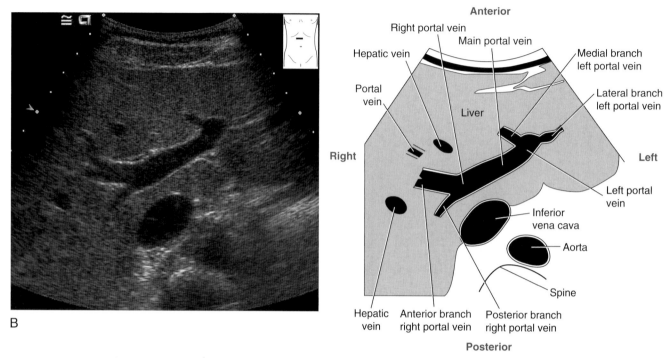

FIGURE 12-5, cont'd   **B,** Another transverse scanning plane image that shows the main portal vein as it branches into right and left portal veins. Further branching from both right and left portal veins is evident in this image.

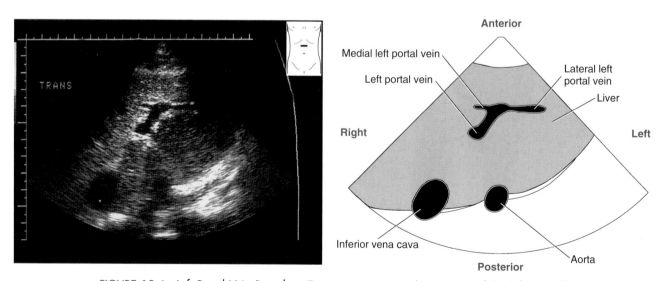

FIGURE 12-6   **Left Portal Vein Branches.** Transverse scanning plane image of the left lobe of the liver demonstrating the left portal vein dividing into its medial and lateral branches.

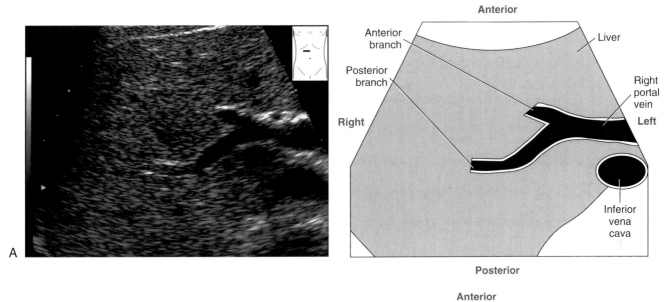

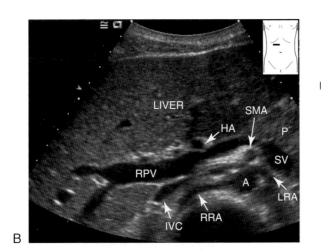

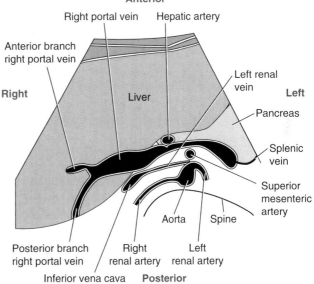

FIGURE 12-7 **Right Portal Vein Branches. A,** Transverse scanning plane image of the right lobe of the liver demonstrating the right portal vein dividing into its anterior and posterior branches. **B,** This transverse plane image clearly shows the vessels and structures near the liver, as well as the right portal vein and its anterior and posterior branches.

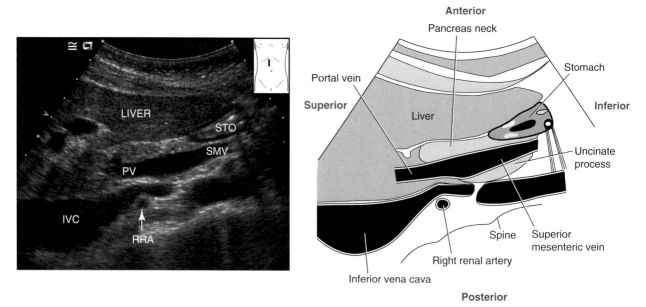

FIGURE 12-8 **Relationship of Superior Mesenteric Vein and Main Portal Vein.** Sagittal oblique scanning plane image, just to the right of the midline of the body, showing a longitudinal section of a portion of the superior mesenteric vein becoming the main portal vein. Observe how the superior mesenteric vein passes between the neck (anteriorly) and uncinate process (posteriorly) of the pancreas. Note the axial section of the right renal artery posterior to the inferior vena cava.

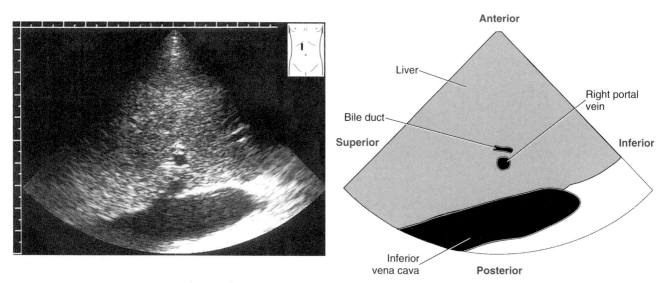

FIGURE 12-9 **Right Portal Vein.** Sagittal scanning plane image showing the circular, short axis section of the right portal vein. Note the long section of anechoic duct directly anterior to the vein.

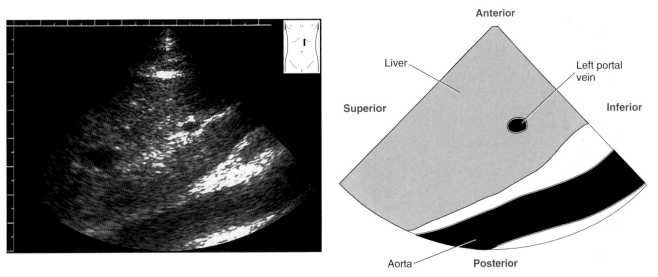

FIGURE 12-10 **Left Portal Vein.** Sagittal scanning plane image showing the circular, short axis section of the left portal vein.

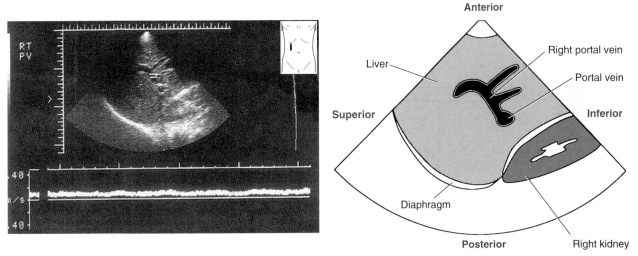

FIGURE 12-11 **Doppler Waveform Right Portal Vein.** Longitudinal section of the right lobe of the liver in a sagittal scanning plane, demonstrating a normal Doppler waveform of the right portal vein. Note the phasic flow (variation) of the Doppler signal in response to respiration. In addition, note that the flow is above baseline. In this case, blood is flowing into the liver, which is normal.

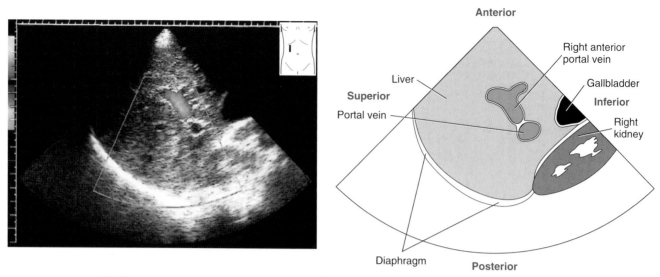

FIGURE 12-12 **Color Doppler Anterior Branch Right Portal Vein.** Color Doppler, sagittal scanning plane image of the anterior branch of the right portal vein.

REFERENCE CHARTS

■ ■ ■ ASSOCIATED PHYSICIANS

- **Surgeon:** Involved in the surgical intervention of various disorders associated with the portal venous system.
- **Internist:** Involved in the diagnosis and medical treatment of disorders related to the portal venous system. For example, an internist may treat a patient whose portal vein hypertension is due to cirrhosis of the liver or a patient who is not a surgical candidate or does not require surgery.
- **Radiologist:** Performs and interprets the various imaging tests used to diagnose diseases related to the portal venous system.

■ ■ ■ COMMON DIAGNOSTIC TESTS

Diagnostic tests may include duplex Doppler sonography, color sonography, venography, computed tomography, and magnetic resonance imaging.

- **Duplex sonography:** Duplex sonography can detect the direction and magnitude of flow within a portal vein. Flow should be toward the liver from the portal vein, and the portal venous system should display phasic flow in response to respiration (see Figure 12-11). This examination and the color-flow examination provide extremely valuable information in a short period and without the use of ionizing radiation. Thus, duplex sonography and color-flow sonography are often used. A sonographer or vascular technologist usually performs this examination. A radiologist interprets the findings.
- **Color-flow sonography:** Color-flow sonography reveals information similar to that derived from duplex sonography. However, color-flow imaging can often

yield this information much faster. A sonographer or vascular technologist usually performs this examination. A radiologist interprets the findings.

- **Direct portal venography:** Although not usually done given today's technological environment, direct portal venography can be carried out by injecting contrast material (dye) into the splenic or portal vein and taking radiographs of the area as the contrast agent is transported throughout the system. This examination provides information related to portal vein anatomy and intraluminal contents. A radiologist, assisted by a radiologic technologist, performs this examination. The radiologist interprets the findings.
- **Computed axial tomography (CT) scan and magnetic resonance imaging (MRI):** CT and MRI can also be done to evaluate the portal vein. In CT, a series of sequential radiographs are taken over the area of interest. The information is stored in a computer, which converts the data into a two- or three-dimensional image. CT is not the best method because it may be difficult to ascertain intraluminal contents. MRI, although not widely used, can often distinguish subtle differences in tissues within the portal system. In MRI, a magnetic field generates data, and a computer converts the information into a diagnostic image. Although MRI is nonionizing, it has several limitations because of the magnetic field. A radiologic technologist performs the CT and MRI examinations. A radiologist interprets the findings.
- **Benefits of sonography:** Clinical data often suggest portal vein pathology. Sonography can easily verify the intraluminal contents and the direction of flow, in addition to indicating other pathologic findings of the abdomen. Thus sonography is often used as a primary diagnostic tool in evaluating the portal venous system.

■ ■ ■ LABORATORY VALUES

Generally, laboratory values do not directly indicate portal vein pathology. A tumor, or cirrhosis of the liver, however, will produce various laboratory and clinical data that could point to portal vein involvement associated with the disorder.

■ ■ ■ VASCULATURE

Superior mesenteric vein + splenic vein → main portal vein
↓
Inferior mesenteric vein → splenic vein
Main portal vein → left portal vein → medial and lateral
  branches
→ right portal vein → anterior and posterior branches

■ ■ ■ AFFECTING CHEMICALS

Nonapplicable

■

CHAPTER 13

Abdominal Vasculature

MARSHA M. NEUMYER

OBJECTIVES

Describe the anatomy of the vasculature of the liver, spleen, mesenteric, and renal systems.

Define the role of duplex scanning and color-flow imaging for evaluation of abdominal vascular disease.

Describe the sonographic appearance of the hepatoportal, mesenteric, and renal vascular systems.

Define the hemodynamic patterns and spectral waveforms found in the normal abdominal vasculature.

KEY WORDS

Doppler Spectral Waveform — Provides information about blood flow velocity, flow direction, presence of flow disturbance or turbulence, and vascular impedance.

Duplex sonography — Real-time imaging and pulsed Doppler capabilities used either simultaneously or sequentially.

Hepatofugal — Flow direction away from the liver.

Hepatopetal — Flow direction toward the liver.

High-resistance vessels — Arteries with low or reversed flow in diastole that supply organs that do not demand constant blood perfusion.

Low-resistance vessels — Arteries supplying organs that demand constant forward blood flow or perfusion.

Spectral Broadening — An increase in returned echoes proportional to an increase in turbulence or flow disturbance.

Systolic Window — Relatively signal-free area between the arterial Doppler shift signal and the baseline during the systolic portion of a Doppler spectral display.

■ ■ ■ NORMAL MEASUREMENTS

Anatomy	Measurement	Anatomy	Measurement
Average Diameter of Abdominal Arteries		**Average Diameter of Abdominal Veins**	
Aorta	2.0 to 2.5 cm	IVC	25 to 35 mm
Celiac artery	0.70 cm	Renal veins	4.0 to 6.0 mm
SMA	0.60 cm	Hepatic veins	4.0 to 7.0 mm
IMA	0.30 cm	SMV	6.0 to 7.0 mm
Renal arteries	0.40 to 0.50 cm	Splenic vein	4.0 to 6.0 mm
		Portal vein	13 mm

Images in this chapter are courtesy Penn State Hershey Vascular Noninvasive Diagnostic Laboratory, Hershey, Pennsylvania.

Since its introduction more than 40 years ago as a fairly complex technology that combined gray-scale imaging for characterization of tissues and blood vessels and pulsed Doppler for assessment of flow dynamics, vascular **duplex sonography** has evolved dramatically. Initially used for noninvasive evaluation of the superficial arteries and veins, outstanding technical advancements have facilitated extension of this modality into the deep vessels of the abdomen. In current clinical practice, duplex technology is complemented by color, power, and harmonic and real-time compound imaging for examination of the hepatoportal, mesenteric, and renal vascular systems. In extended, advanced practice, investigators are exploring the use of 3- and 4-dimensional and volume imaging for use in selected vascular cases.

THE ABDOMINAL ARTERIAL SYSTEM
Location

The abdominal arterial system consists of the segment of the aorta from the level of the diaphragm to the aortic bifurcation and its branches, the celiac axis/artery (and its branches, the common hepatic, splenic, and left gastric arteries), and the superior mesenteric, inferior mesenteric, renal (and renal parenchyma vessels), and common iliac arteries (Figure 13-1).

The abdominal aorta commences at the aortic opening of the diaphragm, lying slightly to the left and anterior to the vertebral column (Table 13-1). It terminates on the body of the fourth lumbar vertebra, at which point it bifurcates into the common iliac arteries. The vessel diameter tapers slightly from its proximal to distal segments.

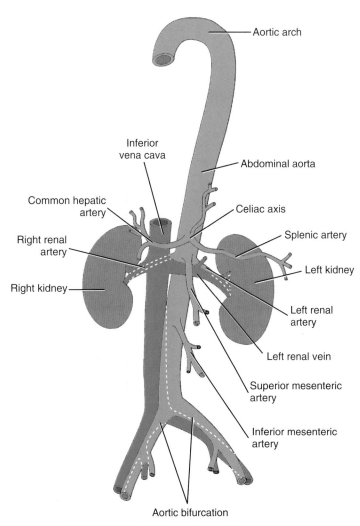

FIGURE 13-1   Abdominal arterial system.

■ ■ ■ **Table 13-1** Location of Abdominal Aorta and Branches Routinely Visualized With Ultrasound

	Aorta (can be tortuous)	Celiac Artery	Left Gastric Artery (very tortuous)	Splenic Artery (tortuous)
Anterior to	Spine	Aorta	Celiac artery, splenic artery, CHA	Celiac artery, pancreas tail, superior pole lt kidney
Posterior to	Lt renal vein, SMA, splenic vein, pancreas body/tail, celiac artery, splenic artery, CHA, lt gastric artery, inferior duodenum, stomach, peritoneum, liver	Lt gastric artery, peritoneum, liver	Liver, peritoneum	Liver, lt gastric artery stomach, peritoneum
Superior to		SMA, pancreas body, splenic vein	Celiac artery, splenic artery, SMA, CHA	Pancreas body, splenic vein, SMA
Inferior to	Diaphragm	Diaphragm, EGJ	Diaphragm	Diaphragm
Medial to	Splenic artery, lt renal artery, lt kidney, lt ureter, lt adrenal gland, pancreas tail, ascending duodenum, lt crus of diaphragm	Splenic artery, cardiac end of stomach		Spleen
Lt lateral to	Spine, IVC, rt renal artery, rt kidney, rt adrenal gland, rt crus of diaphragm, CHA, PHA, GDA	Liver, caudate lobe, CHA	Celiac artery	Celiac artery, lt gastric artery, CHA, aorta
Rt lateral to				

	Common Hepatic Artery	Proper Hepatic Artery	Gastroduodenal Artery	Superior Mesenteric Artery
Anterior to	Celiac artery, IVC	Portal vein	IVC, CBD, pancreas neck/head	Aorta, lt renal vein
Posterior to	Liver, lt gastric artery, peritoneum	Common duct, peritoneum	Liver, peritoneum	Splenic vein, pancreas body, liver, SMV, peritoneum
Superior to	Pancreas neck/head, SMA	GDA		Renal arteries, renal veins, common iliac arteries, common iliac veins
Inferior to		Rt and lt hepatic arteries, porta hepatis	PHA	Diaphragm, celiac artery, splenic artery, lt, gastric artery
Medial to	PHA, common duct, portal vein	Common duct, rt and lt hepatic arteries, porta hepatis, cystic duct	Duodenum	Splenic vein, pancreas tail, lt ureter
Lt lateral to				SMV, IMV, PSC, IVC
Rt lateral to	Celiac artery, splenic artery	CHA	CHA, SMA, SMV, splenic vein, pancreas head	

■ ■ ■ Table 13-1 Location of Abdominal Aorta and Branches Routinely Visualized With Ultrasound—cont'd

	Rt Renal Artery	Lt Renal Artery	Rt Common Iliac Artery	Lt Common Iliac Artery
Anterior to	Rt crus of diaphragm	Lt crus of diaphragm	Rt common iliac vein, proximal IVC, spine	Lt common iliac vein, spine
Posterior to	IVC, rt renal vein, peritoneum, PSC, pancreas head/uncinate	Lt renal vein, peritoneum, pancreas tail, splenic vein	Peritoneum, small intestine, rt ureter	Peritoneum, small intestines, lt ureter
Superior to	Common iliac arteries, common iliac veins, rt ureter	Common iliac arteries, common iliac veins, lt ureter		
Inferior to	SMA, celiac artery, rt adrenal gland	SMA, celiac artery, lt adrenal gland, splenic artery	SMA, renal arteries and veins	
Medial to	Rt kidney	Lt kidney	Rt common iliac vein, proximal IVC, psoas major muscle	SMA, renal arteries and veins
Lt lateral to		Aorta, SMA		Psoas major muscle
Rt lateral to	Aorta, SMA		Lt common iliac vein, lt common iliac artery	Lt common iliac vein, rt common iliac artery, rt common iliac vein

CBD, Common bile duct; **CHA,** common hepatic artery; **EGJ,** esophageal gastric junction; **GDA,** gastroduodenal artery; **IMV,** inferior mesenteric vein; **IVC,** inferior vena cava; **PHA,** proper hepatic artery; **PSC,** portal splenic confluence; **SMA,** superior mesenteric artery; **SMV,** superior mesenteric vein.

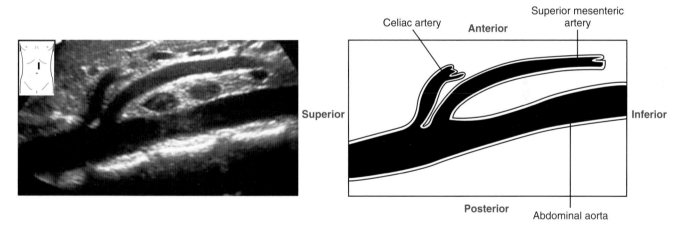

FIGURE 13-2   Gray-scale image of a longitudinal section of the abdominal aorta and the origins of the celiac and superior mesenteric arteries from the anterior wall of the aorta.

The abdominal aorta is bordered anteriorly by the stomach, pancreas, celiac axis, splenic vein, and superior mesenteric artery and vein. It is bordered on its right by the inferior vena cava (IVC) and on its left by the splenic vein and tail of the pancreas.

The celiac and superior mesenteric arteries originate from the anterior wall of the aorta, and the inferior mesenteric artery (IMA) originates from the left antero-lateral wall (Figure 13-2). The celiac artery is bordered on its left side by the cardiac end of the stomach and rests on the superior border of the pancreas. It is located 1 to 3 cm below the diaphragm at about the level of the twelfth thoracic and first lumbar vertebrae. The celiac divides into three major branches—the

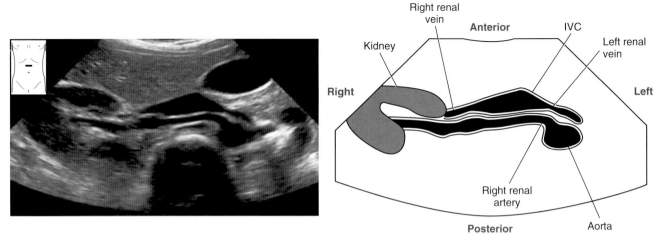

FIGURE 13-3 Transverse gray-scale image of the right kidney demonstrating the length of the right renal artery as it courses behind and inferior to the inferior vena cava.

common hepatic, splenic, and left gastric arteries—approximately 1 to 2 cm from its origin. The celiac artery and its branches supply blood to the stomach, liver, spleen, and small intestine.

From its origin at the celiac axis, the common hepatic artery courses along the superior border of the pancreatic neck and head. Between the duodenum and the anterior surface of the head of the pancreas, it gives rise to the gastroduodenal artery. Coursing superiorly, it becomes the proper hepatic artery and gives rise to the right gastric artery before entering the porta hepatis. Interrogation of the hepatic artery and its branches is best achieved using color-flow imaging and a coronal oblique image plane. Within the liver, the proper hepatic artery branches into the right and left hepatic arteries, which divide into the segmental and subsegmental hepatic artery branches. These branches course parallel to the bile ducts and portal vein branches.

The left gastric artery courses along the lesser curvature of the stomach, sending branches to the anterior and posterior segments of the stomach and esophagus.

The splenic artery is tortuous as it courses along the anterosuperior margin of the pancreas body and tail to terminate within the hilum of the spleen. The splenic artery is best visualized from a transverse scanning plane superior to the body of the pancreas. Using the spleen as an acoustic window and a lateral approach, the distal segment of the artery can be interrogated in the splenic hilum.

The superior mesenteric artery (SMA) originates from the anterior wall of the aorta 1 to 2 cm inferior to the origin of the celiac axis. At its origin, the SMA lies between the aorta (posteriorly) and the splenic

vein and body of the pancreas (anteriorly). Its proximal segment runs between the pancreas and the transverse portion of the duodenum. This artery anastomoses to the celiac artery by way of the superior and inferior pancreaticoduodenal arteries, which serve as major collateral pathways in the presence of occlusive disease of the SMA or celiac artery. The SMA supplies blood to the jejunum, ileum, cecum, ascending and transverse colon, portion of the duodenum, and the pancreatic head.

The inferior mesenteric artery (IMA) originates from the aortic wall approximately 4 cm superior to the aortic bifurcation. The IMA lies anterolateral to the distal abdominal aorta at its origin. It then descends to the left iliac fossa, anterior to the left common iliac artery, to enter the pelvis as the superior hemorrhoidal artery. This vessel lies in close proximity to the aorta along the first several centimeters of its course. The artery supplies blood to the descending and sigmoid flexures of the colon and the greater part of the rectum.

The left and right renal arteries originate from the lateral wall of the aorta approximately 1 to 1.5 cm below the SMA, just posterior to the renal veins. In their proximal segment the renal arteries follow the crus of the diaphragm. The right renal artery is longer than the left because it must pass behind the IVC and right renal vein to enter the hilum of the right kidney (Figure 13-3). The left renal artery originates from the aortic wall somewhat higher than the right, posterior to the left renal vein.

Before entering the hilum of the kidney, each renal artery divides into four or five branches, the greater number of which most often lie between the renal vein and the ureter. The vessels further branch to form the interlobar and arcuate arteries, which pass between the

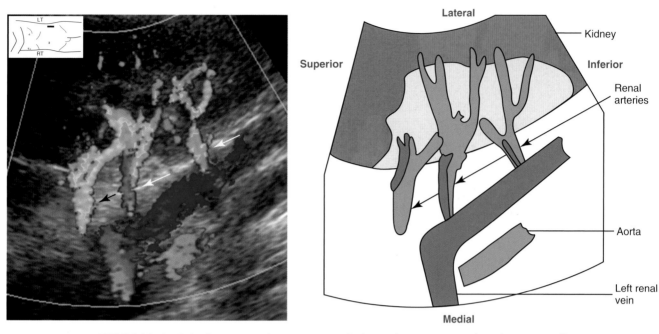

FIGURE 13-4 Color-flow image demonstrating multiple renal arteries arising from the aortic wall and entering the renal hilum.

medullary pyramids of the renal parenchyma (see Urinary System, Chapter 17).

Duplicated and/or accessory renal arteries are noted, originating from the aortic wall in approximately 20% of the population (Figure 13-4). The accessory renal arteries usually enter the upper or lower poles of the kidney rather than entering the organ at the hilum. Duplicate and accessory polar renal arteries are found more often on the left side than the right.

Size
The average diameters of the aorta and its branch arteries are as follows:

■ ■ ■ NORMAL MEASUREMENTS	
Anatomy	**Measurement**
Aorta	2.0 to 2.5 cm
Celiac artery	0.70 cm
SMA	0.60 cm
IMA	0.30 cm
Renal arteries	0.40 to 0.50 cm

Sonographic Appearance
In addition to the following discussion, the sonographic appearance of the abdominal aorta and its branch arteries is covered in Chapter 10.

The abdominal arteries normally appear as anechoic structures with bright, echogenic walls. This linear wall reflectivity is attributed to the acoustic properties of collagen fibers found in the tunica intima and tunica media. The aorta often displays significant pulsatility, making it easy to distinguish from adjacent structures. The branches of the abdominal aorta consistently demonstrated with ultrasound are the celiac artery (its splenic and common hepatic artery branches), the superior mesenteric artery, renal arteries, and common iliac arteries.

Hemodynamic Patterns
The suprarenal abdominal aorta supplies the largest portion of its blood flow to **low-resistance vessels** that supply the liver, spleen, and kidneys. These organs all have high metabolic rates and demand constant forward blood flow. In contrast, in a fasting patient, the SMA is a **high-resistance vessel** supplying the muscular tissues of the small intestine, cecum, and colon. Blood flow through the suprarenal aorta therefore meets little resistance to runoff, and forward flow is noted throughout the cardiac cycle (Figure 13-5, *A*). The peak aortic systolic velocity decreases with age, perhaps as a result of decreased vessel wall compliance. The infrarenal aortic blood supply is principally to the high-resistance peripheral arterial system of the lower extremities and lumbar arteries. The pressure wave noted in this segment of the aorta therefore

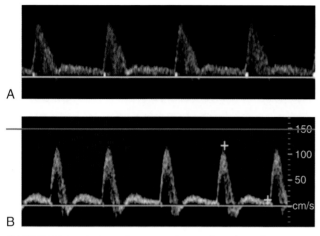

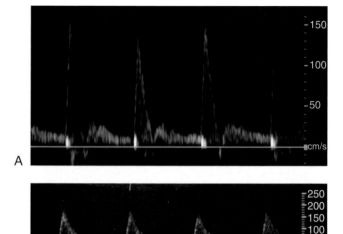

FIGURE 13-5 **A,** Doppler spectral waveform from the suprarenal abdominal aorta. Note forward diastolic flow. **B,** Doppler spectral waveform from the infrarenal aorta, demonstrating the triphasic velocity waveform consistent with a vessel feeding a high-resistance vascular bed.

FIGURE 13-7 **A,** High-resistance velocity spectral waveform recorded from the fasting superior mesenteric artery. **B,** Postprandially, the superior mesenteric artery diastolic flow component increases in response to the metabolic demands imposed by digestion.

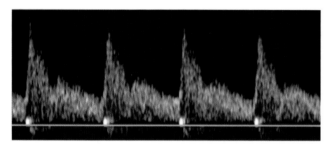

FIGURE 13-6 Doppler velocity waveform from the celiac axis. Note constant forward diastolic flow.

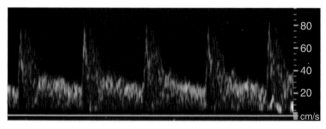

FIGURE 13-8 Doppler spectral waveform from a normal renal artery. The high diastolic flow component is consistent with a vessel feeding a low-resistance end organ.

resembles the velocity waveforms recorded from peripheral arteries (Figure 13-5, *B*). (See Vascular Technology, Chapter 32).

The celiac axis supplies low-resistance end organs—the liver and spleen—through its branch vessels—the hepatic, left gastric, and splenic arteries. Like the flow patterns seen in the suprarenal aorta, constant forward flow is documented throughout the vascular tree supplied by the celiac artery (Figure 13-6).

The SMA supplies the tissues of the pancreas, small intestine, and colon. Flow in the SMA varies, depending on the activity of these organs and their metabolic status. In the fasting state, there is relatively high resistance to arterial flow to the tissues of the gut (Figure 13-7, *A*). After ingestion of a meal, remarkable changes occur in the flow patterns in the SMA, reflecting the metabolic demands imposed by the digestive process. Increases occur in the diameter of the SMA, peak systolic and end-diastolic velocities, and volume flow to the small bowel. Constant forward flow should be observed

throughout the cardiac cycle, reflecting the flow demands of the postprandial vascular bed (Figure 13-7, B).

The kidneys, like the brain, eyes, liver, and spleen, are low-resistance organs that demand constant blood flow to moderate their metabolic activity. Hemodynamic flow patterns in normal renal arteries that supply healthy kidneys demonstrate high diastolic flow (Figure 13-8). In patients with chronic renal disease, the vascular resistance of the kidney increases. This increase in renovascular resistance of the end organ may be expressed in the flow patterns from the renal artery as a decrease in the diastolic flow component.

Doppler Velocity Spectral Analysis

The Doppler velocity waveform from the suprarenal abdominal aorta normally demonstrates an absence of reversed diastolic flow, reflecting the low vascular resistance of its end organs (see Figure 13-5, *A*). In contrast, the signals from the infrarenal aorta are multiphasic, which is consistent with a vessel feeding a high-resistance peripheral arterial tree (see Figure 13-5, *B*). Occasionally, a biphasic flow pattern is present. The absence of a forward diastolic flow cycle reflects the relative decrease in arterial wall compliance or elasticity. This flow pattern may be seen in the elderly population and in patients with medial calcification of the arterial wall. Peak systolic velocity normally ranges from 40 to 100 cm/sec.

The Doppler spectral waveforms from the celiac, hepatic, and splenic arteries demonstrate forward diastolic flow compatible with high flow demands of the liver and spleen (see Figure 13-6). Peak systolic velocity in the celiac artery normally ranges from 98 to 105 cm/sec, whereas the common hepatic and splenic arteries demonstrate velocity ranges that are slightly lower. The splenic artery is frequently tortuous, and *spectral broadening* may be noted in the quasi-steady waveform recorded from this vessel.

In the fasting state the Doppler spectral waveform from the SMA demonstrates low diastolic flow; there may be a brief period of reversed flow during early diastole (see Figure 13-7, *A*). Peak systolic velocity normally ranges from 97 to 142 cm/sec in the fasting state. Postprandially, the peak systolic velocity increases in the normal artery, and a twofold to threefold increase in end-diastolic flow may be documented (see Figure 13-7, *B*). Because of the collateral potential expressed in the mesenteric arterial system, disease in one of the three major mesenteric arteries can result in increased flow and velocity in the others.

The inferior mesenteric artery may be difficult to accurately identify by duplex or color-flow imaging. In the fasting state, its Doppler spectral waveform mimics that of the fasting SMA, exhibiting low diastolic flow. Age-matched peak systolic velocities have not been well validated for the inferior mesenteric artery but most often range from 93 to 189 cm/sec. Postprandially, little immediate change occurs in the diastolic flow value.

The signature Doppler waveform from the renal arteries resembles that from other vessels that feed organs with high flow demand (see Figure 13-8). The normal waveform from the proximal renal artery may demonstrate a clear systolic window, with minimal spectral broadening of velocities evident in the mid to distal segments of the vessel. This increase in spectral bandwidth occurs because the sample volume size used to monitor the flow is normally large in relation to the lumen of the vessel, or the sample volume may have been increased in size during the study to encompass the entire lumen of a poorly visualized artery. Normally, the renal artery peak systolic velocity is less than 100 cm/sec.

Because the normal kidney has high metabolic demands and low vascular resistance, the Doppler spectral waveform from the interlobar and arcuate arteries of the renal medulla and cortex should demonstrate significant diastolic flow (Figure 13-9, *A*).

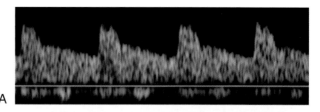
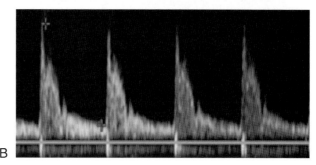

FIGURE 13-9 **A,** Doppler velocity waveform recorded from normal renal parenchyma. **B,** Diastolic flow component of the renal parenchymal Doppler velocity signal decreases as renovascular resistance increases due to intrinsic renal pathology.

With increased renovascular resistance caused by intrinsic renal pathology, the end-diastolic flow component decreases throughout the vascular tree of the kidney, and the velocity waveform becomes markedly pulsatile (Figure 13-9, *B*).

THE ABDOMINAL VENOUS SYSTEM
Location
The abdominal venous system consists of the IVC from the level of its origin at the union of the common iliac veins to the diaphragm, and its tributaries and the portal venous system (Figure 13-10). Because the hepatic artery shares a partnership with the venous circulatory supply of the liver, it will be considered in the discussion of the abdominal venous system.

The IVC is formed by the confluence of the common iliac veins, which drain the lower extremities and pelvis. It normally courses superiorly through the retroperitoneum, lying on the right side of the body just anterolateral to the vertebral processes. The IVC lies medial to the right kidney and posterior to the liver before coursing through the diaphragm to enter the right atrium of the heart (Table 13-2).

Although the normal IVC diameter is less than 2.5 cm, there is often a slight increase in diameter above the entry level of the renal veins because of the increased volume of blood returned from the kidneys. Body habitus, respiration, and right atrial pressure influence the diameter of the IVC.

A number of anatomic anomalies have been recognized. The most common of these include duplication

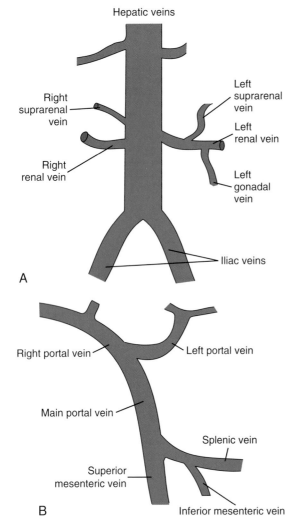

FIGURE 13-10   **A,** Abdominal venous system showing major branches. **B,** Portal venous system.

of the entire length or short segments of the IVC, segmental absence of portions of the vessel, and anatomic relocation of the suprarenal segment, infrarenal segment, or entire length of the IVC to the left of the aorta.

Although the IVC gives rise to multiple tributaries, only those accessible to sonographic evaluation and included as part of the vascular ultrasound examination of the hepatoportal and renal systems will be discussed.

The renal veins return blood from the kidneys to the systemic circulation, emptying into the IVC immediately superior to the level of the renal arteries. The left renal vein is longer than the right renal vein, coursing anterior to the aorta to lie between the aortic wall and the SMA (Figure 13-11). The left renal vein receives the left gonadal and suprarenal veins (see

Figure 13-10, *A*). These smaller veins are not included in the routine evaluation of the renal venous system. The right renal vein is shorter than the left renal vein and may receive the right suprarenal vein.

The hepatic veins empty into the IVC superior to the location of the renal veins. Normally, there are three major hepatic veins—right, middle, and left—that give rise to multiple branches within the parenchyma of the liver (Figure 13-12). The right and left hepatic veins empty the right and left lobes of the liver, respectively, and the middle hepatic vein drains the caudate lobe.

The portal vein and its branches are intraabdominal vessels. The portal vein is formed by the confluence of the superior mesenteric and splenic veins (see Figure 13-10, *B*). It is located posterior to the neck of the pancreas, where the splenic vein can be found just medially (Table 13-3). The splenic vein may receive the inferior mesenteric vein before emptying into the portal vein. The superior mesenteric vein (SMV) returns blood from the small intestine and segments of the large intestine, where it courses superiorly, parallel with the inferior mesenteric vein. The main portal vein courses superiorly and laterally to the right for several centimeters before entering the liver through the porta hepatis. It divides into the left and right portal veins (Figure 13-13). The left portal vein courses horizontally to supply the left lobe of the liver, giving rise to several primary medial and lateral branches. The right portal vein courses to the right lobe of the liver and gives rise to anterior and posterior branches.

The hepatic artery is one of the three primary branches of the celiac trunk. From its origin, it courses superiorly and right laterally to enter the porta hepatis (Figure 13-14, *A*) with the portal vein and common bile duct (Figure 13-14, *B*). It branches into the right and left trunks, which have multiple subdivisions that carry arterial blood flow to the right and left lobes of the liver.

Size

The size of the abdominal veins varies with respiration. The diameters indicated below are those associated with expiration:

■ ■ ■ NORMAL MEASUREMENTS	
Anatomy	**Measurement**
IVC	25 to 35 mm
Renal veins	4.0 to 6.0 mm
Hepatic veins	4.0 to 7.0 mm
SMV	6.0 to 7.0 mm
Splenic vein	4.0 to 6.0 mm
Portal vein	13 mm

■ ■ ■ **Table 13-2** Location of Inferior Vena Cava and Tributaries Routinely Visualized With Ultrasound

	Inferior Vena Cava (IVC)	Hepatic Veins	Rt Renal Vein
Anterior to	Spine, rt crus of diaphragm, rt psoas major muscle, rt renal artery, rt adrenal gland	IVC	Quadratus lumborum muscle, rt renal artery
Posterior to	Pancreas head/uncinate process, transverse duodenum, portal vein, CBD, posterior surface of liver, hepatic veins		Pancreas head
Superior to		Renal veins	Common iliac veins
Inferior to	Diaphragm	Diaphragm	SMA, rt adrenal gland
Medial to	Rt renal vein, rt kidney, rt ureter, rt adrenal gland		Rt kidney
Lt lateral to			
Rt lateral to	Lt renal vein, aorta, caudate lobe liver		IVC

	Lt Renal Vein	Rt Common Iliac Vein	Lt Common Iliac Vein
Anterior to	Aorta, lt renal artery	Psoas major muscle	Psoas major muscle
Posterior to	Pancreas body/tail	Rt common iliac, artery	Lt common iliac artery
Superior to	Common iliac veins		Renal veins
Inferior to	SMA, lt adrenal gland	Renal veins	Lt common iliac artery
Medial to	Lt kidney		Rt common iliac vein and artery
Lt lateral to	IVC		
Rt lateral to		Lt common iliac vein and artery, rt common iliac artery	

IVC, Inferior vena cava; **SMA**, superior mesenteric artery.

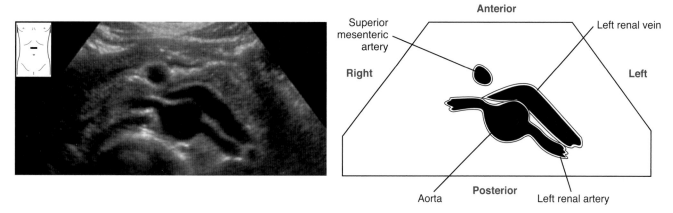

FIGURE 13-11 Transverse image of an axial section of the abdominal aorta demonstrating its posterior relationship to the long section of left renal vein and axial section of the superior mesenteric artery.

Sonographic Appearance

In addition to the following discussion, the sonographic appearance of the abdominal veins is covered in Chapter 11, The Inferior Vena Cava, and Chapter 12, The Portal Venous System.

The IVC normally appears on ultrasound images as an anechoic structure whose diameter varies with changes in respiration. Deep inspiration causes increased abdominal pressure and impedes venous return from the abdomen. This results in dilation of the IVC. Dilation can also occur in the presence of congestive heart failure, tricuspid regurgitation, or any condition that results in increased right atrial pressure.

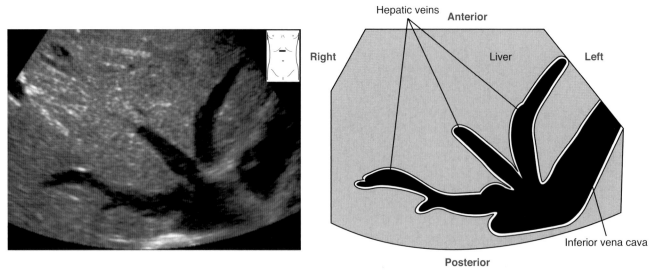

FIGURE 13-12 Subcostal longitudinal gray-scale image of the right, middle, and left hepatic veins at their confluence with the inferior vena cava.

■ ■ ■ **Table 13-3** Location of the Portal Venous System Routinely Visualized With Ultrasound

	Main Portal Vein	Splenic Vein	Superior Mesenteric Vein	Inferior Mesenteric Vein
Anterior to	IVC, pancreas uncinate process	Lt kidney, lt renal vein, lt renal artery, SMA, rt renal artery	Pancreas/inferior head/ uncinate process, IVC, rt ureter, inferior duodenum	Lt common iliac vessels, lt psoas major muscle
Posterior to	Pancreas neck, superior duodenum, CHA, PHA, common duct, peritoneum	Pancreas neck/body/ tail, peritoneum	Pancreas neck, peritoneum	Pancreas body, peritoneum
Superior to	Pancreas head, SMV, IMV, splenic vein	SMV, IMV		
Inferior to	Porta hepatis, rt portal vein branch, lt portal vein branch	Splenic artery, portal vein	Splenic vein, portal vein	Splenic vein, portal vein
Medial to	Cystic duct	Spleen, portal vein	Pancreas head, duodenum	SMV, portal vein, pancreas head
Lt lateral to		IVC, pancreas head		Splenic vein
Rt lateral to	SMV, IMV, splenic vein, pancreas head, aorta celiac artery	SMA, aorta	IMV, splenic vein, SMA	

CHA, Common hepatic artery; IMV, inferior mesenteric vein; IVC, inferior vena cava; PHA, proper hepatic artery; SMV, superior mesenteric vein.

The hepatic veins normally appear sonographically as anechoic structures, which lack echogenic walls. Their diameter may appear small within the parenchyma of the liver, but it increases in the region of the caval confluence.

Several approaches can be used to interrogate the hepatic veins sonographically. Most often, these veins can be insonated from a subcostal approach or from a right intercostal approach. Most often all three branches can be visualized; occasionally, only two branches are seen from the subcostal approach (sometimes referred to as the "bunny sign").

The main portal vein can be interrogated from a right intercostal approach with the transducer angled toward the porta hepatis. Within the porta hepatis, the portal vein is closely associated with the hepatic artery and the common bile duct. Color-flow imaging will facilitate definition of the course of the vein, its branches, and the direction of flow. It should be noted that the hepatic veins are boundary formers coursing longitudinally toward the IVC, whereas the portal veins branch horizontally and are oriented toward the porta hepatis.

The walls of the main portal vein and its branches are echogenic because of the collagen content found in

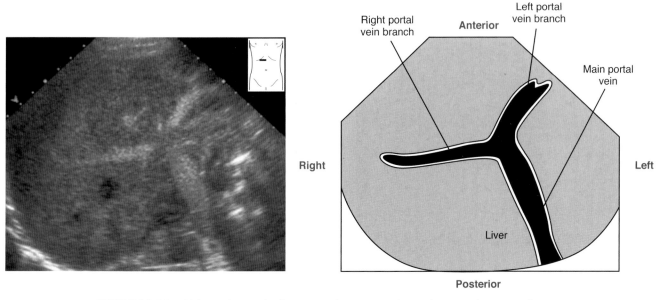

FIGURE 13-13 Oblique, longitudinal, intercostal, contrast-enhanced gray-scale image of main, right, and left portal veins. (Courtesy Edward Grant, M.D.)

the intimal and medial layers of the vein wall. This feature is in sharp contrast to the sonographic appearance of the hepatic vein walls.

The diameters of the left and right portal veins are greater at their origin in the region of the porta hepatis; minimal changes in diameter are noted during respiration. Normally, the diameter of the main portal vein is less than 13 mm in the segment just anterior to the IVC. The diameter increases during expiration and decreases during inspiration as a result of variation in the volume of blood entering the visceral arterial system and the volume outflow through the systemic venous channels.

Longitudinal sections of the renal veins appear sonographically as anechoic tubular structures extending from the renal hila to the posterolateral walls of the IVC. Patency and flow direction in the renal veins is facilitated by using a combination of color and spectral Doppler.

Hemodynamic Patterns and Doppler Spectral Display

The IVC and its tributaries drain the lower extremities, large and small intestines, kidneys, and liver. In contrast to other systemic veins, the portal venous system supplies, rather than empties, a major organ system.

The IVC demonstrates complex flow patterns in its proximal segment as a result of variations in intraabdominal pressure associated with respiration and regurgitation of blood from the right atrium during atrial systole (Figure 13-15, *A*). Distally, the IVC flow pattern reflects the phasic flow patterns seen in the peripheral veins (Figure 13-15, *B*). Color-flow imaging reveals

directional variations associated with respirophasicity in the distal segment of the vein and reflected right atrial pulsations proximally. Velocities are variable but remain low throughout the length of the vessel.

In contrast, the hepatic veins exhibit pulsatility, a reflection of cardiac and respiratory activity (Figure 13-16). Characteristically, the normal hepatic venous flow pattern is similar to that seen in the proximal IVC. The right, middle, and left hepatic veins should demonstrate three phases of flow. The first two are toward the heart and represent reflections of right atrial and ventricular diastole. The third phase is represented by systolic flow reversal and is caused by contraction of the right atrium. This flow pattern yields a W-shaped waveform as a result of changes in central venous pressure, respiration, and compliance of the liver parenchyma. Normal flow direction is **hepatofugal**, or away from the liver. Flow should be found throughout all segments of the right, middle, and left hepatic veins without significant disturbance at the hepatocaval confluence.

Intraabdominal pressure effects associated with respiration are transmitted through the liver to the portal and splanchnic veins, causing an undulating flow pattern in the portal venous system (Figure 13-17). The portal vein and its tributaries are responsible for approximately 70% of the oxygenated blood supply of the liver. Normally the high-volume portal venous flow pattern is characterized by minimally phasic, slightly disordered flow with low peak and mean velocities (20-30 cm/sec) in the supine, fasting patient. Flow direction should be **hepatopetal**, or toward the liver. Portal venous flow normally accelerates during

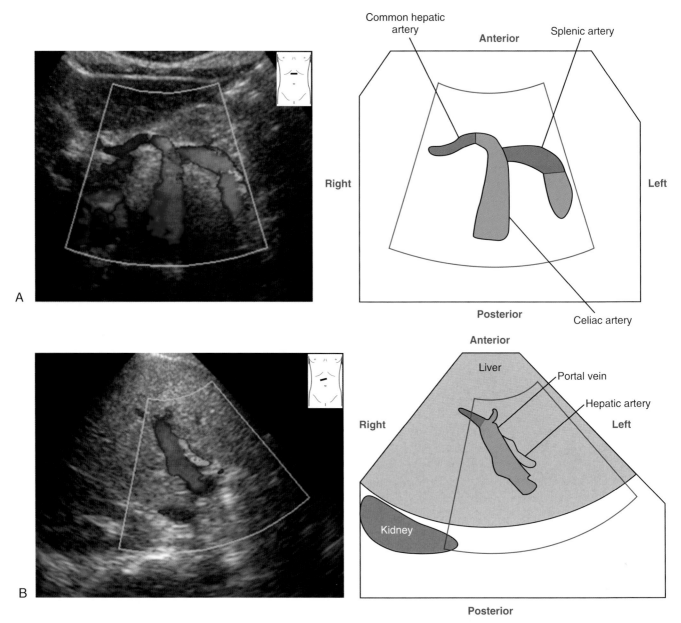

FIGURE 13-14 **A,** Color-flow image of a longitudinal section of the hepatic artery at its origin from celiac artery bifurcation. **B,** Color-flow image of hepatic artery as it courses with portal vein in the porta hepatis.

expiration and decelerates during inspiration. Portal venous flow is affected by posture, exercise, and dietary state. Exercise and postural changes usually cause a decrease in portal venous flow, whereas eating will increase flow as a result of splanchnic vasodilation and hyperemia. To control variations in flow, patients should be examined in the supine or left lateral decubitus position after an 8-hour fast.

The renal veins carry blood from tributaries within the renal medulla and cortex and empty into the IVC. Their flow patterns are influenced by the systemic circulation. For this reason, they do not exhibit

pulsatility associated with atrial or ventricular contraction (Figure 13-18).

The hepatic artery is normally responsible for approximately 30% of the oxygenated blood supply to the liver. Because the liver is a low-resistance end organ, the Doppler spectral waveform pattern from the hepatic artery is characterized by constant forward flow throughout the cardiac cycle (Figure 13-19). Peak systolic velocity is normally less than 100 cm/sec. When portal venous flow is compromised, velocity most often increases in the hepatic artery as a result of collateral compensatory mechanisms.

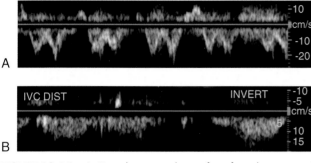

FIGURE 13-15   **A,** Doppler spectral waveform from the proximal inferior vena cava. **B,** Doppler spectral waveform from the distal inferior vena cava.

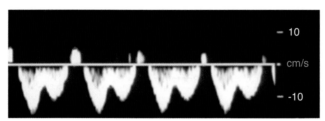

FIGURE 13-16   Doppler spectral waveform from a hepatic vein exhibiting the influence of cardiac and respiratory activity on its waveform pattern.

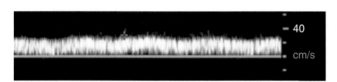

FIGURE 13-17   Doppler spectral waveform from the portal vein demonstrating the minimally phasic flow pattern associated with this vessel.

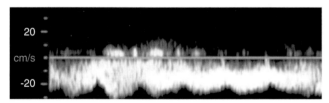

FIGURE 13-18   Doppler spectral waveform from a renal vein exhibiting the influence of the systemic venous circulation.

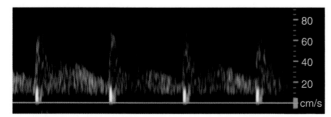

FIGURE 13-19   Doppler spectral waveform pattern from the low-resistance hepatic artery.

REFERENCE CHARTS

■ ■ ■   ASSOCIATED PHYSICIANS

- **Vascular surgeon:** Specializes in the surgical and/or endovascular treatment of abdominal vascular disorders.
- **Gastroenterologist:** Specializes in the treatment of disorders involving the gastrointestinal system.
- **Nephrologist:** Specializes in treatment of disorders involving the kidneys.
- **Interventional vascular radiologist:** Specializes in the endovascular treatment of abdominal vascular disorders.

■ ■ ■   COMMON DIAGNOSTIC TESTS

- **Vascular angiography:** A contrast medium is injected into an artery or vein, and radiographic films are taken at specific intervals to observe blood flow patterns in vessels and organ vasculature. Performed by interventional vascular radiologists and vascular surgeons, assisted by radiologic technologists. Interpreted by interventional vascular radiologists and vascular surgeons.
- **Computed tomography angiography:** A contrast medium is injected intravenously while x-ray data are acquired continuously during a single breath hold or as a bolus-tracking method. The acquired data are reconstructed and displayed as axial slices or in 3-dimensional format. Performed by interventional vascular radiologists and vascular surgeons, with assistance by radiologic technologists. Interpreted by interventional vascular radiologists and vascular surgeons.
- **Magnetic resonance angiography:** There are three types of magnetic resonance angiography (MRA). The first type is unenhanced, meaning it uses no contrast agent. The second type, an enhanced MRA, employs the contrast agent gadolinium and is not useful for imaging vessels less than 1 mm in diameter. The third type of MRA is referred to as phase-sensitive imaging. This method acquires paired images in either 2 or 3 directions. Each pair has a different sensitivity to flowing blood. The collected images are combined to create a 3-dimensional image. Performed and interpreted by interventional vascular radiologists.

■ ■ ■   LABORATORY VALUES

Nonapplicable

■ ■ ■   VASCULATURE

See Chapters 10 through 12 for discussions of the abdominal aorta, inferior vena cava, portal vein, and related structures.

■ ■ ■   AFFECTING CHEMICALS

Nonapplicable

CHAPTER 14

The Liver

MARILYN DICKERSON PRINCE

OBJECTIVES

Identify the principal functions of the liver.
Describe the location of the liver.
Describe the size of the liver.
Describe and identify the vasculature of the liver.
Identify the ligaments, segments, and fissures of the liver.

Describe the sonographic appearance of the liver.
Differentiate between carbohydrate, protein, and fat metabolism in the liver.
Describe the associated physicians, diagnostic tests, and laboratory values related to the liver.

KEY WORDS

Bare Area — Only area of the liver not covered by peritoneum.

Caudate Lobe — Smallest lobe of the liver, bordered by fossa for the inferior vena cava (IVC), falciform ligament, and lesser omentum.

Common Hepatic Artery — Branch of the celiac axis that supplies the liver and divides into the GDA and PHA.

Coronary Ligament — Anterosuperior surface of liver that runs superiorly, then posteriorly on the right to the anterior leaf of the coronary ligaments.

Couinaud's Liver Segmentation — Division of liver segments based on hepatic or portal venous anatomy; used for dividing the liver into 8 segments.

Epiploic Foramen of Winslow — Communication between the greater and lesser sacs of the peritoneum.

Falciform Ligament — Divides right and left lobes; ends at the ligamentum teres or round ligament inferiorly.

Gastrohepatic Ligament — Portion of the lesser omentum that extends across the transverse fissure for the ligamentum venosum at the porta hepatis of the lesser curvature of the stomach.

Glisson's Capsule — Tight, fibrous capsule covering the liver.

Greater Omentum — Fold of omentum that extends from the lesser curvature of the stomach and covers the intestines.

Greater Sac — Protective, thin layer that encloses most of the abdominal organs.

Hemiliver — Right or left half of the liver; a division based on Couinaud's liver segmentation system.

Hepatoduodenal Ligament — Portion of the lesser omentum that extends as the right free border of the gastrohepatic ligament to the proximal duodenum and the right flexure of the colon.

Left Hepatic Vein — One of three main veins draining the liver via the IVC; drains the left lobe.

Left Portal Vein — Branch of the main portal vein that marks the anterior border of the caudate lobe and carries blood from the gastrointestinal tract to the left lobe.

Left Triangular Ligament — Anterosuperior surface of the liver that runs superiorly, then posteriorly on the right to the left triangular ligament.

Lesser Omentum — Double layer of omentum that extends from the liver to part of the duodenum.

Lesser Sac — Small sac posterior to the stomach and anterior to the pancreas and part of the transverse colon; also known as the omentum bursa.

Ligamentum Venosum — Marks the left anterolateral border of the caudate lobe; travels within the transverse fissure.

Main Lobar Fissure — Echogenic line connecting the neck of the gallbladder to the right portal vein; also referred to as the plane associated with the Rex-Cantlie (RC) line in Couinaud's liver segmentation system. The RC line runs from the gallbladder fossa to the IVC along the plane of the main lobar fissure.

Main Portal Vein — Formed by the splenic, superior, and inferior mesenteric veins; drains blood from the gastrointestinal tract to the liver to be processed.

Middle Hepatic Vein — One of 3 main veins draining the liver via the IVC; drains a portion of the right and medial left lobes of the liver.

Morison's Pouch — Space between the posterior subphrenic and posterior subhepatic space; should be free of fluid.

Papillary Process — Normal variant of the caudate lobe. Process can extend distally from the lobe and mimic a lesion.

Porta Hepatis — Area of the hilus where portal vein and hepatic artery enter and common bile duct exits.

Portal Confluence — Union of the splenic, superior, and inferior mesenteric veins near the head of the pancreas that forms the portal vein before entering the liver.

Portal Triad — Portion of the portal vein, biliary duct, and hepatic artery that are disbursed throughout the liver; can be seen microscopically.

Proper Hepatic Artery — Division of the common hepatic artery that supplies the liver.

Quadrate Lobe — "Fourth" lobe of the liver, which is actually the medial portion of the left lobe.

KEY WORDS—cont'd

Reidel's Lobe — Normal variant of the right lobe in which the right lobe extends caudally into the abdomen and toward the iliac crest.

Right Hepatic Vein — One of 3 main veins draining the liver via the IVC; drains the right lobe of the liver.

Right Lobe — Largest lobe of the liver, occupying most of the right hypochondrium.

Right Portal Vein — Branch of the main portal vein that carries blood from the gastrointestinal tract to the right lobe of the liver.

Right Triangular Ligament — Helps form the boundary of the bare area of the liver.

Round Ligament (Ligamentum Teres) — Terminal end of the falciform ligament.

Subhepatic Space — Located posteriorly and inferiorly; forms part of Morison's pouch.

Subphrenic Space — Located posteriorly and inferiorly; forms part of Morison's pouch.

Transverse Fissure — Fissure that conveys the ligamentum venosum.

■■■ NORMAL MEASUREMENTS

Anatomy	Measurement
Liver Size	
Liver weight	Adult males: 1400 to 1800 g Adult females: 1200 to 1400 g
Right lobe	Midclavicular linear measurement: 13 to 17 cm
Left lobe	Highly variable

The liver is a powerhouse among abdominal organs, the largest parenchymal organ in the body. Its bulky mass displaces gas-filled components of the digestive system and provides an acoustic window for visualization of upper abdominal and upper retroperitoneal structures. Liver structures include the portal veins; the hepatic veins, arteries, and ducts; and the hepatic ligaments and fissures. On ultrasound images, many of these structures help divide the liver into easily identifiable segments.

LOCATION

The liver occupies a major portion of the right hypochondrium. Normally, it extends inferiorly into the epigastrium and laterally into the left hypochondrium. Superiorly it reaches the dome of the diaphragm, and posteriorly it borders the bony lumbar region of the muscular posterior abdominal wall (Table 14-1). The bulk of the liver lies beneath the right costal margin (Figure 14-1).

The superior surface, anterior surface, and a portion of the posterior surface of the liver are in contact with the diaphragm (Figure 14-2). The anterosuperior surface of the liver fits snugly into the dome of the diaphragm, separated from the overlying pleural cavities and pericardium. On the right, it rises to the level of the fourth rib interspace on full expiration. The thin edge of the superior surface of the left lobe reaches the level of the fifth rib on full expiration. The anterosuperior surface runs superiorly, then posteriorly, to the anterior leaf of the coronary ligaments on the right. On the left, it runs posteriorly to the left triangular ligament. The right anterosuperior surface of the liver is closest to the

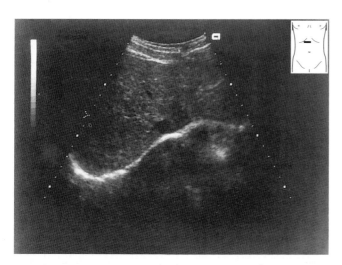

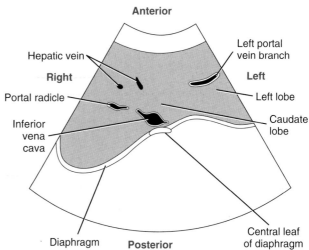

FIGURE 14-1   Transverse scanning plane image showing an axial section of the diaphragmatic undersurface and the posterosuperior liver surface.

■ ■ ■ **Table 14-1**   Location of the Liver Routinely Visualized With Ultrasound

	Lt Lobe	Lt Medial Lobe (inferior liver surface)	Caudate Lobe (posterior liver surface)	Rt Lobe
Anterior to	Stomach, EGJ, celiac artery, lt gastric artery, proximal CHA, splenic artery, aorta, SMA, pancreas body/tail, splenic vein, lt renal vein, fissure for ligamentum venosum (on liver's posterior surface), caudate lobe, diaphragm, spine	Porta hepatis, pylorus, superior portion duodenum, transverse colon, GDA	Diaphragm	Hepatic flexure, rt kidney, rt adrenal gland, descending duodenum, diaphragm
Posterior to	Xiphoid process, 7th and 8th costal cartilages	Anterior liver margin	Porta hepatis, fissure for ligamentum venosum, liver lt lobe	6th to 10th ribs
Superior to	Stomach, bowel, lt kidney, lt adrenal gland	Rt kidney, rt adrenal gland	Splenic vein	Rt kidney
Inferior to	Diaphragm		Diaphragm	Diaphragm
Medial to	Stomach, lt lateral abdominal wall, spleen	GB, fossa	IVC	Rt lateral abdominal wall
Lt lateral to	IVC, falciform ligament (on liver's superior surface), liver rt lobe, fissure for ligamentum teres (on liver's inferior surface), lt medial lobe, spine			
Rt lateral to		Fissure for ligamentum teres, lt lateral lobe, liver	Aorta	Aorta, falciform ligament (on liver's superior surface), liver lt lobe, lt medial lobe (on liver's inferior surface)

CHA, Common hepatic artery; **EGJ,** esophageal gastric junction; **GB,** gallbladder; **GDA,** gastroduodenal artery; **IVC,** inferior vena cava; **PHA,** proper hepatic artery; **SMA,** superior mesenteric artery.

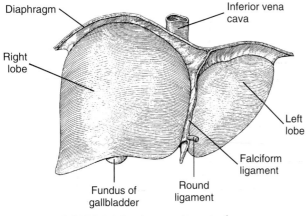

FIGURE 14-2   Anterior Liver Surface.

anterolateral abdominal wall and is palpable most often when the organ is enlarged.

The liver is enclosed by a tight, fibrous capsule known as **Glisson's capsule** and is largely covered by the peritoneum of the **greater sac**. A portion of the posterior surface of the liver is without a peritoneal covering and is called the *bare area*. This portion is in direct contact with the diaphragm.

Right Posterosuperior Surface
The major relations of the right posterosuperior surface are the right posterior fibers of the diaphragm, the upper posterior abdominal wall, the right kidney, and the right adrenal gland. The inferior segment of this surface below the inferior leaf of the coronary ligament communicates with the upper end of the right lumbar paracolic gutter and the visceral surface of the liver (Figure 14-3).

The bony and muscular posterior abdominal wall protects the posterior surface of the liver. The border between the anterior aspect of the liver and the visceral surface is the inferior margin.

Inferior (Visceral) Surface

The inferior or visceral surface of the liver rests on the upper abdominal organs. The inferior (visceral) surface of the liver is marked by indentations from organs in contact with its surface, including the gallbladder, pylorus, duodenum, right colon, right hepatic flexure of the colon, right third of the transverse colon, right adrenal gland, and right kidney.

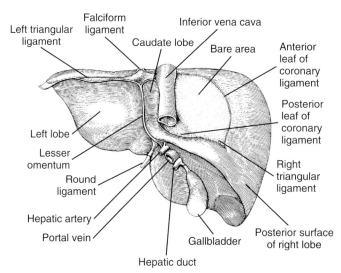

FIGURE 14-3 **Posterior Liver Surface.** Posterior liver surface outlining the boundaries of the bare area.

Right-Sided Inferior Indentations

Right-sided inferior indentations occur at the right hepatic flexure of the colon, the right kidney and adrenal gland, the first part of the duodenum, and the gallbladder.

Left Side of Inferior Surface

The left side of the inferior surface contains a gastric indentation, and the posterior surface is marked by the groove that surrounds the inferior vena cava (IVC) (Figure 14-4; see also Figure 14-3).

The anterior midportion of the inferior surface is the medial portion of the left lobe of the liver, which is also referred to as the **quadrate lobe** of the liver. The left lateral boundary of this portion is the falciform ligament, usually noted near the midline of the body (Figure 14-5; see also Figures 14-2 and 14-3).

Posterior Midportion of Inferior Surface

The posterior midportion of the inferior surface, below the porta hepatis, marks the location of the caudate lobe (Figure 14-6). The posterior portions of the left and caudate lobes form a portion of the anterior boundary of the lesser sac. The lesser sac lies anterior to the pancreas and posterior to the stomach.

Right Lobe

The **right lobe** of the liver lies close to the anterolateral abdominal wall (Figure 14-7 and Table 14-2; see Table 14-1). The right lobe is related to the right lateral undersurface of the diaphragm along the right midaxillary line from the seventh to the eleventh ribs. On the lateral right side, the liver is related to the diaphragmatic recess and the descending fibers of the diaphragm.

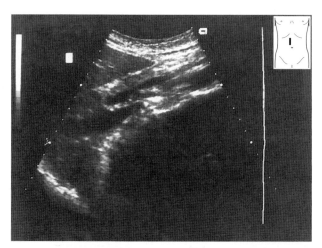 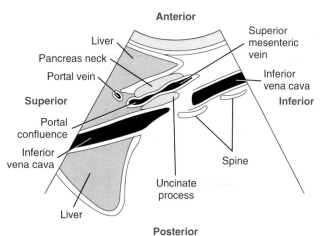

FIGURE 14-4 Sagittal scanning plane image showing a longitudinal section of the left inferior margin of the left hepatic lobe. Note posteriorly how the liver surrounds the IVC.

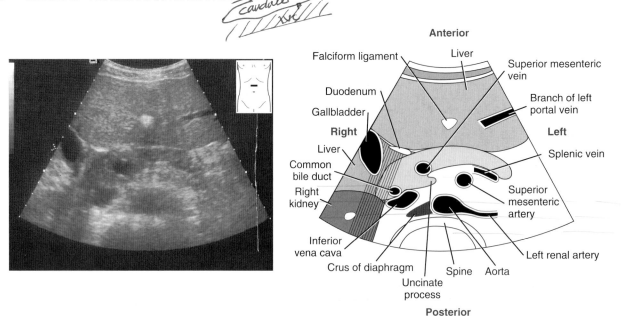

FIGURE 14-5 **Transverse Scanning Plane Image of the Midepigastrium.** The falciform ligament appears in short axis as a triangular-shaped, bright, echogenic focus demarcating the lateral border of the quadrate (medial left) lobe.

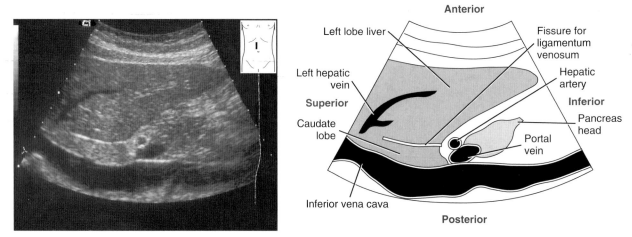

FIGURE 14-6 Parasagittal scanning plane image just to the right of the midline of the body that demonstrates the liver's caudate lobe posterior to the left hepatic lobe and a longitudinal section of the thin, bright ligamentum venosum. The left hepatic vein is seen coursing toward the inferior vena cava.

Left Lobe

The left lobe of the liver is closely related to the undersurface of the diaphragm. It varies in size and shape and may extend deeply into the left upper quadrant. The free inferior margin of the left lobe is closely related to the gastric body and antrum of the stomach. It frequently lies anterior to the body of the pancreas, the splenic vein, and the splenic artery (see Tables 14-1 and 14-2).

Caudate Lobe

The smallest lobe, the caudate, is related to the lumbar region of the posterior abdominal wall and to the lower posterior thoracic wall (see Tables 14-1 and 14-2). The **caudate lobe** is covered by the peritoneum of the **lesser sac.** The anterior boundary of the caudate lobe is marked by the posterior surface of the **left portal vein,** and the posterior boundary is the IVC. The lateral margin of the caudate lobe projects into the superior recess of the

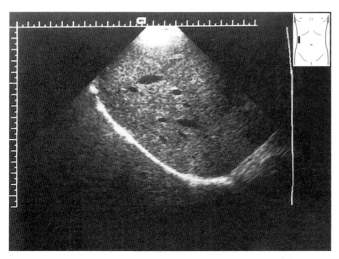

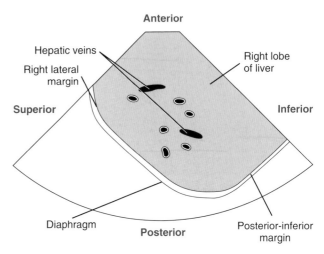

FIGURE 14-7 Longitudinal section of the right lateral margin of the liver illustrating the base of the liver pyramid. Note by the location of the transducer how the right lobe of the liver lies close to the anterolateral abdominal wall.

■ ■ ■ **Table 14-2** Lobar Liver Anatomy With Landmarks

Lobe	Identified by ...	Identified by ...	Identified by ...	Comments
Right	RL lies close to anterolateral abdominal wall	RL lies close to right lateral undersurface of the diaphragm	Diaphragmatic recess on the right lateral side	Largest lobe
Left	LL lies close to gastric body and antrum of the stomach	Anterior to body of pancreas	Anterior to the splenic vein and splenic artery	May extend deep into the left upper quadrant; can vary in size and shape
Quadrate	Anterior midportion of the inferior surface of the LL	Medial portion of the LL	Left lateral boundary is the left intersegmental fissure, which divides the LL into medial and lateral segments. The falciform ligament and ligamentum teres are located within this fissure	Some categorizations do not consider this a lobe
Caudate	Posterior midportion of the inferior liver surface, below porta hepatis, lies between RL and LL	Anterior boundary marked by posterior surface of LPV. Posterior boundary marked by IVC	Separated from LL by proximal portion of LHV and fissure for the ligamentum venosum—the fissure also contains a portion of the lesser omentum	Smallest lobe

lesser sac, also called the *omental bursa*. The caudal border forms the cephalad margin of the **epiploic foramen of Winslow**, the opening between the greater sac of the peritoneal cavity in the abdomen, which encloses the abdominal organs, and the lesser sac. The omental bursa is bordered anteriorly by the stomach, posteriorly by the pancreas, and posteriorly by part of the transverse colon (Table 14-3).

The IVC courses through the bare area of the liver, which lies between the leaflets of the anterior inferior and posterior superior coronary ligaments. The right kidney and right adrenal gland also lie near the bare area of the liver, laterally and inferiorly. The boundaries of the bare area include the falciform ligament, right anterior inferior and right posterior superior coronary ligaments, right triangular ligament, gastrohepatic

■ ■ ■ **Table 14-3** Peritoneal Divisions

Division	Also Called	Functions
Greater sac	Abdominal cavity	Encloses most of the abdominal organs; enclosed organs called "intraperitoneal"
Lesser sac	Omental bursa	Small sac bordered anteriorly by the stomach, posteriorly by the pancreas and a portion of the transverse colon
Epiploic of Winslow	Omental foramen, epiploic foramen	Passageway between greater and lesser sacs just inferior to the liver
Lesser omentum	Gastrohepatic omentum, small omentum	Double peritoneum extends from liver to lesser curvature of stomach and beginning of duodenum
Greater omentum	Gastrocolic omentum	Large fold of peritoneum that extends from stomach, passes anteriorly to the colon and small intestine

ligament, left anterior and left posterior coronary ligaments, and left triangular ligament (see Figure 14-3).

SIZE

In men the liver weighs between 1400 and 1800 g, and in women it weighs between 1200 and 1400 g. The length of the right lobe and the size of the lateral segment of the left lobe determine the contours of the liver.

The right lobe is larger than the left, containing approximately two thirds of the parenchymal tissue. Along the midclavicular line, the normal longitudinal measurement of the right lobe is 13 cm or less, although this measurement has also been stated to be 15 to 17 cm. (Refer to the Normal Measurements box at the beginning of this chapter.)

The left lobe is more varied in size. It may be atrophic if interference with the left portal venous supply occurs as the ductus venosus closes at birth. A larger left lobe helps in visualization of the pancreas and left upper quadrant.

GROSS ANATOMY

The liver is divided into 3 lobes: a right lobe, a left lobe, and a caudate lobe. The right and left lobes are subdivided into 4 segments: anterior and posterior segments on the right and lateral and medial segments on the left. The caudate lobe is a midline structure on the posterior aspect of the liver that separates a portion of the right and left hepatic lobes. The caudate lobe is separated from the left hepatic lobe by the proximal portion of the left hepatic vein and the fissure for the ligamentum venosum (see Figure 14-6). This fissure contains the ligamentum venosum and a portion of the lesser omentum, a double layer of peritoneum that extends from the liver to the lesser curvature of the stomach and the beginning of the duodenum. It is also called the gastrohepatic or small omentum. It is related to the greater omentum, which is a great fold of peritoneum that hangs from the stomach and covers the intestines (see Table 14-3).

The anterior midportion of the inferior surface of the liver is sometimes called the quadrate lobe. It is not an anatomically distinct lobe but is more correctly identified as the medial segment of the left lobe. The left intersegmental fissure divides the medial and lateral segments of the left hepatic lobe. The falciform ligament and the ligamentum teres (round ligament) are located within this fissure. The inferior surface of the liver presents a characteristic H pattern of anatomic lobar segmentation (Figure 14-8, Table 14-4). The anterior portion of the H depicts the gallbladder on the right, dividing the anterior right lobe from the medial left lobe. On the left anteriorly, the ligamentum teres divides the medial from the lateral left lobe. Posteriorly on the right, the IVC separates the right lobe and the caudate lobe, whereas on the left the ligamentum venosum divides the caudate from the lateral left lobe. The crossbar of the H depicts the porta hepatis.

The hepatic veins drain blood from the segments and lobes of the liver. They are interlobar and intersegmental. The right hepatic vein separates and drains the anterior and posterior segments of the right lobe. The left hepatic vein separates and drains the medial and lateral segments of the left lobe of the liver. The middle hepatic vein separates and drains the right and the medial left liver lobes (Figures 14-9 and 14-10, Table 14-5). The hepatic veins subdivide into superior and inferior groups. The smaller inferior veins drain the caudate lobe and the posteromedial portion of the right lobe.

The portal veins course within and supply the hepatic lobes and segments. Although the hepatic veins usually divide the liver segments, the left portal vein serves as an intersegmental boundary between the medial and lateral segments of the left lobe on caudal transverse scans of the left hepatic lobe.

The branching patterns of the portal triads, which consist of the portal vein, the hepatic artery, the bile ducts, and their divisions, are central to the functional segmentation of the hepatic lobes, originally described by Couinaud. One can appreciate the

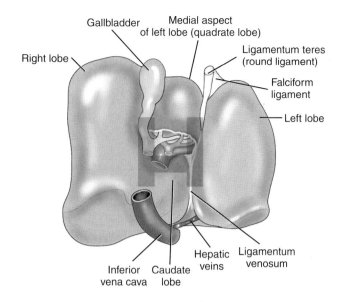

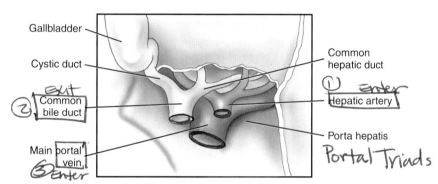

FIGURE 14-8   The inferior surface of the liver depicting the H pattern of lobar segmentation.

Table 14-4 H Pattern of Anatomic Lobar Segmentation

Part of the "H"	Depicts the ...
Anterior portion of the H, toward the right	Gallbladder on the right, dividing the anterior right lobe from the medial aspect of the left lobe
Anterior portion of the H, toward the left	Ligamentum teres divides the medial and the lateral portion of the left lobe
Posterior portion of the H, toward the right	IVC separates the right lobe from the caudate lobe
Posterior portion of the H, toward the left	Ligamentum venosum divides the caudate lobe from the lateral left lobe

Table 14-5 Liver Division by Hepatic Veins

Hepatic Vein	Separates and Drains the ...
Right hepatic vein	Anterior and posterior segments of the right lobe
Left hepatic vein	Medial and lateral segments of the left lobe
Middle hepatic vein	Right lobe and medial left lobe

abundant quantity of portal triads in liver parenchyma when examining a liver biopsy sample microscopically. One research study reported that from an approximate 1.8-cm liver tissue sample, an average of 11 portal triads were found. Portal dyads, which contain any 2 of

the triad structures, were also found in the samples, indicating that portion of the tissue did not capture the entire triad.

The pattern of anatomic segmentation provides the basis for surgical resections of the liver. **Couinaud's liver segmentation** is based on venous anatomy, with either hepatic or portal veins dividing the liver (Tables 14-6 and 14-7 and Figure 14-11). When using the portal vein as the dividing basis, there is always a central portal vein within the segment, whereas a hepatic vein will course at its periphery in the plane between adjacent portal divisions. Segments are thus defined by the portal

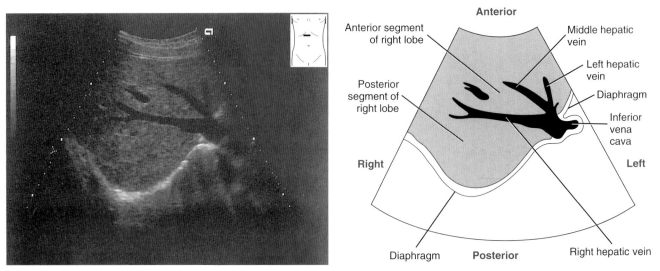

FIGURE 14-9 Transverse scanning plane image demonstrating the hepatic veins draining into the inferior vena cava. Anterior and posterior segments of the right hepatic lobe are prominently displayed. Recall that the right hepatic vein separates the anterior liver segments 5 and 8 from the posterior segments 6 and 7.

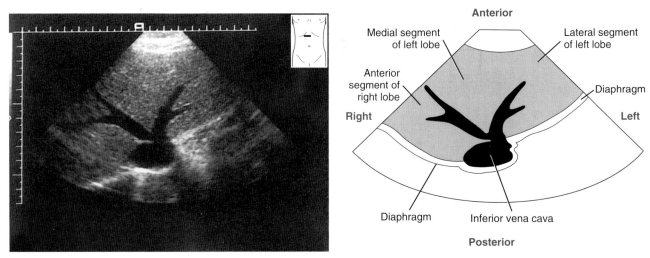

FIGURE 14-10 Transverse scanning plane image showing a section of the hepatic veins and inferior vena cava forming the "bunny sign."

■ ■ ■ **Table 14-6** Couinaud's Liver Segmentation		
Rex-Cantlie line	Runs from gallbladder fossa to IVC and passes through portion of caudate lobe; this is the plane we refer to for the main lobar fissure	Divides liver into right and left hemiliver (liver halves); hemilivers further divided into anterior and posterior segments
Right hemiliver	Anterior and posterior segments divided into …	Inferior and superior segments
Left hemiliver	Anterior segment only divided into …	Superior and inferior segments

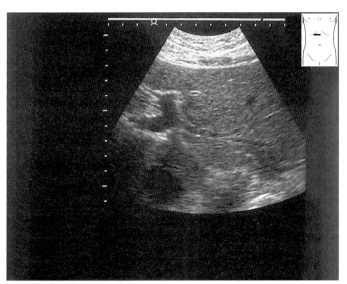

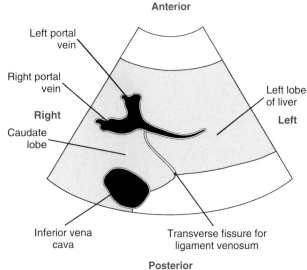

FIGURE 14-11 Transverse scanning plane image showing the left portal vein, demonstrating Couinaud's liver segments 1 through 4. The umbilical portion of the left portal vein branches to liver segments 2, 3, and 4. Note the caudate lobe (segment 1) anterior to the inferior vena cava and posterior to the left portal vein at this level.

Couinaud's Segment	Liver Portion	Identified by ...
Segment 1	Caudate	Bordered posteriorly by IVC and anteriorly by LPV
Segments 2 to 4	Left hemiliver	Segments 2 and 3 found to the left of the ligamentum venosum and falciform ligament
Segments 5 to 8	Right hemiliver	Segments 5 and 8 are anterior; segments 6 and 7 are posterior

Note: Each of the 8 segments has a distinct portal triad independent of the other segments.

venous branches that lead into them and by the hepatic veins that separate them.

The liver is divided into a right and left **hemiliver** via a plane known as the *Rex-Cantlie line*, which runs from the gallbladder fossa toward the IVC and passes through a portion of the caudate lobe. This is the plane we refer to for the **main lobar fissure**. Each hemiliver is further subdivided into an anterior and posterior segment. On the right, the anterior and posterior segments are each subdivided into inferior and superior segments, whereas on the left, only the left anterior segment is divided into superior and inferior segments.

The caudate lobe represents segment 1 (Figure 14-12). The caudate lobe is bordered posteriorly by the IVC and anteriorly by the left portal vein. Moving in a counterclockwise direction, segment 1 is separated from segment 2 by the ligamentum venosum. The left hemiliver contains segments 2 through 4. Segments 2 and 3 are found to the left of the ligamentum venosum and the falciform ligament.

The falciform ligament separates segment 3 from segment 4. Segment 4 is separated from segment 1 by the left portal vein, and the middle hepatic vein and the main lobar fissure separate segments 5 and 8. The right hepatic vein separates anterior segments 5 and 8 from posterior segments 6 and 7 (see Figure 14-9). Segments 5 through 8 are part of the right hemiliver. Each of these 8 segments of the liver is distinct in having a central portal triad independent of the other segments, thus providing an important factor in segmental hepatic surgical resections.

The portal system supplies 75% of total blood flow to the liver and has 3 main tributaries to its confluence: the splenic vein, the superior mesenteric vein, and the inferior mesenteric vein, which may join the splenic vein on its course to the **portal confluence** (union of the splenic and superior and inferior mesenteric veins that form the portal vein before entering the liver).

The **main portal vein** enters the porta hepatis and divides into left and right branches (Figures 14-13 and 14-14; see Figure 14-11). These veins then branch into medial and lateral divisions on the left and anterior and posterior divisions on the right, and they become

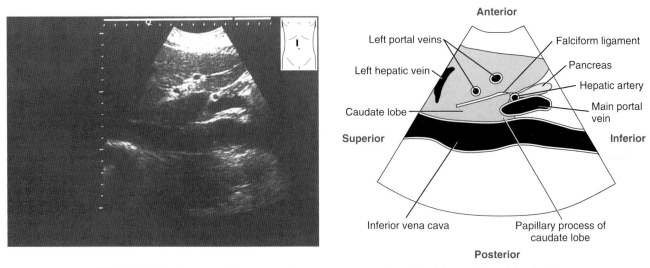

FIGURE 14-12 Parasagittal scanning plane image just to the right of the midline of the body, demonstrating the origin of the main portal vein. Note the papillary process of the caudate lobe.

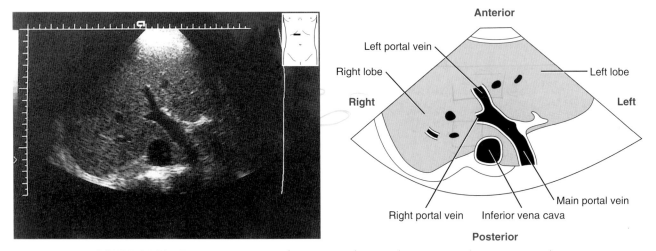

FIGURE 14-13 Transverse scanning plane image showing the main portal vein entering the porta hepatis just anterior to the inferior vena cava and then dividing into right and left branches.

intrasegmental. The main and **right portal veins** traverse and supply the bulk of the liver centrally with blood from the gastrointestinal tract for processing. The left portal vein ascends anteriorly, proximal to the falciform ligament. In patients with severe portal hypertension the left portal vein enters the falciform ligament and communicates with the recanalized ligamentum teres, which had been the postnatally obliterated umbilical vein. The caudate lobe is supplied with blood from the right and left portal veins.

The liver is supplied via the **common hepatic artery,** a branch of the celiac axis of the aorta. The common hepatic artery pursues a horizontal course to the right and branches into the gastroduodenal (GDA) artery and proper hepatic artery (PHA). The **proper hepatic artery** courses superiorly, supplying the liver via the right,

middle, and left hepatic arteries. The cystic artery feeds the gallbladder after it branches from the right hepatic artery. The right gastric artery, which supplies the right side of the lesser curvature of the stomach, can originate from the gastroduodenal artery, common hepatic artery, or proper hepatic artery.

Peritoneal ligaments connect the liver to upper abdominal structures. The coronary ligament connects the posterosuperior surface of the liver to the diaphragm at the margins of the bare area. The bare area separates and lies between the right posterior **subphrenic space** above the posterior **subhepatic space (Morison's pouch)** below (Figure 14-15). The upper layer of the coronary ligament extends from the superior liver surface to the inferior surface of the diaphragm. The lower layer extends from the posterior surface of the right lobe of

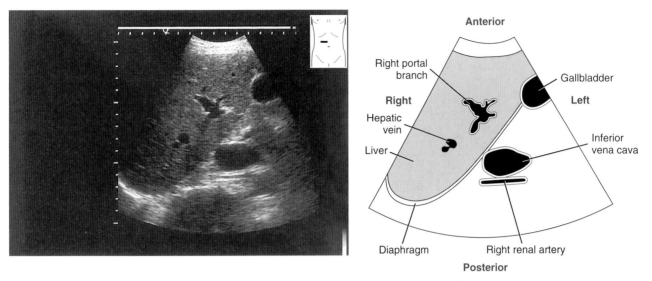

FIGURE 14-14 Transverse scanning plane image showing the right portal vein. Note the longitudinal section of the right renal artery coursing posteriorly to the axial section of the inferior vena cava.

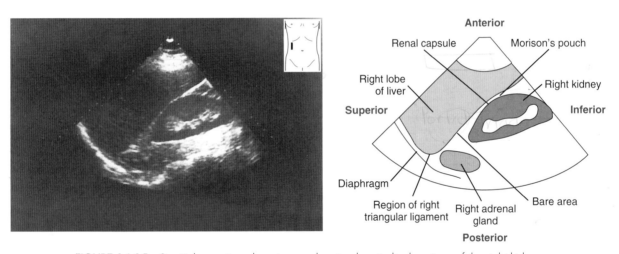

FIGURE 14-15 Sagittal scanning plane image showing longitudinal sections of the right kidney and right adrenal gland in contact with the bare area of the liver. Observe how the anterior kidney surface is separated from the posterior liver surface by Morison's pouch, a peritoneal space that is not specifically appreciated sonographically unless it is abnormally filled with fluid. The bright, thin, curved line seen between the liver and kidney is the fibrous renal capsule.

the liver to the right kidney, the right adrenal gland, and the IVC.

The right triangular ligament is formed by an extension of the coronary ligament inferiorly to the right. It begins at the right margin of the bare area and connects the posterior surface of the right lobe to the right undersurface of the diaphragm. The posterior subphrenic and posterior subhepatic spaces, separated by the bare area medially, become continuous, lateral to the right triangular ligament.

The left triangular ligament is an extension of the falciform ligament to the left. As the falciform ligament passes over the liver dome, it divides into 2 leaflets. The left leaflet forms a portion of the left triangular ligament. The right leaflet merges with the coronary ligament. It connects the posterior surface of the left lobe to the left aspect of the diaphragm. The triangular and coronary ligaments are not normally visualized on ultrasound examinations.

The falciform ligament connects the liver to the anterior abdominal wall and to the diaphragm. The attachment extends from the superior surface of the liver at the umbilical notch to the inferior surface at the porta hepatis (Figure 14-16). The right, anterior, and superior

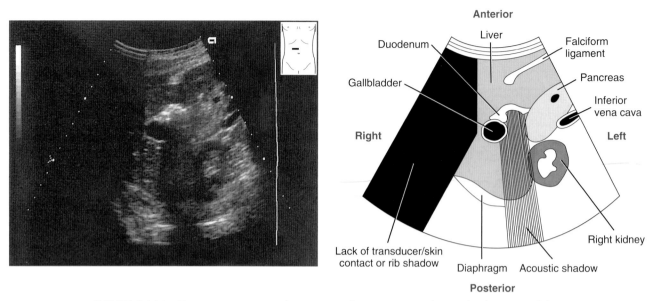

FIGURE 14-16   Transverse scanning plane image demonstrating a longitudinal section of the falciform ligament coursing toward the anterior abdominal wall. Observe the characteristic sickle shape.

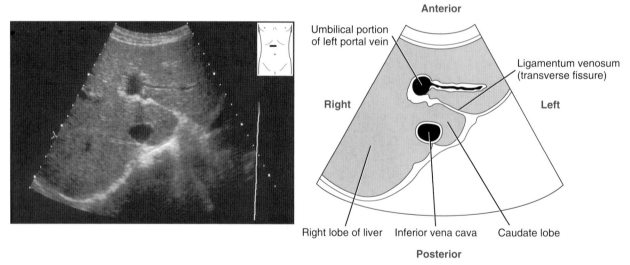

FIGURE 14-17   Transverse scanning plane image that shows the transverse fissure (ligamentum venosum) coursing toward the left portal vein, marking the anterior border of the caudate lobe.

surfaces unite to form the convex upper surface of the liver. The posterior surface is a continuation of that surface.

The lesser omentum is a mesentery or double layer of peritoneum that joins the lesser curvature of the stomach and the proximal duodenum to the liver. The lesser omentum contains the gastrohepatic and **hepatoduodenal ligaments**.

The gastrohepatic ligament is the portion of the lesser omentum that extends across the **transverse**

fissure (fissure for the ligamentum venosum) of the liver at the porta hepatis to the lesser curvature of the stomach. The lesser omentum separates the lesser sac from the gastrohepatic recess.

The ligamentum venosum marks the left anterolateral border of the caudate lobe (Figure 14-17). The lateral segment of the left lobe is separated from the caudate lobe by the fissure for the ligamentum venosum. The ligamentum venosum is a remnant of the fetal ductus venosus, which shunted oxygenated blood

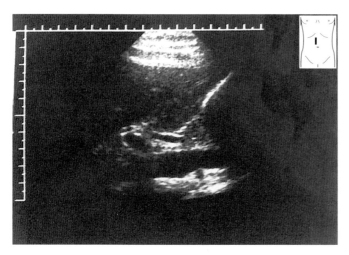

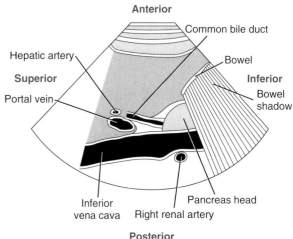

FIGURE 14-18 Sagittal scanning plane image demonstrating a longitudinal section of the common bile duct coursing inferiorly to the head of the pancreas (this is at the level of the hepatoduodenal ligament).

from the umbilical vein to the IVC. The transverse fissure for the ligamentum venosum contains the gastrohepatic ligament.

The hepatoduodenal ligament is the portion of the lesser omentum that extends as the right free border of the gastrohepatic ligament to the proximal duodenum and the right hepatic flexure of the colon. The hepatoduodenal ligament marks the right ventral border of the lesser omentum. Portions of the common bile duct and the hepatic artery are often visualized on transverse scanning plane images at the level of the hepatoduodenal ligament, just superior to the head of the pancreas and adjacent to the porta hepatis. The **porta hepatis** is the opening of the liver through which the portal veins and hepatic arteries enter and the hepatic ducts exit. The common bile duct and hepatic artery course anteriorly to the portal vein in the portal triad at this level. The common bile duct is the anterolateral vessel. It then passes posteriorly to the duodenum and enters the pancreas (Figure 14-18).

PHYSIOLOGY

The liver is a primary center of metabolism, supporting multiple body systems and activities. In support of the digestive and excretory systems the liver metabolizes fats, carbohydrates, and proteins and forms bile and urea. The hepatic parenchyma is composed of hepatocytes, interspersed with Kupffer cells, and organized into lobules approximately 1 by 2 mm in size. Typically, there are approximately 1 million lobules within the liver. Peripherally around each lobule are several portal triads, each containing portal venules, bile ductules, and hepatic arterioles. Portal venules carry blood from the gastrointestinal tract for cleansing and synthesis to the hepatocyte. Bile ductules carry substances including

waste material from the hepatocyte. This substance will eventually comprise bile and be stored in the gallbladder until activated by food in the duodenum (see Chapter 15). Hepatic arterioles carry oxygenated blood to the hepatocyte for nourishment.

Kupffer cells protect the hepatocytes by engulfing toxic or harmful substances, including ethanol from alcohol ingestion. The importance of this cell function is still being studied. One research study reports that the activation of Kupffer cells may reduce liver damage from hepatocarcinoma, ethanol ingestion, or other toxic agents. The amazing durability of the liver, despite the repeated onslaught of harmful substances or presence of disease, may be due in part to the activity of the Kupffer cells.

Principal functions of the liver may be categorized as metabolic, protective, secretory, formative, or miscellaneous.

Metabolic Functions of the Liver

Metabolic functions of the liver involve uptake of body nutrients, such as carbohydrates, amino acids or proteins, fats, and vitamins. The liver serves as a storage site for these substances, performs metabolic conversions of these substances into nutrients, and subsequently releases them into the blood and bile vessels.

The liver absorbs intestinal splanchnic and venous blood received from the portal veins—which drain the digestive tract, the pancreas, and the spleen—and receives a second supply of arterial blood from the hepatic artery and a branch of the superior mesenteric artery. The liver is a dual circulatory system, receiving blood from the gastrointestinal tract via the portal vein for processing and receiving blood for organ function from the proper hepatic artery and its branches.

The venous blood contains products of digestion, such as amino acids and glucose. The liver uses glucose to metabolize carbohydrates. For carbohydrate metabolism, the liver breaks down, stores, and manufactures simple sugars, which the body uses as a primary source of energy.

- Carbohydrate metabolism in the liver involves the processes of glycogenesis, the formation and storage of glycogen, a polysaccharide; glycogenolysis, the conversion of glycogen into its essential nutrient, glucose; and the release of glucose into the bloodstream. Diabetes mellitus is a commonly identified disease characterized by high levels of glucose measured in the blood.
- Protein metabolism results in the synthesis of amino acids into proteins. Proteins serve a variety of functions in the structure and metabolism of the body. Structural proteins are found in hair, muscle, and connective tissue. Enzymes such as those that act as biologic catalysts in metabolic reactions are proteins, as are molecules such as hemoglobin, which transport vital nutrients.
- Fat metabolism in the liver is a process involving the synthesis of fatty acids from carbohydrates. Fat is absorbed from fatty acids and desaturated in the liver. Ketones are intermediary products formed during this process. Fat metabolism results in the formation of cholesterol and phospholipids. Phospholipids are structural components of cell membranes that protect a cell's contents from its environment.

Cholesterol is a major component of the bile that is secreted by the liver and serves to emulsify fats. Cholesterol is a steroid present in many food products, such as eggs, dairy products, oils, fats, and meats; it is present in all tissues, most abundantly in nervous and glandular tissue and the brain.

The presence of cholesterol in the bile is a result of its solubility in the presence of bile salts and the phospholipid lecithin. These substances, along with the bile pigments bilirubin (reddish) and biliverdin (greenish), are the primary components of bile. If either the lecithin or bile salts are deficient, cholesterol may precipitate, or separate, out of the solution and form gallstones, which may accumulate in the gallbladder or obstruct the common bile duct. In patients with bile duct obstruction, excessive bile pigments may appear in the blood and result in jaundice, a yellow discoloration of the skin, sclerae of the eyes, and mucous membranes. Approximately 1 pint of bile is secreted each day.

The secretion of bile is a major secretory function of the liver. Bile is secreted continuously by the liver and passes from the liver through the hepatic ducts into the common bile duct and empties into the duodenum as food is digested. When the duodenum is empty, bile backs up into the gallbladder, where the organic substances are concentrated and stored.

Additional metabolic functions of the liver include the storage of minerals and vitamins, formation of vitamin A, metabolism of steroid hormones, and degradation and detoxification of drugs such as alcohol and barbiturates.

Detoxification of Poisonous and Harmful Substances

Another protective function of the liver is the detoxification of poisonous and harmful substances absorbed by the intestine. This process may include the conversion of harmful substances, such as ammonia, a waste product of protein metabolism, into useful or excretable substances, such as the amino acid arginine and urea. Arginine is a useful amino acid, and urea is a waste product that is excreted.

Synthesizing Blood Proteins

The liver synthesizes the blood proteins *albumin*, *fibrinogen*, *prothrombin*, and *globulins*. The synthesis of blood plasma proteins, which include albumin and various globulins, is a formative function of the liver. Prothrombin and fibrinogen are blood-clotting factors. The synthesis of heparin, an anticoagulant, also takes place in the liver.

Additional Liver Functions

The liver stores vitamins and other metabolic substances. It also regulates blood volume and acts as a reservoir for blood that is released as it regulates blood volume and blood flow through the body. Additionally, the liver serves as a major source of body heat as a result of the many hepatocellular chemical reactions that take place within it.

SONOGRAPHIC APPEARANCE

The normal liver should appear homogeneous and moderately echogenic throughout. A boundary between the left and right hepatic lobes can be imagined along a line coursing posteriorly from the gallbladder fossa to the groove for the IVC. This line is the main lobar fissure. This fissure is identified sonographically along a right lateral, sagittal oblique scanning plane and extends a short but variable distance between the long axis section of the neck of the gallbladder and the axial or short axis section of the right portal vein. The main lobar fissure appears as a thin, bright line connecting the gallbladder neck to the portal vein (Figure 14-19).

Many landmark structures are visible on a sagittal scanning plane image showing the long axis of the IVC. Cephalad (superiorly) to caudad (inferiorly), one should see, anterior to the IVC, the following structures: the right atrium, the central leaf of the diaphragm superior to the left hepatic lobe, the middle hepatic vein as

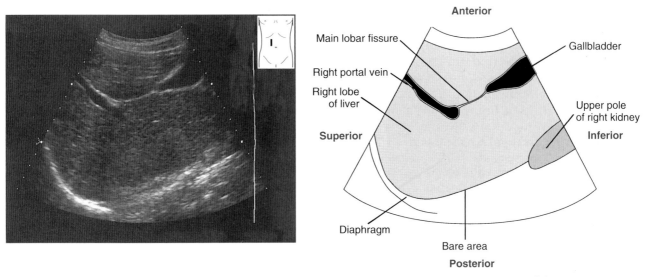

FIGURE 14-19 Sagittal scanning plane image that shows how the longitudinal section of the main lobar fissure appears as an echogenic line connecting the neck of the gallbladder to the right portal vein.

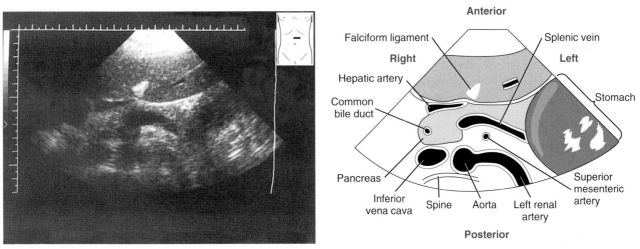

FIGURE 14-20 Transverse scanning plane image of the midepigastrium. Note the axial section of the falciform ligament and its characteristic pyramidal shape. This echogenic focus is also referred to as the round ligament or ligamentum teres at this level.

it enters the vena cava, the caudate lobe of the liver separated from the lateral left lobe by the ligamentum venosum, the extrahepatic main portal vein in cross-section, and the head of the pancreas in cross-section. The superior mesenteric vein may be seen coursing toward its junction with the splenic vein at the portal confluence. The left portal vein may be visualized on its C-shaped superior course, proximal to the falciform ligament.

Ligaments and fissures are demonstrated as highly echogenic because of the presence of collagen and fat within and around these structures. The attachment of the falciform ligament from the upper surfaces of the liver to the diaphragm and the upper abdominal wall appears to divide the right and left lobes. It represents the lower margin of peritoneum surrounding the ligamentum teres, or round ligament, of the liver. The falciform ligament is highly echogenic, appearing sickle shaped in longitudinal sections and pyramidal in axial sections (Figure 14-20). Falciform

The **round ligament (ligamentum teres)** is the obliterated umbilical vein, a fibrous cord that extends upward from the diaphragm to the anterior abdominal wall. On transverse scans, it most often is identifiable coursing within the lower margin of the falciform ligament. These structures lie close to the anterior midline surface of the body and within the near field of the transducer. They are displayed on the upper midportion of the screen.

The echogenic falciform ligament courses anteroinferiorly from the left portal vein toward the umbilicus. Transverse scans through the liver frequently demonstrate an echogenic focus in the area of the falciform ligament. This structure correlates the sonographic appearance of the falciform ligament with its appearance on computed tomographic (CT) scans, although it may be prominent enough to raise the suspicion of a solid mass. The presence of a recanalized umbilical vein within the falciform ligament should be looked for in patients with portal hypertension.

The main portal vein is visualized at its origin, posteroinferior to the neck of the pancreas. Identification of the porta hepatis is possible by identifying the main portal vein anterior to the IVC and then moving slightly cephalad. The main portal vein can be seen entering the porta hepatis, where it divides into a smaller, more anterior and more superior left portal vein and a larger, more posterior and more inferior right portal vein. Portal veins are surrounded by bright echogenic walls due to the thick collagenous tissue in the walls. Portal veins decrease in size as they approach the diaphragm. The Doppler flow signal of a portal vein is normally continuous, monophasic, and exhibits low velocity, usually between 20 and 40 cm/s. Abnormally prominent pulsatility may be observed in patients with right heart failure, tricuspid regurgitation, fistula between a hepatic and portal vein, or portal hypertension.

The junction of the right and left portal veins is noted on a superiorly angled transverse scanning plane image just inferior to the plane that demonstrates the convergence of the 3 hepatic veins on the IVC. This level also identifies the location of the union of the left and right hepatic ducts to form the proximal portion of the common duct, the common hepatic duct. The common hepatic duct can be followed medially, anterior to the right portal vein. This is the recommended location for measuring the common hepatic duct. Any measurement greater than 5 mm raises the possibility of biliary obstruction.

The hepatic veins increase in size as they drain toward the diaphragm and IVC. Any large vein in the liver near the diaphragm may be considered a hepatic vein. Normal Doppler flow signals in the hepatic veins demonstrate a triphasic waveform. There are several (additional) features that distinguish hepatic veins from portal veins. Hepatic veins course between lobes and segments, whereas portal veins course within segments. Hepatic veins drain toward the right atrium and usually have indistinct, anechoic borders, except near the IVC, where the venous walls appear more reflective. The positions of the hepatic veins can therefore be used to identify the segments of the liver and provide precise descriptions of focal abnormalities.

Identification of hepatic segments is important in localizing potentially resectable lesions of the liver. Lesions of this type include primary hepatic neoplasms, single metastatic lesions, and some nonmalignant hepatic abnormalities (Figure 14-21).

Posterior to the IVC on parasagittal scans, the anechoic right renal artery is seen in short axis, anterior to the right linear crus of the diaphragm noted with very low-level echoes. Any other solid-appearing mass

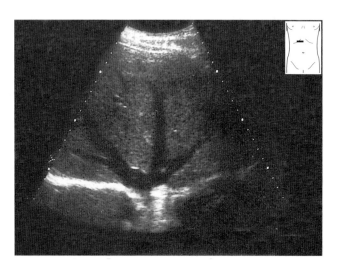
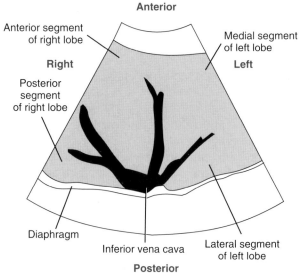

FIGURE 14-21 Transverse scanning plane image demonstrating longitudinal sections of the hepatic veins draining into the axial section of the inferior vena cava; providing sonographic segmentation of the hepatic lobes.

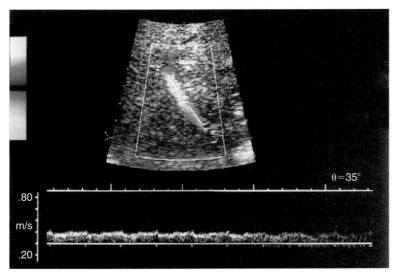

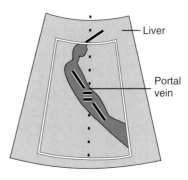
Liver

Portal vein

θ=35°

.80

m/s

.20

FIGURE 14-22 Color-flow Doppler image showing the characteristic waveform of a normal portal vein. Note that the blood flow is in the direction of the liver toward the transducer.

posterior to the IVC and inferior to the liver suggests the presence of enlarged lymph nodes or adrenal lesions.

SONOGRAPHIC APPLICATIONS

Ultrasound examinations of the liver are indicated for the following:

- Suspected liver enlargement
- Suspected hepatic or perihepatic masses
- Suspected abscesses
- Suspected obstructive or metastatic lesions
- Cystic, solid, and complex masses, which are routinely identifiable because they can distort the smooth contour of the liver
- Abnormal lesions, which are usually hyperechoic or hypoechoic compared with the appearance of normal liver parenchyma
- Pleural effusions, which may be visualized in the subdiaphragmatic (subphrenic) region superior to the liver capsule
- Ascites, identifiable when fluid collects in the subcapsular or intraperitoneal spaces surrounding the liver

fluid in abdomen

Duplex abdominal and color-flow Doppler are used to assess the following:

- Vascular structures of the liver and porta hepatis, such as the portal vein, hepatic arteries and veins, and the splenic artery and vein (Figures 14-22 and 14-23). The presence, direction, and blood flow velocity in a sample volume are evaluated with these examinations.
- Portal hypertension
- Portal or hepatic vein thrombosis
- Preoperative and postoperative hepatic surgery. For example, in some patients with cirrhotic liver disease and variceal hemorrhages, interventional

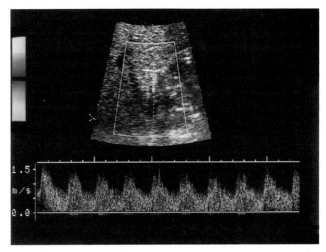

1.5

m/s

0.0

FIGURE 14-23 Color-flow Doppler image demonstrating the characteristic arterial waveform of the normal hepatic artery.

radiologists surgically place a permanent shunt between the hepatic vein and intrahepatic portal vein to prevent bleeding of gastroesophageal varices. This placement is designed to divert blood around the liver, thereby relieving portal hypertension by reducing portal vein pressure. The procedure is known as placement of a TIPS (transjugular intrahepatic portosystemic) shunt. Color Doppler ultrasound evaluation of the direction and flow of the portal vein in a patient with a TIPS shunt is commonly performed before and after the procedure (Figures 14-24 to 14-26). Preoperative screening helps determine whether a patient is a candidate for a TIPS shunt. The portal vein, hepatic artery, and hepatic veins are evaluated for patency and flow direction. A TIPS shunt is contraindicated in any patient with portal vein

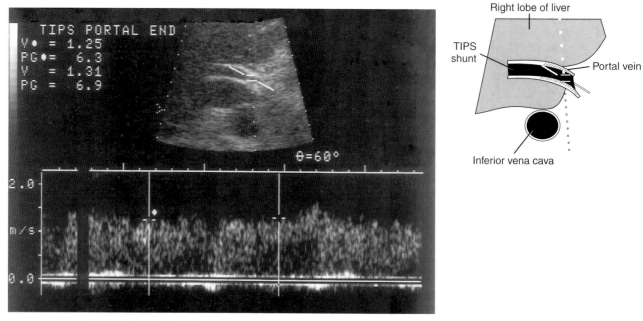

FIGURE 14-24 Oblique transverse scanning plane image of a liver section to evaluate the proximal portal end of the TIPS shunt after placement.

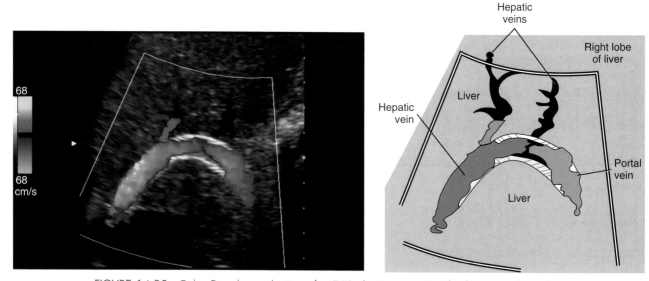

FIGURE 14-25 Color Doppler evaluation of a TIPS shunt connecting the hepatic vein to the intrahepatic portal vein. Note that the color blue represents flow away from the transducer (hepatic vein) and the color red represents flow moving toward the transducer (portal vein).

thrombosis. The postoperative evaluation assesses how well the patient responds to the treatment.

• Tumor invasion of the portal vein, which may be observed in cases of hepatocellular carcinoma and with metastases. To differentiate tumor invasion from portal vein thrombosis, color Doppler can be used to demonstrate tumor vascularity presenting with low-resistance arterial signals within the portal vein lesion.

• Donors for partial liver transplant and in patients before and after liver transplant. Complications in complete and partial liver transplant patients can include hepatic artery thrombosis, pseudoaneurysm and rupture, and/or hepatic vein stenosis. Acute liver

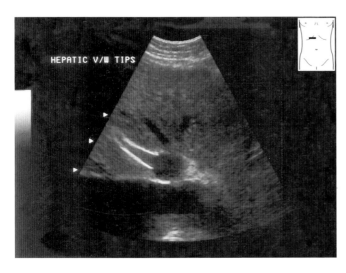
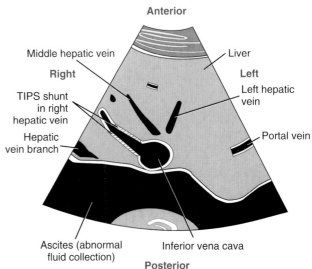

FIGURE 14-26 Transverse scanning plane image showing an axial section of the liver at the level of the hepatic veins draining into the inferior vena cava. Observe the highly reflective terminal end of the TIPS shunt within the right hepatic vein.

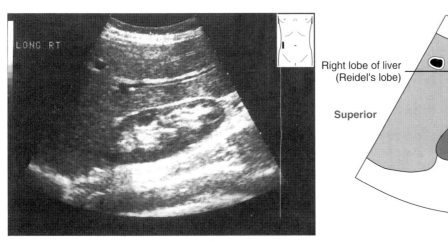
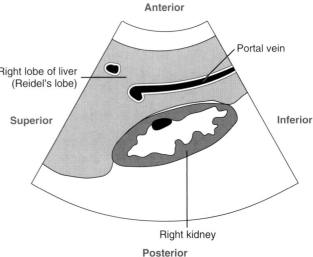

FIGURE 14-27 Sagittal scanning plane image of a woman with Reidel's lobe, a tongue-like extension of the right lobe of the liver. This Reidel's lobe extends inferiorly to the iliac crest.

failure can be caused by acute rejection or hepatic artery thrombosis. Biliary complication has also been noted in up to 10% of adult liver transplant patients; it is more frequent in pediatric liver transplant patients. Other complications include fluid collections and post-transplant lymphoproliferative disorder.

NORMAL VARIANTS

- **Reidel's lobe**: A tongue-like inferior extension of the right lobe, as far caudally as the iliac crest (Figure 14-27). It has the same sonographic appearance as normal liver parenchyma. On ultrasound this variant can be identified when liver tissue extends well below the inferior pole of the right kidney during normal respiration.
- **Distal papillary process of the caudate lobe**: May be confused with an enlarged lymph node or another extrahepatic lesion. This process appears as a rounded prominence on the anteroinferior aspect of the caudate, or it may appear as a separate structure. It has the same sonographic appearance as normal liver parenchyma.
- **Elongated left lobe**: Has a tip that can extend left laterally, all the way to the spleen. The sonographic appearance is the same as the normal liver.

REFERENCE CHARTS

■■■ ASSOCIATED PHYSICIANS

- **Gastroenterologist:** Specializes in treating diseases of the gastrointestinal tract, including the stomach, small and large bowel, gallbladder, and bile ducts.
- **Internist:** Specializes in studying the physiology and pathology of internal organs and diagnosing and treating disorders of those organs.
- **Oncologist:** Specializes in the study and treatment of tumors and malignancies.
- **Radiologist:** Specializes in the diagnostic interpretation of imaging modalities that assess the liver.
- **Surgeon:** Utilizes operative procedures to treat diseases, trauma, and organ deformity.
- **Vascular specialist:** Studies and treats disorders of blood vessels.

■■■ COMMON DIAGNOSTIC TESTS

- **Computed tomography (CT):** This x-ray examination utilizes a narrow collimated beam of x-rays that rotate around the patient in a continuous 360-degree arc in order to image the body in cross-sectional slices. The image is created by a digital computer that calculates attenuation or tissue absorption of the x-ray beams. Very small differences in density of body structures may be demonstrated and are displayed on x-ray film. The examination is performed by radiologic technologists who specialize in computed tomography and is interpreted by radiologists.
- **Angiography:** This examination utilizes x-rays to visualize the internal structure of the heart and blood vessels after the injection of a contrast medium into an artery or vein. The contrast material is inserted into a peripheral artery via a catheter, which is then threaded through the vessel to a visceral site. Angiograms are performed by radiologists and assisted by radiologic technologists. The examination is interpreted by the radiologist.
- **Magnetic resonance imaging (MR, MRI):** The MR scanner surrounds the patient with powerful electromagnets that create a magnetic field. Hydrogen atoms in the patient's body are disturbed by this field. The atoms' protons become aligned in the direction of the magnetic field's poles. The computers process and measure the speed and volume with which the protons return to their normal state and display a diagnostic image of striking clarity on a monitor. Intravenous contrast materials may be given to enhance image definition. MR produces cross-sectional and sagittal soft tissue images. The examinations are performed by registered radiologic technologists and interpreted by radiologists. Physicists assist radiologists in the MR laboratory because of the complexity of the MR equipment.
- **Radionuclide scintigraphy:** Scintigraphy utilizes a gamma camera to detect radioactive substances given intravenously or by mouth. Scintigraphy commences when the radioisotope reaches optimum activity in the part being examined. For liver studies this begins immediately after injection. A technetium sulfur colloid is the radionuclide used in liver studies. Recording devices convert voltage impulses received from the scanner into a paper or x-ray film record of a series of dots that reflect the radiation intensities received. Abnormalities are indicated by an absence of activity. The examinations are performed by certified nuclear medicine technologists. They are interpreted by radiologists or nuclear physicians.
- **Liver biopsy:** A needle is inserted into the RUQ to remove a sample of liver tissue for microscopic evaluation. This examination assesses severity of liver cell damage and is performed by a radiologist.

■■■ LABORATORY VALUES

Test	Normal	Increase	Decrease
LIVER FUNCTION TESTS			
Albumin	3.3 to 4.5 g/dL	Hemolytic anemia	Liver damage
Bilirubin	Adult indirect ≤1.1 mg/dL	Jaundice, liver damage, obstruction	
	Adult direct <0.5 mg/dL		
Alkaline phosphatase (ALP)	1.5 to 4.5 BU/dL	Metastases	
	0.8 to 2.9 BLB	Obstruction	
	Unit	Lesions	
		Jaundice	
AST (SGOT)	5 to 30 U/L	Hepatitis	
		Liver injury	
		Jaundice	
		Cholestasis	
		Myocardial infarction	
		Muscle disease	
		Cirrhosis	
		Metastases	
		Fatty liver	
		Lymphoma	

▪▪▪ LABORATORY VALUES—cont'd

Test	Normal	Increase	Decrease
ALT (SGPT)	6 to 37 U/L	Jaundice	
		Hepatitis	
Beta globulin	0.7 to 1.2 g/dL	Fatty liver	Liver disease
			Cancer
Cholesterol	140 to 200 mg/dL	Gamma globulin	0.5 to 1.6 g/dL
Lactic dehydrogenase (LDH)	100 to 225 U/L	Liver disease	
	180 to 280 U/L	Cancer	
Protein	6.6 to 7.8 g/dL	Chronic liver disease	
Prothrombin			
Time (PTT)	11 to 15 seconds	Liver disease	
1—Forward			
2—Reverse			

▪▪▪ VASCULATURE

Vessel	Branch of	Supplies
ARTERIAL SYSTEM		
Common hepatic artery	Celiac artery	Liver
Proper hepatic artery	Common hepatic	Liver
Right hepatic artery	Proper hepatic	Right lobe
		Right caudate
Left hepatic artery	Proper hepatic (may arise from left gastric artery)	Left lobe
		Quadrate lobe
		Left caudate

Vessel	Tributary to	Drains
VENOUS SYSTEM		
Central veins	Hepatic veins	Sinusoids
Right hepatic vein	Inferior vena cava	Right lobe
Middle hepatic vein	Inferior vena cava	Right lobe
		Caudate lobe
Left hepatic vein	Inferior vena cava	Left lobe
		Quadrate lobe

Vessel	Tributary to	Drains
PORTAL SYSTEM		
Main portal vein		Gastrointestinal tract
Superior mesenteric vein	Portal vein	Gastrointestinal tract
Inferior mesenteric vein	Splenic vein	Gastrointestinal tract
Splenic vein	Portal vein	Spleen
	Pancreas	

▪▪▪ AFFECTING CHEMICALS

Alcohol and other substances, such as certain prescription medications, can be harmful to the liver.

CHAPTER 15

The Biliary System

YONELLA DEMARS, REVA ARNEZ CURRY, AND BETTY BATES TEMPKIN

OBJECTIVES

Describe the gross anatomy of the biliary system.
Describe the basic function of the biliary system.
Describe the ultrasound appearance of the biliary system.

Describe diagnostic tests that may be used to examine the biliary system.

KEY WORDS

Ampulla of Vater (Hepatopancreatic Ampulla) — Dilatation or opening formed by the common bile duct and pancreatic duct(s) as they enter the duodenum, where they empty bile and pancreatic enzymes that assist in the digestive process.

Bile Ducts — Drain the liver of bile.

Bilirubin — A bile pigment. Green when oxidized.

Body — Refers to the middle and main portion of the gallbladder.

Cholecystectomy — Surgical removal of the gallbladder.

Cholecystitis — Condition in which the gallbladder is inflamed. Presents sonographically with edematous, thickened gallbladder walls.

Cholecystokinin (CCK) — Peptide hormone that stimulates the gallbladder to contract and the sphincter of Oddi to relax and increases hepatic production of bile. An injectable form can be used to stimulate the gallbladder during sonographic examination for a type of function test.

Choledochal (Choledochus) Cyst — Normal, localized dilatation of the common bile duct.

Choledocholithiasis — Presence of gallstones in the biliary tract.

Cholelithiasis — Formation or presence of gallstones, which are calcifications in the gallbladder or biliary duct.

Common Bile Duct (CBD) — Distal portion of the biliary duct or common duct. Transports bile from the level of the cystic duct, inferomedially toward the head of the pancreas, and then enters the duodenum and empties the bile to aid in digestion.

Common Duct (CD)/Biliary Duct — Formed by the union of right and left intrahepatic ducts. Serves to transport bile (fluid that aids digestion; manufactured in the liver) from approximately the level of the liver hilum, inferiorly to the gallbladder (stores and concentrates bile) and duodenum to assist digestion. Its proximal portion is called the *common hepatic duct*; distal portion is called the *common bile duct.*

Common Hepatic Duct (CHD) — Proximal portion of the biliary duct or common duct. Transports bile (fluid that aids digestion; manufactured in the liver) inferiorly to the cystic duct that directs the flow of bile it receives directly into the gallbladder. Continues inferiorly as the distal portion of the common duct known as the *common bile duct.*

Cystic Duct — Directs the flow of bile it receives from the common hepatic duct directly into the neck of the gallbladder.

Extrahepatic — Outside of or not enclosed by liver tissue.

Fundus — Refers to the inferior, widest portion of the gallbladder.

Gallbladder — Bile reservoir on the posteroinferior surface of the liver. Has three descriptive divisions: fundus, body, and neck. The fundus is the "bottom" of the pouch. The middle and main portion of the gallbladder is the body, and the narrower area leading into the cystic duct is the neck.

Gallbladder Fossa — Indentation located on the posteroinferior portion of the right lobe of the liver where the gallbladder is situated.

Hartmann's Pouch — A small sacculation (outpouching) in the area of the gallbladder neck. Named after Henri Hartmann, a French surgeon (1860–1952). The term *infundibulum* is also applied to this sacculation, which some consider an abnormality and others consider just an oddity.

Hepatic Ducts (Right, Left) — Right and left intrahepatic ducts or tubules that direct the bile produced in the liver to the biliary duct. The ducts join at approximately the level of the liver hilum to form the biliary duct or common duct (CD).

Hepatic Portal System — System responsible for venous drainage of the gastrointestinal tract, including the spleen, pancreas, and gallbladder. Blood is conveyed from these organs via the portal vein to the liver. The portal vein subdivides until the blood reaches the hepatic sinusoids. Blood therefore passes through two sets of "exchange" vessels: the capillaries within the organs of the gastrointestinal tract, the spleen, pancreas, and gallbladder, and the hepatic sinusoids. From the sinusoids, blood converges into hepatic veins and finally the inferior vena cava (IVC) before returning to the heart.

Hilum — Indention, depression, or pit on an organ forming a doorway or area of entrance and exit for vessels, ducts, and nerves; sometimes called *hilus.*

Infraduodenal Common Bile Duct — Portion of the common bile duct inferior to the duodenum.

Intraduodenal Common Bile Duct — Portion of the common bile duct within the duodenum.

KEY WORDS—cont'd

Intrahepatic — Completely or partially enclosed in liver tissue.

Liver Function Tests — A collection of laboratory tests that indicates how the liver is functioning or performing.

Neck — Refers to the narrow portion of the gallbladder that is connected to the cystic duct.

Polyps — Protruding growth or mass from a mucous membrane.

Porta Hepatis — Also known as the liver hilum or doorway giving entrance and exit to hepatic vessels, ducts, and nerves.

Portal Triad — Intrahepatic bile ducts run alongside portal veins and hepatic arteries in a portal triad, surrounded by connective tissue and radiating through the lobes and segments of the liver. Intrahepatic ducts join to form right and left hepatic ducts that join near the porta hepatis to form the biliary duct or common duct. The distal portion of the common duct, the common bile duct along with the main portal vein and proper hepatic artery, form an extrahepatic portal triad.

Portal Vein — The gateway through which blood returning from the gastrointestinal tract and accessory organs passes before returning to the heart.

Proper Hepatic Artery — Branch of the common hepatic artery; supplies the gallbladder and the liver.

Retroduodenal Common Bile Duct — Portion of common bile duct that runs behind the duodenum.

Sphincter of Oddi (Oddi's Muscle) — A muscle sheath surrounding the CBD (joined at times by the pancreatic duct) at the ampulla of Vater. Aids in regulating bile flow into the duodenum.

Spiral Valves of Heister — A series of mucosal folds within the lumen of the cystic duct.

Supraduodenal Common Bile Duct — Portion of common bile duct superior to the duodenum.

■ ■ ■ NORMAL MEASUREMENTS

Anatomy	Measurement
Gallbladder	8 to 12 cm long 3 to 5 cm diameter
Gallbladder wall	3 mm thick
Right and left hepatic ducts	0.5 to 2.5 cm long (left is longer than right) 0.1 to 0.2 cm diameter
Common hepatic duct	2.0 to 6.5 cm long 0.1 to 0.2 cm diameter
Common bile duct	5 to 15 cm long 0.1 to 0.7 cm diameter
Cystic duct	0.5 to 0.8 cm long 0.1 to 0.4 cm diameter

The biliary system is intimately associated with the liver and pancreas. It consists of the **gallbladder**, acting as a reservoir for bile, and the **bile ducts** that drain the liver of bile. The bile duct and pancreatic duct(s) may join and form one duct or remain separate and enter the duodenum together, where they empty bile and pancreatic enzymes to assist the digestive process. The pancreas and associated ducts are the focus of Chapter 16.

The basic function of the biliary system is to drain the liver of bile and then store the bile until it is needed to aid digestion. As mentioned, the gallbladder acts as the storage receptacle for bile, and the various ducts provide a place to which the bile flows. The gallbladder concentrates the bile by secreting mucus and absorbing water. For a review of bile production, see the discussion of the liver in Chapter 14.

LOCATION
Gallbladder

The **gallbladder fossa** (or indentation) is located on the posteroinferior portion of the right lobe of the liver where the gallbladder is situated (Table 15-1). This fossa or bed is closely related to the main lobar fissure of the liver (Figure 15-1). Typically, the gallbladder is not totally surrounded by hepatic tissue; however, it is possible for this to occur. An **intrahepatic** gallbladder will be totally (or almost totally) enclosed in liver tissue.

Due to its long mesentery, the gallbladder will change location as the patient changes position. A gallbladder found to be just at the inferior border of the right lobe of the liver with the patient supine may then be found to have shifted closer to the midline when the patient is placed on the left side with the right side raised. This patient repositioning is known as the *left lateral decubitus* (LLD) or *left lateral oblique* (LLO) positions.

Some imagers believe that by simply bending the right arm 90 degrees at the elbow and then placing that hand over the midline, the location of the gallbladder may be estimated—with the gallbladder being in the area of the wrist. This method is not particularly accurate but it does give a rough idea of the location of the gallbladder.

Bile from the liver reaches the gallbladder through the hepatic ducts, the proximal portion of the common duct (the common hepatic duct), and the cystic duct.

Hepatic Ducts

The left and right intrahepatic ducts join at approximately the level of the liver **hilum** (also called the **porta hepatis**, or doorway) to form the **biliary duct** or **common duct (CD)**. The *proximal portion* of the CD is referred to as the common hepatic duct; the *distal portion* is the common bile duct (Figure 15-2).

■ ■ ■ **Table 15-1** Location of Gallbladder and Biliary Tract Routinely Visualized With Ultrasound

	Rt and Lt Hepatic Ducts	Common Hepatic Duct	Cystic Duct	Common Bile Duct	Gallbladder (location variable)
Anterior to	Portal vein, rt branch hepatic artery	PHA, portal vein, IVC	Portal vein	PHA, portal vein, IVC	Superior portion rt kidney
Posterior to	Liver, peritoneum	Liver, peritoneum	Liver, peritoneum	Liver, superior portion duodenum, peritoneum, GDA	Peritoneum (inferior surface, fundus), transverse colon (fundus)
Superior to	CHD, CBD, cystic duct, duodenum, pancreas	Cystic duct, CBD, GDA	CBD	Superior portion duodenum, pancreas head	
Inferior to		Rt and lt hepatic ducts, liver	CHD	CHA, cystic duct, superior portion duodenum	Rt branch portal vein, liver's main lobar fissure, rt lobe liver, ninth costal cartilage (fundus)
Medial to	Liver rt lateral lobe	Cystic duct, liver rt lateral lobe	Liver rt lateral lobe, GB neck	Cystic duct, duodenum	
Lt lateral to					
Rt lateral to	CHA, liver caudate lobe, duodenum, pancreas	CHA, GDA	CHD, CBD	Pancreas head, terminal pancreatic duct, PHA, CHA, superior portion duodenum	Cystic duct (neck), rt branch portal vein

CBD, Common bile duct; **CHA,** common hepatic artery; **CHD,** common hepatic duct; **GB,** gallbladder; **GDA,** gastroduodenal artery; **IVC,** inferior vena cava; **PHA,** proper hepatic artery.

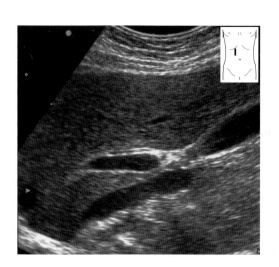
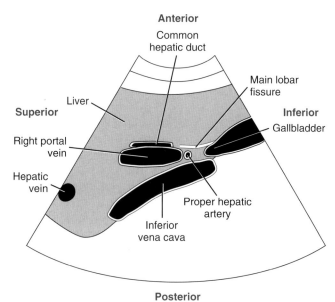

FIGURE 15-1 **Main Lobar Fissure.** Note the location of the gallbladder and how it relates to the main lobar fissure.

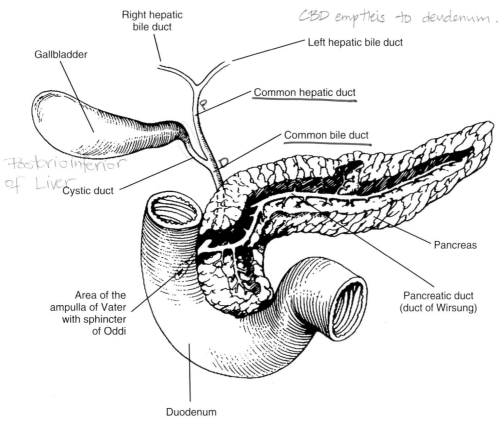

Gallbladder and biliary tract, including the pancreatic duct, and the duodenum.

■ ■ ■ **FIGURE 15-2** Biliary System

Biliary Structure	Location
Gallbladder (GB)	• On posteroinferior surface of the liver • Right kidney may be noted posterior to GB • Near main lobar fissure • Follow main portal vein toward the right to help locate • Easier to locate when distended
Cystic duct (CD)	• Extends from GB neck and meets CHD where CBD begins • Located on posteroinferior surface of liver
Right and left hepatic ducts	• Intrahepatic • Drain right and left lobes of the liver • Located on posterior medial surface of the liver toward the liver hilum • Join at the level of the liver hilum (also known as porta hepatis) to form the biliary duct or common duct
Common hepatic duct (CHD)	• Proximal portion of the common duct • Located on posterior surface of liver • Becomes the common bile duct after receiving the cystic duct from the gallbladder
Common bile duct (CBD)	• Distal portion of the common duct • Extends inferiorly from the union of the CHD and cystic duct to enter the duodenum near the head of the pancreas • Parts of CBD can be described in relationship to the duodenum (i.e., supra-, retro-, infra-, and intraduodenal portions) • Enters duodenum at the ampulla of Vater through sphincter of Oddi muscle • Pancreatic duct from the pancreas can join the CBD in entering the duodenum at the ampulla of Vater

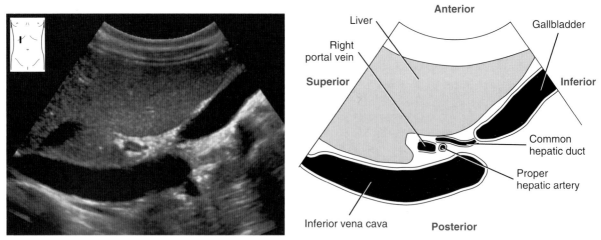

FIGURE 15-3 **Common Hepatic Duct and Right Portal Vein Relationship.** Sagittal scanning plane image demonstrating a longitudinal section of the common hepatic duct seen just anterior to the longitudinal section of the right portal vein and axial section of the proper hepatic artery. The common hepatic duct is often mistaken as the common bile duct, which is located more inferiorly and is more closely associated with the main portal vein.

Common Hepatic Duct (CHD)

The **common hepatic duct (CHD)** extends inferiorly from the liver hilum to the level of the gallbladder neck, where it meets the cystic duct (see Figure 15-2). It is anterior to the right portal vein and proper hepatic artery (Figure 15-3).

Cystic Duct

The **cystic duct** connects the gallbladder to the CHD. It directs the flow of bile it receives from the CHD, directly into the gallbladder.

Common Bile Duct (CBD)

The **common bile duct (CBD)** is the distal or inferior potion of the common duct. It is a continuation of the CHD but decribed separately based on its location and association with adjacent anatomy that is different from the anatomy associated with the CHD. From its origin at the level of the CHD and cystic duct, the CBD runs inferiorly along the right border of the lesser omentum, along the hepatoduodenal ligament; passes posterior to the first portion of the duodenum; passes through or lies on the back of the posterolateral portion of the pancreas head; and enters the posteromedial aspect of the descending portion of the duodenum and terminates. It is anterior and slightly right lateral to the main portal vein and right lateral to the proper and common hepatic arteries (Figure 15-4; see also Figure 15-2).

When referring specifically to the CBD, anatomists use terms that relate its location to the duodenum: *supraduodenal, retroduodenal, infraduodenal, intraduodenal.* The part of the CBD superior to the duodenum is the **supraduodenal** section. As the name implies, the portion posterior to the duodenum is the **retroduodenal** section; the **infraduodenal** portion is inferior to the duodenum; and the part of the CBD within the duodenum is the **intraduodenal** portion (Figure 15-5, *A* and *B*).

The infraduodenal portion of the CBD is the portion previously mentioned that may be located within a groove on the posterolateral portion of the head of the pancreas or pass directly through the head. At this point the CBD either joins the pancreatic duct(s) to form a single duct or remains separate and enters the **ampulla of Vater** (or **hepatopancreatic ampulla**, an opening into the duodenum), where the intraduodenal CBD empties bile to assist in the digestive process. A muscle sheath—known as the **sphincter of Oddi**, or **Oddi's muscle**—surrounds the CBD at the ampulla of Vater. The sphincter of Oddi aids in regulating bile flow into the duodenum.

SIZE
Gallbladder

The overall length of the normal gallbladder is highly variable, depending on the amount of bile within and any existing normal variant. There are times when the gallbladder is simply difficult to see, not because of some structural variation, but because of physiology. For example, a patient who has fasted (not eaten) since midnight prior to an ultrasound examination may present with a bile-filled, easily visualized gallbladder. A patient who has eaten, causing the gallbladder to partially or completely empty to aid digestion, may present with a partially bile-filled, small gallbladder or, a collapsed, bile-free gallbladder, that may appear as nonexistent at first. However, when a patient has fasted correctly for the exam and a bile-filled gallbladder is

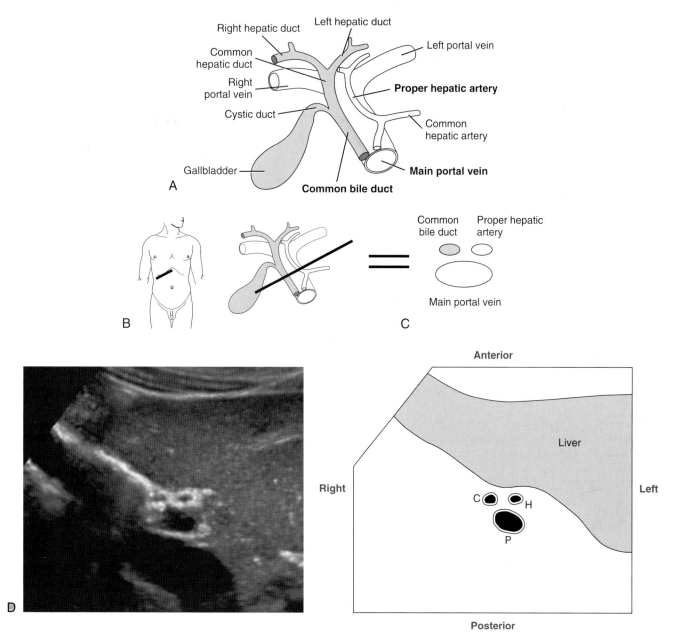

FIGURE 15-4   Portal Vein, Hepatic Artery, and Common Duct Relationship. **A,** Observe how the common duct (common hepatic duct and common bile duct) is anterolateral to the proper hepatic artery. Notice that the proximal common duct, the common hepatic duct, is anterior to the right portal vein branch, and the distal portion of the common duct, the common bile duct, is anterior to the main portion of the portal vein. **B,** In an oblique transverse scanning plane image at approximately the angle of the solid line (approximately the same level as the right costal margin angle), one should see the relationship demonstrated in *C*. **C,** Note that the common bile duct and proper hepatic artery have approximately equal diameter. **D,** Oblique transverse scanning plane image demonstrating "Mickey's Sign," formed by the appearance of the axial sections of the extrahepatic portal triad. *C,* Common bile duct; *H,* proper hepatic artery; *P,* main portal vein.

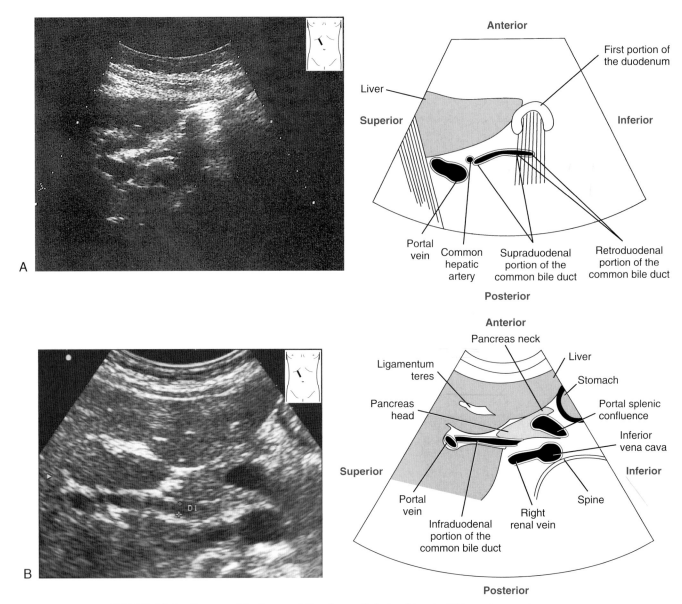

FIGURE 15-5 **Common Bile Duct and Duodenum Relationship. A,** Obliqued sagittal scanning plane image showing a longitudinal section of the supraduodenal and retroduodenal segments of the common bile duct. **B,** Longitudinal section of the infraduodenal segment of the common bile duct in an oblique sagittal scanning plane.

visualized, it is found to have a normal length of approximately 8 to 9 cm in the majority of patients, although some reports have cited gallbladder length as much as 12 cm as measured from the neck to the fundus. Figure 15-6 shows a fully distended gallbladder. The normal gallbladder is approximately 3 to 5 cm in diameter and holds up to approximately 40 mL of bile. To put this amount in perspective, a teaspoon typically holds approximately 5 mL of fluid; therefore the gallbladder holds approximately 8 teaspoons of fluid. Recall that 2.5 cm equals 1 inch; this provides a better picture of the sizes involved when visualizing the biliary system. With

experience, the sonographer discovers that the gallbladder has a wide variety of shapes, sizes, and locations.

The walls of the gallbladder are generally only a few millimeters thick, up to approximately 3 mm. This wall thickness is important to note. Certain conditions, such as **cholecystitis** (inflammation of the gallbladder), may cause the walls to appear edematous and perhaps even greatly thickened. Localized thickening of the gallbladder wall may indicate the presence of a mass or other condition that would call for further investigation. As would be expected, the wall thickness is slightly less when the gallbladder is full or distended (the walls are

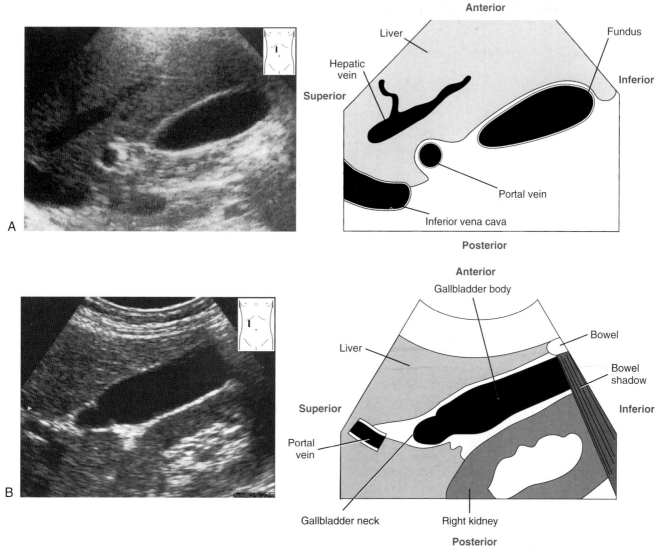

FIGURE 15-6 Distended Gallbladder. A, Gallbladder fundus. Sagittal scanning plane image demonstrating a longitudinal section of the fundus. Notice the proximity of the axial section of the portal vein and longitudinal section of the inferior vena cava; **B,** Gallbladder body and neck. Longitudinal section of the body and neck seen in a sagittal scanning plane. Note the long section of the right kidney seen immediately posterior to the gallbladder.

stretched) as compared with an empty gallbladder, when the walls are slightly thicker.

Common Hepatic Duct (CHD)

The length and inside diameter of the CHD are variable. Schwartz reports a CHD length of 3 to 4 cm, whereas Oikarinen gives a length of 2 to 6.5 cm for the common hepatic duct and 0.5 to 2.5 cm for the right and left hepatic ducts, with the left hepatic duct typically longer than the right. The diameter of the right and left hepatic ducts has been reported at between 0.1 and 0.2 cm.

A fairly widely accepted upper limit for the inner diameter of the CHD is 4 mm. One study has reported the diameter to range from approximately 1 to 7 mm in the normal patient, depending on age, previous surgery, and gallbladder function or disease. It is typical for an individual sonographic practice to set an acceptable upper limit on duct size based on criteria used by referring physicians, especially surgeons. Soto and Castrillon report that the CHD should be measured at the level of the right hepatic artery where it crosses between the CHD and the portal vein. They also report that it's a good rule of thumb to consider it normal for the extrahepatic duct to dilate approximately 1 mm per decade of life. Thus, the upper limits of a CHD in a geriatric patient is 10 mm.

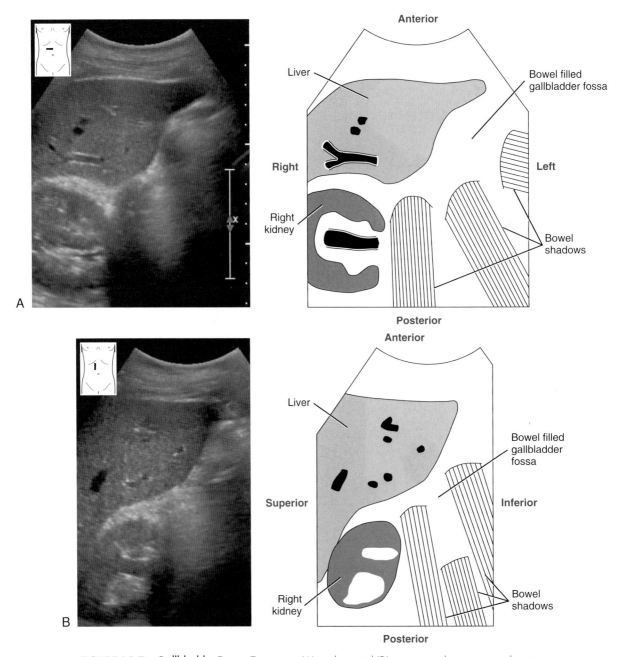

FIGURE 15-7 **Gallbladder Fossa.** Transverse (A) and sagittal (B) scanning plane images showing an empty gallbladder fossa after cholecystectomy. Notice how bowel has filled the space where the gallbladder would normally be located.

Cystic Duct

The diameter of the cystic duct is approximately 3 mm. The length is highly variable, ranging from 1.0 to 3.5 cm. An average length of 4 cm has been reported at surgery. The apparent large difference in these figures is common and holds little significance on sonography.

Common Bile Duct (CBD)

The length of the CBD is also highly variable. A range in length of 8 to 11.5 cm has been suggested, although lengths of up to 17 cm have been reported. The diameter has been reported to be 1 to 7 mm in the normal patient and up to 10 mm in a patient after **cholecystectomy** (surgical removal of the gallbladder), although larger diameters have been reported. As discussed, individual practices will set an upper limit that is appropriate to their particular patient population. Figure 15-7 shows the fossa of a patient who has undergone a cholecystectomy.

GROSS ANATOMY
Gallbladder

The gallbladder is perfused by the hepatic artery, a branch of the celiac artery, which is a branch of the

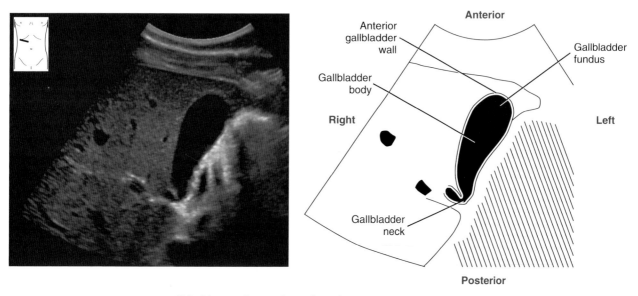

FIGURE 15-8 *Gallbladder Fundus, Body, and Neck.* Transverse oblique scanning plane image showing all three gallbladder sections in a longitudinal orientation. The fundus is the bottom portion; the body the middle; the neck the narrow portion adjacent to the body.

abdominal aorta. The hepatic artery, or *common hepatic artery*, as it is often called, divides into the proper hepatic and gastroduodenal arteries. The **proper hepatic artery** supplies the gallbladder and the liver. The cystic artery may, on occasion, originate directly from the common hepatic artery or, rarely, from the gastroduodenal artery, but it usually originates from the right branch of the proper hepatic artery. It passes posterior to the CHD and anterior to the cystic duct. At this point, it travels inferiorly and divides into superficial and deep branches.

Venous drainage of the gallbladder is by way of the **hepatic portal system**. The gallbladder is drained by tributaries of the hepatic portal venous system, which carry blood to the inferior vena cava. The *portal circulatory route* is the term used to describe venous blood that passes through two capillary exchange systems before reaching the heart. "Portal" comes from the Latin word *porta*, which means "gateway." The **portal vein** is the gateway through which blood returning from the gastrointestinal tract and accessory organs passes before returning to the heart.

This system includes all the veins draining the gastrointestinal tract, including the spleen, pancreas, and gallbladder. Blood is conveyed from these organs via the portal vein to the liver. The portal vein subdivides until the blood reaches the hepatic sinusoids. Blood therefore passes through two sets of "exchange" vessels: the capillaries within the organs of the gastrointestinal tract, the spleen, pancreas, and gallbladder, and the hepatic sinusoids. From the sinusoids, blood converges into hepatic veins and finally the inferior vena cava before returning to the heart.

There are three distinct layers to the gallbladder wall: the inner *mucosa*; the middle *fibromuscular* layer; and the outer *serous* layer. Inside the gallbladder are many minute, inward folds or *rugae*. These folds aid in concentrating the bile through absorption of water and secretion of mucus.

The gallbladder may be descriptively divided into three major sections: *fundus, body,* and *neck.* The shape of the normal gallbladder has been likened to that of a pear, which has a narrow "neck" and a round "bottom" (Figure 15-8). The **fundus** is the bottom portion (refer to Figure 15-6, *A*). The middle and main portions of the gallbladder are called the **body**, and the narrower area leading into the cystic duct is the **neck** (refer to Figure 15-6, *B*).

Hepatic Ducts

Surrounded by a sheath of connective tissue, intrahepatic bile ducts and hepatic arteries accompany portal veins in **portal triads** that radiate throughout the lobes and segments of the liver. The intrahepatic ducts unite to form the **right** and **left** main **hepatic ducts**. As noted, the right and left main ducts join at approximately the level of the liver hilum to form the CHD, the proximal portion of the CD (refer to Figure 15-2).

Biliary Ducts

The cystic duct, CBD, and part of the CHD are **extrahepatic** biliary ducts (not enclosed by liver tissue). They are lined with subepithelial connective tissue and some smooth muscle fibers.

Cystic Duct

The lumen of the cystic duct contains a series of mucosal folds, the spiral valves of Heister. Even though this area of folds is called a valve, it is a misnomer. There does not seem to be any valve or flow control action; bile flows freely in both directions through the cystic duct. Pressure differences in the biliary system, along with the stimulated contraction of the gallbladder, seem to govern the flow of bile. The spiral valves of Heister prevent the cystic duct from overdistending or collapsing.

PHYSIOLOGY

Bile is produced by the liver and carried to the gastrointestinal system by the biliary tract. The sphincter of Oddi, located in the duodenum, regulates the passage of bile into the duodenum and at the same time prevents reflux of gastrointestinal fluids into the biliary system. When closed, the sphincter of Oddi forces the gallbladder to fill with bile. When fats and amino acids are ingested, the duodenal mucosa releases cholecystokinin (CCK), a peptide hormone. CCK stimulates the gallbladder to contract and the sphincter of Oddi to relax, and it increases hepatic production of bile. An injectable form of CCK has been used to stimulate the gallbladder during sonographic examination for a type of function test.

The gallbladder is actually more than just a storage area for bile. Related blood vessels and lymphatics concentrate the stored bile through absorption of water and inorganic salts. Bile in the gallbladder is much more concentrated than hepatic bile. Bile is composed mostly of water (82%) and bile acids (12%). The remaining constituents include cholesterol, bilirubin (bile pigment), proteins, electrolytes, and mucus.

SONOGRAPHIC APPEARANCE

Much of the biliary system is readily appreciated on sonography. It is especially common for the gallbladder, CHD, and CBD to be imaged. In the absence of disease, the other portions of the biliary system may prove difficult to appreciate because they are so small.

Gallbladder

The sonographic appearance of a longitudinal section of the normal, distended gallbladder is that of an anechoic or nearly anechoic pear-shaped structure with thin, bright walls in the right upper quadrant of the abdomen. As mentioned, there is variation in shape and size of the gallbladder. The longitudinal appearance of the normal gallbladder has also been compared to a partially filled water balloon because it is slightly more oval than round (Figure 15-9, A). An axial view of the normal gallbladder at the level of the body will show an almost round to oval-shaped, anechoic structure

with reflective walls (Figure 15-9, B and C). An axial section of the gallbladder should not be mistaken for axial sections of the inferior vena cava or aorta.

It is important to identify whether or not the gallbladder is distended. A nonfasting patient will not have a distended gallbladder. The nondistended gallbladder may be mistaken for bowel or pathology (Figure 15-10, A and B). In the "empty" gallbladder the walls are thicker and may appear more irregular, with the central portion containing a few random echoes.

The walls of a distended gallbladder tend to be well defined, regular, and echo-dense (Figure 15-10, C). As mentioned, normal gallbladder wall thickness is usually 3 mm or less (Figure 15-11). The wall may be difficult to measure when the gallbladder is in a partially distended, normal state or if pathology is present. Inadequate examination may lead to a false diagnosis of thickened walls or cholecystitis (the presence of a thickened gallbladder wall).

Four landmarks may be helpful in locating the gallbladder: the *portal vein*, *right kidney*, *duodenum*, and *main lobar fissure.*

- **Portal vein.** From its origin posterior to the pancreas neck, the longitudinal main portal vein can be followed as it courses toward the liver (Figure 15-12). It will reveal the gallbladder to be just inferior to the level of the right portal vein branch. Moreover, the right portal vein must be located to visualize the CHD (see Figure 15-1). In a transverse scan of the midepigastrium, finding the main portal vein (or portal-splenic confluence) and following it to the right will reveal (in typical order of appearance) the anechoic longitudinal portal vein; mid-gray longitudinal pancreas head section; anechoic to reflective and gassy long section of the duodenum; mid- to low-gray axial section of liver; longitudinal or axial (depending on its position) anechoic gallbladder section; and again, axial liver (Figure 15-13). This common relationship is important because during a scan, each anechoic structure can be eliminated as a possible gallbladder.
- **Right kidney.** An axial section of the superior/midportion of the right kidney may also be typically noted with the gallbladder immediately anterior and to the left (see Figure 15-9). Further, the anechoic, axial section of the inferior vena cava can be visualized just posterior to the head of the pancreas and could be mistaken for an extremely posteriorly lying (or floating) gallbladder.
- **Duodenum.** Whether anechoic or gassy, the duodenum serves as an excellent landmark because it is usually sandwiched between the gallbladder (laterally) and pancreas head (medially) (see Figure 15-13).
- **Main lobar fissure.** The thin, reflective, main lobar fissure may be demonstrated between the portal

Text continued on p. 242

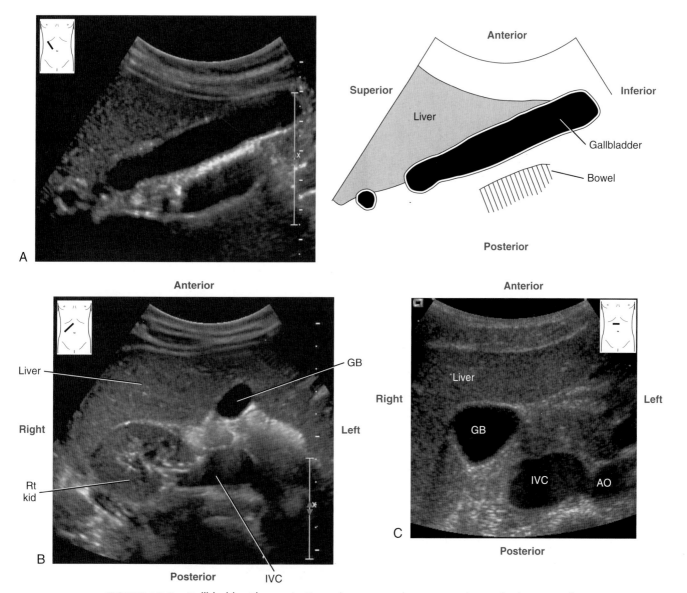

FIGURE 15-9 **Gallbladder Shape. A,** Sagittal scanning plane image; longitudinal section of the gallbladder. Notice its oblong shape. **B,** Oblique transverse scanning plane image; axial body/middle section of the gallbladder (GB) anterior, and the right kidney and inferior vena cava (IVC), posterior. **C,** Another axial section of the body of the gallbladder (GB) in a different patient. Notice the shape of the gallbladder and its anechoic, bile-filled lumen. Observe the posterior through transmission. Also note the similarly shaped, anechoic, axial sections of the inferior vena cava (IVC) and aorta (AO), which should not be confused with the gallbladder.

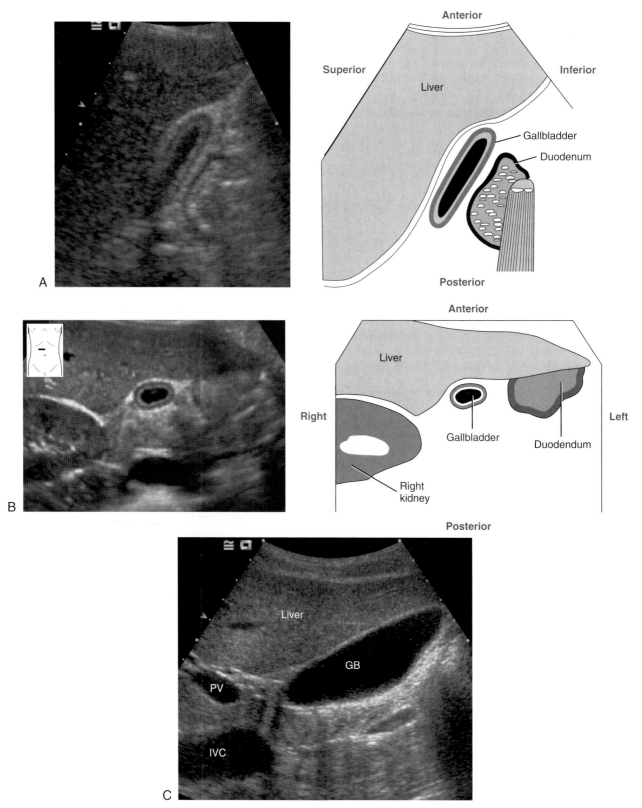

FIGURE 15-10 **Nondistended/Distended Gallbladder. A,** Sagittal scanning plane image; longitudinal section of the gallbladder that is nondistended or contracted. **B,** Transverse scanning plane image; axial body/middle section of the same nondistended gallbladder. Observe how the walls are prominent and could appear thickened due to its contracted state. Note that it's slightly more oval than round. **C,** Sagittal scanning plane image; longitudinal section of a distended gallbladder (GB). Notice how the walls of a normal, distended gallbladder appear well-defined, smooth, and echo dense. *IVC,* Inferior vena cava; *PV,* portal vein.

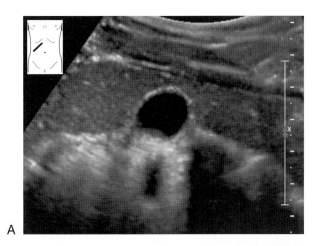

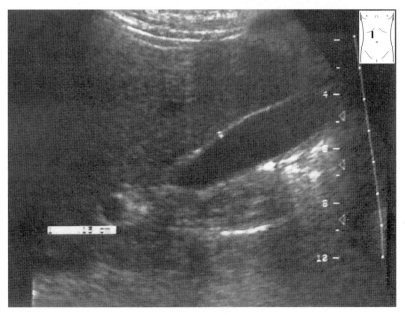

FIGURE 15-11 **Gallbladder Wall Thickness.** The thickness of the normal gallbladder wall is usually less than 3 mm. Cholecystitis and carcinoma are just two examples of pathologic states that may alter the thickness and appearance of the gallbladder wall. Care must be taken when adjusting technique to resolve actual wall thickness and not misrepresent the walls by setting the gain or power settings too high. Image **A** shows an oblique transverse scanning plane image demonstrating the correct place to measure the anterior gallbladder wall. Note measurement caliper placement. Image **B** shows a sagittal scannning plane image also demonstrating the anterior gallbladder wall measurement.

vein and the gallbladder. It helps to form the "bed" in which the gallbladder lies (Figure 15-14). The main lobar fissure is considerably more difficult to consistently appreciate than the portal vein, but it is of value. Reference to all the landmarks will make locating the gallbladder easier.

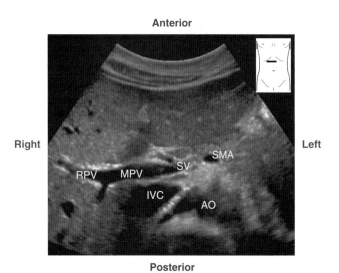

Anterior

Right

Left

Posterior

FIGURE 15-12 **Main Portal Vein.** The main portal vein (MPV) is a useful landmark when locating the gallbladder. This transverse scanning plane image shows that following the longitudinal MPV from its origin to the liver will reveal the right portal vein (RPV) branch, which is typically at a level just superior to the gallbladder. *AO,* Aorta; *IVC,* inferior vena cava; *SMA,* superior mesenteric artery; *SV,* splenic vein.

At times, regardless of scanning technique, the gallbladder simply will not be visualized. Nonvisualization may occur for a number of reasons:

- If the gallbladder fails to develop (agenesis), there will be nothing to image. However, this cause of nonvisualization is rare.
- A small, tubelike (vermiform or wormlike) gallbladder may appear as a bile duct and be missed on sonography.
- As previously noted, an empty or contracted gallbladder may be small and can be overlooked.
- The gallbladder is obscured or hidden by bowel gas.

The fundus of the gallbladder can be challenging to visualize because of its close proximity to bowel. Bowel often creates a shadow that partially obscures the fundus (Figure 15-15). Thus, changing patient position or transducer position may be necessary to examine the entirety of the fundus. Floating gallstones, **polyps** (protruding masses from the inner wall of the gallbladder), and other masses may be present in the fundus of the gallbladder and easily missed on casual examination.

A small sacculation (outpouching) may be seen in some patients in the area of the gallbladder neck (Figure 15-16). This has been called **Hartmann's pouch** after Henri Hartmann (1860–1952), a French surgeon. The term *infundibulum* is also applied to this dilatation of the gallbladder neck area. Some consider this sacculation an abnormality, whereas others consider it an oddity. It must be carefully screened to detect coexisting abnormalities, such as cholelithiasis (gallstones).

Shadows and other minor distortions related to the edge of the gallbladder walls and distal to the spiral

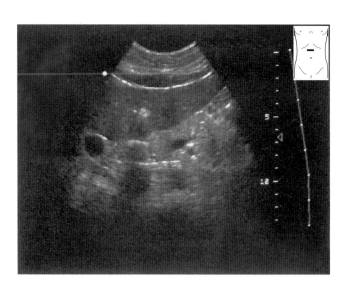

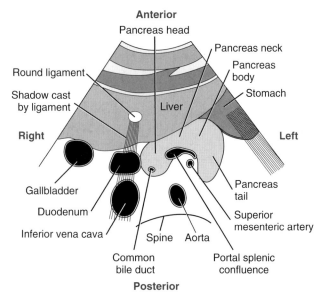

FIGURE 15-13 **Relationship of Gallbladder, Duodenum, and Pancreas.** A transverse scanning plane image through the mid-epigastrium may reveal the above relationship. Notice how the gallbladder is lateral to the duodenum, which is just lateral to the head of the pancreas.

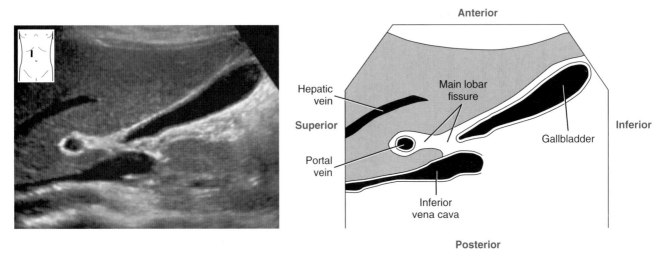

FIGURE 15-14 **Main Lobar Fissure and Gallbladder Relationship.** The main lobar fissure helps to form the "bed" in which the gallbladder lies and serves as a useful landmark to help locate the gallbladder.

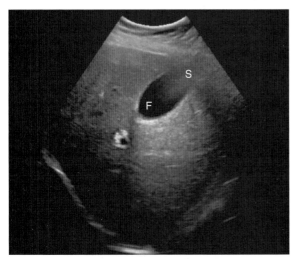

FIGURE 15-15 **Bowel Shadows.** The fundus of the gallbladder can be challenging to examine because of its close proximity to bowel. Bowel often creates a shadow (S) that partially obscures the fundus (F). Changing patient position or transducer position can help visualize the entirety of the fundus.

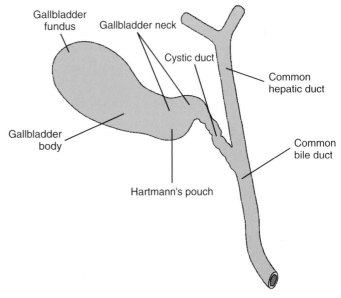

FIGURE 15-16 **Hartmann's Pouch.** A dilatation located in the area of the neck of the gallbladder is called *Hartmann's pouch*. This slight sacculation is also known as the *infundibulum*.

valves of Heister are common. High-frequency sound produces a particularly striking shadow from these areas because it is more easily reflected than the lower frequencies (Figure 15-17). Each shadow must be explored to determine whether it is natural or associated with disease. An acoustic shadow should be followed to its origin to learn whether it begins slightly more anteriorly and interrupts the representation of the wall. If it interrupts the wall, the shadow may indicate abnormal anatomy and deserves further study.

Ductal System

In the average patient, bile ducts other than the common duct are small and usually not appreciated sonographically. The common duct is larger in diameter and can be seen on ultrasound closely associated with the portal venous system. Its longitudinal section may be noted as two bright, parallel lines separated by just 1 mm or so of anechoic bile. Because of its small diameter, axial sections of the common duct appear very small, round, and anechoic with reflective walls.

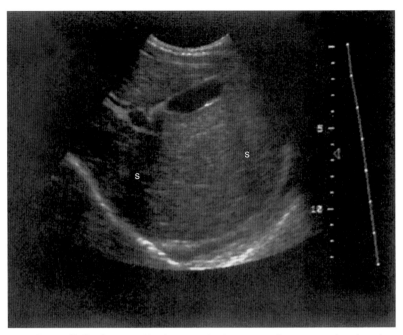

FIGURE 15-17 **Wall Shadowing.** Shadows and other minor distortions related to the edge of the gallbladder walls and distal to the spiral valves of Heister are common. High-frequency sound produces a particularly striking shadow from these areas because it is more easily reflected than the lower frequencies. *S,* Shadowing.

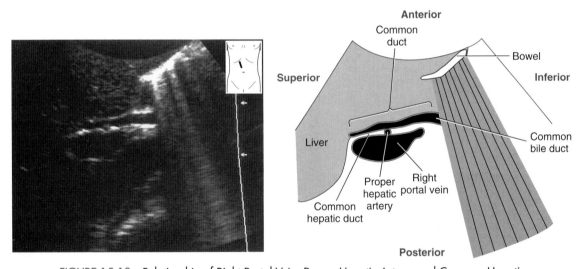

FIGURE 15-18 **Relationship of Right Portal Vein, Proper Hepatic Artery, and Common Hepatic Duct.** Slightly oblique, sagittal scanning plane image showing a longitudinal section of the common duct. An axial section of the proper hepatic artery is seen between the common hepatic duct portion of the common duct (anteriorly) and right portal vein (posteriorly).

As previously discussed, the proximal common duct, the CHD, is located anterior to the right portal vein; it is not uncommon to see a portion of the proper hepatic artery running between them (Figure 15-18). The CHD is often mistaken for the CBD, which is generally more closely associated with the main portal vein than the right branch. However, there are always variations, so it

is possible to see the CBD and the right portal vein at the same time.

As noted, the distal CBD is located anterior and slightly right lateral to the main portal vein. In an oblique sagittal scanning plane, a longitudinal section of the supraduodenal CBD can be seen coursing superior to inferior, between an axial section of the common hepatic artery and the first portion of the duodenum. The small, round, anechoic axial section of the common hepatic artery is visualized at the superoanterior edge of the CBD, and the duodenum is seen inferiorly (see Figure 15-5, *A*). Depending on the contents of the duodenum, it may be possible to follow the supraduodenal CBD inferiorly and visualize a long section of the retroduodenal CBD. In some cases, patients drink water to fill up the duodenum (obliterating any reflective gas) to make a passable window for the sound waves and expose the retroduodenal portion of the duct. A longitudinal section of the infraduodenal CBD can be seen medial to the first portion of the duodenum, running inferiorly to the posterolateral edge of the axial section of the pancreas head (see Figure 15-5, *B*). In many cases the long section of the gastroduodenal artery can be visualized running parallel and anterior to the long section of the infraduodenal CBD. Generally, the intraduodenal CBD is not routinely visualized.

In a transverse scanning plane, an axial section of the infraduodenal CBD is routinely noted on the posterolateral border of the pancreas head, posterior to a small axial section of the gastroduodenal artery. The contrast between the small, round anechoic duct and artery and the midgray appearance of pancreatic parenchyma makes it easier to detect the small diameter structures (Figure 15-19).

Because of the appearance of the shape that its axial sections form together, the extrahepatic portal triad has become known as "Mickey's Sign" or the "Mickey Mouse Sign." The CBD is the right "ear" of the famous mouse, the proper hepatic artery the left "ear," and the larger main portal vein is the "face" (see Figure 15-4, *C* and *D*.)

SONOGRAPHIC APPLICATIONS

For most physicians, sonography is the method of choice for examining the biliary system. Some specific applications of sonographic examination of the biliary system include:

- Assessment for possible obstruction of the biliary ductal system
- Presence of stones in the gallbladder (**cholelithiasis**)
- Presence of stones in the ductal system (**choledocholithiasis**)
- Ruling out masses associated with the biliary system
- Postsurgical follow-up evaluation (e.g., cholecystectomy)

Indications for Examinations

Clinical indications that are normally used as reasons for an ultrasound examination of the biliary system and right upper quadrant (RUQ) include:

- RUQ pain
- Positive Murphy's sign (RUQ pain) on physical examination

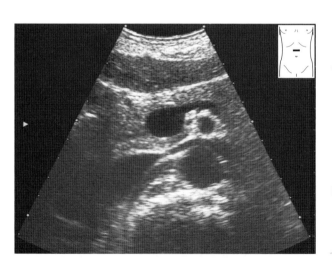 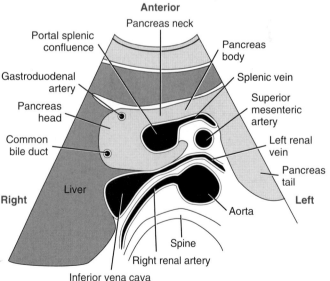

FIGURE 15-19 Relationship of Infraduodenal Common Bile Duct, Pancreas Head, and Gastroduodenal Artery. Transverse scanning plane image of the mid-epigastrium demonstrating an axial section of the infraduodenal common bile duct on the posterolateral border of the pancreas head, posterior to an axial section of the gastroduodenal artery.

- Nausea
- Vomiting
- Pain radiating to the right shoulder or scapula
- Jaundice or abnormal liver function tests (LFTs)
- Loss of appetite
- Intolerance to fatty foods or dairy products

NORMAL VARIANTS

The biliary system may not develop normally, which can cause different types of deviations to occur. Deviations are of special interest to the sonographer because they may challenge adequate examination. For example, what appears to be a septated gallbladder (a gallbladder with divisions or septations) may simply be a gallbladder folded onto itself. If the patient's position is changed, the gallbladder may unfold to reveal no septation (Figure 15-20).

Other variations may be considered pathologic or may contribute to the development of disease. For instance, a gallbladder attached to the liver by a particularly long mesentery can mimic a "floating" gallbladder that is prone to torsion (twisting) as opposed to a gallbladder that is partially embedded in liver tissue.

Gallbladder

Congenital abnormalities of the gallbladder are relatively common:

- **Floating gallbladder:** low position in the abdomen

- **Hypoplasia:** underdevelopment; relatively rare but must be ruled out as possible reason for nonvisualization on sonography and other imaging modalities
- **Agenesis:** complete failure of the gallbladder to develop; relatively rare but must be ruled out as possible reason for nonvisualization on sonography and other imaging modalities
- **Duplicated gallbladder:** with or without duplication of the cystic duct
- **Double gallbladder (rare):** two gallbladders are present; however, only one is functioning
  Variations in gallbladder shape are very common:
- **Bilobed:** hourglass-shaped
- **Septated:** characterized by one or more internal divisions of the gallbladder; septations tend to be associated with gallstone formation resulting from the stasis of gallbladder contents; they may make it difficult to identify cholelithiasis (gallstones)
- **Junctional fold:** fold seen at the body and neck. Hartmann's pouch may fold back on itself at the neck, creating a pouch for stones to collect, which could cause obstruction.
- **Phrygian cap:** the most common variation in gallbladder shape. In this case, the gallbladder fundus is partially folded onto itself, so that it appears similar to the Phrygian cap worn by the early Roman freed slaves and later by French revolutionaries as a symbol of liberty. This looks similar to a Smurf's hat (Figure 15-21).

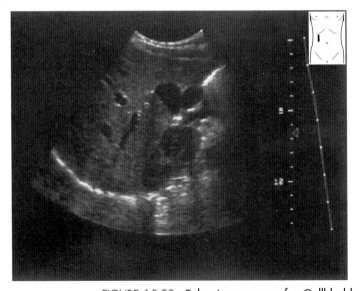
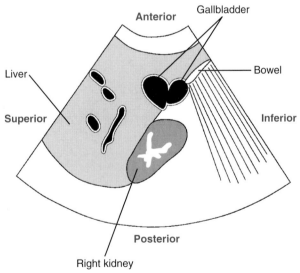

FIGURE 15-20 **False Appearance of a Gallbladder Variation.** In this sagittal scanning plane image, it appears that a septation is present in the gallbladder. However, when the patient's position was changed, the gallbladder was observed folded onto itself (a normal variation) and *not* abnormally septated. Clearly, it is imperative that the patient be placed in at least two different positions during sonographic examination of the gallbladder and biliary tract to rule out normal variations from abnormalities.

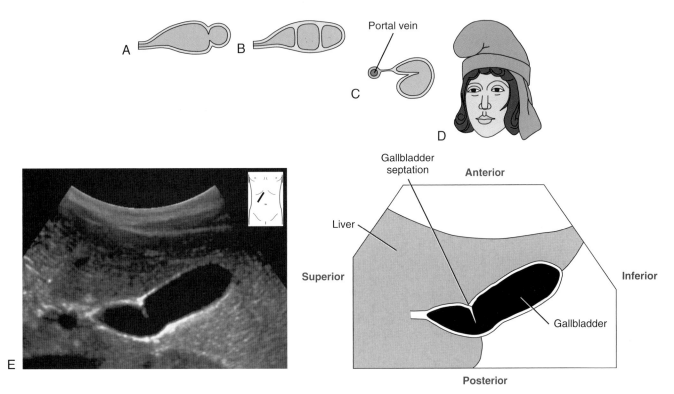

FIGURE 15-21 *Typical Gallbladder Shape Variations.* **A,** Bilobed gallbladder. **B,** True septated gallbladder. **C,** Gallbladder folded onto itself in what has been called the Phrygian gallbladder, named after the shape of a Phrygian cap seen in *D.* **D,** The Phrygian cap was worn by early Roman freed slaves and later by French revolutionaries as a symbol of liberty. **E,** Example of a gallbladder septation.

Biliary Ducts

- Variations in the extrahepatic biliary ducts are frequently seen and may appear in almost any combination. For example, the cystic duct may join the CHD at almost any point from the porta hepatis to the duodenum. With a low juncture, the cystic duct may run parallel to the CHD for some distance.

- Accessory hepatic ducts are also fairly common; on sonographic examination, they may present as an "extra" tubular structure. Such variations should not be an obstacle; following them to their origin will differentiate them from similar appearing structures.

- A more easily recognized variation is the **choledochal (or choledochus) cyst.** Of the three types—congenital cystic dilation, intraduodenal (choledochocele), and congenital diverticulum—the first is the most common. A choledochal cyst is a localized dilatation of the CBD. When caused by a congenital diverticulum, it may appear as a separate or loosely connected structure to the CBD. The choledochocele (or intraduodenum) is formed by a section of the CBD that has entered the duodenum and enlarged. This is similar to the process involved in the formation of a ureterocele.

- Biliary atresia (congenital closure) may be diffuse or focal in the extrahepatic ducts, or it may be intrahepatic. Diffuse extrahepatic biliary atresia is the most common.

REFERENCE CHARTS

■ ■ ■ ASSOCIATED PHYSICIANS

- **Surgeon:** Involved in the diagnosis of biliary disease, as well as surgical intervention.
- **Internist:** Involved in the diagnosis and medical treatment of biliary disease.
- **Radiologist:** Performs and interprets the various imaging tests used to diagnose biliary disease.

■■■ DIAGNOSTIC TESTS

- **Oral cholecystogram (OCG):** A contrast material (dye) is ingested by the patient the night before the test. Information on structure and function of the gallbladder is obtained. This test is performed by a radiologist assisted by a radiologic technologist and is interpreted by the radiologist.
- **Nuclear medicine (HIDA scan):** A minute amount of a radiopharmaceutical is injected. It passes through the bloodstream to the liver, then to the biliary system, and eventually into the duodenum. Functional information is the primary focus of this test, and some structural information is also obtained. This test is performed by a nuclear medicine technologist and interpreted by the radiologist.
- **Computed axial tomography (CT scan):** A radiologic examination in which cross-sectional x-ray images of the biliary system and other abdominal structures are obtained. A contrast medium may be administered to differentiate between disease and normal anatomy. Structural information is the primary focus of this test, but some functional information may be obtained. It is performed by a radiologic technologist and interpreted by the radiologist.
- **Cholangiography:** A contrast material is injected into the biliary system either by catheter (i.e., T-tube cholangiogram) or by needle (transhepatic cholangiogram) under radiographic guidance. This yields structural information about the entire biliary system, especially about obstruction. It may be performed before, during, or after surgery. Surgeons, radiologists, and radiologic technologists are involved in the procedure, and it is interpreted by the radiologist.
- **Endoscopic retrograde cholangiopancreatography (ERCP):** In this endoscopic, radiographically guided examination, the ampulla of Vater is cannulized through a tube inserted into the patient's upper gastrointestinal tract. Contrast material is then injected to fill and delineate the pancreatic and bile ducts. Information on obstructive processes is the objective. This type of endoscopy is usually performed by the gastroenterologist, who is assisted by the radiologist. The gastroenterologist interprets the endoscopic results, and the radiologist interprets the radiologic findings.
- **Hepatobiliary scintigraphy:** A radionuclide imaging study that evaluates both liver function and the biliary sytem. It traces the production of bile and its pathway through the biliary system into the small intestine. It detects bile leaks, biliary atresia, and/or neonatal hepatitis. Hepatobiliary scintigraphy also provides functional information that US, CT, or MR cannot.
- **Endoscopic ultrasonography (EUS):** Involves an endoscope and ultrasound probe to visualize the GI tract. EUS requires expert skills and specific equipment. This test is usually only available at tertiary care facilities. This is commonly used for patients with biliary obstruction, to stage malignancies affecting the biliary tracts and to assist in image-guided interventions.

■■■ LABORATORY VALUES

Serum bilirubin (adult)	Direct (conjugated): <0.5 mg/dL Indirect (unconjugated): ≤1.1 mg/dL Urine: negative Elevated if there is obstruction, excess amount of red blood destruction, or malfunction of liver cells
Serum bilirubin (infant)	1 to 12 mg/dL
Urobilinogen	Fecal: 50 to 300 mg/24 hours Urine: *Men:* 0.3 to 2.1 Ehrlich units/2 hours
Serum alkaline phosphatase	Elevated in cases of hepatic jaundice, abscess, cirrhosis, carcinoma, or obstruction
Alanine aminotransferase (ALT)	Elevated in cases of acute cirrhosis, hepatic metastasis, and pancreatitis
White blood cell count	Elevated in cases of infection (cholecystitis, cholangitis, etc.)
Aspartate aminotransferase	Elevated with liver cell injuries
Carcinoembryonic antigen	Cancer indicator
Lactic acid dehydrogenase	Elevated in cases of hepatitis, cirrhosis, and obstructive jaundice
Prothrombin time (PT)	Clotting time is longer in patients with acute cholecystitis, cancer, cirrhosis, and obstruction

Collectively, these laboratory tests or liver function tests are used to help in the diagnosis of hepatobiliary diseases. These tests are a great indicator for physicians to determine how the liver is functioning. Elevations in certain labs allows for a quick and more accurate diagnosis.

■■■ VASCULATURE

BLOOD SUPPLY
Common hepatic artery → proper hepatic artery → cystic artery → gastroduodenal artery

VENOUS DRAINAGE
Cystic veins → hepatic veins → IVC
The gallbladder neck is drained via the cystic veins.
The gallbladder body and fundus are drained via hepatic sinusoids.

■■■ AFFECTING CHEMICALS

Nonapplicable

CHAPTER 16

The Pancreas

REVA ARNEZ CURRY AND BETTY BATES TEMPKIN

OBJECTIVES

List the gross anatomy of the pancreas.

Explain the function of the pancreas.

Draw the epigastric vessels that surround the pancreas.

Draw the blood supply to the pancreas.

Describe the scanning plane used and the sonographic appearance of the pancreas in axial views, using vascular landmarks and adjacent anatomy.

Describe the scanning plane used and the sonographic appearance of the pancreas in longitudinal views, using vascular landmarks and adjacent anatomy.

Describe the relationship of the pancreas, duodenum, and biliary system.

■

KEY WORDS

Acini Cells — Produce pancreatic juice that is composed of enzymes to help digest fats, proteins, carbohydrates, and nucleic acids.

Alpha Cells — Cells that account for 15% to 20% of pancreatic endocrine tissue and produce the hormone glucagon.

Ampulla of Vater — Dilatation in the second portion of the duodenum, where the common bile duct and pancreatic duct(s) enter to discharge substances that aid in the digestive process.

Beta Cells — Constitute 60% to 70% of the pancreatic endocrine cells that produce insulin.

Common Bile Duct (CBD) — Distal portion of the biliary tract that transports and then discharges bile (that was manufactured in the liver) into the duodenum as needed to aid the digestive process.

Delta Cells — Cells that account for approximately 5% of pancreatic endocrine tissue that produces the hormone somatostatin.

Duct of Santorini — Pancreatic accessory duct that enters the duodenum approximately 2 cm superior to the duct of Wirsung.

Duct of Wirsung — Main pancreatic duct. Transports and discharges pancreatic juice into the duodenum through the ampulla of Vater to aid the digestive process.

Endocrine — Produces and secretes hormones directly into the bloodstream with a ductal system.

Epsilon Cells — Cells that account for less than 1% of pancreatic endocrine cells, and produce the hormone ghrelin, which may affect blood sugar regulation.

Exocrine — Produces and transports pancreatic juice via ducts to aid in digestion.

Gamma Cells — Pancreatic Polypeptide (Pp) cells that comprise less than 5% of pancreatic endocrine cells and may affect blood sugar regulation.

Gastroduodenal Artery — First branch of the common hepatic artery. Courses along the anterolateral aspect of the pancreas head just right lateral to the pancreas neck, where it divides into anterior and posterior superior pancreaticoduodenal branches. Supplies blood to the head of the pancreas and the duodenum.

Glucagon — Hormone produced by alpha cells in the pancreas that causes the release of glucose to meet the immediate energy needs of the body.

Insulin — Hormone produced by beta cells in the pancreas that causes glycogen formation from glucose in the liver.

Islets of Langerhans — Groups of alpha, beta, and delta endocrine cells in the pancreas that produce insulin.

Pancreatic Arcades — Vascular connections between the pancreaticoduodenal, hepatic, splenic, and superior mesenteric arteries that supply blood to the head of the pancreas.

Pancreatic Body — Bordered right laterally by the pancreas neck, left laterally by the pancreas tail, anteriorly by the posterior wall of the stomach, and posteriorly by the splenic vein. Considered the largest portion of the pancreas.

Pancreatic Head — Lies right lateral to the superior mesenteric vein; cradled in the C-loop of the duodenum; directly anterior to the inferior vena cava.

Pancreatic Juice — Composed of enzymes produced by acini cells in the pancreas that help digest fats, proteins, carbohydrates, and nucleic acids.

Pancreatic Neck — Situated between the pancreatic head and body immediately anterior to the superior mesenteric vein. At a slightly higher level, it lies anterior to the portal splenic confluence.

Pancreatic Splenic Artery — Section of the artery located within the pancreas.

Pancreatic Tail — Left lateral to the pancreas body and aorta and extends to the hilum of the spleen. Situated between the stomach anteriorly and left kidney posteriorly. The splenic vein runs along its posterosuperior surface. May lie higher, lower, or on an even level with the body.

Pancreaticoduodenal Arteries — Arteries that supply the head of the pancreas and part of the duodenum with blood. Part of the pancreatic arcades (the vascular connections between the hepatic, splenic, and superior mesenteric arteries that also supply blood to the head of the pancreas).

Continued

Portal Splenic Confluence — Area just posterior to the neck of the pancreas, where the splenic vein meets the superior mesenteric vein. Together, these veins form the portal vein.

Portal Vein — Formed by the confluence of the splenic vein and superior mesenteric vein just posterior to the neck of the pancreas.

Prehilar Splenic Artery — Section of the artery before it enters the hilum of the spleen.

Prepancreatic Splenic Artery — Section of the artery before it leaves the pancreas.

Somatostatin — Hormone produced by alpha cells in the pancreas that inhibits the production of insulin and glucose.

Sphincter of Oddi — Muscle surrounding the ampulla of Vater that controls the flow of pancreatic juice from the pancreas and bile from the biliary tract into the duodenum.

Splenic Artery — Supplies the body and tail of the pancreas with blood. From its origin at the celiac axis it runs along the superior edge of the pancreas body and tail parallel to the splenic vein.

Splenic Vein — Along with tributaries of the superior mesenteric vein, serves as the venous drainage for the pancreas.

Superior Mesenteric Vein — Along with tributaries of the splenic vein, serves as venous drainage for the pancreas.

Suprapancreatic Splenic Artery — First 3-cm section of the artery as it originates from the celiac axis.

Uncinate Process — Posteromedial projection of the pancreas head that lies directly posterior to the superior mesenteric vein and directly anterior to the inferior vena cava or in some cases, due to its size, the abdominal aorta.

■■■ NORMAL MEASUREMENTS

Anatomy	Measurement
Total length of pancreas	12 to 18 cm
AP measurement of head	2 to 3 cm
AP measurement of neck	1.5 to 2.5 cm
AP measurement of body	2 to 3 cm
AP measurement of tail	1 to 2 cm

The pancreas has been and continues to be a most interesting challenge to imaging using sonography. Its close relationship to the stomach, duodenum and proximal jejunum of the small intestine, transverse colon of the large intestine, and their contents may affect sound beam transmission and obscure pancreatic structures. This is especially true for patients who have been poorly prepped. Despite these obstacles, sonography has become useful for the evaluation and early detection of diseases of the pancreas.

LOCATION

The pancreas is descriptively divided into 5 parts: head, uncinate process, neck, body, and tail. When describing the location of the pancreas (Table 16-1), we move from the head and uncinate process on the right, through the neck and body, to the tail on the left. The pancreas is situated in the epigastrium and left hypochondrium. Position of the gland is variable, but it usually lies at the level of the first or second lumbar vertebra, extending from the C-loop of the duodenum to the splenic hilum. It lies horizontally across or anterior to the aorta and is shaped like an upside-down U (the ends of the U appear to have been pulled outward). The pancreas has also

been described as dumbbell-, tadpole-, sausage-, and comma-shaped, with the head being the larger portion.

Most of the pancreas is retroperitoneal; however, a small portion of the head is surrounded by peritoneum. Posterior to the pancreas are connective prevertebral tissue, the inferior vena cava, aorta, and diaphragm. Anterior to the pancreas are the stomach and transverse colon.

The pancreas is closely related to the biliary tract and portal venous system. The main pancreatic duct, also called the **duct of Wirsung**, usually joins the common bile duct (see Chapter 15 for a description of the biliary tree) before both vessels enter the duodenum at the **ampulla of Vater**, a dilatation in the second portion of the duodenum (Figure 16-1). An accessory pancreatic duct, called the **duct of Santorini**, enters the duodenum approximately 2 cm superior to the duct of Wirsung. The **portal splenic confluence** is the area just posterior to the neck of the pancreas, where the **splenic vein** meets the **superior mesenteric vein**; together, these veins form the **portal vein** (Figure 16-2). The inferior mesenteric vein courses from inferior to superior as it drains the large intestine via several smaller branches. This vessel most often empties blood into the splenic vein; however, there is considerable variance regarding where the inferior mesenteric vein joins the portal system.

SIZE

The length of the pancreas ranges between 12 cm and 18 cm, or 6 to 8 inches. It is approximately 2.5 cm thick, 3 to 5 cm wide, and weighs between 60 g and 80 g. It is important to note the overall contour of the gland along with its size. Is the contour smooth, well defined, and without localized enlargement that appears to be out of place compared with the rest of the gland? This is important because a portion of the gland may be

■ ■ ■ **Table 16-1** Location of the Pancreas Head, Uncinate, Neck, Body, and Tail Routinely Visualized With Ultrasound

	Head	Uncinate Process (variable size)	Neck	Body	Tail
Anterior to	IVC, CBD	IVC	SMV, uncinate process	Splenic vein, SMA, lt renal vein, lt adrenal gland, aorta	Splenic vein, lt kidney
Posterior to	Peritoneum (except for small enclosed portion), superior duodenum (partially overlaps), GDA	SMV, pancreas neck, peritoneum	Peritoneum, liver	Stomach, liver, peritoneum (except for posterior surface)	Stomach, splenic artery (portion[s]), lateral lt lobe liver, bowel portion
Superior to	Duodenum C-loop			Duodenojejunal flexure (inferior surface)	
Inferior to	Liver, superior duodenum, CHA, PHA	Liver, superior duodenum, CHA, PHA	Liver, pylorus, CHA, PHA, portal vein	Celiac artery, splenic artery, CHA	Liver lt lateral lobe
Medial to	Duodenum C-loop, GDA, CBD	Pancreas head	Pancreas head, GDA	Pancreas tail	Spleen
Lt lateral to				Pancreas neck, GDA, SMV	Lt renal artery, lt renal vein, SMA, aorta, pancreas body
Rt lateral to	SMV, uncinate process, splenic vein, pancreas neck, aorta	SMA	Pancreas body		

CBD, Common bile duct; CHA, common hepatic artery; GDA, gastroduodenal artery; IVC, inferior vena cava; PHA, proper hepatic artery; SMA, superior mesenteric artery; SMV, superior mesenteric vein; UP, uncinate process.

enlarged, yet it may actually be within normal limits. Therefore an assessment of glandular contour is essential when evaluating size.

Anteroposterior measurements of the head, neck, body, and tail vary widely. The *head* ranges between 2 and 3 cm, although some heads sized at up to 4 cm have been noted. It has been questioned whether the *uncinate process* (a medial extension of the head) contributes to these wide ranges. The size of the *neck* is between 1.5 and 2.5 cm; the *body* is between 2 and 3 cm; and the *tail* is between 1 and 2 cm.

According to one reference, the "top normal" measurements for the adult pancreas were 3 cm for the head, 1 cm for the neck, 2.2 cm for the body, and 2.8 cm for the tail. One study on pancreatic imaging showed that the most reliable measurements of the head, body, and tail were taken in the morning after overnight fasting, as opposed to taking measurements after the patient had eaten and/or later in the day.

Figure 16-3 shows the correct caliper placement to measure each segment of the pancreas. Note how the epigastric vessels serve as distinctive landmarks. The splenic vein should be seen in its entirety to accurately measure the tail. As with many abdominal organs, the size of the pancreas gland normally decreases with age.

GROSS ANATOMY
Head

The **pancreatic head** lies to the right of the superior mesenteric vein. It is cradled in the C-loop of the duodenum, directly anterior to the inferior vena cava. Two vessels may be identified at the head of the pancreas: the common bile duct along the posterolateral portion and the gastroduodenal artery anterolaterally.

The **common bile duct (CBD)** is the distal portion of the biliary tract that courses inferomedially from the level of the gallbladder neck, running posterior to the first part of the duodenum and then either passing directly through the pancreatic head or running along a groove on its posterolateral surface to meet with the main pancreatic duct. Joined together or separately, the ducts enter the duodenum at the ampulla of Vater (see Figure 16-1). The common bile duct transports and then discharges bile (manufactured in the liver) into the duodenum as needed to aid the digestive process.

The **gastroduodenal artery** is the first branch of the common hepatic artery, which originates from the celiac axis. It courses along the anterolateral aspect of the pancreas head just right lateral to the pancreas neck, where it divides into the anterior and posterior

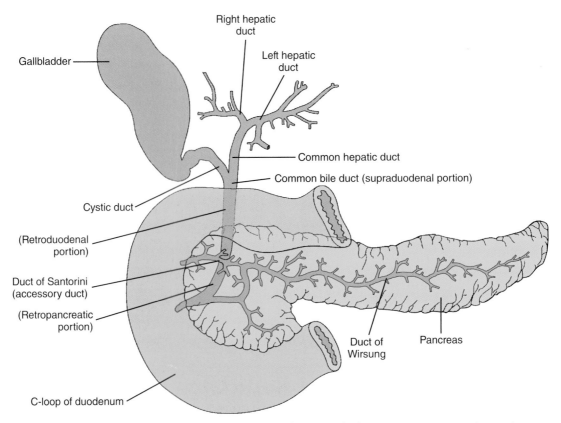

FIGURE 16-1 **Relationship of the Pancreas, Duodenum, and Biliary System.** Note that the head of the pancreas is partially surrounded by the C-loop of the duodenum. The union of the main pancreatic duct and distal common bile duct is illustrated.

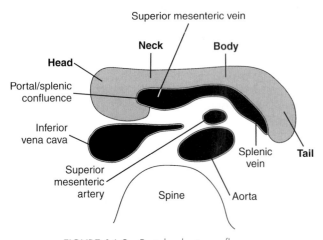

FIGURE 16-2 Portal splenic confluence.

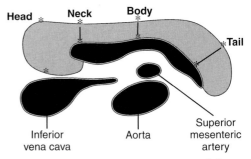

FIGURE 16-3 **Anteroposterior Measurement of the Pancreas.** Correct caliper placement for measuring the anteroposterior dimension of the head, neck, body, and tail of the pancreas.

superior pancreaticoduodenal branches. It supplies blood to the head of the pancreas and the duodenum (Figure 16-4).

The **uncinate process** is a posteromedial projection of the pancreas head that lies directly posterior to the superior mesenteric vein and directly anterior to the inferior vena cava or in some cases, due to its size, the aorta.

One way to visualize this area is to draw an imaginary line from the middle of the portal splenic confluence to the middle of the inferior vena cava on a transverse image of the mid epigastrium. The tissue located to the right of the imaginary line is most likely the uncinate process (Figure 16-5).

Neck

Structurally, the **pancreatic neck** is located between the pancreatic head and body. It is situated immediately

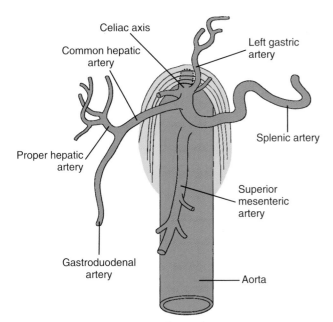

FIGURE 16-4 **Celiac Axis and Branches.** Note the gastroduodenal artery as it courses inferiorly to the first branch of the proper hepatic artery.

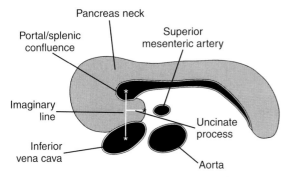

FIGURE 16-5 **Uncinate Process.** A line drawn from the middle of the portal splenic confluence to the middle of the inferior vena cava to locate the uncinate process.

anterior to the superior mesenteric vein; slightly superior to that level, it lies anterior to the portal splenic confluence. Some sonographers do not consider the neck to be an individual structure but, rather, include it as part of either the head or the body.

Body

The **pancreatic body** lies anterior to the aorta, superior mesenteric artery, and splenic vein. The splenic vein runs along the posterior superior surface of the body and tail, closely following the shape of the gland (see Figure 16-2). The pancreas body is bordered right laterally by the neck, left laterally by the tail (although it is not certain exactly where the body ends and the tail begins), and anteriorly by the posterior wall of the stomach. The body is considered the largest portion of the pancreas.

Tail

The **pancreatic tail** lies left lateral to the pancreas body and aorta and extends to the hilum of the spleen. It is situated between the stomach anteriorly and left kidney posteriorly. The splenic vein runs along its posterosuperior surface. The tail may lie higher, lower, or on an even level with the body.

VASCULAR ANATOMY

The arterial supply of the pancreas includes blood from the **pancreaticoduodenal arteries** (branches of the gastroduodenal artery and superior mesenteric artery) and branches of the splenic artery. The superior and inferior pancreaticoduodenal arteries supply a portion of the duodenum and along with the **pancreatic arcades**—the vascular connections between the hepatic, splenic, and superior mesenteric arteries—supply the head of the pancreas.

The pancreatic branches of the **splenic artery** supply the body and tail of the pancreas with blood. As it originates from the celiac axis, the splenic artery runs along the superior edge of the pancreas body and tail parallel to the splenic vein. The splenic artery is normally tortuous and can course anteriorly to the lateral portion of the tail. It descriptively consists of four sections (Figure 16-6):

- **Suprapancreatic:** The first 3 cm of the splenic artery as it originates from the celiac axis. The dorsal pancreatic artery originates from this section.
- **Pancreatic:** Within the pancreas. The pancreatic magna, or great artery, originates from this section.
- **Prepancreatic:** Before it leaves the pancreas. The caudal pancreatic artery originates from prepancreatic or prehilar sections.
- **Prehilar:** Before it enters the spleen.

The venous drainage of the pancreas is through tributaries of the splenic vein and superior mesenteric vein.

PHYSIOLOGY

The pancreas is a (digestive **exocrine**) and (hormonal **endocrine**) gland. Approximately 90% of the gland is exocrine and 10% endocrine: Only 2% of the gland's weight is composed of endocrine tissue.

The exocrine function (via ducts) is carried out by the **acini cells** of the pancreas, which can produce up to 2 L of pancreatic juice per day. Acini cells resemble grape clusters, with small areas of endocrine tissue interspersed between. **Pancreatic juice** is composed of enzymes that help digest fats, proteins, carbohydrates, and nucleic acids. Pancreatic enzymes that aid in digestion include amylase, which digests carbohydrates; lipase, which digests fat; trypsin, chymotrypsin, and carboxypeptidase, which digest proteins; and nucleases, which digest nucleic acids. The largest component of

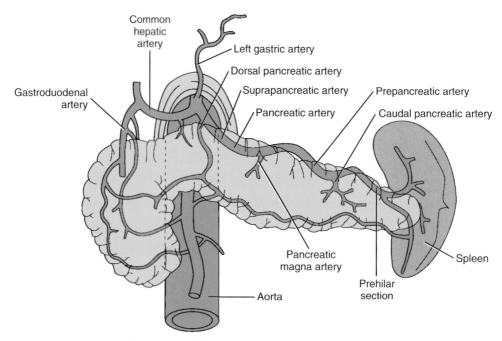

FIGURE 16-6 **Arterial Anatomy of the Pancreas.** The suprapancreatic, pancreatic, prepancreatic, and prehilar sections of the splenic artery are shown. Note the origin of the dorsal pancreatic, pancreatic magna, and caudal pancreatic arteries from the splenic artery.

■ ■ ■ **Table 16-2** Components of Pancreatic Juice

Components of Pancreatic Juice Enzyme	Acts on
Amylase	Carbohydrates
Lipase	Fats
Trypsin, chymotrypsin, carboxypeptidase	Proteins
Nucleases	Nucleic acids
Sodium bicarbonate	Hydrochloric acid

pancreatic juice is sodium bicarbonate, a substance needed to neutralize hydrochloric acid produced in the stomach. Cells lining the pancreatic duct produce bicarbonate (Table 16-2).

Chyme (partially digested food) in the duodenum stimulates the release of hormones, which act on pancreatic juice formation. These hormones are cholecystokinin, gastrin, acetylcholine, and secretin. The first three stimulate acini cells to produce digestive enzymes; secretin stimulates production of sodium bicarbonate. Intercalated ducts drain pancreatic juice from the acini cells into intralobular connecting ducts and, finally, into the main pancreatic duct.

Pancreatic juice moves into the duodenum through the main pancreatic duct, the duct of Wirsung, a vessel approximately 2 mm in diameter. In approximately 77% of cadavers, the duct of Wirsung meets the common bile duct before both ducts enter the duodenum through the ampulla of Vater. As previously mentioned,

an accessory duct, the duct of Santorini is a normal variant that enters the duodenum approximately 2 cm superior to the main duct (see Figure 16-1). The **sphincter of Oddi**, a muscle surrounding the ampulla, relaxes to allow pancreatic juice (and, if the gallbladder has been stimulated, bile) to flow into the duodenum.

The **endocrine** portion of the pancreas is located in the **alpha**, **beta**, **delta**, **gamma**, and **epsilon** cells in the **islets of Langerhans**. Beta cells comprise 60% to 70% of the endocrine cells and produce **insulin**, a hormone that causes glycogen formation from glucose in the liver. It also enables cells with insulin receptors to take up glucose. Hence, blood glucose level decreases. Alpha cells account for 15% to 20% of endocrine tissue and produce **glucagon**, a hormone that causes the opposite effect—cells release glucose to meet the immediate energy needs of the body. Glucagon also stimulates the liver to convert glycogen to glucose, thus increasing blood glucose levels. Delta cells constitute approximately 5% of endocrine tissue and produce a substance called **somatostatin**. This hormone inhibits the production of insulin and glucagon. Gamma cells secrete pancreatic polypeptide (PP) and comprise less than 5% of endocrine cells. Epsilon cells constitute less than 1% of endocrine tissue. The exact function of gamma and epsilon cells is not clearly understood. One research study on 24 human fetal pancreases documented the occasional product of PP and ghrelin together. Studies have documented the release of PP in hypoglycemia, when food is ingested and in response to "sham" eating,

■ ■ **Table 16-3** Endocrine Cells and Pancreatic Hormones

Type of Cell	Hormone	Action
Beta	Insulin	Glucose → Glycogen
Alpha	Glucagon	Glycogen → Glucose
Delta	Somatostatin	Alpha/beta inhibitor
Gamma	Pancreatic polypeptide	Related to blood sugar regulation
Epsilon	Ghrelin	Related to blood sugar regulation

when food is chewed but not swallowed. Pancreatic hormones produced by alpha, beta, gamma, delta, and epsilon cells are released in minute quantities directly into the bloodstream (Table 16-3).

SONOGRAPHIC APPEARANCE

When evaluating the pancreas, the sonographer must examine the texture, contour, shape, and size of the gland. Echo texture of the normal pancreas varies and can appear homogeneous to heterogeneous depending on the amount of interlobular fat that is present. Generally the pancreas appears more echo-dense or hyper-echoic compared to the appearance of the normal liver. The borders of the pancreas are usually well defined with a smooth, curvilinear contour. Shape and size of the pancreas were discussed earlier in the chapter.

The main pancreatic duct (duct of Wirsung) is best seen longitudinally in a transverse scanning plane, within the central portion of the pancreas. Two thin reflective lines separated by about 2 mm of anechoic pancreatic juice may be visualized running the entire length of the pancreas, or only a section or two may be visible at one time depending on the exact orientation of the duct and whether the scanning plane is slightly obliqued. When identifying the duct, care must be taken not to confuse it with the splenic vein, splenic artery, or posterior stomach wall. The close proximity of these structures and similar sonographic appearance can make it a challenge to differentiate them from one another. If there is a question, the splenic vein can be differentiated by following the vessel to its portal vein junction. The splenic artery can be followed back to its origin at the celiac axis, and having the patient drink fluid (if not restricted) will distend the stomach, making it easily identifiable (it also serves to obliterate any view obscuring gas in the stomach as well as provides a clear sonic "window," making imaging of the epigastrium easier).

Transverse Scanning Plane Images Showing Longitudinal Pancreas

The pancreas essentially transverses the abdomen, with the head on the right, the neck and body through the midline, and the tail on the left. Therefore the long axis and other longitudinal sections of the pancreas are seen in transverse scanning plane images. Since the pancreas is surrounded by epigastric vessels (*gastroduodenal artery, common bile duct, inferior vena cava, superior mesenteric vein, portal splenic confluence, portal vein, splenic vein, superior mesenteric artery, aorta*), these vessels serve as excellent landmarks.

Head (Inferior Vena Cava, Gastroduodenal Artery, Common Bile Duct)

As previously noted, the head sits directly in front of (or anterior to) the inferior vena cava, and portions of the common bile duct and gastroduodenal artery run along the right lateral border of the head. The inferior vena cava appears just posterior to the head and uncinate process as a round or oval anechoic structure with thin, smooth walls. Depending on the breathing technique being used, the inferior vena cava can appear very wide or narrow. The common bile duct (seen posterolaterally) and the gastroduodenal artery (seen anterolaterally) appear as two small, anechoic structures with bright walls. As seen in Figure 16-7, longitudinal sections of the pancreas head and axial sections of the inferior vena cava, common bile duct, and gastroduodenal artery are visualized in transverse scanning plane images.

Neck (Superior Mesenteric Vein, Portal Splenic Confluence, Inferior Vena Cava)

As discussed, a portion of the superior mesenteric vein is directly posterior to the inferior level of the neck of the pancreas, and the portal splenic confluence (splenic vein joins the superior mesenteric vein to form the portal vein) is directly posterior to a more superior level of the neck. Just medial to the pancreas head, the neck and uncinate process are separated by the superior mesenteric vein. These vessels appear anechoic with reflective borders and are relatively easy to differentiate because the confluence is larger. The gland is thinner at the neck and merges into the pancreas body (Figure 16-8).

Body and Tail (Splenic Vein, Superior Mesenteric Artery, Aorta)

The pancreas body is located anterior to the splenic vein, superior mesenteric artery, and aorta. It has been described as projecting more anteriorly than the other segments of the pancreas, thus serving as a shelf for the stomach (Figure 16-9). The splenic vein clearly denotes the body and tail of the pancreas and can be seen (coursing from the hilum of the spleen) closely following along the posterosuperior margin of the tail and body, to its confluence with the superior mesenteric vein (forming the portal vein) behind the neck of the

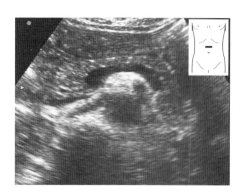
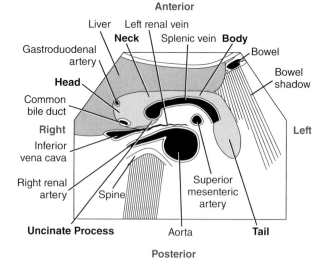

Anterior

Liver — Left renal vein

Gastroduodenal artery — **Neck** — Splenic vein — **Body** — Bowel — Bowel shadow

Head

Common bile duct

Right — Left

Inferior vena cava

Right renal artery — Spine — Superior mesenteric artery

Uncinate Process — Aorta — **Tail**

Posterior

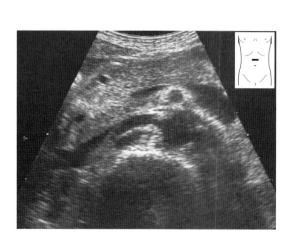
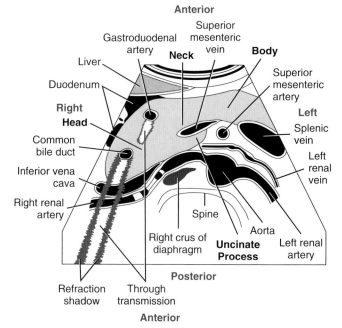

Anterior

Gastroduodenal artery — Superior mesenteric vein — **Neck** — **Body**

Liver — Superior mesenteric artery

Duodenum

Right — **Left**

Head — Splenic vein

Common bile duct — Left renal vein

Inferior vena cava — Spine — Aorta

Right renal artery

Right crus of diaphragm — **Uncinate Process** — Left renal artery

Posterior

Refraction shadow — Through transmission

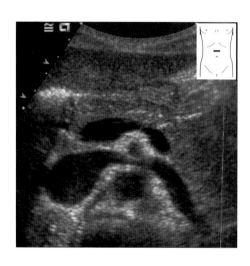
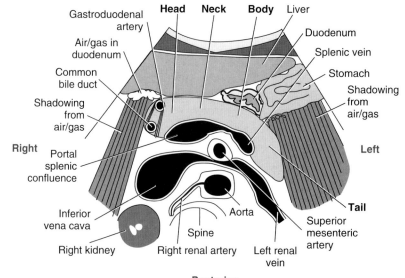

Anterior

Gastroduodenal artery — **Head** — **Neck** — **Body** — Liver

Air/gas in duodenum — Duodenum

Common bile duct — Splenic vein

Shadowing from air/gas — Stomach — Shadowing from air/gas

Right — **Left**

Portal splenic confluence

Inferior vena cava — Aorta — **Tail**

Right kidney — Spine — Right renal artery — Left renal vein — Superior mesenteric artery

Posterior

FIGURE 16-7 **Longitudinal Pancreas Head.** *Transverse scanning plane images of the mid-epigastrium highlighting longitudinal sections of the pancreas head. Note the appearance and proximity of surrounding structures. Observe the anechoic, axial sections of the common bile duct (posteriorly) and gastroduodenal artery (anteriorly) along the right lateral margin of the head.*

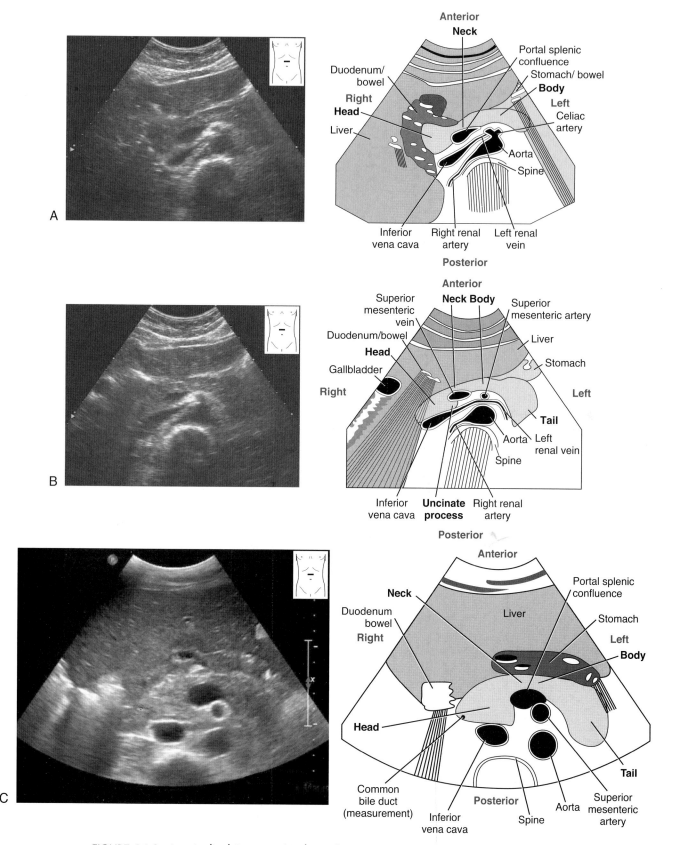

FIGURE 16-8 Longitudinal Pancreas Neck. Mid-epigastric transverse scanning plane images highlighting longitudinal sections of the neck of the pancreas and associated adjacent structures. Notice how compact the anatomy is and how closely related the pancreas is to adjacent epigastric vessels, duodenum and bowel, and the stomach. **A** is the level where the portal splenic confluence is directly posterior to the neck. In **B,** a level slightly inferior to the level in A, observe how the uncinate process is always present when the superior mesenteric vein is visualized. This is the level where the superior mesenteric vein is sandwiched between the neck (anteriorly) and uncinate (posteriorly). In **C,** the neck is easy identifiable just anterior to the portal splenic confluence. Note the calipers indicating the common bile duct measurement, and observe how the pancreas serves as a shelf for the stomach (seen anteriorly).

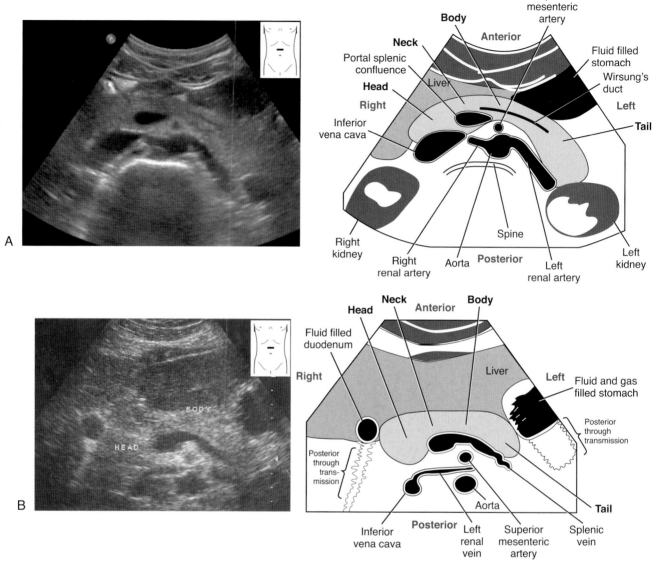

FIGURE 16-9 Longitudinal Pancreas Body. A, B, and C are transverse scanning plane images of the mid-epigastrium, highlighting longitudinal sections of the pancreas body. Notice how the body lies anterior to, and in the same plane with, the aorta and superior mesenteric artery, medial to the neck and tail, and posterior to the stomach and liver. In **A**, observe the anechoic, longitudinal section of Wirsung's duct (main pancreatic duct) in the central portion of the body and part of the tail. Also notice how the fluid-filled stomach helps to delineate the anterior margins of the body and tail. Parts **B** and **C** (located on the next page) clearly demonstrate how the splenic vein runs along the posterior surface of the body.

pancreas. The splenic vein presents with bright walls and anechoic lumen (Figures 16-10 and 16-11).

Sagittal Scanning Plane Images Showing Axial Pancreas

Sagittal scanning plane images of the pancreas show the gland in axial sections. Once again, the epigastric vessels (*gastroduodenal artery, common bile duct, inferior xvena cava, superior mesenteric vein, portal splenic confluence, portal vein, splenic vein, superior mesenteric artery,*

aorta) serve as excellent landmarks for identifying the pancreas.

Head (Inferior Vena Cava, Gastroduodenal Artery, Common Bile Duct)

Figure 16-12 shows axial sections of the pancreas head, which are situated between the homogeneous midgray liver anteriorly and the longitudinal section of the anechoic inferior vena cava posteriorly.

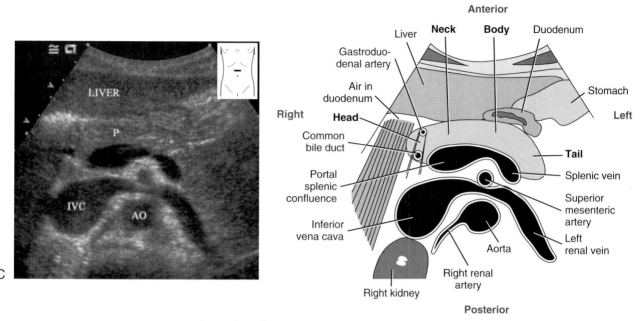

FIGURE 16-9, cont'd **C,** The splenic vein runs along the posterior surface of the body.

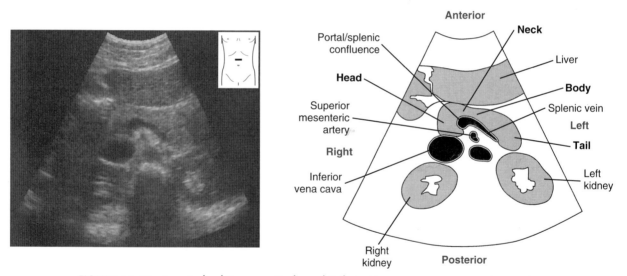

FIGURE 16-10 **Longitudinal Pancreas Body and Tail.** In this transverse scanning plane image of the mid epigastrium, it is easy to appreciate the anechoic longitudinal section of the splenic vein following along the curvilinear shape of the posterior surface of the pancreas body and tail. Notice how the splenic vein enlarges at the confluence, marking the entrance of the superior mesenteric vein. (Image courtesy Jeanes Hospital, Philadelphia, Pennsylvania.)

Neck (Superior Mesenteric Vein, Portal Vein, Inferior Vena Cava)

As previously noted, just medial to the pancreas head, the neck and uncinate process are separated by the superior mesenteric vein. Figure 16-13 demonstrates what this anatomic relationship looks like in a sagittal scanning plane. Moving slightly more medial may move away from the uncinate process, depending on its size, which is variable. However, another section of the

pancreas neck and superior mesenteric vein should be viewable (Figure 16-14).

Body and Tail (Splenic Vein, Superior Mesenteric Artery, Aorta)

Slightly medial to the pancreas neck, the body of the pancreas is situated between the splenic vein (posteriorly) and the stomach and liver (anteriorly). The normal pancreas body is anterior to, and in the same plane as,

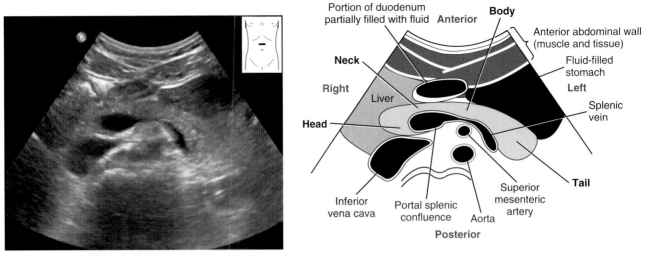

FIGURE 16-11 **Longitudinal Pancreas Body and Tail.** Mid-epigastric transverse scanning plane image showing a longitudinal section of the pancreas body and tail. Observe how the splenic vein hugs their posterior surface along its course to the confluence, making it an excellent vascular landmark.

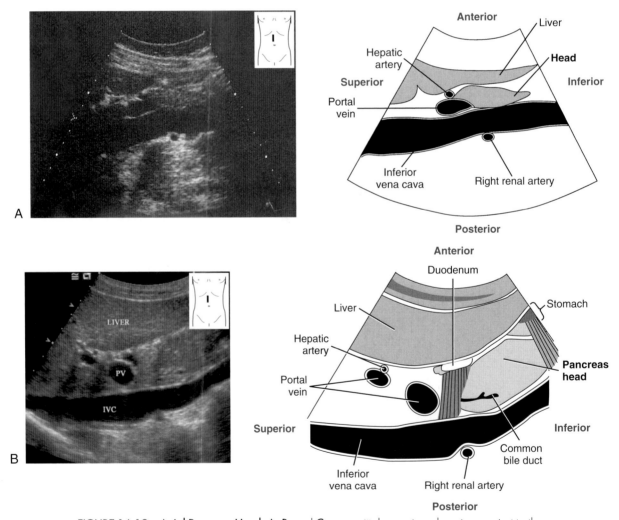

FIGURE 16-12 **Axial Pancreas Head.** A, B, and C are sagittal scanning plane images just to the right of the midline, highlighting axial sections of the pancreas head. A demonstrates an axial section of the pancreas head sandwiched between the liver (anteriorly) and inferior vena cava (posteriorly). Observe the anechoic, axial sections of the portal vein and hepatic artery just superior to the head. Notice how the small, anechoic, axial section of the right renal artery is posterior to the inferior vena cava and head of the pancreas. In B, the head of the pancreas is clearly demonstrated just anterior to the anechoic, longitudinal section of the inferior vena cava and posterior to the liver. The small, anechoic, longitudinal structure in the posterior portion of the head is the common bile duct. Observe a portion of the duodenum, axial sections of the portal vein and hepatic artery superior to the head. (A, Image courtesy Jeanes Hospital, Philadelphia, Pennsylvania.)

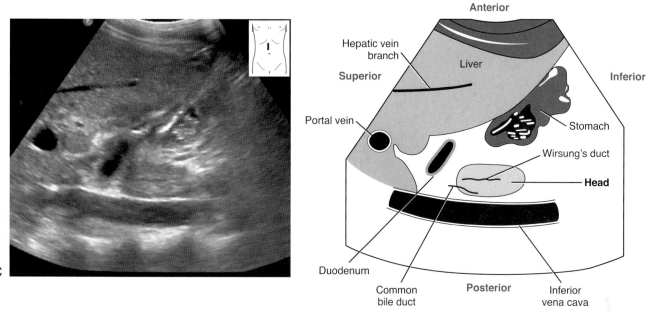

FIGURE 16-12, cont'd   In **C,** the axial section of the head is seen immediately anterior to the long, anechoic section of the inferior vena cava. Observe the long, anechoic section of Wirsung's duct (main pancreatic duct) in the central portion of the head and the long, anechoic section of the common bile duct posteriorly. Also note the food and fluid in the stomach and duodenum anterior and superior to the head of the pancreas.

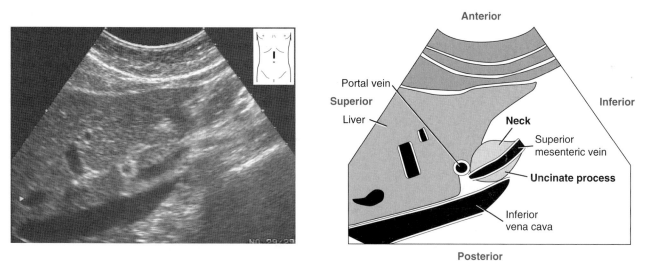

FIGURE 16-13   **Axial Pancreas Neck.** Sagittal scanning plane image just medial to the level of the head of the pancreas. Note the axial sections of the pancreas neck (anteriorly) and uncinate process (posteriorly) separated by the anechoic, longitudinal section of the superior mesenteric vein. Note how the uncinate process sits directly anterior to, or in front of, the longitudinal, anechoic section of the inferior vena cava. The level where the pancreas neck is anterior to the superior mesenteric vein and uncinate process is a level slightly inferior to the level of the portal splenic confluence.

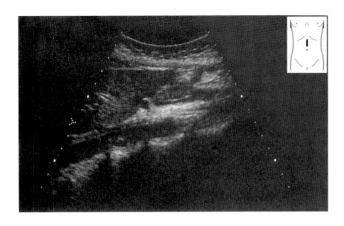
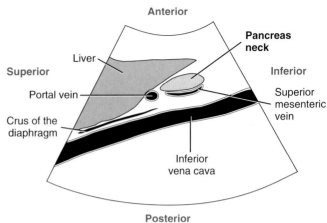

FIGURE 16-14 **Axial Pancreas Neck.** Sagittal scanning plane image of the abdomen at the level of the neck of the pancreas. Note the axial section of the midgray neck located immediately anterior to the anechoic long section of the superior mesenteric vein. (Image courtesy Jeanes Hospital, Philadelphia, Pennsylvania.)

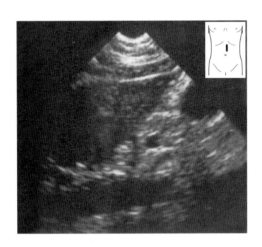
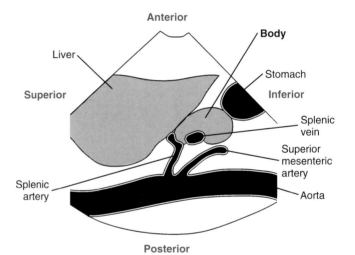

FIGURE 16-15 **Axial Pancreas Body.** Sagittal scanning plane image of the abdomen just to the left of the midline, showing an axial section of the body of the pancreas inferior to the anechoic, long section of the celiac axis/splenic artery, immediately anterior to the anechoic axial section of the splenic vein, anterior to the anechoic long sections of the superior mesenteric artery and aorta, and posterior to portions of the liver and fluid-filled stomach.

the superior mesenteric artery and abdominal aorta (Figures 16-15 and 16-16).

The body of the pancreas merges left laterally into the tail. Again, the best vascular landmark to help identify the tail is the anechoic splenic vein running along its posterosuperior surface. The tail can also be identified anterior to the left kidney (Figures 16-17 and 16-18).

SONOGRAPHIC APPLICATIONS

Uses of pancreatic sonography include the following:
- Structural measurements
- Associate distal biliary tree measurements
- Identification of pancreatic masses
- Identification of epigastric masses
- Main pancreatic duct measurements
- Adjacent associated biliary masses
- Associated biliary obstruction
- Diagnosis and follow-up evaluation of acute and chronic pancreatitis
- Diagnosis and follow-up evaluation of pancreatic pseudocysts
- Endoscopic pancreatic ultrasound for identification of pancreatic lesions on patients whose CT results were inconclusive

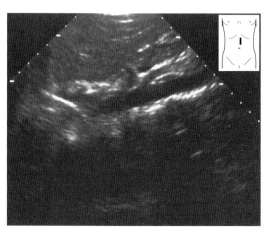

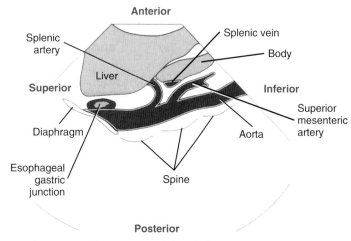

FIGURE 16-16 **Axial Pancreas Body.** Sagittal scanning plane image of the abdomen just to the left of the midline, showing another axial section of the body of the pancreas inferior to the anechoic long section of the celiac axis/splenic artery, immediately anterior to the anechoic axial section of the splenic vein, anterior to the anechoic long sections of the superior mesenteric artery and aorta and posterior to a portion of the liver.

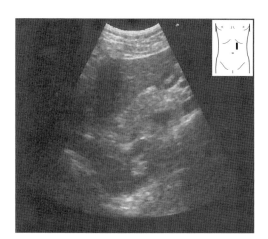

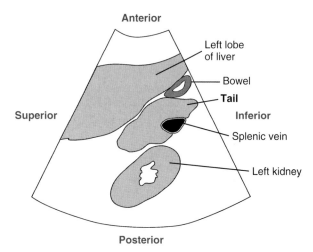

FIGURE 16-17 **Axial Pancreas Tail.** Sagittal scanning plane image of the abdomen slightly left lateral to the aorta. An axial section of the tail of the pancreas is noted between the liver (anteriorly) and left kidney (posteriorly). Note the portion of bowel anteroinferiorly to the tail and the axial section of the anechoic splenic vein along the tail's posterior margin. (Image courtesy Jeanes Hospital, Philadelphia, Pennsylvania.)

NORMAL VARIANTS

- **Annular pancreas:** A condition in which a ring of pancreatic tissue surrounds the second portion (C-loop) of the duodenum.
- **Ectopic (heterotopic, aberrant) pancreas:** Tissue that has no vascular or structural connection to the body of the pancreas. Because ectopic tissues may be as small as 1 cm in size, the condition can be difficult to detect with sonography.
- **Partial duplication of the pancreas tail:** Rare variation. Sonographically, the tail may appear to be grossly enlarged (see Figure 16-18).

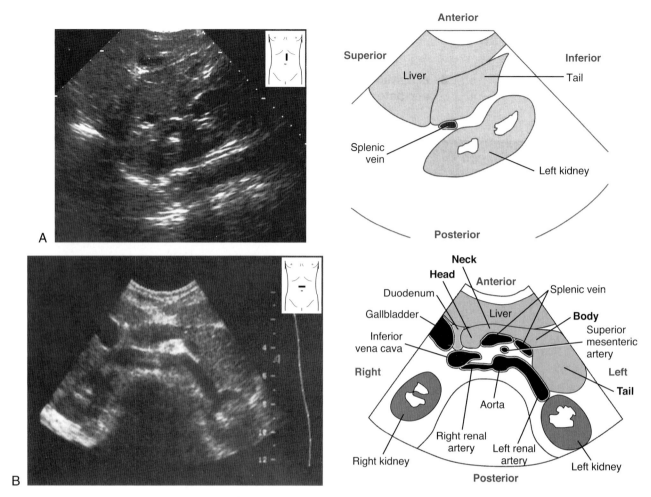

FIGURE 16-18 **Pancreas Tail. A,** Sagittal scanning plane image of the abdomen, just to the left of the midline, showing an axial section of the pancreas tail situated between a long section of the left lobe of the liver (anterosuperiorly) and long section of the left kidney (posteriorly). Note the anechoic axial section of splenic vein between the tail and left kidney. **B,** Transverse scanning plane image of the mid epigastrium, demonstrating an enlarged tail of the pancreas. This patient has a congenital malformation in which the tail is partially duplicated.

REFERENCE CHARTS

■ ■ ■ ASSOCIATED PHYSICIANS

- **Internist:** Involved in diagnosing and treating pancreatic disease.
- **Radiologist:** Interprets/diagnoses imaging modality tests used to evaluate the pancreas and related diseases.
- **Surgeon:** Involved in surgery of the pancreas.

■ ■ ■ COMMON DIAGNOSTIC TESTS

- **General radiography:** Except for the appearance of calcifications, plain radiography is not very revealing for pancreatic disease. An upper gastrointestinal (UGI) series, a study in which the patient swallows barium to outline the stomach and duodenum, detects pancreatic masses or enlargement through displacement of the C-loop of the duodenum by the mass. The UGI series is performed by a radiologist assisted by a radiologic technologist. The radiologist interprets the findings.

- Endoscopic retrograde cholangiopancreatico-duodenography (ERCP): A tube is placed into the duodenum via the esophagus and stomach. Within the tube are fiberoptics to allow visualization of the anatomy and a means for inserting a catheter. The catheter tip is placed in the end of the common bile duct (or the pancreatic duct, depending on the anatomic configuration). A contrast medium is injected into the biliary system, which visualizes structures in retrograde order (in the reverse direction). This examination is usually performed and interpreted by a radiologist and/or gastroenterologist assisted by a radiologic technologist.
- Computed axial tomography (CT) scan: An x-ray beam passes through the patient to be detected by a series of devices that provide an electrical signal to a computer. The computer then arranges the data into a sectional image of the body. Structural and some functional information is obtained. A contrast material may or may not be administered. This examination is performed by a radiologic technologist, and the findings are interpreted by a radiologist.
- Magnetic resonance imaging (MRI): Images are similar in format to those of a CT scan; however, the images are generated using a strong magnetic field instead of radiation. An MRI technologist or a radiologic technologist performs the examination, and a radiologist interprets the findings.
- Angiography: A contrast material is injected into an epigastric vessel to visualize the vascularity of the pancreas of a suspected lesion. This examination is performed by a radiologist assisted by a radiologic technologist. The radiologist interprets the findings.

■ ■ ■   **LABORATORY VALUES**

SERUM TESTS

Amylase	60–80 units
Lipase	1.5 U/mL
Glucose (fasting)	65–110 mg/dL
(all sugars)	80–20 mg/dL

URINE TESTS

Amylase (2 hr)	35–260 units/hr
Alkaline phosphatase	<3.5 U/8 hr

■ ■ ■   **VASCULATURE**

Arterial supply to the head and neck of the pancreas:
Gastroduodenal artery → pancreaticoduodenal arteries → pancreatic arcades
Arterial supply to the body and tail of the pancreas:

Pancreatic splenic artery → suprapancreatic splenic artery → pancreatic splenic artery → prepancreatic splenic artery → prehilar splenic artery

■ ■ ■   **AFFECTING CHEMICALS**

Prolonged alcohol ingestion over a period of years (alcoholism) is toxic to the pancreas.

CHAPTER 17

The Urinary and Adrenal Systems

REVA ARNEZ CURRY AND BETTY BATES TEMPKIN

OBJECTIVES

Describe the function of the urinary and adrenal system.

Explain the blood supply of the kidneys and adrenal glands.

Explain the function of the nephron.

List the hormones and laboratory values associated with the kidneys and adrenal glands, and explain the function of each.

Describe the location of the kidneys, ureters, urethra, urinary bladder, and adrenal glands.

Describe the size of the kidneys, ureters, urethra, urinary bladder, and adrenal glands.

Describe the sonographic appearance of the urinary and adrenal systems.

Describe associated physicians, diagnostic tests, and laboratory values for the kidneys and adrenal glands.

■

KEY WORDS

Adrenal Cortex — Outer layer of the adrenal gland; contains 3 zones that produce steroid hormones, also called *corticoids*.

Adrenal Medulla — Inner layer of the adrenal gland that produces epinephrine and nor-epinephrine hormones.

Aldosterone — Hormone produced by the adrenal cortex that acts on the distal convoluted tubule, which increases water reabsorbed into the bloodstream.

Antidiuretic Hormone (ADH) — Hormone released from the posterior pituitary gland to increase the amount of water returned to the bloodstream from the distal collecting tubules.

Bowman's Capsule — Receives plasma solute from the glomerulus and routes it to the proximal convoluted tubule.

Collecting System — Consists of the infundibulum and renal pelvis, which receive urine from the renal pyramids and convey it to the ureter, which carries the urine to the urinary bladder.

Columns of Bertin — Bands of cortical tissue separating the medullary pyramids from each other.

Erythropoietin Hormone — Hormone released by the kidneys in response to a decrease in oxygen. Erythropoietin acts on bone marrow, causing more red blood cells, the carriers of oxygen, to be produced.

Filtration — First step in urine formation. Filtration takes place in the glomerulus.

Gerota's Fascia — Surrounds the kidney and perirenal fat. Anchors the kidneys and limits any infection arising from them.

Glomerulus — A network of vessels that filters blood to produce a plasma solute, also called *nephric filtrate*, which is received by Bowman's capsule on its way to the proximal convoluted tubule.

Infundibulum — Portion of the renal sinus that contains the minor and major calyces.

Loop of Henle — Where filtration and reabsorption occur.

Lower Urinary Tract — Consists of the urinary bladder and urethra.

Major Calyces — Portion of the infundibulum in the renal sinus that receives urine from the minor calyces and then conveys it to the renal pelvis.

Medullary Pyramids (Renal Pyramids) — Comprise the renal medulla and contain the loops of Henle (*renal loops*), where filtration and reabsorption occur. Convey urine to the minor calyces.

Minor Calyces — Portion of the infundibulum in the renal sinus that receives urine from the medullary pyramids and then conveys it to the major calyces. Form the peripheral border of the renal sinus.

Morison's Pouch — Peritoneal space separating the right kidney from the liver. Also known as the *subhepatic recess* or *hepatorenal recess*.

Nephron — Functional unit of the kidney.

Perinephric Space (Renal Space) — Part of the retroperitoneal space within the renal fascia that contains the kidney, perirenal fat, adrenal gland, and proximal ureter.

Renal — Pertaining to the kidney, a part of the urinary system.

Renal Corpuscle — Structure that includes Bowman's capsule and glomerulus of the nephron.

Renal Cortex — Outer portion of renal parenchyma that contains the renal corpuscle and the proximal and distal convoluted tubules of the nephron.

Renal Hilum — Medial portion of the renal sinus, where the renal artery enters the kidney and the renal vein and ureter exit.

Renal Lobes — Portions of the kidney that consist of a single pyramid, bordered on both sides by interlobar arteries and veins, with cortical tissue at their base.

Renal Medulla — Inner portion of renal parenchyma composed of 8 to 18 medullary pyramids.

Renal Parenchyma — One of the two major areas of the kidney. Consists of the cortex and the medulla.

Renal Pelvis — Upper expanded end of the ureter that receives urine from the major calyces.

KEY WORDS—cont'd

Renal Sinus — Makes up the central portion of the kidney. Houses the renal artery and vein, fatty fibrous tissue, nerves, and lymphatics but is primarily composed of the collecting system and the renal hilum.

Renal Tubule — Structure that comprises the proximal convoluted tubule, loop of Henle, distal convoluted tubule, and collecting duct. Together with the renal corpuscle, the renal tubule comprises the nephron.

Renin — Hormone released by the juxtaglomerular apparatus in the nephron in response to decreased blood volume. Renin acts on angiotensinogen in the blood to increase systemic pressure.

Trigone — Portion of bladder wall defined by imaginary lines that form a triangle that corresponds to or joins the orifices of the ureters and urethra.

Tubular Reabsorption — Process by which substances in the plasma solute that are useful to the body are reabsorbed in the bloodstream.

Tubular Secretion — Process in which waste substances are secreted into the distal convoluted tube for excretion in urine.

Upper Urinary Tract — Composed of the kidneys and ureters.

Ureters — Begin in the kidney as the renal pelvis to transport urine to the urinary bladder.

Urethra — Consists of a membranous, hollow canal that conveys urine from the bladder to the outside.

Urinary Bladder — An elastic, muscular sac that collects urine from the ureters before it is excreted through the urethra.

Zona Fasciculata — Middle portion of the adrenal cortex that produces glucocorticoids, including cortisol that regulates glucose metabolism.

Zona Glomerulosa — The outermost portion of the adrenal gland; produces mineralocorticoids that regulate sodium and potassium levels.

Zona Reticularis — The innermost portion of the adrenal cortex that supplements sex hormones produced by the ovaries and testes.

■■■ NORMAL MEASUREMENTS

Structure	Length	Diameter	Depth (Thickness)
Adult kidney	9 to 12 cm	4 to 6 cm	2.5 to 4.0 cm
Neonatal kidney	3.5 to 5.0 cm	2 to 3 cm	1.5 to 2.5 cm
Ureters	28 to 34 cm	6 mm	NA
Distended urinary bladder wall	NA	NA	3 to 6 mm
Female urethra	4 cm	NA	NA
Male urethra	20 cm	NA	NA

NA, Not applicable.

The urinary system includes two kidneys, a ureter for each kidney, a urinary bladder, and a urethra. The kidneys and ureters make up the **upper urinary tract**, and the urinary bladder and urethra form the **lower urinary tract**.

The kidneys (also called *renals*) are excretory organs that maintain the body's chemical equilibrium through the excretion of urine, a waste product. Each kidney has a ureter that carries the urine to the urinary bladder for temporary storage. Urine is excreted from the bladder to outside the body through the urethra, a membranous canal.

Detoxification, blood pressure regulation, and the maintenance of the correct balance of pH, minerals, iron, and salt levels in the blood are functions of the urinary system.

LOCATION

Upper Urinary Tract: Kidneys, Ureters
Kidneys

The kidneys are retroperitoneal organs that lie one on each side of the spine between the peritoneum and the back muscles. The kidney has a lateral convex and a medial concave border. The liver displaces the right kidney inferiorly (Table 17-1); hence it is located lower than the left kidney and has a slightly shorter ureter.

The kidneys lie in the lower thoracic and lumbar area, between the twelfth thoracic and fourth lumbar vertebrae (Figure 17-1). Deep inspiration causes the kidneys to descend.

Anterior to the right kidney are the right lobe of the liver, second part of the duodenum, hepatic flexure of the colon, and jejunum or ileum of the small bowel (Figure 17-2). **Morison's pouch** (also called the *hepatorenal recess* or *subhepatic recess*) is a peritoneal space separating the right kidney and the liver. One of the most dependent peritoneal spaces in the abdomen, Morison's pouch has the potential to abnormally fill with fluid. The right adrenal gland is situated anterosuperior and slightly medial to the right kidney. Table 17-2 describes portions of the right kidney covered by these structures.

Table 17-1 Location of the Urinary System and Adrenal Glands Routinely Visualized With Ultrasound

	Rt Kidney	Rt Ureter	Lt Kidney	Lt Ureter	Urinary Bladder	Rt Adrenal Gland	Lt Adrenal Gland
Anterior to	Psoas major muscle (medial portion of superior pole), quadratus lumborum muscle (inferior pole), transversus abdominus muscle (lateral portions of superior pole and midsection of kidney), 12th rib (superior pole), transverse process 1st lumbar vertebra (superior pole), diaphragm	Psoas major muscle, rt common iliac artery and vein	Psoas major muscle (medial portion of superior pole), quadratus lumborum muscle (inferior pole), transversus abdominus muscle (lateral portions of superior pole and midsection of kidney), 11th and 12th ribs (superior pole), transverse process 1st lumbar vertebra (superior pole), diaphragm	Psoas major muscle, Lt common iliac artery and vein	Seminal vesicles (in males), vagina (in females), posterior cul-de-sac (in females), rectum	Diaphragm, rt kidney (medial portion of superior pole)	Lt kidney (medial portion of superior pole)
Posterior to	Liver rt lobe, 2nd portion duodenum (midsection of kidney), hepatic flexure colon (lateral portion of inferior pole), jejunum/ileum small bowel inferior pole), rt adrenal gland (narrow medial portion of superior pole), peritoneum, GB (in some cases, superior pole)	Peritoneum, descending duodenum, terminal ileum, ductus deferens (in males), uterine artery (in females), fundus urinary bladder	Pancreas tail (midsection of kidney), Lt adrenal gland (medial portion of superior pole), spleen (lateral portion of superior pole), stomach (superior pole), jejunum (inferior pole), splenic flexure colon (lateral portion of inferior pole), splenic artery (mid-section of kidney)	Peritoneum, colon, ductus deferens (in males), uterine artery (in females), fundus urinary bladder	Peritoneum, symphysis pubis	IVC, liver rt lobe, duodenum (inferior portion in some cases), peritoneum	Stomach, splenic artery, peritoneum (superior anterior surface), pancreas body (inferior anterior surface)
Superior to	Rt ureter, rt iliac crest, rt common iliac artery and vein	Rt common iliac artery and vein, urinary bladder	Lt ureter, lt iliac crest, Lt common iliac artery and vein	Lt common iliac artery and vein, urinary bladder	Prostate gland (in males)	Rt kidney, rt renal artery and vein	Lt kidney, lt renal artery and vein
Inferior to	Diaphragm, liver rt lobe, rt adrenal gland	Rt kidney, rt renal artery and vein	Diaphragm, spleen (lateral portions of superior pole and midsection of kidney)	Lt kidney, lt renal artery and vein	Aorta, IVC, rt and lt common iliac arteries and veins	Liver rt lobe, diaphragm	Spleen, diaphragm
Medial to	Rt lateral abdominal wall		Lt lateral abdominal wall, spleen		Rt and lt ureters, rt and lt common iliac arteries and veins	Rt kidney (medial portion of superior pole)	Lt kidney (medial portion of superior pole), spleen
Lt lateral to			Lt renal artery, lt renal vein, lt ureter, aorta, lt common iliac artery and vein, lt adrenal gland	Aorta, spine			Aorta, celiac artery, spine
Rt lateral to	Rt renal artery, rt renal vein, rt ureter, IVC, rt common iliac artery and vein	IVC, spine				Spine	

AGL, Adrenal gland; GB, gallbladder; IVC, inferior vena cava; UB, urinary bladder.

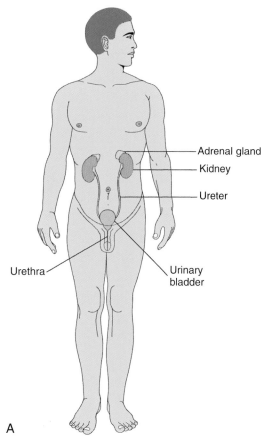

Adrenal gland
Kidney
Ureter
Urethra
Urinary bladder

A

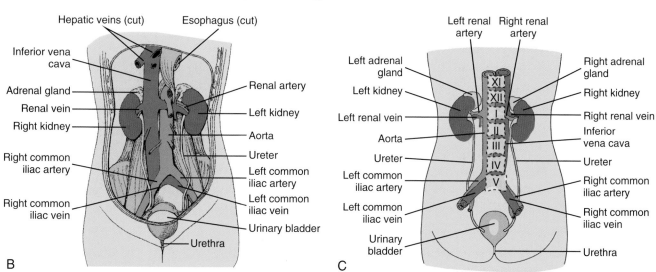

Hepatic veins (cut)   Esophagus (cut)

Inferior vena cava

Adrenal gland
Renal vein
Right kidney

Right common iliac artery

Right common iliac vein

Renal artery
Left kidney
Aorta
Ureter
Left common iliac artery
Left common iliac vein
Urinary bladder
Urethra

B

Left renal artery   Right renal artery

Left adrenal gland
Left kidney
Left renal vein
Aorta
Ureter
Left common iliac artery
Left common iliac vein
Urinary bladder

Right adrenal gland
Right kidney
Right renal vein
Inferior vena cava
Ureter
Right common iliac artery
Right common iliac vein
Urethra

C

FIGURE 17-1 **The Urinary Tract. A,** Adrenal glands, kidneys, ureters, urinary bladder, and urethra. **B,** Frontal view of the urinary system shows how the ureters cross the iliac vessels anteriorly. **C,** Posterior view shows the urinary tract from behind. Note frontal placement of the ureters.

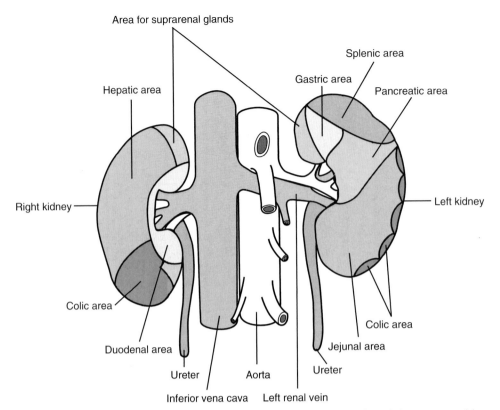

FIGURE 17-2 **Frontal View of the Kidneys.** Delineates the portions of the kidneys covered by the overlying adrenal glands, liver, duodenum, hepatic flexure, jejunum, stomach, splenic flexure, spleen, and pancreatic tail (see Tables 17-2 and 17-3).

■ ■ ■ **Table 17-2**   Anterior Structures That Cover the Right Kidney

Structure	Portion of Kidney Covered
Right adrenal	Superior-medial
Right lobe of liver	Lateral
Second part of duodenum	Medial
Hepatic flexure of colon and jejunum or ileum of small bowel	Inferior

■ ■ ■ **Table 17-3**   Anterior Structures That Cover the Left Kidney

Structure	Portion of Kidney Covered
Tail of pancreas	Medial
Left adrenal gland	Superior-medial
Spleen	Superior-lateral
Jejunum	Inferior
Stomach	Superior
Splenic flexure of colon	Lateral

■ ■ ■ **Table 17-4**   Structures Posterior to Kidneys

Structure	Portion of Kidney Covered
Diaphragm	Superior
Psoas muscle	Medial
Transversus muscle	Lateral
Quadratus lumborum muscle	Between lateral and medial portions

Anterior to the left kidney are the tail of the pancreas, the spleen, the jejunum, the stomach, and the splenic flexure of the colon (see Figure 17-2). The left adrenal gland is situated anterosuperior and slightly medial to the left kidney. Table 17-3 describes portions of the left kidney covered by these structures.

Posterior to both kidneys are the diaphragm, the psoas muscle, the transversus muscle, and the quadratus lumborum muscle (Figure 17-3). Table 17-4 lists structures posterior to the kidneys.

Ureters

The **ureters** are retroperitoneal structures that begin as an expanded area, the renal pelvis, in the hilum of each kidney. The ureters extend inferiorly along the psoas muscle. They travel from the renal hilum into the abdominopelvic cavity, and finally enter the urinary bladder posteriorly (see Figure 17-1, *C*).

The right ureter is posterior to the duodenum, terminal ileum, and right colic, ileocolic, and gonadal vessels.

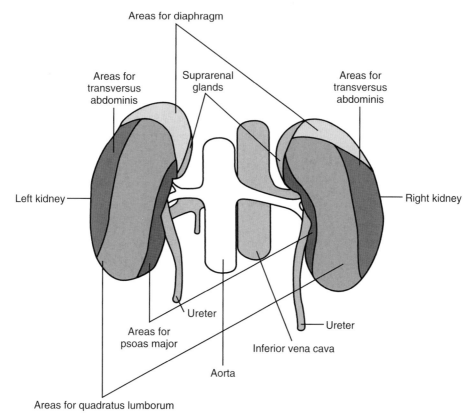

FIGURE 17-3 **Posterior View of the Kidneys.** Delineates the portions of the kidneys covered by the overlying diaphragm, quadratus lumborum, psoas, and transversus muscles (see Table 17-4).

The left ureter is posterior to the colon and the left colic and left gonadal (testicular or ovarian) vessels.

The abdominal portions of both ureters pass anteriorly to the psoas muscle and the bifurcation of the common iliac arteries. The pelvic portions of the ureters pass posteriorly to the ductus deferens in the male and uterine artery in the female.

Lower Urinary Tract: Urinary Bladder, Urethra
Urinary Bladder
Both ureters empty posteriorly into the urinary bladder, a retroperitoneal organ that is posterior to the symphysis pubis. The male urinary bladder is anterior to the seminal vesicles and the rectum and superior to the prostate gland. The ductus deferens, on its superior, slightly lateral course fromn the scrotum, crosses the ureter anteriorly, before descending into the prostate gland (Figure 17-4). The female urinary bladder is anterior to the vagina, posterior cul-de-sac, and rectum (Figure 17-5).

Urethra
The urethra is a membranous canal that conveys urine out of the urinary bladder. It exits inferiorly via the neck of the urinary bladder. The male urethra is much longer than the female urethra and also functions as a pathway for seminal fluid.

SIZE
The normal adult kidney is approximately 9 to 12 cm in length, 2.5 to 4 cm in depth, and 4 to 6 cm in diameter. The left kidney is slightly longer. In one study the left kidney had a median length of 11.2 cm, and the right kidney had a length of 10.9 cm. Another study reported that kidneys are longer in the male, with an average length of 12.4 cm; the average is 11.6 cm in females. One study showed that renal length increases slightly, 6.8% on the right and 6.6% on the left, after oral hydration. This may mean that when renal measurements are critical, the hydration state of the patient should be considered. The kidney may shrink due to atrophic changes associated with age, circulatory insufficiency, or renal disease. If only one kidney is present (i.e., congenital absence of a kidney), it may be larger than normal as a result of hypertrophy necessary to accommodate the increased workload.

The neonatal kidney measures 3.3 to 5.0 cm in length, 1.5 to 2.5 cm in depth, and 2 to 3 cm in diameter. The pediatric kidney is proportionately larger than the adult kidney and may extend inferiorly to the iliac crest. The left pediatric kidney has been noted to be approximately the same length as the pediatric spleen, with a 1.25 or greater spleen-to-left-kidney ratio indicating a possibility of splenomegaly.

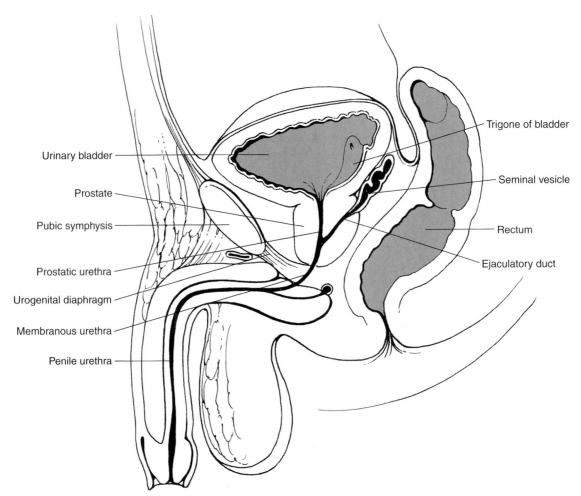

FIGURE 17-4 **Lower Urinary Tract in the Male.** Note the three different parts of the male urethra.

The adult ureters are hollow, narrow tubes ranging from 25 to 30 cm in length. The diameter ranges between 4 and 7 mm. In a cadaver the diameter is a uniform 5 mm throughout the length. The ureters transport urine to the bladder through peristaltic action. The urinary bladder is a symmetric hollow organ whose size depends on the quantity of contained urine. The wall of a distended bladder will normally measure 3 to 6 mm, depending on the degree of bladder distention. A moderately full adult bladder contains approximately 500 mL of urine. The bladder capacity in children over 1 year of age can be calculated by the child's age + 2 × 30 to determine the approximate mL capacity. The adult male urethra is 20 cm in length; the adult female urethra is considerably shorter, measuring approximately 3.5 cm in length.

GROSS ANATOMY
Upper Urinary Tract: Kidneys, Ureters
Kidneys
The kidney is descriptively divided into upper, middle, and lower portions. It has several protective coverings that cushion and protect the entire organ (Figure 17-6).

First, it is covered with a tough, fibrous capsule that is closely applied but not adherent to the parenchyma. Second, a layer of perirenal fat surrounds the encapsulated kidney and is continuous with the fat in the renal sinus. The third layer, the renal fascia or **Gerota's fascia**, surrounds the kidney and perirenal fat. Gerota's fascia is surrounded by yet another layer of fat, called *pararenal fat*. This layer is especially thick posterior to Gerota's fascia. The renal fascia anchors the kidneys and limits any infection arising from them. The double layer of renal fat (perirenal and pararenal) accommodates kidney movement during respiration. Listed below are some common alternative names given to the tissues that cover the kidneys:

- Perinephric fat = adipose capsule = packing fat of Zuckerkandl
- Perirenal fascia = perinephric fascia = fascia of Gerota
- Pararenal fat = pararenal body
- Renal capsule = true capsule = fibrous capsule

The kidney is composed of two distinct areas, the peripheral *parenchyma* and central *sinus*. A dissected view of the kidney is shown in Figure 17-7.

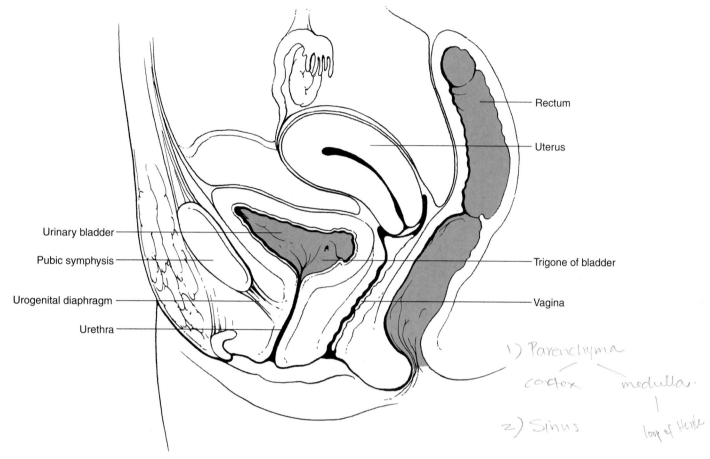

FIGURE 17-5 Lower Urinary Tract in the Female.

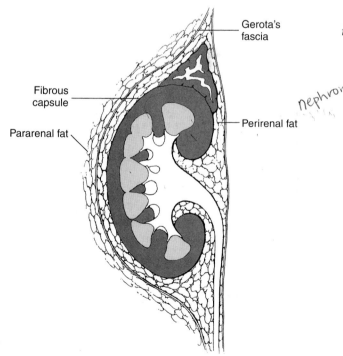

FIGURE 17-6 **Four Layers Surrounding the Kidney.** Fibrous capsule, perirenal fat, Gerota's fascia, and pararenal fat.

Renal parenchyma consists of two areas, the *cortex* and *medulla*:

- The **renal cortex** is the outer portion of the parenchyma (see Figure 17-7). It contains the renal corpuscle and the proximal and distal convoluted tubules of the nephron, the **functional unit of the kidney.**
- The inner portion of the parenchyma is called the **renal medulla**; it consists of 8 to 18 **medullary pyramids**, which contain the *loops of Henle* (also called *renal loops*), where **filtration and reabsorption** occur (Figure 17-8).
- The medullary pyramids are triangular structures with a narrow tip, called the *apex*, and a broad base. The apex of a pyramid sits within a minor calyx located in the renal sinus. From the apex, the pyramid expands and extends laterally to its base, which abuts the renal cortex. Pyramids are separated from each other by bands of cortical tissue called **columns of Bertin.** Therefore the base and sides of each pyramid are surrounded by the cortex (see Figure 17-7). Pyramids are also one of the components that comprise a renal lobe. **Renal lobes** are referred to as those portions of the kidney

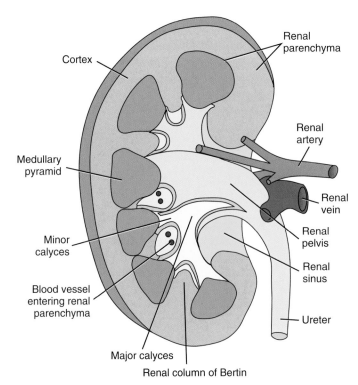

FIGURE 17-7 *Section of Internal Kidney Anatomy.* Notice how the number of medullary pyramids equals the number of minor calyces and also how the minor calyces form the border of the renal sinus. Observe how the ureter begins in the kidney as the renal pelvis.

that consist of a single pyramid, bordered on both sides by interlobar arteries and veins, with cortical tissue at its base (Figure 17-9).

The **renal sinus** is the central portion of the kidney. It houses the renal artery and vein, fatty fibrous tissue, nerves, and lymphatics but is primarily composed of the *collecting system* and the *renal hilum:*

- The **collecting system** consists of the *infundibulum* and *renal pelvis:*
  - The **infundibulum** is composed of the *minor* and *major calyces.* The 8 to 18 renal pyramids convey urine to an equal number of **minor calyces**, which form the peripheral border of the renal sinus (see Figure 17-7). There are usually 2 to 3 **major calyces** that receive urine from the minor calyces.
  - The **renal pelvis** is the upper expanded end of the ureter that receives urine from the major calyces.
- The **renal hilum** is the medial portion of the renal sinus, where the renal artery enters the kidney and the renal vein and ureter exit (see Figure 17-7).

Ureters

The ureters begin in the kidney as the renal pelvis. They are composed of three layers of tissue: an inner mucosal layer, a medial layer of longitudinal and circular smooth muscle, and an outer fibrous layer. Ureteral peristalsis transports urine to the urinary bladder. Urine is carried into the urinary bladder between intervals of several seconds and several minutes, depending on the state of hydration or fluid balance in the body. Blood is supplied to the ureters by branches from the renal, internal spermatic, hypogastric, and inferior vesical arteries.

Lower Urinary Tract: Urinary Bladder, Urethra
Urinary Bladder

The ureters enter the urinary bladder posteriorly at the **trigone** area, the portion of bladder wall defined by imaginary lines that form a triangle that corresponds or joins the orifices of the ureters and urethra. The **urinary bladder** is an elastic, muscular sac that collects urine from the ureters before it is excreted through the urethra. It consists of four layers of tissues: an inner mucosa, a submucosa, the muscularis, and the outer serosa. The mucosa folds when the bladder is empty, and it distends and becomes smooth when the bladder is full. The muscularis layer is composed of three layers of smooth muscle called the *detrusor muscle.* The outermost layer of the bladder, the serosa, is located at the superior portion of the bladder. It is an extension of pelvic peritoneum (Figure 17-10).

The inferior portion of the urinary bladder consists of a posterior base (the trigone area) and the neck,

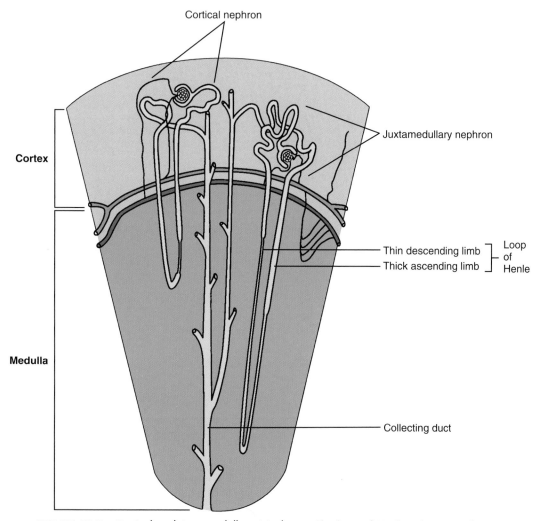

FIGURE 17-8 **Cortical and Juxtamedullary Nephrons.** The loop of Henle is longer in the juxtamedullary nephron.

which communicates with the urethra. The inferolateral surfaces of the bladder meet anteriorly and are in contact with the pelvic floor muscles.

The anterior portion of the urinary bladder lies behind the pubic bone and the symphysis pubis. Only the superior portion of the urinary bladder is covered by an extension of peritoneum. The location of the superior portion is variable, depending on the amount of urine in the bladder (Figure 17-11).

The urinary bladder is anchored to the pelvis by ligaments that extend anteriorly from the bladder neck and attach to the pubic bones. These ligaments are called *pubovesical* in the female, and *puboprostatic* in the male. Lateral ligaments extend to fuse with the tendinous arch of the obturator internus muscles.

Blood is supplied to the urinary bladder by the superior, middle, and inferior vesicles derived from the anterior trunk of the hypogastric ("internal iliac") artery. The obturator and inferior gluteal arteries also supply small visceral branches to the bladder, and additional branches in the female are derived from the uterine and vaginal arteries.

Urethra

The **urethra** consists of a membranous, hollow canal that conveys urine from the bladder to the outside. The male urethra is approximately 20 cm in length, compared with the female urethra, which is approximately 3.5 cm in length. The male urethra is composed of three parts. The first portion, the prostatic urethra, receives secretions from the prostate gland. The second part is the short, membranous urethra, which pierces the urogenital diaphragm. The third, and longest, portion is the penile urethra, which extends the entire length of the

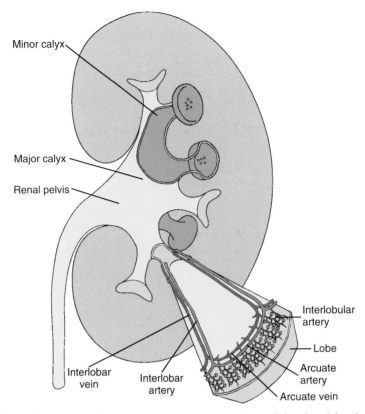

FIGURE 17-9   **Renal Lobe.** Note that the lobe is triangular and bordered by the interlobar vasculature. The arcuate and interlobular vessels and the surrounding cortical tissue form the base of the lobe.

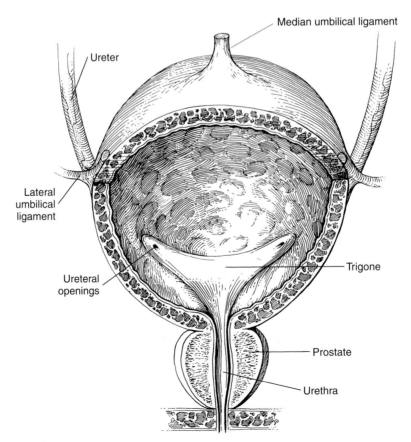

FIGURE 17-10   **Urinary Bladder.** Note the triangular area, the trigone, where the ureters enter. Also shown is the lateral umbilical ligament.

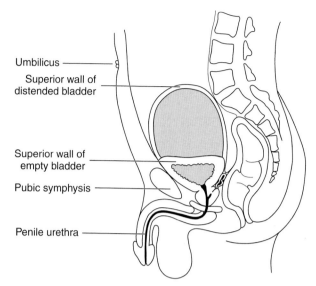

Umbilicus

Superior wall of
distended bladder

Superior wall of
empty bladder

Pubic symphysis

Penile urethra

FIGURE 17-11 **Urinary Bladder.** Difference between the appearance of an empty and distended urinary bladder. Note how the superior portion of the distended bladder moves toward the umbilicus.

penis (see Figure 17-4). The female urethra is composed of the membranous urethra, which also pierces the urogenital diaphragm (see Figure 17-5).

PHYSIOLOGY

As the primary excretory organs (see Chapter 5), the kidneys' principal functions are urine production and homeostasis (maintenance of normal body physiology). The kidneys function independently to excrete metabolic waste products and maintain blood volume. A unilateral condition, such as complete obstruction, congenital absence of a kidney, trauma, or removal of a kidney, will not affect the remaining kidney's ability to function; the healthy kidney will accommodate the increased workload. Failure of both kidneys, however, will lead to uremia, a toxic and fatal condition if untreated.

The kidneys filter approximately 1600 mL of blood per minute and, depending on the state of hydration, produce on average 150 mL of urine daily. The excreted urine is 95% water and 5% nitrogenous waste and inorganic salts. Nitrogenous waste consists of the byproducts of metabolism. The amount of nitrogenous waste is measured by blood urea nitrogen (BUN) and creatinine (Cr), laboratory tests that measure the kidneys' ability to get rid of waste (see *Laboratory Values* in the Reference Charts section at the end of this chapter).

The functional unit of the kidney is the **nephron**. There are over a million microscopic nephrons in each kidney. The nephron functions by moving metabolic products from areas of high concentration to areas of low concentration. This is accomplished through osmosis, the passive transport of cellular material. Another method is active transport, which uses cellular energy to move material from one area to another.

There are two types of nephrons, juxtamedullary and cortical, which are named for their location in the kidney and the length of their loops. Juxtamedullary nephrons originate in the inner third of the renal cortex and have longer loops of Henle than cortical nephrons, which are located in the outer two thirds of the renal cortex (see Figure 17-8).

The nephron consists of a **renal corpuscle**, which includes Bowman's capsule and the glomerulus, and a **renal tubule** (proximal convoluted tubule, loop of Henle, distal convoluted tubule, collecting duct) (Figure 17-12). The medulla contains the loop of Henle and collecting duct. The renal cortex contains the glomerulus, Bowman's capsule, and the proximal and distal convoluted tubules.

Blood reaches the nephron in the following manner. Blood enters the kidney through the *renal artery*, a branch of the aorta. The renal artery forms *interlobar arteries*, which travel between the renal pyramids. The interlobar arteries branch into *arcuate* arteries, located at the base of the renal pyramids. From the arcuate arteries, the interlobular arteries travel into the renal cortex. The interlobular arteries branch into *afferent arterioles*, which carry blood into the glomerulus of the nephron. Blood from the efferent arterioles supplies the peritubular capillaries, which in turn supply the proximal and distal convoluted tubules and the vasa recta. The vasa recta are a series of intertwining capillary loops that surround the juxtamedullary nephron. Through osmotic pressure, the vasa recta trap salt and urea in the medulla and move water back into the blood. This mechanism is called the *countercurrent multiplier system* and helps the kidneys maintain homeostasis. Blood from the peritubular capillaries drains into the interlobular veins, which in turn drain into arcuate veins. The arcuate veins drain into the interlobar veins, which convey blood back to the renal veins. The renal veins carry blood to the inferior vena cava.

How the Nephron Works

- **Filtration:** This is the first step in urine formation. It takes place in the **glomerulus**. As blood enters the glomerulus, afferent arterioles carrying the blood branch into capillaries. As the vessels narrow, the blood pressure in the vessels increases. Most capillaries have a blood pressure of approximately 25 mm Hg (mercury). However, in the glomerulus the pressure is 60 to 90 mm Hg. This higher blood pressure forces a plasma-like fluid from the blood to filter into **Bowman's capsule**. This "nephric filtrate" contains water, salt, glucose, urea, and amino acids. Proteins

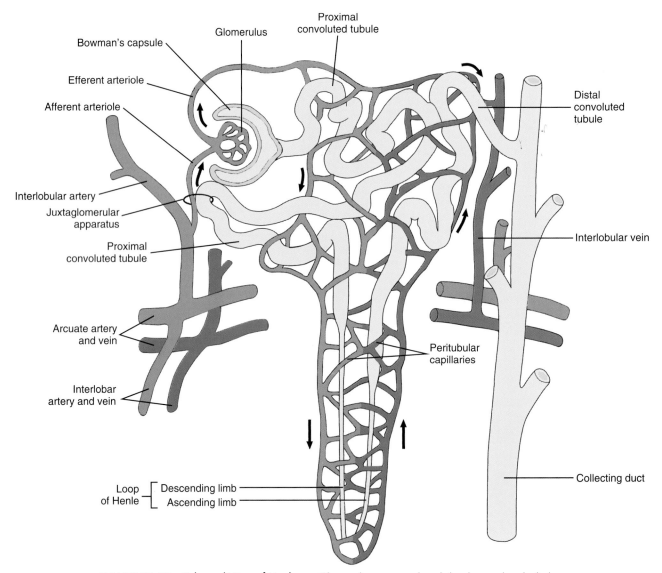

FIGURE 17-12 **Enlarged View of Nephron.** Glomerulus, proximal and distal convoluted tubules, loop of Henle, and collecting duct are shown. Note juxtaglomerular apparatus.

and cells, which are too large to pass through the semipermeable walls of the glomerular capillaries, remain in the blood.

○ Osmotic pressure forces water to return to the blood. This pressure is created by the difference in protein content of the fluid in the proximal convoluted tubule and the plasma in the glomerular capsule. The protein concentration in the proximal convoluted tubule is 2 to 5 mg/100 mL compared with the capsule concentration of 6 to 8 mg/100 mL. This concentration gradient creates osmotic pressure, which returns water from the proximal convoluted tubule back to the plasma in the glomerular capsule, where it is returned into the blood.

○ The fluid that enters the glomerulus is called *ultrafiltrate.* The volume of filtrate produced per minute is 115 mL for women and 165 mL for men. This means that the body's entire blood volume is filtered approximately every 40 minutes. During this process, 99% of the blood volume is returned and 1% is excreted.

• **Tubular reabsorption**: This is the process by which substances in the plasma solute that are useful to the body are reabsorbed into the bloodstream. These substances include water, glucose, vitamins, amino acids, bicarbonate ions, and chloride salts of magnesium, sodium, calcium, and potassium. Reabsorption takes place in the proximal convoluted tubule and the descending and ascending **loop of Henle.**

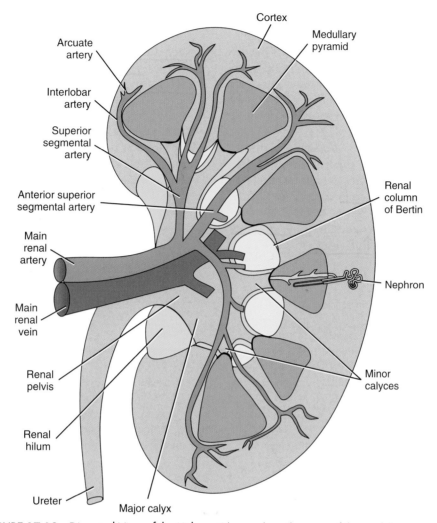

Cortex

Medullary pyramid

Arcuate artery

Interlobar artery

Superior segmental artery

Anterior superior segmental artery

Main renal artery

Main renal vein

Renal pelvis

Renal hilum

Ureter

Major calyx

Renal column of Bertin

Nephron

Minor calyces

FIGURE 17-13 **Dissected View of the Kidney.** Observe how the apex of the medullary pyramid lies within the minor calyx and how several minor calyces empty urine into a single major calyx. Also, notice how the urine would empty from all of the major calyces into the renal pelvis and down the ureter on its way to the urinary bladder.

Approximately 65% of the salt and water in the ultrafiltrate is reabsorbed from the proximal convoluted tubule, and 20% is reabsorbed from the loop of Henle. The amount of reabsorption of the remaining ultrafiltrate depends on hormonal influence and takes place in the distal convoluted tubule. Tubular reabsorption takes place through active transport and expends a large amount of energy. It has been estimated that 6% of total calories consumed by the body at rest (no physical activity) may be required for tubular resorption.

Tubular secretion: This is the process whereby waste substances, including ammonia, drugs, hydrogen, and potassium, are secreted into the distal convoluted tubule. The secretion process is controlled through active transport. Urine exits the distal convoluted tubule into the collecting tubule or duct. The collecting ducts convey urine to the renal pyramids. The apex of the pyramid lies within the minor calyx, which is part of the collecting system for urine. Several minor calyces empty urine into each major calyx; several major calyces empty urine into the renal pelvis (Figure 17-13). The urine is emptied from the renal pelvis into the ureter and, by peristalsis, is carried to the urinary bladder.

Protective Mechanisms That Preserve Nephron Function

The kidneys are sensitive to changes in blood volume and have the capacity to alter it to maintain homeostasis. This is necessary because the kidneys need a large volume of blood for urine production and to nourish the cells lining the nephron. The latter are especially sensitive to anoxia (lack of oxygen), and a prolonged decrease in blood oxygen may result in irreversible cellular death. Thus, there are several protective mechanisms that enable the kidneys to regulate blood volume and guard against anoxia; these mechanisms are discussed below and summarized in Table 17-5.

↑ Blood Volume

- **Antidiuretic hormone (ADH):** A decrease in blood volume stimulates receptors in the left atrium of the heart and the lungs. This activates the release of ADH from the posterior pituitary gland. ADH increases the quantity of water returned from the distal collecting tubule to the bloodstream. As a result, urine volume decreases and blood volume increases.

↑ Blood Volume.

- **Aldosterone hormone:** Another hormone that affects blood volume is aldosterone, which is produced by the adrenal cortex and acts on the distal convoluted tubule. A decrease in blood volume stimulates the release of aldosterone. Aldosterone causes salt and water to be reabsorbed from the nephron into the bloodstream, which increases blood volume.
- **Juxtaglomerular apparatus:** This system is located at the point where the afferent and efferent arterioles and distal convoluted tubule come into contact (Figure 17-14). Granular cells in the afferent arteriole detect a decrease in blood volume. The granular cells release renin, which acts on angiotensinogen in the blood to increase systemic pressure. Cells in the distal convoluted tubule in contact with the afferent and

■ ■ ■ **Table 17-5** Affecting Chemicals/Hormones—Hormones Associated With the Urinary System

Hormone	Stimulated by	Released by	Effect
Antidiuretic hormone (ADH)	Decrease in blood volume	Posterior pituitary gland	Increases water reabsorption in distal collecting tubules
Aldosterone	Decrease in blood volume	Adrenal cortex	Increases salt and water reabsorption in the distal collecting tubules
Renin	Decrease in blood volume	Granular cells in the afferent arteriole	Acts on angiotensinogen in the blood to increase systemic pressure
Erythropoietin	Decrease in oxygen	Kidneys	Increases red blood cell production

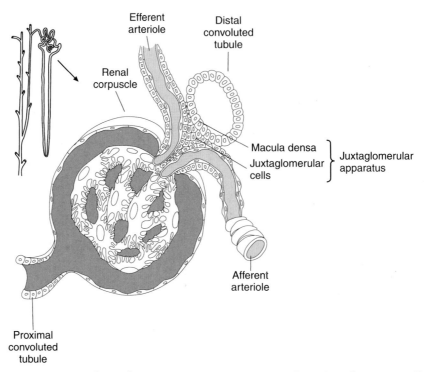

FIGURE 17-14 **Juxtaglomerular Apparatus.** Note granular cells in the afferent and efferent arterioles. The macula densa are located in the distal convoluted tubule.

efferent arterioles are called *macula densa* (see Figure 17-14). It is believed that the macula densa can inhibit renin secretion when the blood volume returns to normal.

- **Erythropoietin hormone**: The kidneys release this hormone in response to a decrease in oxygen (e.g., due to hemorrhage). Erythropoietin acts on bone marrow, causing red blood cells to be produced. It also causes mature red blood cells stored in the bone marrow to be released into the bloodstream. This mechanism increases the number of red cells in the blood, thus enhancing the ability of the blood to carry oxygen.

- Another protective mechanism takes place during prolonged anoxia. Blood is shunted from the outer cortex to the inner cortex to maintain renal function. The kidneys are also able to decrease resistance in the renal capillary bed (increasing the blood supply to the kidneys) when systemic pressure drops.

SONOGRAPHIC APPEARANCE
Upper Urinary Tract: Kidneys, Ureters
Kidneys
The normal kidney appears heterogeneous with a smooth contour. In longitudinal sections the normal adult kidney appears as an elliptical structure (Figure 17-15). Axial or short axis sections of the normal adult kidney appear rounded and broken medially by the renal hilum. The renal vein and artery can be visualized in the hilar region (Figure 17-16). Figures 17-17 through 17-20 show longitudinal sections of the right and left kidneys. Axial views of both kidneys are seen in Figures 17-21 through 17-24.

A detailed description of the sonographic patterns of normal renal anatomy follows:

- **Renal capsule**: This fibrous capsule appears as a thin, continuous, highly reflective line visualized along the periphery of the kidney; it is hyperechoic relative to adjacent renal cortex (see Figure 17-16).

- **Renal cortex**: This presents as midgray or medium- to low-level homogeneous echoes that are less than or equal to the density of the liver or spleen. As discussed, the extensions of cortex seen between the medullary pyramids are the columns of Bertin (see Figure 17-16). The discrete, echogenic dots that may be seen at the corticomedullary junction are the arcuate vessels; they serve as a marker for evaluation of cortical thickness.

- **Renal medulla**: Consists of the medullary pyramids, which appear as triangular, round, or blunted anechoic areas when urine filled and are otherwise not visible. They are 1.2 to 1.5 cm thick. Anechoic pyramids have a distinctive and readily identifiable appearance; their echo-free presentation is in sharp contrast to the highly echogenic sinus and medium-gray cortex (see Figure 17-18).

Text continued on p. 286

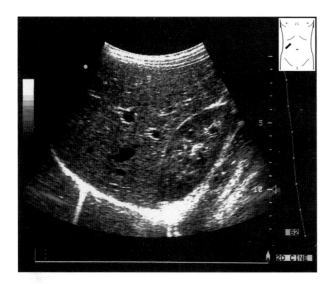

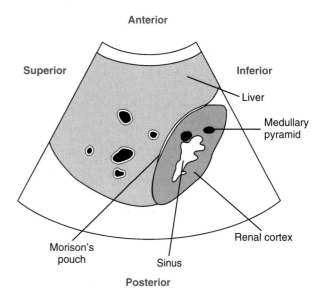

FIGURE 17-15 **Longitudinal Right Kidney.** Sagittal scanning plane image showing a longitudinal section of the right kidney. The liver is superoanterior to the kidney. The curvilinear, highly echogenic line between the liver and right kidney is the renal capsule and site of Morison's pouch, a peritoneal space that has the potential to abnormally fill with fluid. Note the anechoic medullary pyramids along the periphery of the bright, centrally located renal sinus.

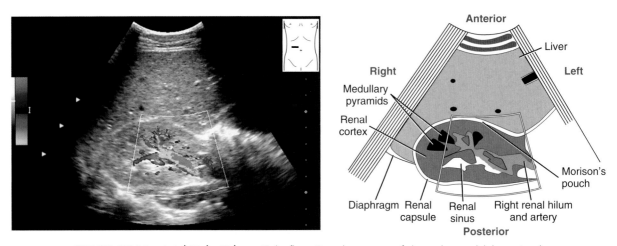

FIGURE 17-16 **Axial Right Kidney.** Color-flow Doppler image of the right renal hilum. Axial section of the right kidney shows the renal hilum where the renal artery enters the kidney and the renal vein and ureter exit.

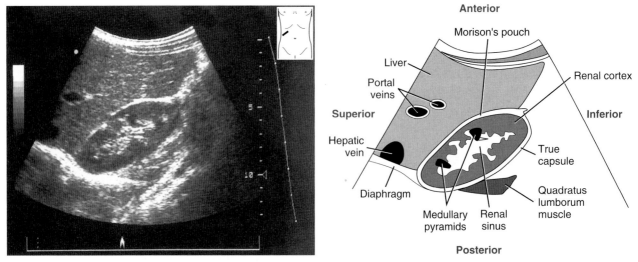

FIGURE 17-17 **Longitudinal Right Kidney.** Longitudinal section of the right kidney and liver, which is seen anteriorly. A low-gray section of the quadratus lumborum muscle can be identified posterior to the kidney. The renal sinus and true capsule appear highly reflective and in sharp contrast to the homogeneous midgray shades of the renal cortex and liver parenchyma. Note how the kidney appears hypoechoic relative to the liver.

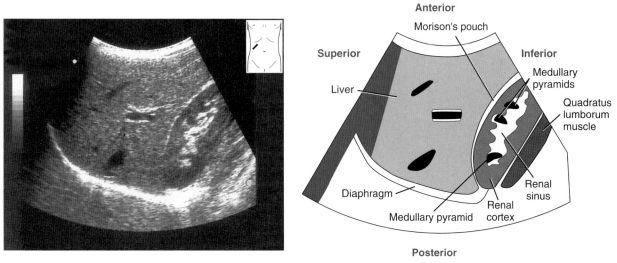

FIGURE 17-18 Longitudinal Right Kidney. Sagittal scanning plane image that shows a longitudinal section of the right kidney posteroinferior to the liver. The renal sinus appears bright and prominent with irregular borders that are marked by several anechoic medullary pyramids. Note the triangular shape of the urine-filled pyramids. The renal cortex appears homogeneous and smooth in contour.

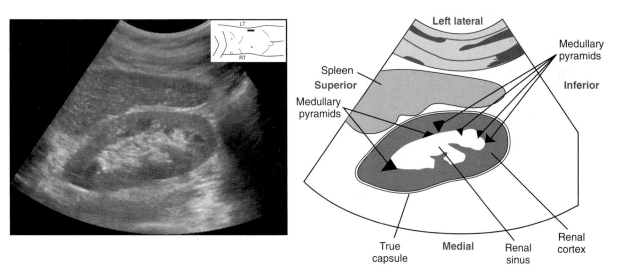

FIGURE 17-19 Longitudinal Left Kidney. Coronal scanning plane image showing a longitudinal section of the superior and mid portions of the left kidney. Note the spleen superiorly.

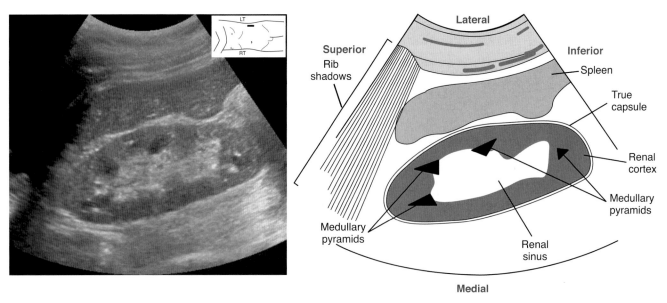

FIGURE 17-20 **Longitudinal Left Kidney.** Coronal scanning plane image demonstrating the long axis section of the left kidney. Note the well-defined renal sinus and its hyperechoic appearance relative to the renal parenchyma.

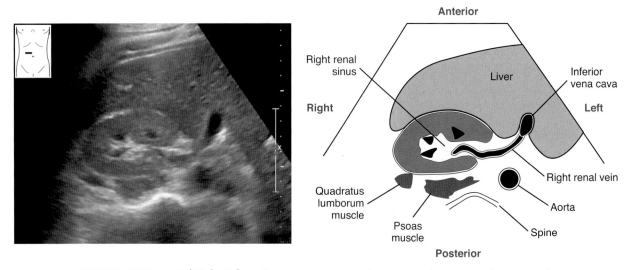

FIGURE 17-21 **Axial Right Kidney.** Transverse scanning plane image showing axial sections of the right kidney, liver, inferior vena cava, aorta, psoas and quadratus lumborum muscles, and longitudinal sections of the right renal vein and portion of the pancreas head and view of the right kidney and liver. Notice how the kidney is sandwiched between the liver (anteriorly) and musculature (posteriorly).

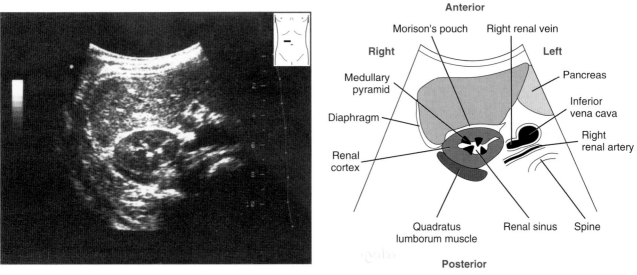

FIGURE 17-22 Axial Right Kidney. Transverse scanning plane image demonstrating an axial section of the right kidney. Notice the distinctive shape of the short axis section of the kidney and its location between the anterior liver and posterior quadratus lumborum muscle. Observe how the homogeneous columns of Bertin extend between the anechoic pyramids to meet the renal sinus. Note the portion of anechoic right renal vein and inferior vena cava just medial to the kidney.

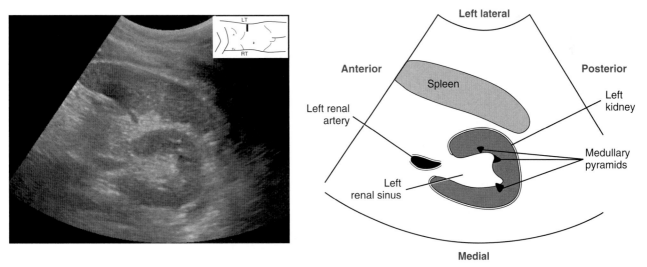

FIGURE 17-23 Axial Left Kidney. Axial section of the left kidney and spleen. Observe the anechoic portion of left renal artery entering the renal hilum. Note the anechoic pyramids lateral to the highly reflective sinus.

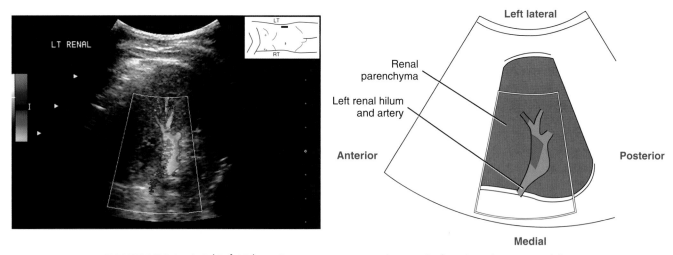

FIGURE 17-24 **Axial Left Kidney.** Transverse scanning plane, color-flow Doppler image of the renal hilum of the left kidney.

- **Renal sinus:** This presents as the bright, echo-dense, *echogenic* ovoid central portion of the kidney with irregular borders (see Figures 17-17 and 17-18). The sinus is markedly echogenic due to the dense fat and fibrous tissue it contains. It also houses the collecting system, lymphatics, and renal vessels. The renal pelvis and infundibulum of the collecting system are not seen if collapsed; otherwise they are urine filled and appear anechoic. In most cases, normal lymphatics are not appreciated sonographically.
- **Renal vasculature:** Renal vasculature appears as anechoic lumens surrounded by bright walls, which can be followed to their origin (Figure 17-25).
Renal Doppler may be used to assess arterial and venous blood flow in kidneys. It is also used in assessing blood flow in renal transplant patients. However, research has shown that renal Doppler alone cannot effectively evaluate transplant patients for signs of acute rejection. Further, renal Doppler has been used to detect vascularity in renal tumors and atriovenous malformations.
- **Renal measurements:** Correct caliper placement for renal measurements is demonstrated in Figure 17-26. Compare the size of the adult kidneys shown in Figure 17-26 with the kidney size in the fetus, neonate, and child shown in Figure 17-27. Normal renal length in children can range from approximately 4.48 cm in the neonate to the normal adult size of 9 to 16 cm by the time the child reaches adolescence.
Next, compare the sonographic appearance of the adult kidneys shown in Figure 17-26 with the kidney's sonographic appearance shown in Figure 17-27. Notice how the renal cortex in the normal pediatric kidney is hyperechoic relative to the cortex in the adult kidney. Also, the medullary pyramids in the pediatric kidney

are more visible than the pyramids in the adult kidney. The pediatric medullary pyramids are so readily distinguishable that a novice sonographer could mistake them for cystic masses within the kidney if not familiar with their normal sonographic presentation.

Ureters
The ureters are not normally identifiable with ultrasound. However, "ureteral jets," or the effect of the urine entering the urinary bladder through the ureteral orifices, can be observed on real-time examination (Figure 17-28).

Lower Urinary Tract: Urinary Bladder, Urethra
Urinary Bladder
In a short axis or axial section the bladder appears somewhat squared by the laterally lying psoas muscles (see Figure 17-28). In a longitudinal section the posterior surface of the bladder may be somewhat indented by an anteverted uterus or an enlarged prostate (Figure 17-29). The size and shape of the bladder vary depending on the quantity of urine stored. Nevertheless, the distended bladder should appear symmetric.

The bladder lumen is not visible if it is collapsed; otherwise, it appears anechoic. The distended bladder wall appears as a smooth, bright outline that is hyperechoic relative to the anechoic, urine-filled lumen.

The anechoic appearance of the urine in the bladder provides an excellent medium to visualize urinary bladder filling. Squirts of urine can be seen entering the posterior portion of the bladder through the ureteral orifices in the trigone area. As mentioned, this action, called ureteral jets, can be seen in as little as 20 minutes after ingestion of large amounts of water in a well-hydrated patient (see Figure 17-28).

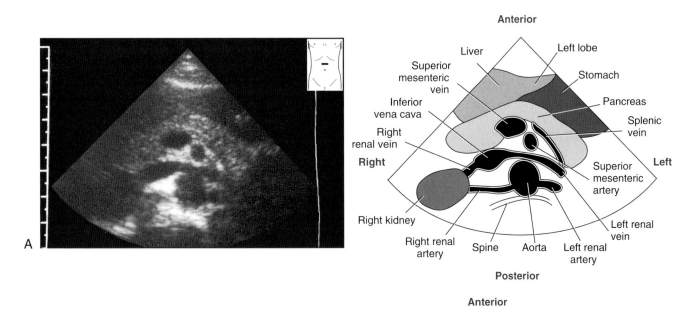

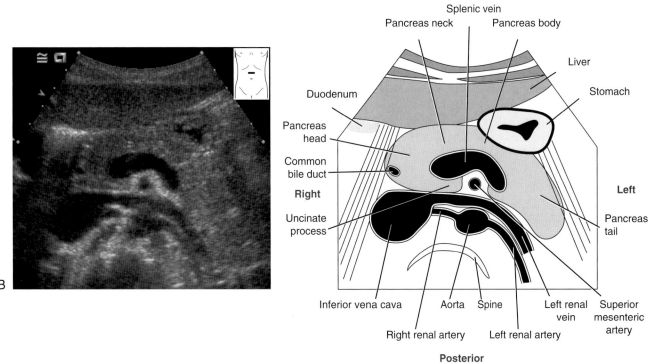

FIGURE 17-25 **Renal Vasculature. A,** Transverse scanning plane image of the mid-epigastric region. Note the renal veins anterior to the renal arteries. **B,** Renal vasculature well defined in a different patient.

Urethra

When visualized, the urethra appears hyperechoic relative to adjacent structures.

The Adrenal Glands

The adrenal glands are only briefly discussed in this section, because in the adult they are difficult to visualize with ultrasound. Nevertheless, their close proximity to the kidneys makes them sonographically significant.

The adrenal glands are much more readily detected sonographically in fetuses and young children. This has been attributed to adrenal size. The infant adrenal is proportionally larger than the adult adrenal. At birth,

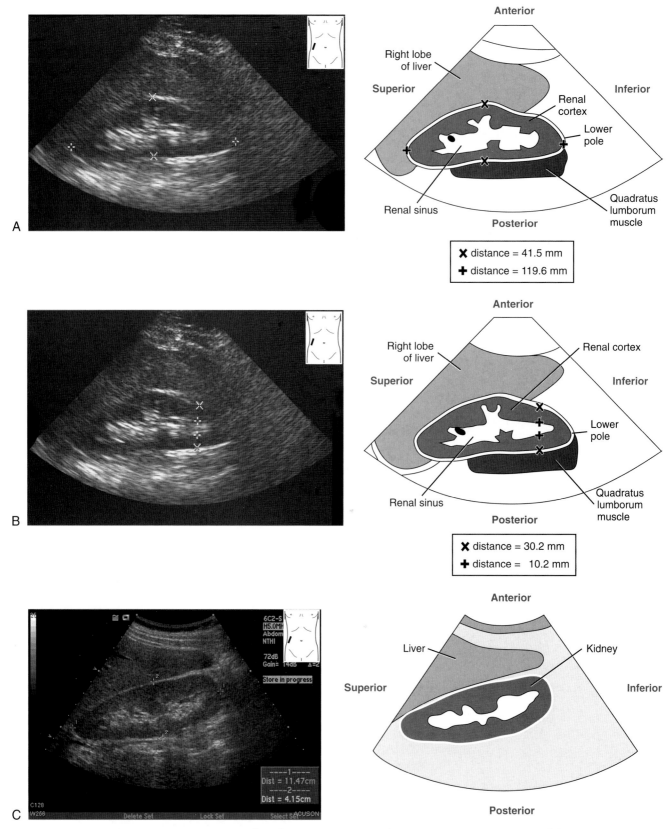

FIGURE 17-26   Long Axis Right Kidney. A, Long axis and anteroposterior measurements of the right kidney. The length (superior to inferior) and anteroposterior dimensions are measured and are within normal limits. **B,** Longitudinal section of the right kidney demonstrating the renal sinus measurement compared with the anteroposterior measurement. The anteroposterior renal sinus measurement is approximately one third that of the anteroposterior measurement. Note that a cortical thickness measurement can be obtained by subtracting the anteroposterior renal sinus measurement from the anteroposterior kidney measurement. **C,** Long axis and anteroposterior measurements of the right kidney in a different patient.

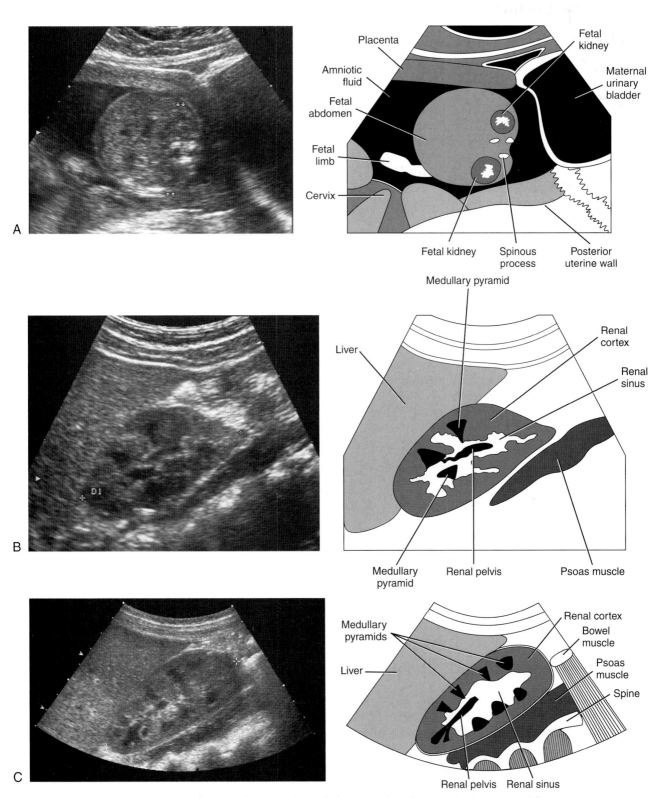

FIGURE 17-27 **Pediatric Kidneys.** Pediatric kidneys in chronologic order by age in different patients. **A,** Fetal kidneys. **B,** A 3-week-old neonate. **C,** A 7-year-old child.

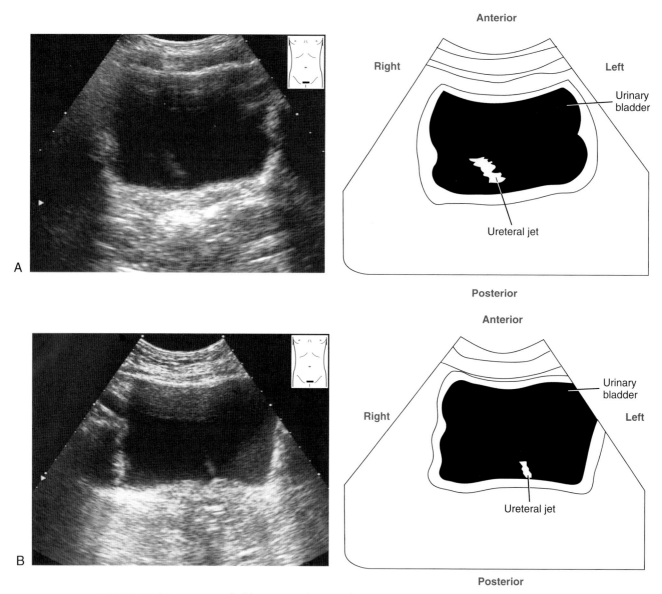

FIGURE 17-28 **Urinary Bladder.** *Ureteral jets* is the term used to describe the sonographic appearance of urine entering the filling bladder. The ureteral jets are visualized in motion as the urine squirts into the bladder from the ureter(s). They appear barely echogenic yet hyperechoic relative to the anechoic appearance of the urine and are therefore identifiable. **A,** Transverse scanning plane image of the pelvis. Ureteral jet identified in the posterior portion of the bladder, where the ureteral orifices are located. Note the symmetry of the bladder. **B,** Same patient; ureteral jet noted posteriorly from the left ureter.

the adrenal is one third the size of the kidney, whereas in the adult it is one thirteenth the size of the kidney. Normally, the adult adrenal glands appear as small, indistinct, low-gray structures that are hypoechoic relative to adjacent anatomy. In some cases, only the highly reflective fat that surrounds them is seen. In the neonate the adrenals are characterized by a thin, hyperechoic core surrounded by a thick, anechoic zone.

This section will take a brief look at the anatomy and physiology of the adrenal gland. The adrenals are paired endocrine organs located at the superior and medial border of the kidneys. They are approximately 2 inches in length, 1.1 inch in diameter, and 0.4 inch in depth. The glands are enclosed with the kidneys in Gerota's fascia and are surrounded by fat. Each gland consists of an outer cortex and an inner medulla (Figure 17-30). The cortex and medulla function independently; thus the adrenal is actually 2 hormonal glands in 1.

The **adrenal cortex** contains 3 areas called zones. Each zone produces steroid hormones, commonly

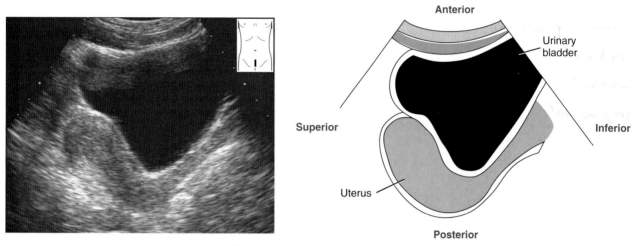

FIGURE 17-29 Urinary Bladder. Sagittal scanning plane image of the pelvis showing longitudinal sections of the distended bladder, uterus, and vagina. Observe how the posterior surface of the bladder is somewhat indented by the uterus. Notice the smooth bladder contour and the bright appearance of the bladder wall, which is hyperechoic relative to the midgray appearance of the uterus and anechoic appearance of the urine-filled bladder lumen.

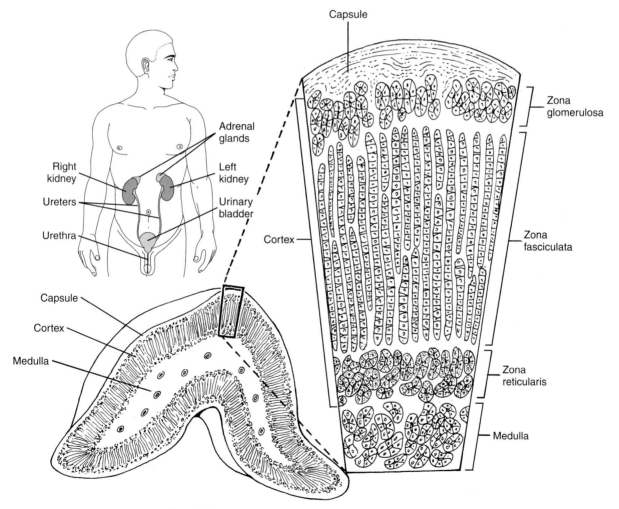

FIGURE 17-30 Adrenal Gland. Cross-section of an adrenal gland demonstrating the capsule, cortex, and medulla. The cortex is descriptively divided into zones, the zona glomerulosa, zona fasciculata, and zona reticularis.

Column of Burtin?
cortex?
Sinus?
Trigone area?

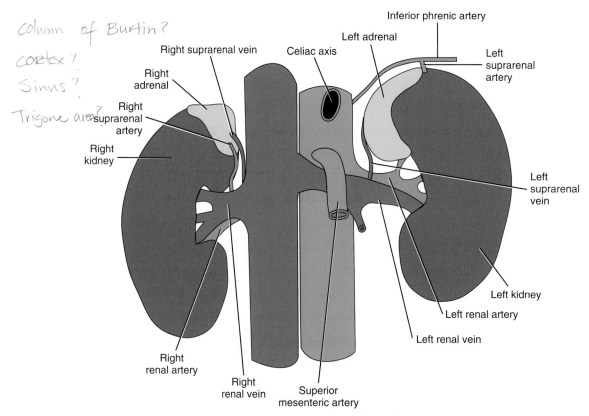

FIGURE 17-31 Adrenal vasculature.

called *corticoids*. The zone at the outermost portion of the cortex is called the *zona glomerulosa*. It produces mineralocorticoids, of which the most important is **aldosterone**; aldosterone regulates sodium and potassium levels. The next zone is called the *zona fasciculata*. It produces glucocorticoids. Cortisol is its primary substance; it regulates glucose metabolism. The innermost zone is called the *zona reticularis*. It supplements the sex hormones produced by the reproductive organs, the ovaries and testes.

The **adrenal medulla** is composed of chromaffin cells, which secrete epinephrine and norepinephrine. The adrenals produce four times as much epinephrine as norepinephrine. These hormones are responsible for the "fight-or-flight" response. Their effects include an increase in heart and respiratory rates and dilatation of the coronary blood vessels.

The adrenals are supplied with blood from the suprarenal arteries (Figure 17-31). The right suprarenal artery originates slightly inferior to the superior mesenteric artery and slightly superior to the right renal artery. The left suprarenal artery is a branch of the inferior phrenic artery, which arises directly from the aorta. The origin of the inferior phrenic artery is more superior than the origin of the right suprarenal artery. The left phrenic artery originates slightly inferior to the celiac axis and

slightly superior to the origin of the superior mesenteric artery.

The adrenals are drained by the suprarenal veins (see Figure 17-31). The left suprarenal vein drains into the left renal vein, which then drains into the inferior vena cava. The right suprarenal vein drains directly into the inferior vena cava.

SONOGRAPHIC APPLICATIONS
Sonography is used to evaluate several aspects of the urinary system. Common considerations include the following:
- Renal size
- Detection and composition of renal masses and cysts
- Urinary system obstruction
- Renal abscess
- Renal hematoma
- Enlarged ureters
- Urinary bladder masses
- Renal transplantation
- Doppler evaluation of renal blood flow abnormalities
- Ultrasound-guided biopsies of renal parenchyma or masses
- Ultrasound-guided fluid aspirations

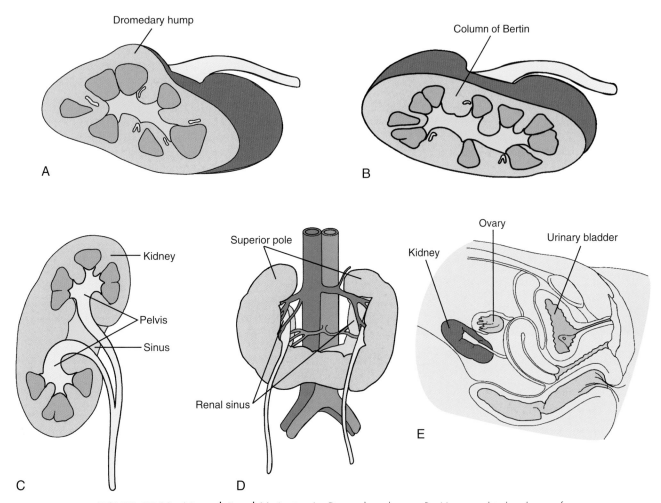

FIGURE 17-32 **Normal Renal Variants. A,** Dromedary hump. **B,** Hypertrophied column of Bertin. **C,** Double collecting system. Includes double renal pelvis and partially bifid ureter. **D,** Horseshoe kidney, connected at the lower poles. **E,** Pelvic kidney.

NORMAL VARIANTS

The following urinary system normal variants can be observed on ultrasound:

- **Dromedary hump:** Consists of localized bulge(s) on the lateral border of the kidney. It has the same sonographic appearance as a normal renal cortex (Figure 17-32, A). *mostly seen on left side*
- **Hypertrophied column of Bertin:** Occurs in varying degrees of size and may indent the renal sinus of the kidney. It has the same sonographic appearance as the normal renal cortex (Figure 17-32, B).
- **Double collecting system:** Occurs when the renal sinus is divided (Figure 17-32, C). Each sinus has a renal pelvis. A bifid (double) ureter may also be present.
- **Horseshoe kidneys:** Occurs when the kidneys are connected, usually at the lower poles (Figure 17-32, D). It has the same sonographic appearance as

normal renal tissue. However, the junction between the two kidneys can be visualized on sonography.
- **Renal ectopia:** Occurs when one or both kidneys occur outside the normal renal fossa. Locations include the lower abdominal and pelvic region (Figure 17-32, E). Other ectopic locations (e.g., intra-thoracic) are rare.

REFERENCE CHARTS

■ ■ ■   ASSOCIATED PHYSICIANS

- **Urologist:** Specializes in surgical diseases of the urinary system in the female and genitourinary tract in the male.
- **Nephrologist:** Specializes in diseases of the kidney.
- **Radiologist:** Specializes in the diagnostic interpretation of imaging modalities that assess renal disease.

■■■ COMMON DIAGNOSTIC TESTS

- **Intravenous pyelogram (IVP):** A radiologic examination in which a contrast medium ("dye") is injected into a vein and then x-ray films are taken at specific intervals to observe kidney function and urinary system anatomy. This test is performed by a radiologic technologist and radiologist. The examination is interpreted by the radiologist.
- **Computed axial tomography (CT) scan:** A radiologic examination in which cross-sectional x-ray images of the kidneys and other urinary system structures are obtained to assess anatomy. A contrast medium may be administered to differentiate between pathology and normal anatomy. This test is performed by a radiologic technologist and radiologist. The examination is interpreted by the radiologist. Some diagnostic labs are using spiral CT for improved imaging of renal vascular anatomy in live renal donor patients.

■■■ LABORATORY VALUES

RENAL
- **Blood urea nitrogen (BUN):** Used to assess renal function and measure the kidneys' ability to get rid of waste.
  - Normal BUN is 26 mg/dL.
  - Elevation of this value may indicate renal disease.
- **Creatinine (Cr):** Used to assess renal function and measure the kidneys' ability to get rid of waste.
  - Normal Cr is 1.1 mg/dL.
  - Elevation of this value may indicate renal disease.
- **Glomerular filtration rate:** Measures how well the kidneys remove waste and excess fluid from the blood. Normal GFR is 90 mL/min; lower values may indicate disease.
- **Specific gravity:** A measure of how much dissolved material is present in the urine. The higher the quantity of dissolved solutes, the higher the specific gravity. For example, specific gravity is higher when the kidneys must preserve water (e.g., during exercise) to compensate for water lost in sweat. The volume of urine therefore is decreased.
  - Normal range of specific gravity is 1.101 to 1.025. (The specific gravity of distilled water, which has no solutes, is 1.000.)

ADRENAL
- **Aldosterone:** A measure of adrenal function, 4 to 31 ng/dL value in the upright position. Aldosterone values are affected by salt intake and posture. Levels are higher when salt intake is reduced or when the patient is in the upright position. Levels are lower with increased salt intake or when the patient is in the supine position.
- **DHEA-S:** Blood is drawn between 12 and 1 PM and 4 and 5 PM. Abnormal levels may be related to early puberty, infertility, and abnormal testosterone or estrogen production. Normal range is 2.0 to 10.0 ng/mL. The ideal value is 7.0 to 8.0 ng/dL.
- **Serum cortisol:** Measures adrenal hormonal levels. Blood tests are taken at 8 AM and 4 PM. Ideally the 8 AM value should be halved at the 4 PM reading. Normal reading is 7 to 25 mcg/dL.

■■■ VASCULATURE

Aorta → renal artery → interlobar artery → arcuate artery → interlobular artery → afferent arterioles → glomerulus → efferent arteriole → peritubular capillaries → proximal and distal convoluted tubules and vasa recta → interlobular vein → arcuate vein → interlobar vein → renal vein → inferior vena cava

■■■ AFFECTING CHEMICALS/HORMONES

See Table 17-5.

CHAPTER 18

The Spleen

KACEY DAVIS AND REVA ARNEZ CURRY

OBJECTIVES

Describe the function of the spleen.
Describe the location of the spleen.
Define size relationships of the normal spleen.
Describe gross anatomy of the normal spleen.

Describe the sonographic appearance of the normal spleen.
Describe the associated physicians, diagnostic tests, and laboratory values relevant to the normal spleen.

KEY WORDS

Culling — Removal of abnormal red blood cells from the blood by the spleen.

Erythrocyte — Red blood cell.

Hematopoiesis — Produces erythrocytes, as well as white blood cells, in the developing fetus. In the adult, red blood cell production is performed only in cases of severe hemolytic anemia.

Hemoglobin — Oxygen-carrying and iron-containing pigment of red blood cells.

Phagocytosis — Removal of worn-out and abnormal red blood cells and platelets from the bloodstream by phagocyte cells in the spleen.

Pitting — Removal of nuclei from old red blood cells by the spleen without destroying the cell.

Red Pulp — Along with white pulp, comprises spleen parenchyma. Red pulp is where

worn-out red blood cells and bloodborne pathogens are destroyed. Consists of splenic sinuses and splenic cords.

Reticuloendothelial System — Has the responsibility of phagocytosis (engulfing and destroying) of damaged or old cells and their debris, foreign materials, and pathogens, taking them out of the circulating blood. Reticuloendothelial cells are found in the spleen, as well as in the Kupffer cells of the liver, lymph nodes, alveoli, brain, blood vessels, and mucous membranes.

Splenic Artery (SA) — Arises from the celiac axis of the abdominal aorta and travels laterally toward the left to supply the spleen with oxygen-rich blood.

Splenic Hilum — This portion of the spleen, located medially, is where the vasculature enters and exits.

Splenic Vein (SV) — Conveys venous blood from the spleen; running medially along the gastrolienal ligament to its confluence with the superior mesenteric vein posterior to the neck of the pancreas to form the portal vein.

White Pulp — Along with red pulp, comprises spleen parenchyma. White pulp is where immune functions take place. Consists of lymphatic tissue containing lymphocytes and monocytes that continually produce and are active in ingesting and digesting harmful pathogens that enter the bloodstream.

■■■ NORMAL MEASUREMENTS

Anatomy	Measurement
Spleen long axis	8 to 13 cm
Spleen anteroposterior diameter	7 to 8 cm
Spleen thickness	3 to 4 cm
Splenic volume	60 to 200 mL
Splenic index	107 to 314 cm^3

The spleen is an intraperitoneal organ that lies in the left upper quadrant of the abdominal cavity. It is part of the **reticuloendothelial system**. This system has the responsibility for phagocytosis (engulfing and destroying) of damaged or old cells and their debris, foreign materials, and pathogens, taking them out of the circulating blood. The spleen is composed primarily of lymph tissue. Although the spleen is a component of

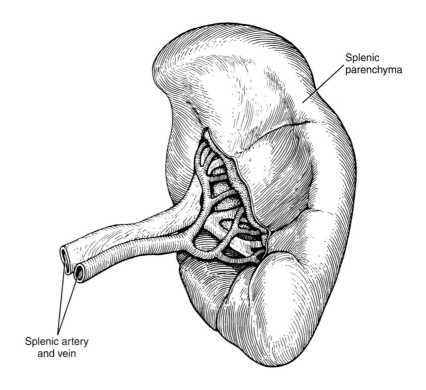

Splenic parenchyma

Splenic artery and vein

Splenic artery (SA)	• Branch of the celiac artery.
	• Branches of SA before reaching the spleen:
	• Pancreatic branches from the initial portion of the splenic artery.
	• Short gastric branches, which supply superior portion of the greater curvature of the stomach.
	• Left gastroepiploic, which supplies middle portion of the greater curvature of the stomach.
	• Branches of the SA after reaching the spleen:
	• 2 to 3 lobar arterial branches at the splenic hilum.
	• Each lobar artery can further branch into 2 to 4 lobular arterial branches.
	• Lobular arteries branch into smaller splenic arteries, which terminate in tiny capillaries.
	• Tiny capillaries anastomose with venous sinuses. NOTE: The capillaries are permeable, meaning that red blood cells can pass through them. This provides the filtering function of the spleen.
Splenic vein (SV)	• Splenic venous sinuses anastomose with splenic capillaries from splenic arteries.
	• Venous sinuses unite to form venules, which merge to eventually form the splenic vein.
	• Splenic vein exits spleen at the hilum.
	• Courses from lateral to medial along posteroinferior border of pancreas body and tail.
	• Joins superior mesenteric vein to form portal vein at the level of the pancreas neck.

the body's defense system, it is not essential to life and can be removed without adverse effects (Figure 18-1).

LOCATION

The spleen lies in the left hypochondrium, with its longest axis along the tenth rib. It lies posterolateral to the body and fundus of the stomach, posterolateral to the tail of the pancreas, and posterior to the left colic flexure (Figure 18-2, *B* and *C*; Table 18-1). The left kidney is located inferior and medial to the spleen. Posterior to the spleen are the diaphragm, the left lung,

and the eighth, ninth, tenth, and eleventh ribs. The spleen is covered by peritoneum, with the exception of the medially located **splenic hilum**, where the vasculature structures and lymph nodes are located (see Figure 18-2, *C*).

SIZE

The size of the spleen varies among individuals, and at different times it can vary in the same individual. The normal range of measurements for the spleen is 8 to 13 cm in length, 7 to 8 cm in anteroposterior diameter,

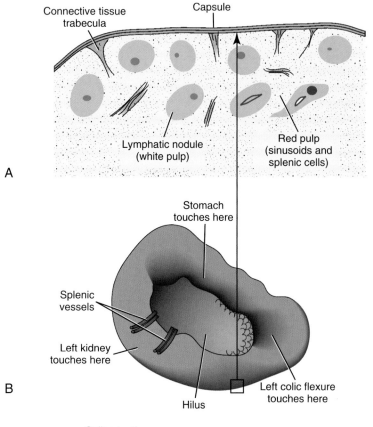

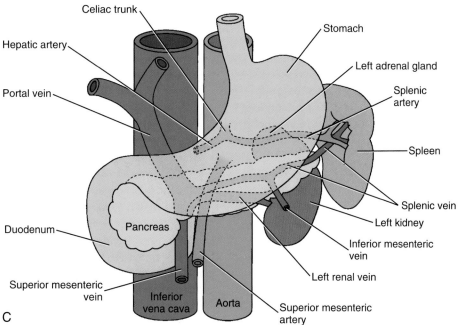

FIGURE 18-2   **A,** Microscopic organization of the spleen. **B,** Medial surface of the spleen.
C, Surrounding splenic anatomic relationships (see Table 18-1).

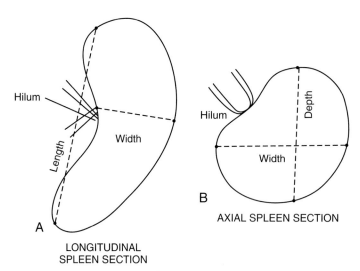

FIGURE 18-3 **A,** Longitudinal section of the spleen with length and width measurements. **B,** Axial section of the spleen with depth and width measurements.

	Spleen
Anterior to	8th, 9th, 10th, 11th ribs, diaphragm, lt lung
Posterior to	Stomach body/fundus, lt colic flexure, peritoneum (except for hilum)
Superior to	Lt kidney
Inferior to	Diaphragm
Medial to	
Lt lateral to	Stomach body/fundus, lt kidney, pancreas tail, splenic artery, splenic vein, inferior mesenteric vein, liver
Rt lateral to	

■ ■ ■ **Table 18-1** Location of the Spleen Routinely Visualized With Ultrasound

and 3 to 4 cm in thickness. Normal splenic volume is 60 to 200 mL, although normal volumes of up to 350 mL have been reported. The normal splenic index is between 107 and 314 cm³. Volume is calculated automatically after measuring the perimeter, area, and longitudinal diameter, whereas the splenic index is the length × width × thickness of the organ.

Another technique to assess normal size is to use calipers, measuring the length and width on a longitudinal section and measuring the width and depth on an axial section (Figure 18-3). There is mixed opinion on which method is best in assessing spleen size, with studies favoring the longitudinal diameter, splenic index, or splenic volume.

The spleen is generally smooth in contour, with a convex superior surface and a concave inferior surface.

As with the gallbladder, the shape of the spleen is just as important as the measurements when assessing normal size. For instance, it is possible to have a normal longitudinal diameter but an enlarged volume, or an enlarged longitudinal diameter with a normal volume. It is important to assess splenic size using department protocols to improve standardization and reduce operator error.

GROSS ANATOMY

The spleen is a highly vascular mass of lymphoid tissues. Considered the largest lymphoid organ, it is ovoid and has a convex superior surface and a concave inferior surface. The spleen is entirely covered by the peritoneum except at the hilum, where all vessels enter and exit.

The **splenic artery (SA)** arises from the celiac axis of the abdominal aorta and travels laterally toward the left to supply the spleen with oxygenated blood. Initially from the celiac axis, the SA size is estimated to be 5.6 mm in diameter. It gives off pancreatic branches that supply the body and tail of the pancreas, short gastric branches that help supply the superior portion of the greater curvature of the stomach, and the left gastroepiploic artery, which supplies the middle portion of the greater curvature of the stomach (Figure 18-4). At the splenic hilar area, the SA branches into 2 to 4 lobar arteries. These further branch into lobular arteries, which further subdivide into smaller splenic arteries, which will eventually terminate in tiny capillaries (see Figure 18-1). These capillaries are permeable and help provide the filtering function of the spleen. In one cadaver study the lobular subdivisions and areas of the spleen were too varied to draw definitive conclusions as to which lobular arteries supplied particular areas of the

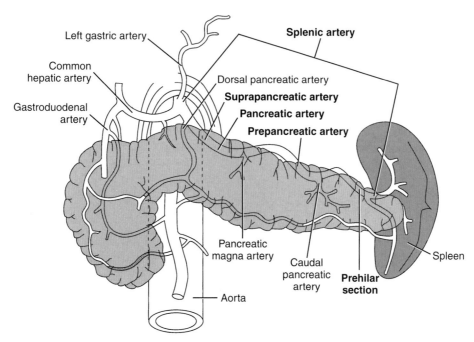

FIGURE 18-4 Suprapancreatic, pancreatic, prepancreatic, and prehilar sections of the splenic artery.

spleen. The same study found that the lobular arteries appear to become more tortuous in older patients.

The splenic capillaries anastomose with tiny splenic venous sinuses, which unite to form splenic venules. The venules merge to eventually form the splenic vein (SV), which conveys venous blood from the spleen at the splenic hilum and courses in a horizontal direction along the gastrolienal ligament to its confluence with the superior mesenteric vein at the pancreas to form the main portal vein.

The spleen's location affords it the protection of the ribs. Consequently, the spleen is usually not palpable unless it is pathologically enlarged.

The spleen is composed of red pulp and white pulp. The white pulp consists of the malpighian corpuscles, small nodular masses of lymphatic tissue that surrounds and follows the smaller splenic arteries. The red pulp, which is looser and more vascular, consists of the splenic sinuses and splenic cords. The sinuses are long, slender channels lined with epithelial cells. The red pulp occupies all of the space not filled by white pulp or splenic cords (see Figure 18-2, A).

PHYSIOLOGY

As part of the reticuloendothelial system, the spleen's main function is to help remove old cells, debris, pathogens, and foreign substances from circulation. Reticuloendothelial cells are found in the spleen, as well as in the Kupffer cells of the liver, lymph nodes, alveoli, brain,

blood vessels, and mucous membranes. In addition, the spleen:

- Produces lymphocytes, monocytes (phagocytes), plasma cells, and antibodies
- Stores iron and metabolites
- Produces red blood cells (this function primarily occurs in the fetus)
- Produces white blood cells throughout life
- Acts as a blood a reservoir
- Regulates platelet and leukocyte life span

Four major functions of the spleen are defense, hematopoiesis, red blood cell and platelet destruction, and service as a blood reservoir.

Defense

Functioning as a defense mechanism, the spleen aids in the destruction and removal of microorganisms by phagocytosis. In the white pulp, lymphocytes and monocytes are continually produced and are active in ingesting and digesting harmful pathogens that enter the bloodstream. These cells are able to recognize foreign harmful substances and turn themselves into antibody-producing plasma cells and memory cells. The plasma cells destroy the invading microorganism by creating antibodies to that particular pathogen. The memory cells "remember" that particular pathogen, and should it attack the body again, the antibodies are quickly activated to destroy it. This is called the *immune response*.

Hematopoiesis

This function produces **erythrocytes**, also called *red blood cells*, as well as white blood cells in the developing fetus. In the adult, however, red blood cell production is performed only in cases of severe hemolytic anemia.

RBC Removal

The spleen inspects passing red blood cells for imperfections and destroys those it recognizes as abnormal. Blood then passes through the red pulp and into the splenic sinuses. This portion of the spleen is a filter that aids in **phagocytosis** of degenerating red blood cells. **Pitting**, the removal of nuclei from old red blood cells without damaging the cells, and **culling**, the removal of abnormal red blood cells, occur. The **hemoglobin** (iron-containing pigment) in these cells is broken down. The iron is either used immediately to produce new red blood cells or is transported via the portal vein to the liver and bone marrow for storage. The globin is used to break down other proteins for use in the body. The most abundant pigment released is hemosiderin. Iron can be stored in hemosiderin until it is needed to make more hemoglobin. Heme, also a pigment, is not needed and is turned into bilirubin and excreted by the liver in bile.

Storage

The ability of the spleen to store red blood cells (blood reservoir) is due to its high smooth-muscle content. The red pulp of the spleen, with its venous sinuses, holds a considerable volume of blood that can be quickly released into the circulatory system if needed. The spleen's average volume of about 350 mL can drop quickly and dramatically after sympathetic stimulation that causes the smooth muscle to constrict. However, if the number of cells stored becomes excessive, splenomegaly (enlargement of the spleen) will develop.

SONOGRAPHIC APPEARANCE

The normal spleen should have a uniform homogeneous and smooth texture (Figure 18-5). It is medium

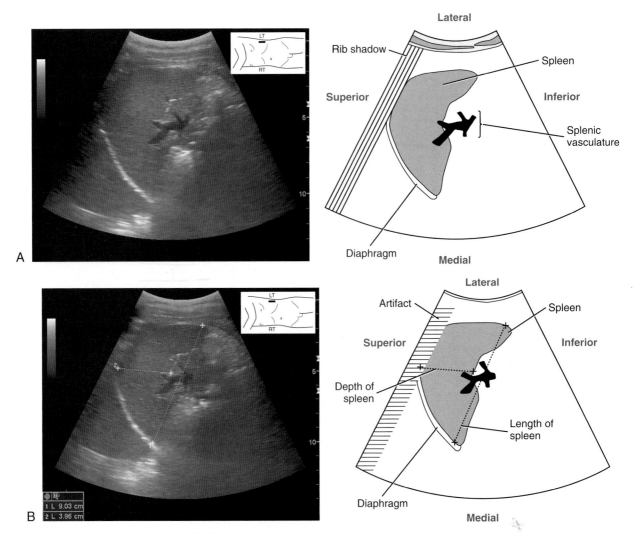

FIGURE 18-5　**Normal Spleen. A,** Longitudinal section. **B,** Longitudinal section with measurements.

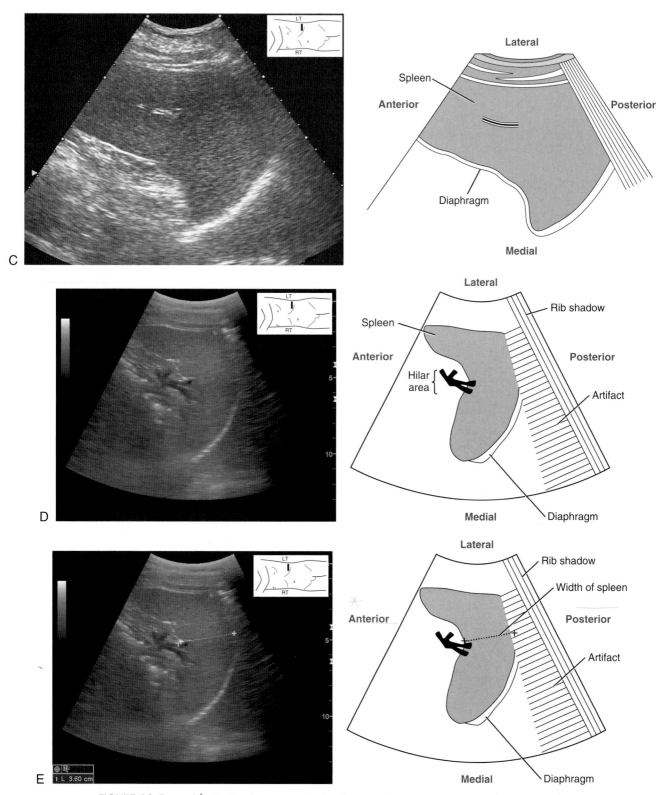

FIGURE 18-5, cont'd **C**, Axial section. **D**, Another axial section. **E**, An axial section with measurements.

hyper to kidney

gray in color and should be the same (isoechoic) or less echogenic (hypoechoic) relative to the liver. Bright reflections may be seen throughout the spleen that represent calcifications of small arterial walls or calcified granulomatous inclusions. The significance of the latter varies according to patient history. The organ may be difficult to visualize as a result of overlying ribs or gas in the adjacent bowel. It is often easiest to scan the spleen intercostally from a lateral approach. In a coronal scanning plane, longitudinal view, the spleen and left kidney can usually be visualized if there is not too much interference from bowel gas (Figure 18-6). The entirety of the spleen is more readily visualized ultrasonically when it is pathologically enlarged. The splenic hilum, however, is usually visualized, making it easy to document splenic vasculature at the hilar area (Figure 18-7).

SONOGRAPHIC APPLICATIONS

- The most common use of sonography in imaging the spleen is to detect enlargement or splenomegaly. Thirty years ago, when articulated arm B scanning was in wide use, the rule of thumb was that if the spleen was visualized anterior to the aorta, it was pathologically enlarged. Today, with real-time scanning, the determination of splenomegaly has become basically a subjective judgment; however, a long axis measurement of the spleen greater than 13 cm indicates splenomegaly. The more experience the sonographer and interpreting physician have, the more accurate their judgment will be.
- Ultrasound can help assess splenic masses, although primary splenic masses are quite rare.
- Ultrasound is also useful in assessing splenic damage from blunt trauma, such as rupture or hemorrhage.

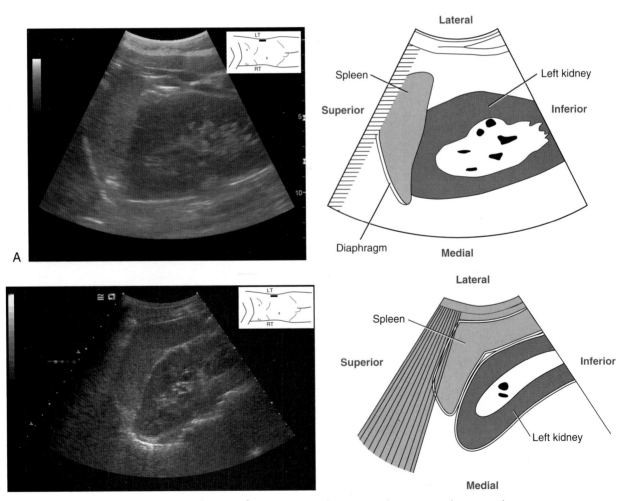

FIGURE 18-6· **Splenic Kidney Interface. A,** Coronal scanning plane image showing a longitudinal section of the normal interface between the spleen and left kidney. **B,** Same view as **A,** but in a different patient.

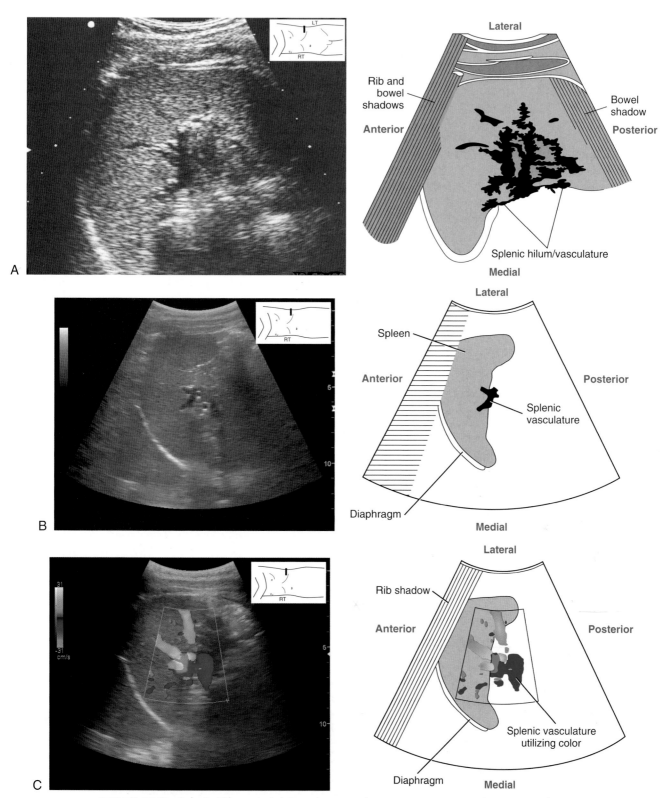

FIGURE 18-7 **Splenic Hilum. A,** Left lateral approach, transverse scanning plane image demonstrating the hilar area in this axial section of the spleen. **B,** Same view as **A,** clearly demonstrating the splenic hilum in a different patient. **C,** Color-flow image of **B.**

NORMAL VARIANTS

Accessory Spleen

Accessory spleen is found in up to 10% of the general population. These islands of tissue are usually less than 1 cm in diameter. More than one accessory spleen may be present, most often near the splenic hilum or attached to the tail of the pancreas (Figure 18-8).

Asplenia *Rare*

This rare congenital abnormality may be associated with a congenital heart defect. If solitary, there are no complications. The liver may be visualized more distinctly to the left of the midline than usual.

Splenomegaly

This pathologic finding is included because it is the most common splenic abnormality. Splenomegaly may be diagnosed sonographically when the long axis of the spleen measures greater than 13 cm. It is most often due to complications of other organic disease. Splenomegaly is noted as a mass in the left upper quadrant. It may be due to recent trauma, portal venous congestion, systemic infection, or a blood disorder such as anemia. One study of 78 patients with an enlarged spleen showed that the diagnosis could be made by palpation alone, defined as palpating the spleen below the costal margin by 0.5 to 2.0 cm, in only 18 patients. In this study, 24 patients were diagnosed with splenomegaly by ultrasound longitudinal diameter alone. This measurement has been shown to correlate fairly well with three-dimensional CT studies. Another 38 patients from the study group were diagnosed by ultrasound volume measurements. The wide range of assessment techniques highlights the care that must be taken when assessing splenomegaly.

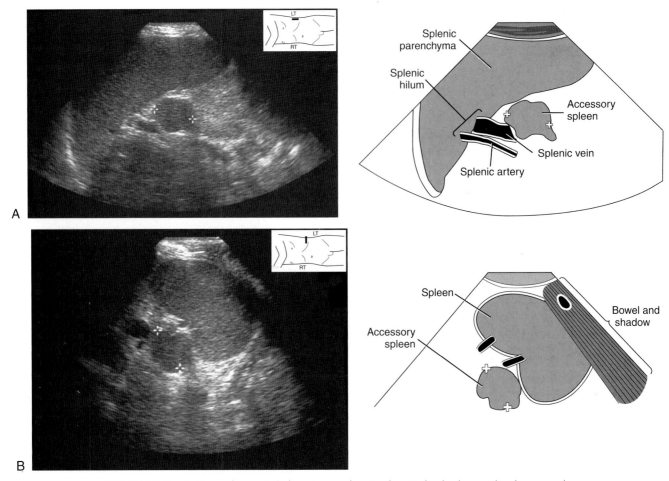

FIGURE 18-8   **A,** Coronal scanning plane image showing longitudinal spleen with splenomegaly and a section of accessory spleen (between calipers). **B,** Transverse scanning plane image from a left approach of same patient showing an axial section of the spleen with splenomegaly and a section of accessory spleen (between calipers).

presence of Bacteria w/in blood System, also
Known as sepsis.

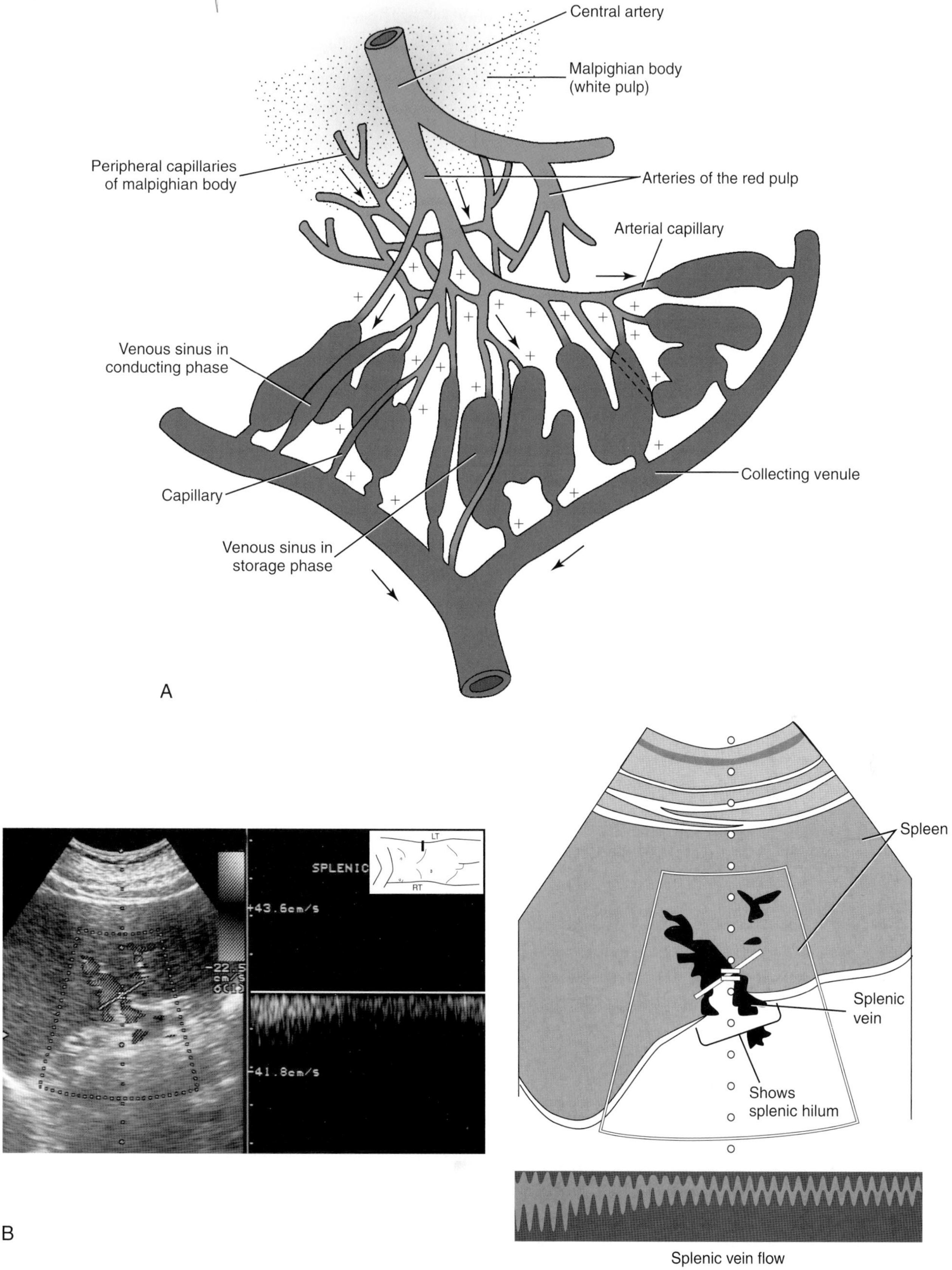

FIGURE 18-9 **A,** Vascular anatomy of the spleen. **B,** Normal splenic hilum showing splenic vein and Doppler tracing.

REFERENCE CHARTS

■ ■ ■ ASSOCIATED PHYSICIANS

- **Family physician:** Often serves as referring physician, coordinating patient care. In this capacity, the physician recommends referral to specialists when necessary.
- **Internist:** Specializes in the diagnosis and treatment of internal disorders.
- **Surgeon:** Specializes in performing surgical procedures.
- **Radiologist:** Specializes in interpreting diagnostic imaging procedures.
- **Hematologist:** Specializes in treating diseases of blood.

■ ■ ■ COMMON DIAGNOSTIC TESTS

- **X-ray:** In this test, ionized electromagnetic waves create photographic images, which are then read and interpreted. It is performed by a radiologic technologist and interpreted by a radiologist.
- **Ultrasound:** Nonionized sound waves generate diagnostic images in this test. The sound waves do not penetrate bone or air. The test is performed by a sonographer and interpreted by a radiologist.
- **Nuclear medicine:** This test involves intravenous injection of radionuclides to create diagnostic images. The radionuclides "tag" specific cells, so that the resulting image is specific to the area of interest. This test is performed by a nuclear medicine technologist and interpreted by a radiologist.
- **Computed axial tomography (CT) scan:** The ionized waves create a cross-sectional x-ray image of the body. This test is performed by a radiologic technologist who is certified for "CT" or "CAT scan." The scan is interpreted by a radiologist.
- **Magnetic resonance imaging (MRI):** This test uses nuclear magnetic resonance to produce images. This test is performed by a radiologic technologist who is certified in "MRI." The scan is interpreted by a radiologist.

■ ■ ■ AFFECTING CHEMICALS

- **Anticoagulants:** These thin the blood in patients whose blood tends to clot abnormally or who are at high risk for developing thromboemboli. Patients receiving such treatment are more likely to experience internal hemorrhage or bleeding from small cuts that does not clot in a normal manner. The patient's hematocrit should be monitored.

■ ■ ■ LABORATORY VALUES

- **Hematocrit:** The hematocrit reading indicates the percentage of red blood cells per volume of blood. Normal values for men are 40% to 54%; for women, 37% to 47%. An abnormally low hematocrit points to internal bleeding.
- **Bacteremia:** The presence of bacteria within the blood system, also known as sepsis. Symptoms include chills, fever, and possibly the presence of abscesses.
- **Leukocytosis:** An increase in the number of circulating leukocytes (above 10,000 per mm^3). This finding is indicative of an infection of the blood. It may occur in hemorrhage, following surgery, in malignancies, during pregnancy, and in toxemia. It can also be due to leukemia.
- **Leukopenia:** An abnormally low number of leukocytes in the blood (below 5000 per mm^3). This may develop as a result of certain drugs, or it can be due to a bone marrow disorder.
- **Thrombocytopenia:** An abnormal decrease in the number of circulating platelets. The normal range is 150,000 to 350,000 per mm^3. The decrease may be due to internal hemorrhage.

■ ■ ■ VASCULATURE

- Figure 18-9; see Figures 18-1 and 18-2, *A.*

CHAPTER 19

The Gastrointestinal System

MARILYN DICKERSON PRINCE

OBJECTIVES

Differentiate the structures of the gastrointestinal tract.

Describe the functions of the gastrointestinal tract components.

Localize anatomical relationships between bowel segments and abdominal organs.

Identify the 5 layers of bowel known as the *gut signature*.

Know the vasculature of the gastrointestinal tract.

Describe the size of the gastrointestinal tract structures.

Describe the location of the gastrointestinal tract components.

Recognize the sonographic appearance of the gastrointestinal tract.

List the ultrasound findings suggestive of appendicitis.

Describe the associated physicians, diagnostic tests, and laboratory values related to the gastrointestinal tract.

■

KEY WORDS

Alimentary Canal — Another name for the gastrointestinal tract.

Brunner's (Duodenal) Glands — Produce alkaline substance that helps neutralize acid contents of the stomach. Perform same function as pyloric glands in the stomach.

Cardiac (Esophageal) Orifice — Marks the junction of the greater and lesser curvature of the stomach and the entrance of the esophagus into the stomach.

Cholecystokinin — Hormone released by stimulation of fat in the intestine; acts to contract the gallbladder and helps with stomach emptying.

Duodenal Bulb — First, or superior, portion of the duodenum.

Gastrin — Hormone released from the stomach that stimulates gastric acid secretion.

Gastrocolic Ligament — Attached to the transverse colon, the apron-like part of the greater omentum.

Gastrophrenic Ligament — Attached to the diaphragm, the posterior segment of the stomach fundus and the esophagus, it marks the superior segment of the greater omentum.

Gastrosplenic Ligament — Connects the greater curvature and fundus of the stomach with the splenic hilum; also known as the *gastrolienal ligament*, it marks the left part of the greater omentum.

Greater Omentum — Attaches the greater curvature of the stomach to the colon and drapes anteriorly over the stomach and intestines.

Gut Signature — Characteristic appearance of the bowel on ultrasound, where up to 5 layers of bowel wall can be visualized.

Haustra — Small pouches or recesses throughout the colon resulting from sacculations caused by the teniae coli — the longitudinal bands or ribbons through which smooth muscle fibers course in the center of the colon.

Hepatic (Right Colic) Flexure — Location where the ascending colon bends right at the liver and becomes the transverse colon.

Lesser Omentum — One of 5 ligamentous structures of mesentery that support the stomach and connect it to the liver. Also known as the *gastrohepatic omentum* or ligament.

Meckel's Diverticulum — Normal variant in 2% to 3% of the population, where a remnant of prenatal yolk stalk projects from the side of the ileum.

Mediastinum — Median portion of the thoracic cavity.

Mesentery — A double fold of the peritoneum that connects bowel segments to the posterior peritoneal wall or to other bowel segments.

Mesothelium — A single-cell layer of tissue covering the bowel wall. May be referred to as the serosal surface but is actually peripheral to the serosal layer.

Mucosa — Innermost layer of bowel; in direct contact with intraluminal contents.

Muscularis propria — Fourth layer of bowel; contains circular and longitudinal fibrous bands.

Parietal Peritoneum — Covers the anterior, posterior, and lateral walls of the peritoneal cavity.

Peristalsis — Forward movement of intestinal contents resulting from muscle contractions.

Peritoneum — Serous membrane that lines the walls of the abdomen and pelvis and covers the internal organs.

Rectouterine Pouch — Deepest fold of the peritoneal cavity in females. Also called the *posterior cul-de-sac*; it forms a space between the rectum and lower uterine segment in females. This is also known as the *pouch of Douglas*.

Secretin — Hormone released from the small bowel that stimulates the secretion of bicarbonate to decrease acid content of the intestine.

Serosa — Outer layer of bowel; located peripherally to muscularis propria layer; a loose layer of connective tissue may be unresolvable from a layer of mesothelium.

Continued

Splenic (Left Colic) Flexure — Location where the transverse colon bends inferiorly at the spleen to descend into the pelvic cavity.

Submucosa — Layer of bowel between the mucosa and muscularis that contains blood vessels and lymph channels.

Suspensory Ligament (Ligament of Treitz) — Fibromuscular band that holds the ascending, fourth portion of the duodenum in place.

Valves of Kerckring (Valvulae Conniventes) — Large folds of mucous membrane that project into the bowel lumen and provide greater absorption areas as the passage of food is slowed.

Visceral Peritoneum — Peritoneum that covers intraperitoneal organs.

■ ■ ■ NORMAL MEASUREMENTS

Anatomy	Measurement
Pharynx	10 cm
Esophagus	23 cm
Stomach	25 to 30 cm (10 to 12 cm diameter, 2 to 4 L capacity)
Pyloric canal	2 to 3 cm (4 cm diameter)
Small intestine (3 parts)	Total length = 6 meters (4 cm diameter) Duodenum 25 cm Jejunum 2.3 m Ileum 3.5 m
Large intestine	2 meters
Duodenum (4 parts)	Total length = 25 cm Duodenal bulb or superior duodenum 3 to 5 cm Descending duodenum 10 cm Transverse duodenum 2.5 to 5 cm Ascending duodenum 2.5 to 5 cm

The gastrointestinal (GI) tract includes the mouth, pharynx, esophagus, stomach, and small and large intestines. It is also known as the alimentary canal (Figure 19-1 and Table 19-1).

The GI tract accounts for a major portion of the digestive system. Food is ingested through the mouth and chewed. The salivary glands in the mouth release enzymes that initiate the breakdown of food particles into small, digestible molecules. The particles are then conveyed through the pharynx and esophagus to the stomach. In the stomach, food is mixed and the principal chemical changes occur; here, food is reduced and converted to chyme.

Most of the digestive processes take place in the small bowel. Carbohydrates, proteins, fats, vitamins, and some fluids including water and electrolytes are digested and absorbed in the small bowel. The large bowel absorbs much of the remaining fluid and finally eliminates the undigested products.

LOCATION

Mouth

The mouth is the origin of the alimentary canal, bound ventrally by the lips, laterally by the cheeks, anteriorly by the hard and soft palate, and posteriorly by the tongue. It communicates posteroinferiorly with the pharynx.

Pharynx

The pharynx is located behind the nose, mouth, and larynx. It extends from the undersurface of the skull to the level of the cricoid cartilage in front and to the intervertebral disk between the fifth and sixth cervical vertebrae behind.

Superiorly, the pharynx contacts the body of the sphenoid and basilar process of the occipital bone; inferiorly, it is continuous with the esophagus. Posteriorly, the pharynx is connected with the cervical portion of the vertebral column and the longus colli muscles. Anteriorly, it forms attachments to the lower jaw, the tongue, the hyoid bone, and the thyroid and cricoid cartilages. Laterally, the pharynx is in contact with the common and internal carotid arteries and the internal jugular veins.

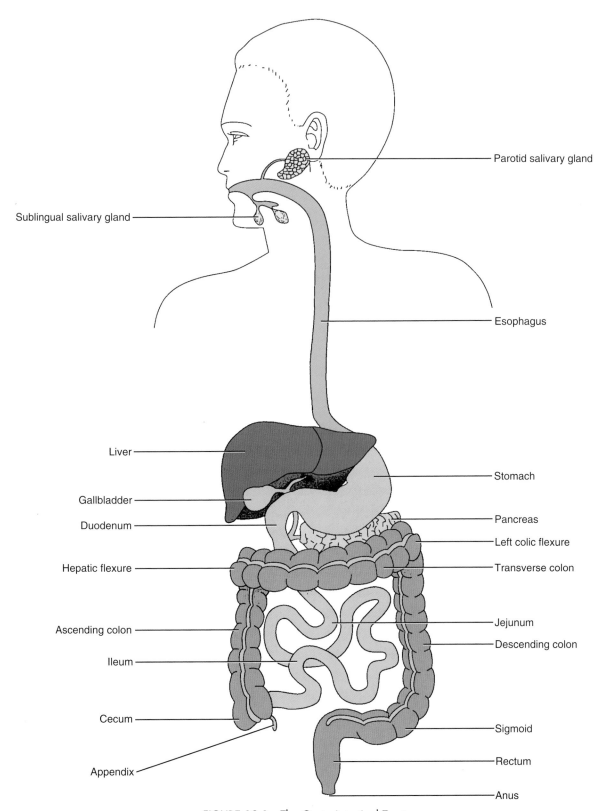

FIGURE 19-1 The Gastrointestinal Tract.

■ ■ ■ **Table 19-1** Location of the Gastrointestinal System Routinely Visualized With Ultrasound

	Esophageal Gastric Junction	Stomach	1st Portion Superior Duodenum	2nd Portion Descending Duodenum
Anterior to	Aorta	Pancreas spleen, lt kidney (superior pole), colon splenic flexure, ascending transverse mesocolon, aorta, lt adrenal gland	GDA, pancreas head, CBD, CHA portal vein	Rt kidney, rt ureter
Posterior to	Liver lt lobe	Anterior abdominal wall, liver lt lobe	GB, liver	Peritoneum, transverse colon, CBD
Superior to	Celiac artery	Pancreas		5th lumbar vertebrae
Inferior to	Diaphragm	Diaphragm, liver lt lobe and medial rt lobe		Colon, GB neck
Medial to		Left costal margin	GB neck	Colon hepatic flexure
Lt lateral to	Spine			
Rt lateral to			Pylorus	Spine, pancreas head

	3rd Portion Transverse Duodenum	4th Portion Ascending Duodenum	Jejunum	Ileum
Anterior to	IVC, aorta	Lt psoas major muscle	Lt psoas major muscle, lt kidney (interior pole)	Rt psoas major muscle, rt iliac vessels, rt kidney (inferior pole), rt ureter
Posterior to	SMV, SMA			
Superior to				
Inferior to		1st lumbar vertebrae		
Medial to			Lt iliac crest	Rt iliac crest, large intestine, cecum
Lt lateral to		Spine, aorta		
Rt lateral to	4th lumbar vertebrae			

	Cecum	Vermiform Process (Appendix)	Ascending Colon	Hepatic Flexure	Transverse Colon
Anterior to	Iliacus muscle, psoas major muscle	Rt iliac vessels	Rt iliac crest, iliacus muscle, quadratus lumborum muscle, rt kidney (lateral portion of inferior pole)	Rt kidney (lateral portion of inferior pole)	Descending duodenum, pancreas, portions of jejunum and ileum
Posterior to	Anterior abdominal wall	Cecum (some cases), ileum (some cases), ileocecal opening (attachment)	Peritoneum	Peritoneum	Peritoneum
Superior to		Cecum (some cases)	Cecum	Ascending colon	Ascending colon, descending colon, small intestine
Inferior to	Ascending colon	Cecum (some cases), ileocecal opening (attachment)	Liver rt lobe (hepatic flexure)		Liver
Medial to					
Lt lateral to					Hepatic flexure
Rt lateral to	Ileum		GB	Transverse colon	Splenic flexure

■ ■ ■ **Table 19-1** Location of the Gastrointestinal System Routinely Visualized With Ultrasound—cont'd

	Splenic Flexure	Descending Colon	Iliac Colon	Sigmoid Colon	Rectum
Anterior to	Lt kidney (lateral portion of inferior pole), spleen (inferior portion)	Lt iliac crest, iliacus muscle, quadratus lumborum muscle	Iliacus muscle, psoas major muscle	Sacrum, external iliac vessels	Sacrum, coccyx
Posterior to	Peritoneum	Peritoneum, some small intestines	Peritoneum	Peritoneum, some small intestines, urinary bladder (in males), uterus (in females)	Peritoneum, prostate gland (in males), vagina (in females), lt piriformis muscle
Superior to	Descending colon	Iliac colon, sigmoid colon	Sigmoid colon	Rectum	Anus
Inferior to	Spleen (splenic flexure)	Spleen	Lt iliac crest, descending colon	Iliac colon	Sigmoid colon
Medial to		Quadratus lumborum muscle		Rt lateral abdominal wall	Sigmoid colon
Lt lateral to	Transverse colon	Psoas major muscle, lt kidney			
Rt lateral to					

CBD, Common bile duct; **CHA**, common hepatic artery; **GB**, gallbladder; **GDA**, gastroduodenal artery; **IVC**, inferior vena cava; **SMA**, superior mesenteric artery; **SMA**, superior mesenteric vein.

Esophagus

The esophagus begins at the level of the cricoid cartilage of the neck, which is the level of the sixth cervical vertebra. The esophagus is a continuation of the pharynx and ends at the stomach, after passing through the left dome of the diaphragm at the tenth thoracic vertebra level. It courses posteriorly to the trachea from the seventh cervical to the fourth thoracic vertebral bodies.

As the esophagus continues through the thorax, it courses through the posterior portion of the middle mediastinum and is in contact with the aorta and its branches, the tracheobronchial tree, the heart, the lungs, and the interbronchial lymph nodes. Descending below the bifurcation of the trachea, it is in contact with the left atrium (base) of the heart.

The esophagus lies anterior to the seventh cervical to eighth thoracic vertebral bodies. It courses inferiorly to the right of and slightly anterior to the descending aorta to enter the left diaphragmatic dome at the level of the tenth thoracic vertebra.

The terminal part of the esophagus lies in a groove on the posterior aspect of the left lobe of the liver. It connects with the cardiac region of the stomach. The entrance of the esophagus into the stomach occurs at the **cardiac (esophageal) orifice**. This orifice marks the juncture of the greater and lesser curvatures of the stomach. The orifice is anterior to and slightly to the left of the abdominal aorta (Figure 19-2).

Above and to the left of the esophageal (cardiac) orifice, the fundus of the stomach curves superiorly toward the left undersurface of the diaphragm. The stomach lies in the left upper quadrant, within the left hypochondrium and epigastric regions. The lower aspect of the stomach lies on the transpyloric plane as it crosses the midline to reach its terminal point at the duodenum of the small intestine. The left hemidiaphragm separates the stomach from the pleura of the left lung and the apex of the heart. The anterior surface of the stomach is in contact with the diaphragm; the thoracic wall formed on the left by the seventh, eighth, and ninth ribs; the left lobe of the liver; and the anterior abdominal wall.

Peritoneum

The **peritoneum** is a serous membrane that covers abdominal and pelvic viscera or internal organs and lines the walls of the abdomen and pelvis. It forms two layers, the **parietal peritoneum** and the **visceral peritoneum**. Parietal peritoneum lines the walls of the abdominal and pelvic cavities, whereas the visceral layer covers the organs. The space between the two layers is the peritoneal cavity. In males the peritoneal cavity is closed, but in females a communication with the exterior exists

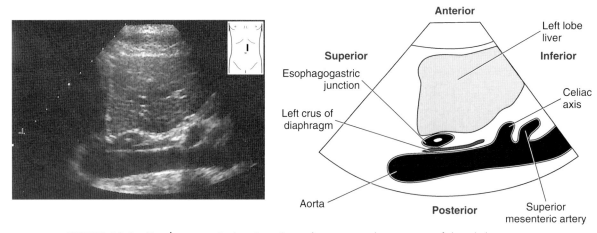

FIGURE 19-2 **Esophagogastric Junction.** Sagittal scanning plane image of the abdomen just to the left of the midline, demonstrating the esophagogastric or esophageal-gastric junction posterior to the left lobe of the liver.

through the uterus, fallopian tubes, and vagina. The peritoneal cavity is divided into two parts, the greater and lesser sacs. The greater sac extends from the diaphragm into the pelvis, while the lesser sac lies behind the stomach and freely communicates with the greater sac through an oval window opening called the *epiploic foramen* (foramen of Winslow).

Abdominal structures and organs are classified into 1 of 2 major categories based on their relationship to the peritoneum: *intraperitoneal* and *retroperitoneal*. Intraperitoneal organs and structures are covered with a visceral peritoneum that separates them from the surrounding peritoneal cavity. Retroperitoneal structures lie behind the peritoneum and are partly covered by visceral peritoneum. Structures within the peritoneum are generally mobile, whereas retroperitoneal structures are relatively fixed in their location.

Intraperitoneal organs include the following:

- Stomach
- 1st part of the duodenum
- Jejunum
- Ileum
- Cecum
- Appendix
- Transverse colon
- Sigmoid colon
- Upper 3rd of rectum
- Liver
- Uterus
- Spleen
- Fallopian tubes
- Ovaries

The retroperitoneal organs are:

- 2nd and 3rd parts of duodenum
- Ascending colon
- Pancreas
- Kidneys
- Descending colon
- Middle 3rd of rectum
- Adrenal glands
- Proximal ureters
- Gonadal blood vessels
- Renal vessels
- Inferior vena cava
- Aorta

Peritoneal ligaments are 2-layered folds of peritoneum that connect internal organs to other organs or to the abdominal walls.

Omenta are 2-layered folds of peritoneum that connect the stomach to other viscera. The greater omentum hangs down from the greater curvature of the stomach, like an apron, on the coils of the small intestine and is then folded back on itself to be attached to the transverse colon, thus draping both the transverse colon and the small intestine. Readily movable, it contains fat and warms the intestine and spreads easily into areas of trauma, often sealing hernias and walling off infections that could cause peritonitis like appendicitis.

The lesser omentum suspends the lesser curvature of the stomach from the fissure of the ligamentum venosum, the fibrous remnant of the ductus venosus of fetal circulation, and connects the lesser curvature of the stomach and the first part of the duodenum to the porta hepatis. The lesser omentum extends from the portal fissure of the liver to the diaphragm, where the layers separate to enclose the end of the esophagus. It also forms 2 ligaments, 1 associated with the liver, the hepatogastric ligament, and the other, the hepatoduodenal ligament, is associated with the duodenum.

Mesenteries are 2-layered folds of peritoneum connecting parts of the intestine to the posterior abdominal wall. Peritoneal folds also form the subphrenic spaces and the paracolic gutters. The peritoneum performs a number of important functions involving abdominal viscera. The peritoneal fluid, which is secreted by the peritoneum into the peritoneal cavity, ensures that the mobile viscera glide easily on one another.

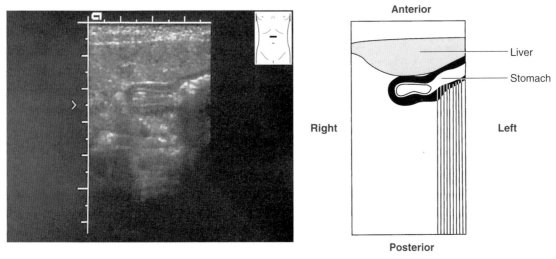

FIGURE 19-3 Stomach. Transverse scanning plane image of the epigastrium, demonstrating the long axis of the pylorus.

The peritoneal coverings of the intestine tend to stick together in infection. The greater omentum, which is commonly on the move, may adhere to other peritoneal surfaces around a focus of infection. Thus many intraperitoneal infections become sealed off and remain localized.

The peritoneal folds play an important role in suspending various organs within the abdominal cavity. They also serve as a means of conveying blood vessels, lymphatics, and nerves to these organs.

Large amounts of fat are stored in the peritoneal ligaments and mesenteries.

Stomach

The stomach is suspended within the peritoneal cavity. The posterior surface of the stomach is related to the diaphragm, the gastric surface of the spleen, the left adrenal gland, the superior portion of the left kidney, the anterior surface of the pancreas, the splenic flexure of the colon, and the ascending layer of the transverse mesocolon. These structures form a shallow bed on which the stomach rests. A small portion of the stomach, proximal to the cardiac orifice and in contact with the diaphragm and left adrenal gland, is not covered by peritoneum.

Posteroinferior to the stomach are the lesser sac, the pancreas, the left adrenal gland, the transverse colon, and the spleen.

The lesser curvature of the stomach marks the right border of the organ, extending between the esophageal (cardiac) and pyloric orifices.

The greater curvature marks the left border, descending in front of the left crus of the diaphragm along the left side of the eleventh and twelfth thoracic vertebrae.

This curvature crosses the first lumbar vertebra as it courses to the right and ascends to the pylorus.

The body of the stomach is in contact on the left with the left costal margin and the anterior abdominal wall. Inferiorly, it descends to the midlumbar vertebral level.

The antrum of the pylorus is near the midline and begins as a slight dilatation at the angular incisure in the lesser curvature. The antrum ascends, blending into the pyloric canal, which lies on the transpyloric plane between the first and second lumbar vertebral bodies.

The pyloric orifice communicates with the duodenum, the first section of small intestine. With the stomach empty, the pylorus is just to the right of the midline at the first lumbar vertebra level (Figure 19-3). A fully distended stomach may cause the pylorus to become situated 5 to 8 cm to the right of midline (Figure 19-4).

Small Bowel

The small bowel or intestine is descriptively divided into 3 portions: duodenum (or superior portion), jejunum, and ileum. It is related anteriorly to the greater omentum and the abdominal wall and is connected to the spine by a fold of peritoneum, the **mesentery**. The small bowel is contained in the central and lower part of the abdominal cavity and is surrounded superiorly and laterally by the large intestine, partly extending below the pelvic brim anterior to the rectum.

Duodenum

The duodenum, or superior portion, is the shortest part of the small intestine, measuring about 25 cm and extending from the stomach to the jejunum. It is a C-shaped, tubular structure typically described in 4

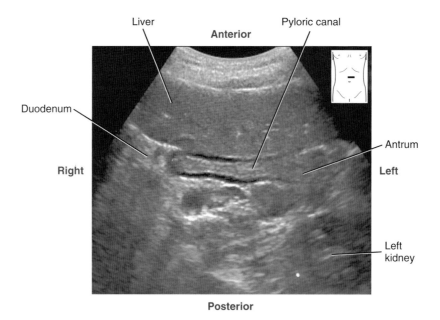

FIGURE 19-4 **Pyloric Canal.** Transverse scanning plane image of the mid epigastrium, showing the stomach wall anterior to the pancreas.

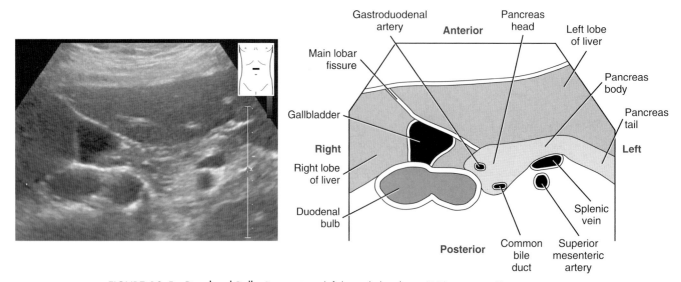

FIGURE 19-5 **Duodenal Bulb.** Patient is in left lateral decubitus (LLD) position. Transverse scanning plane image of the mid epigastrium, showing the duodenum/duodenal bulb.

parts: *duodenal bulb* and *descending, transverse,* and *ascending* portions.

The first portion of the duodenum, the **duodenal bulb,** begins at the pylorus and ends at the medial side of the neck of the gallbladder, posterior to the left lobe of the liver. It is peritoneal initially and supported by the hepatoduodenal ligament. The duodenal first part passes anterior to the common bile duct and the gastroduodenal artery, the common hepatic artery, the hepatic portal vein, the IVC, and the head of the pancreas (Figure 19-5).

The second portion, the descending duodenum, is retroperitoneal and runs posteriorly, parallel and to the right of the spine. It extends from the gallbladder neck, at the level of the first lumbar vertebra, to the body of the fourth lumbar vertebra. The transverse colon crosses anteriorly to the middle third of the descending duodenum and is connected by a small amount of connective tissue. The head of the pancreas is medial to this portion; lateral to it is the hepatic flexure of the colon. About halfway down the medial border of this segment, the descending duodenum receives the common bile duct and the main pancreatic duct via the ampulla of Vater. The secondary pancreatic duct, the duct Santorini, if present, also joins at this location.

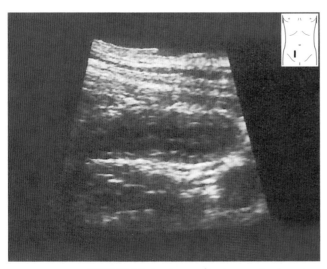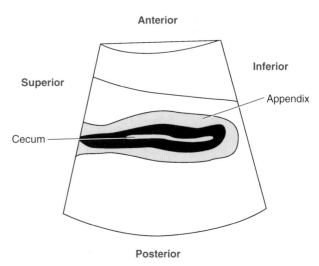

FIGURE 19-6 **Appendix.** Longitudinal section of normal appendix seen in a sagittal scanning plane image of the right lower quadrant. Note that the appendix is not usually identified; this was a false positive.

The gallbladder fundus, right lobe of the liver, coils of small intestine, and the transverse colon lie anterior to this duodenal segment. The hilum of the right kidney and the right ureter are located posteriorly. Lateral to the descending duodenum are the ascending colon, the right colic flexure, and the right lobe of the liver. Medial to it is the head of the pancreas.

The transverse duodenum is the third portion of the duodenum. It has similar length and begins to the right of the fourth lumbar vertebra and passes from right to left on the subcostal plane, inferior to the head of the pancreas, anterior to the great vessels, the right psoas muscle, the right ureter, and diaphragmatic crura, ending in the fourth duodenal portion just to the left of the aorta.

The gallbladder, the right lobe of the liver, and the medial portion of the left lobe of the liver are anterior to the C-shaped duodenum.

The fourth portion is the ascending duodenum. It rises upward on the left side of the spine and aorta to the level of the upper border of the second lumbar vertebra, where it bends ventrally and downward to join the proximal jejunum at the duodenojejunal flexure. The ascending portion lies anterior to the left margin of the aorta and the medial border of the left psoas muscle. This fourth duodenal portion is held in place by the **suspensory ligament (ligament of Treitz)**, a fibromuscular band that courses toward the left from the right crus of the diaphragm. This location marks the landmark anatomical division between the upper and lower GI tracts. The small bowel leaves its retroperitoneal position and becomes intraperitoneal at the level of the suspensory ligament.

Jejunum and Ileum
At the duodenojejunal flexure, the jejunum is contained within the peritoneum. The jejunum occupies the umbilical and left iliac regions. The ileum occupies the umbilical, hypogastric, right iliac, and pelvic regions and terminates in the right iliac fossa by opening into the inner side of the origin of the large bowel, the cecum.

Large Bowel
The large bowel or intestine begins in the right inguinal region and extends from the end of the ileum to the anus. It is descriptively divided into 6 portions: *cecum, ascending colon, transverse colon, descending colon, rectum,* and *anus.* Two flexures are associated with the colon: hepatic (right colic) flexure and splenic (left colic) flexure.

Cecum
The cecum is situated below the ileocecal opening as a blind cul-de-sac. The vermiform appendix opens into the cecum approximately 2 to 3 cm below the opening (Figure 19-6).

Ascending Colon
The ascending colon arises from the right iliac fossa, across the iliac crest, to the visceral surface of the right lobe of the liver. It bends here at the **hepatic (right colic) flexure** and becomes the transverse colon.

Transverse Colon
The transverse colon crosses the abdomen anterior to the duodenum and just below the transpyloric plane.

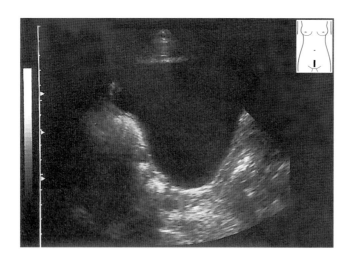

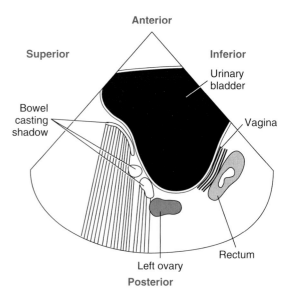

FIGURE 19-7 **Rectum.** Sagittal scanning plane image at the midline of the female pelvis showing the rectum, seen posterior to the vagina.

The pancreas is posterosuperior to the transverse colon. Just inferior to the spleen, the colon bends at the **splenic (left colic) flexure** inferiorly and becomes the descending colon.

Descending Colon
From the splenic flexure, the colon descends on the left side of the abdomen into the left iliac fossa and over the pelvic brim, where it becomes the sigmoid colon.

Sigmoid Colon, Rectum, and Anus
The pelvic sigmoid colon reaches the midline anterior to the sacrum, where it becomes the rectum, which then descends into the pelvic cavity to the level of the pelvic floor (Figure 19-7). The rectum penetrates the levator ani muscle to become the anal canal.

At this point the anal canal crosses the pelvic floor, and the GI tract terminates through the opening of the anus.

SIZE
Pharynx
The pharynx is just under 10 cm in length and is broader in the transverse than in the anteroposterior diameter. The largest portion is opposite the cornua of the hyoid bone; its narrowest portion is at the termination in the esophagus.

Esophagus
The esophagus is a muscular tube approximately 23 cm in length. It is the narrowest part of the alimentary canal and is most contracted at the origin and at the point where it passes through the diaphragm.

Stomach
The size of the stomach varies considerably. In the adult male its capacity is 2 to 4 L. The greatest length of the stomach is from 25 to 30 cm, from the top of the fundus to the bottom of the greater curvature; its widest diameter is 10 to 12 cm. The distance between the 2 openings ranges from 7 to 15 cm.

Pyloric Canal
The pyloric canal is 2 to 3 cm in length.

Small Bowel
The small bowel is approximately 6 m in length and 4 cm in diameter. It decreases in size from the origin to the termination.

Duodenum
The duodenum is the smallest, widest, and most fixed portion of the small intestine, measuring some 25 cm in length. It is subdivided into 4 parts. The superior duodenum (duodenal bulb) is 3 to 5 cm in length, the descending duodenum is approximately 10 cm in length, and the transverse and ascending portions are each 2.5 to 5 cm in length.

Jejunum
The jejunum makes up the upper two fifths of the remaining small intestine, a length of about 2.3 m. Its width is approximately 4 cm.

Ileum
The ileum accounts for the lower three fifths (3.5 m) of the small bowel and is some 3 cm in diameter.

Table 19-2 Peritoneal Ligaments and Omenta of the GI Tract

	Location	Function
Gastrosplenic	A peritoneal fold extending from the greater curvature of the stomach and connecting it to the hilum of the spleen	Contains short gastric vessels and left gastroepiploic vessels
Gastrocolic ligament	Stretches from the greater curvature of the stomach to the transverse colon	Forms part of the anterior wall of the lesser sac
Splenocolic ligament	Connects the spleen and the colon via the splenic capsule and the transverse colon	Made of visceral peritoneum, it is a component of the greater omentum
Greater omentum	A double fold of peritoneum attaching greater curvature of stomach and 1st part of duodenum to the transverse colon	Hangs in front of the intestines like an apron, contains fat; spreads easily to seal off areas of trauma
Lesser omentum	Suspends the lesser curvature of the stomach from the fissure of the ligamentum venosum	Connects lesser curvature of stomach and 1st part of duodenum to the porta hepatis

Large Bowel

The large bowel is nearly 2 m in length, largest at the cecum and gradually diminishing in size to the rectum.

GROSS ANATOMY

The gut is a long, hollow tube composed of multiple layers contained within the abdominopelvic cavity and attached by the mesentery.

Esophagus

The esophagus is the most muscular structure of the GI tract. Its outer muscular layer is composed of longitudinal fibers; its inner muscle layer has a circular axis.

The arteries that supply the esophagus derive from the inferior thyroid branch of the subclavian artery, the descending thoracic aorta, the gastric branch of the celiac axis, and the left inferior phrenic artery of the abdominal aorta.

Stomach

The stomach has 3 parts: the fundus (superiorly), the body (or corpus), which is the major portion of the stomach, and the pylorus. The pylorus is subdivided into 3 regions: the antrum, the pyloric canal, and the pyloric sphincter.

The ligamentous structures of the mesentery that support the stomach include the 3 parts of the greater omentum: the gastrophrenic ligament, the gastrocolic ligament, and the gastrosplenic ligament. These structures help support the surface of the greater curvature. The greater omentum is fat laden and double layered and hangs down from the greater curvature of the stomach, connecting it with the spleen, transverse colon, and diaphragm. It passes inferiorly to the pelvis and loops back, thus creating 4 layers of peritoneum before it attaches to the transverse colon.

The gastrohepatic ligament, a part of the lesser omentum (Table 19-2), supports the lesser curvature of the stomach. The lesser omentum is a fold of peritoneum that connects the lesser curvature of the stomach and the proximal duodenum via the hepatoduodenal ligament to the liver. The lesser omentum is posterior to the left lobe of the liver and is attached in the fissure for the ligament venosum and to the porta hepatis on the inferior surface of the liver.

Arterial flow to the stomach is supplied by the right gastric branch of the proper hepatic artery, the pyloric and right gastroepiploic branches of the hepatic artery, the left gastroepiploic branch, the vasa brevia from the splenic artery, and the left gastric artery off the celiac artery.

Veins of the stomach are generally parallel to the arterial vessels and drain into the portal system.

Small Bowel

The small bowel, like the esophagus, stomach, and the large intestine, has a 2-layered muscular structure within its walls, the muscularis propria, with the outer layer of cells arranged longitudinally and the inner layer of cells following a circular axis. The duodenum, jejunum, and ileum comprise the small intestine.

Duodenum

The C-shaped duodenum is the most proximal portion of the small bowel and is divided into 4 parts: the duodenal (or superior) bulb and the descending, transverse, and ascending portions.

The first portion of the duodenum is not fixed, whereas the remaining portions of the small bowel are bound to the neighboring viscera and the posterior abdominal wall by the extensive peritoneal fold, the mesentery, which allows for free motion. The fan-shaped mesentery contains blood vessels, nerves, lymphatic glands, and fat between its 2 layers.

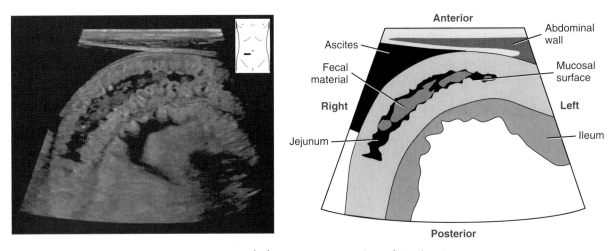

FIGURE 19-8   Valvulae Conniventes (valves of Kerckring).

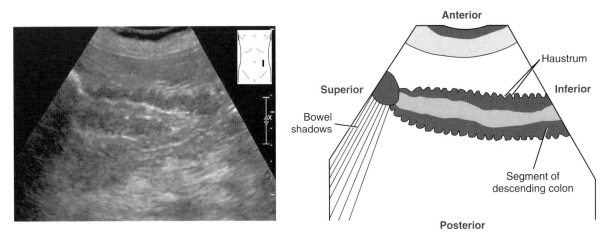

FIGURE 19-9   Haustra. Descending colon segment showing haustra.

Jejunum and Ileum

The jejunum is distinguishable from the ileum by the presence of greater vascularity, the presence of **Brunner's (duodenal) glands** (which are similar to the pyloric glands of the stomach), large and thickly set valvulae conniventes, and larger villi. Duodenal and pyloric glands produce an alkaline substance to reduce the acidity produced by stomach digestion. The **valvulae conniventes (valves of Kerckring)** are large folds of mucous membrane that project into the lumen of the bowel and serve to retard the passage of food and provide a greater absorbing area (Figure 19-8). These folds begin to appear about 3 to 5 cm beyond the pylorus and almost entirely disappear in the lower part of the ileum, which contributes to the narrowing of the ileum as it courses toward the cecum. The ileum connects to the large intestine at the ileocecal orifice.

Large Bowel

The large bowel is both shorter and larger than the small bowel and, as discussed, contains the vermiform appendix; cecum; ascending, transverse, descending, and sigmoid colons; right and left colic flexures; rectum; and anus. The colon has a segmented appearance because of **haustra**, small pouches caused by sacculation (Figure 19-9). The haustra serve to move contents through the colon. A haustrum distends as it fills, which causes muscles to contract and push the contents to the adjacent haustrum.

The celiac, superior, and inferior mesenteric arteries supply the small and large intestines. The celiac artery, arising from the anterior abdominal aorta, supplies the duodenum from its gastric, gastroduodenal, and superior pancreaticoduodenal branches (Figure 19-10).

The superior mesenteric artery (SMA) arises from the anterior surface of the abdominal aorta, passes between

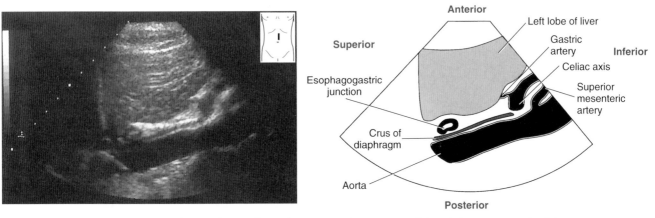

FIGURE 19-10 Gastric Artery. Sagittal scanning plane image of the abdomen just to the left of the midline, demonstrating a longitudinal section of the gastric artery.

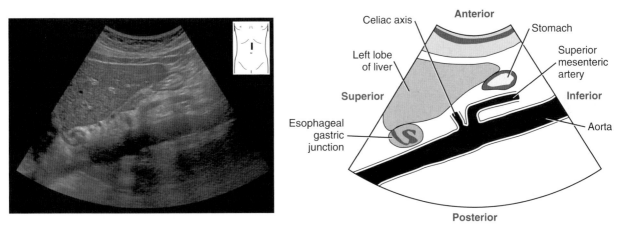

FIGURE 19-11 Superior Mesenteric Artery. Sagittal scanning plane image of the abdomen just to the left of the midline, showing a longitudinal section of the superior mesenteric artery.

the head and neck of the pancreas, and supplies branches to the intestines. The SMA branches to the small bowel include the inferior pancreaticoduodenal, the jejunal, and the ileal arteries (Figure 19-11).

The SMA branches that feed the large intestine include the ileocolic, the right colic, and the middle colic arteries.

The inferior mesenteric artery (IMA) supplies the large intestine from the left border of the transverse colon to the rectum, arising from the anterior surface of the abdominal aorta at the level of the third lumbar vertebra and descending retroperitoneally. Branches of the IMA include the left colic, the sigmoid, and the superior rectal arteries.

Venous return from the small and large intestines empties into the portal system via vessels that parallel the SMA branches. These channels may drain directly into the portal vein, the splenic vein, and the inferior mesenteric vein or the superior mesenteric vein. The superior mesenteric vein courses to the right of the

SMA and joins the splenic vein to form the portal vein, which enters the liver as its major blood supply. This junction is referred to as the *portal vein confluence* (Figure 19-12).

PHYSIOLOGY
Primary functions of the GI tract are the digestion and absorption of nutrients. The GI tract is the largest endocrine organ in the body. When food is eaten, nervous activity, distention, and chemical stimulation of the GI tract result in the release of hormones from endocrine cells scattered throughout the **mucosa** from the stomach to the colon. These hormones influence intestinal absorption and act on the secretion of enzymes, water, and electrolytes. The absorption of water, electrolytes, and nutrients influences the motility and growth of the GI tract.

Several GI hormones are well known. **Gastrin** is an endocrine hormone released from the stomach that stimulates the secretion of gastric acid. **Cholecystokinin**

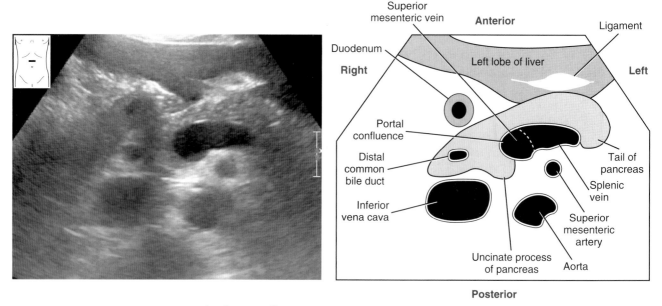

FIGURE 19-12 **Portal Splenic Confluence.** Transverse scanning plane image of the mid epigastrium highlighting the portal vein confluence.

is released by the presence of fat in the intestine and serves to regulate gallbladder contraction and gastric emptying. **Secretin** is released from the small bowel, and as "nature's antacid," it stimulates the secretion of bicarbonate, naturally decreasing the acid content of the intestine.

The digestive system breaks down food products—carbohydrates, fats, and proteins—into small, absorbable nutrients. The GI tract plays a major role in digestion. Food products are reduced to small, absorbable molecules by chemical actions. These actions are initiated by the enzymes present in the juices of the tract.

Food transport and digestion begin in the mouth. The oral cavity, pharynx, and esophagus are coordinated to prepare the food for transport to the stomach. The esophagus has 2 major functions: transport of the food from the mouth to the stomach and prevention of reflux of the GI contents.

The esophagus transports swallowed material from the pharynx to the stomach, using muscular contractions. The lower esophagus acts as a sphincter, controlling the passage of material entering the stomach. Reflux is prevented by closure of the upper and lower esophageal sphincters between swallows.

The stomach performs important functions related to the storage and digestion of food. It holds a large volume of ingested material, thus providing a storage function. Digestion involves the breakdown, or hydrolysis, of nutrients into smaller molecules so that they can be absorbed or transported across the intestinal cell. This process makes the stomach the primary or principle

organ of digestion. Muscles of the stomach contract and mix the material ingested with gastric juice, thereby facilitating the digestive function of the stomach. The stomach contents are then propelled into the duodenum of the small bowel.

Absorption of all major food products takes place in the small bowel. After the products mix with digestive secretions and enzymes, carbohydrates are reduced to monosaccharides and disaccharides, proteins to peptides and amino acids, and fats to monoglycerides and fatty acids. These nutrients are then absorbed through the intestinal mucosa into the bloodstream. They enter the general circulation via the capillaries into the portal system or via the lacteals into the intestinal lymphatics. The remaining contents are moved to the large bowel for elimination.

In the large bowel, intestinal material is transformed from a liquid to a semisolid state by the time it reaches the descending and sigmoid colons, as water and electrolytes are absorbed. Most of the absorption process occurs in the cecum. In the sigmoid and rectum, the material is stored and then eliminated.

SONOGRAPHIC APPEARANCE

Visualization of the bowel can be impeded by the presence of air or gas within the lumen, which will reflect the sound and thus prevent transmission of the beam (Figure 19-13). However, since pathologic processes of the intestinal tract tend to displace air and feces, diseased segments of bowel tend to stand out against normal bowel segments. Furthermore, technological advances in ultrasound imaging have improved the

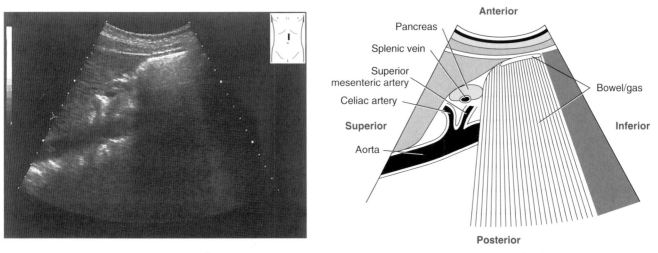

FIGURE 19-13 **Bowel.** Sagittal scanning plane image of the abdomen just to the left of the midline, showing a longitudinal section of the abdominal aorta obscured by overlying gas-filled bowel.

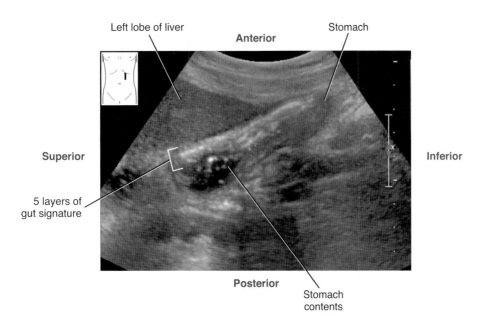

FIGURE 19-14 **Gut Signature.** Longitudinal image of the gut signature, demonstrating five layers of the anterior intestinal wall.

ability to study the bowel wall using transabdominal imaging. The sonographic appearance of bowel varies, depending on its contents and compressibility. The bowel may or may not contain air, gas, feces, or fluid within the lumen.

A localized segment can be suggested by the location of the bowel loop and its relation to the abdominal wall, to viscera, and to the peritoneum. Recall that the peritoneal coverings and folds of the intestine tend to stick together during infectious processes, thus sealing off intraperitoneal infections. This increases the probability of sonographic localization.

The layers of the bowel wall create a characteristic appearance on sonography called a **gut signature**, wherein up to 5 layers can typically be visualized (Figure 19-14). The first, third, and fifth layers are echogenic, and the second and fourth layers are hypoechoic in comparison.

Investigators commonly describe 5 principal layers as visible on both transabdominal and endoscopic ultrasound imaging (Table 19-3). The innermost superficial *mucosal layer* is highly reflective and directly contacts the intraluminal contents and is lined with epithelium having many folds, which increase the absorptive surface

■ ■ ■ **Table 19-3** Gut Signature

Layer	Name	Echogenicity
Innermost	Mucosal	Bright; highly reflective
Second inner	Deep mucosal (muscularis mucosa)	Hypoechoic (compared to mucosal, submucosal, and serosal)
Third middle	Submucosal	Hyperechoic (compared to deep mucosal and muscularis propria)
Fourth outer	Muscularis propria (circular and longitudinal muscle layers)	Hypoechoic (compared to submucosal and serosal)
Fifth outermost	Serosal	Hyperechoic (compared to adjacent structures)

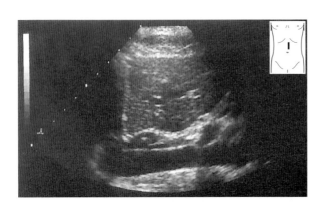
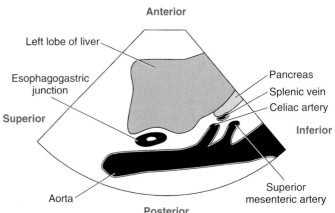

FIGURE 19-15 **Esophagogastric Junction.** Sagittal scanning plane image just to the left of the midline, demonstrating the esophagogastric (EG) junction anterior to the abdominal aorta.

and give the mucosal layer its high echogenicity. The next layer, the *deep mucosal* layer, the muscularis mucosa, appears hypoechoic relative to the mucosal layer. The submucosa beneath it appears hyperechoic compared to the deep mucosal layer and contains blood vessels and lymph channels in connective tissue. The fourth layer, the *muscularis propria*, appears hypoechoic relative to the submucosa and contains both circular and longitudinal layers of fibrous muscle bands that help move intestinal contents forward (peristalsis). The serosa is a thin, loose layer of connective tissue that appears hyperechoic compared to adjacent structures, due to being surrounded by the outermost single-cell layer of mesothelium, or serosal fat covering the intraperitoneal bowel loops.

The bowel wall has an average total thickness of 3 mm if distended and 5 mm if not distended. **Wall thickness up to 7 mm is generally regarded the upper limit of normal.**

Small bowel may appear collapsed or contain fluid, mucus, gas, or other visible contents. The jejunum demonstrates a ladder pattern throughout its length due to its valvulae conniventes. The ileum demonstrates a smaller, more smooth-walled appearance as it courses toward the cecum.

The large bowel gives a similar appearance but is differentiated by its largely fixed locations within the paracolic gutters of the retroperitoneal spaces and the presence of visible haustra.

Esophagus

The esophagus is normally recognized at the esophagogastric (EG) junction on a sagittal scanning plane image just to the left of the midline, which includes a longitudinal view of the abdominal aorta (Figure 19-15). The esophagus appears as a target lesion, surrounded by the crura of the diaphragm; anterior to the aorta; along the posterior aspect of the left lobe of the liver. The normal esophageal wall measures 5 mm. In the neck, it may be seen posterior to the thyroid gland on the left and is usually recognized by its bull's-eye appearance (Figure 19-16). Empty loops of bowel also demonstrate the target (bull's eye) pattern: a thin, hypoechoic sonolucent periphery with a bright, echogenic center of varying size.

Stomach

The stomach can usually be identified by its characteristic location between the free edge of the left lobe of

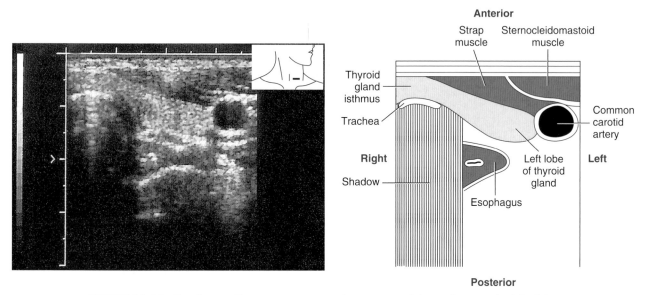

FIGURE 19-16 Esophagus. Transverse scanning plane image of the neck just to the left of the midline, showing an axial section of the esophagus posterior to the left lobe of the thyroid gland.

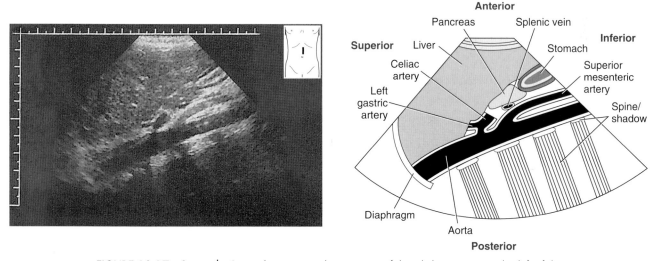

FIGURE 19-17 Stomach. Sagittal scanning plane image of the abdomen, just to the left of the midline, demonstrating the collapsed stomach antrum anteroinferior to the pancreas.

the liver and the anterior surface of the spleen. Normal wall thickness of the stomach measures from 3 to 5 mm (±1 mm). The collapsed antrum of the stomach lies anterior to the pancreas (Figure 19-17) and has a mean thickness of 13.8 mm.

Separation of the fundus of the stomach and the left hemidiaphragm suggests a pathologic process in the subphrenic space, such as an abscess. A large mass in the pancreas will displace the stomach anteriorly and perhaps superiorly. Posterior displacement of the stomach is most probably caused by an enlarged left lobe of the liver, since this lobe is the only structure anterior to the stomach. Splenic enlargement tends to displace the stomach medially.

A fluid-filled stomach appears anechoic with bright walls and therefore may simulate a cystic mass such as a pseudocyst in the left upper quadrant (Figure 19-18). Sonographic visualization of peristalsis helps to identify bowel and thus differentiate it from cystic masses.

Small Bowel

The duodenal bulb is related to the gallbladder and the transverse colon near the hepatic flexure. It is anterior and lateral to the head of the pancreas. The duodenum, the gallbladder, and the portal confluence form a triad that helps to localize the head of the pancreas. Gas in the duodenum, however, may mimic mass lesions

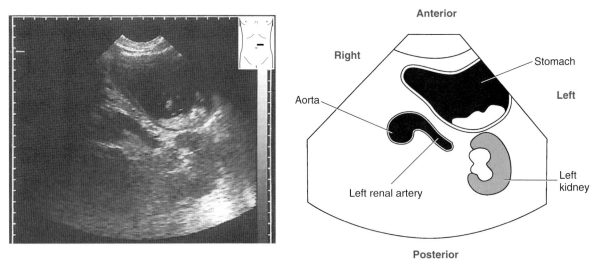

FIGURE 19-18 **Stomach.** Transverse scanning plane image of the epigastrium, just to the left of the midline, showing the fluid-filled stomach anterior to the left kidney.

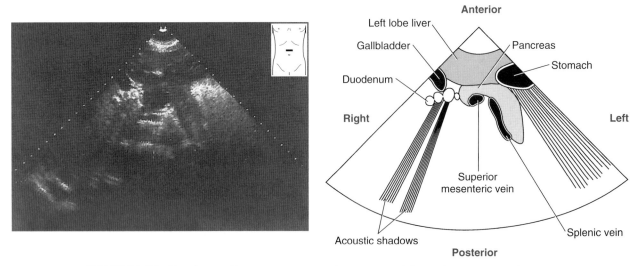

FIGURE 19-19 **Duodenum.** Transverse scanning plane image of the mid epigastrium, showing gas in the duodenum mimicking stones in the gallbladder or a mass in the head of the pancreas.

or pseudomasses in the pancreas or a stone-filled gallbladder (Figure 19-19).

A distended gallbladder can indent the superolateral aspect of the duodenal bulb and the descending duodenum. The distal third part of the duodenum is the only segment of the bowel that extends posterior to the SMA and the SMV. The proximal portion of the jejunum is inferior to the body and tail of the pancreas and anterior to the left kidney (Figure 19-20).

Large Bowel

The collapsed transverse colon may be seen on longitudinal views of the abdomen, inferior to the pancreas and stomach (Figure 19-21). It lies beneath the anterior abdominal wall, throughout its course, and passes anterior to the left kidney as it bends caudally to form the splenic flexure (Figure 19-22).

The right colic flexure is inferior to the right lobe of the liver and at a lower level than the left colic flexure, which is inferior to the spleen. The right colic (hepatic) flexure may produce artifacts simulating gallbladder disease if it is gas filled, and the left colic (splenic) flexure may mimic the left kidney.

The sigmoid colon is anterior to the external iliac vessels and the sacrum. In females, it is posterior to the posterior surface of the mid and fundal segments of the uterus and the superior part of the vagina (Figure 19-23). In males, the sigmoid colon is identified posterior to the

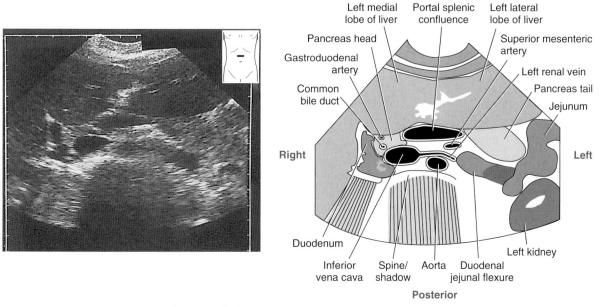

FIGURE 19-20 **Duodenojejunal Flexure.** Transverse scanning plane image of the mid epigastrium, demonstrating the duodenojejunal flexure posterior to the body and tail of the pancreas. The jejunum is that portion of small bowel located anterior to the left kidney.

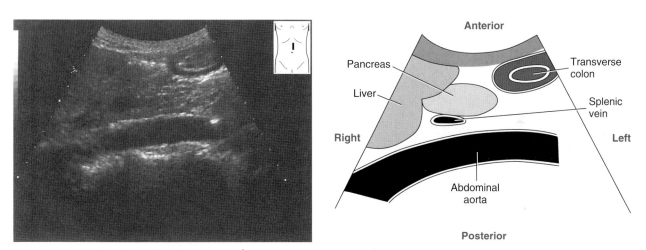

FIGURE 19-21 **Transverse Colon.** Compressed section of the transverse colon noted on a sagittal scanning plane image of the abdomen, just to the left of the midline. The axial section of transverse colon is seen anterior to the longitudinal section of the aorta and inferior to the axial section of the pancreas.

urinary bladder (Figure 19-24). In either sex, the sigmoid may be visualized superior to the bladder.

The rectum is posterior to the lower uterine segment and the vagina in the female, with the peritoneum over its anterior surface extending to the uterine surface. This forms the **rectouterine pouch**, also called the pouch of Douglas or posterior cul-de-sac. The rectum is identified posterior to the prostate gland, the seminal vesicles, and the bladder in the male; it is anterior to the levator

ani muscles in both the male and female pelvis (Figure 19-25).

SONOGRAPHIC APPLICATIONS

Ultrasound helps to narrow the differential diagnosis of bowel disorders by visualization of the bowel wall and its layers.

- **Thickening of the bowel wall:** This most common feature of bowel disease may be diffuse,

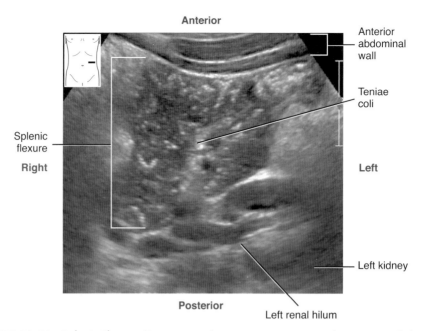

FIGURE 19-22 **Splenic Flexure.** Transverse colon courses posterior to the anterior abdominal wall and anterior to the left kidney as it bends caudally to form the splenic flexure.

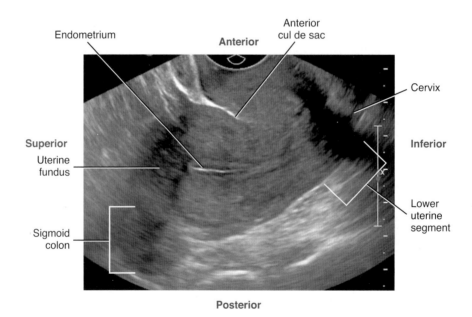

FIGURE 19-23 **Sigmoid Colon.** The sigmoid colon in a female patient may be localized posterior to the fundal and mid segments of the uterus, as seen in this transvaginal image.

circumferential, or segmental. Thickening of the bowel wall occurs with infiltration, inflammation, edema, or tumor growth, thus allowing for sonographic recognition of the pathologic process. Causes of wall thickening include pyloric stenosis, hematoma, intussusception, tumor, appendicitis, and edema. Submucosal edema with thickening demonstrates decreased echogenicity of the bowel wall.

• **Neoplasms:** May demonstrate decreased-to-intermediate echogenicity. Differential diagnosis of gastric lesions may include adenocarcinoma of the stomach, lymphoma, leukemia, Crohn's disease, intussusception, and metastases. The most common cancer of the colon is primary adenocarcinoma, although leiomyosarcomas, metastases, and lymphomas have also been reported. Malignant lesions are often associated

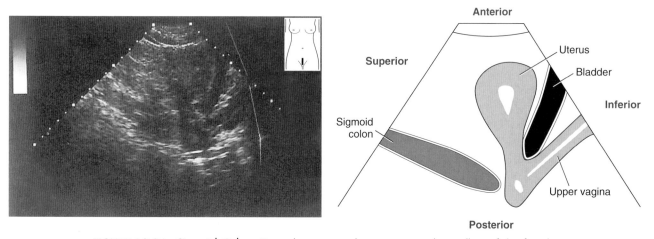

FIGURE 19-24 **Sigmoid Colon.** Sagittal scanning plane image at the midline of the female pelvis, showing a longitudinal section of the sigmoid colon, superior and posterior to the uterus and vagina.

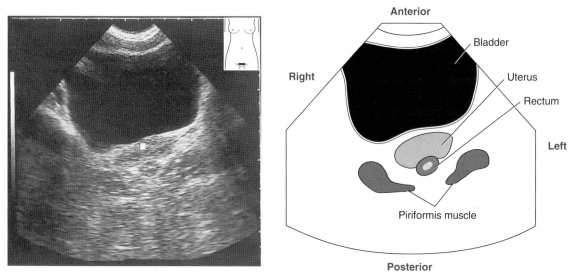

FIGURE 19-25 **Rectum.** Transverse scanning plane image at the midline of the female pelvis, showing an axial section of the rectum posterior to the uterus and anterior to the piriformis muscles.

with cases of adult intussusception, which are localized more than 75% of the time in the small bowel.

- **Ulceration of bowel:** Caused by inflammation. Edema, which is primarily accumulated in loose connective tissues, may appear as the first sign of inflammation in the bowel wall (Figure 19-26). Deep or submucosal inflammation, such as that found in Crohn's disease, causes thickening of the bowel wall. Concentric, focal thickening of the gut walls that presents with the sonographic findings of a hypoechoic rim, a homogeneous thickness, and a central echogenic area that is tubular shaped longitudinally ("pseudokidney sign") and doughnut shaped ("doughnut sign") on axial sections may be

observed with inflammation, lymphoma, edema, neoplasm, and intussusception.

- **Intussusception:** A bowel abnormality that occurs when a proximal bowel segment, called the *intussusceptum*, invaginates into the lumen of a distal bowel segment, called the *intussuscipiens*. When intussusception occurs, a strangulating obstruction results from compression and angulation of the mesenteric vessels of the invaginated bowel. Although intussusception is more commonly found idiopathically in children, with a peak incidence among those ages 5 through 9, it may be found to have an underlying abnormality in either children or adults. In older children, **Meckel's diverticulum**, duplication

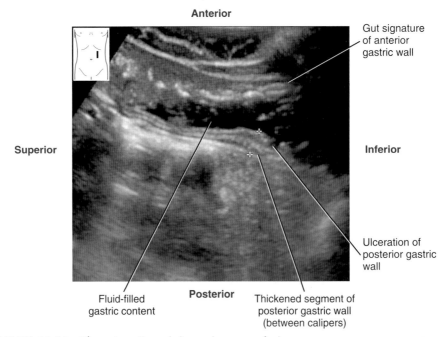

Anterior

Gut signature of anterior gastric wall

Superior

Inferior

Ulceration of posterior gastric wall

Fluid-filled gastric content

Posterior

Thickened segment of posterior gastric wall (between calipers)

FIGURE 19-26 **Ulceration.** Transabdominal image of ulceration in a posterior gastric wall segment. The ulceration is suggested inferiorly.

cysts, intestinal polyps and lymphomas, and cystic fibrosis have been associated with intussusception. In adults, malignant lesions are more commonly associated with this abnormality. Benign colonic tumors such as lipomas or polyps and inflammatory disease of the colon or appendix may also cause intussusception. With all lesions, peristalsis is thought to propel the intraluminal mass forward and drag the attached bowel wall segment along with it.

- **Serosal inflammation:** May indent or displace the bowel. Appendicitis is an inflammatory process that exerts such an effect on the cecum. Normal bowel loops demonstrate peristalsis and are compressible; an inflamed appendix does not exhibit peristalsis and is not compressed. The normal appendix is rarely visualized, except occasionally in a thin patient or when it is surrounded by ascites. Appendicoliths and periappendiceal abscesses can also be visualized.

Most disease processes of the bowel result in stiffening of the diseased segments, which leads to less compressible segments with reduced peristalsis. The graded compression technique, initially described by Puylaert, is used to assess for non-compressible bowel and involves the use of a linear footprint, high-frequency transducer to displace gas-filled bowel loops while applying moderate compression. Ultrasound is commonly used as the initial exam in the emergency room assessment of RLQ pain to exclude acute appendicitis. Ultrasound findings of a non-compressible, blind-ending tubular structure that measures greater than 6 mm in outer wall to outer wall diameter and lacks peristalsis in the long axis and demonstrates the target appearance in cross-section are suggestive of appendicitis, particularly when increased blood flow is suggested in the structural wall using color Doppler.

- **Dilated bowel:** Occurs when it is obstructed and when ileus occurs. Ileus causes paralysis of bowel loops. Peristalsis is absent in the affected loop or loops of bowel, which results in gas accumulating in the paralyzed loop. Localized ileus commonly occurs near an inflammatory process.
- **Obstructed bowel:** Prevents gas from passing through the GI tract and builds up proximal to the obstructed loop. The portion of bowel distal to the obstruction becomes decompressed.
- **Malrotation of the bowel:** Can be assessed with Doppler imaging. Malrotation of the bowel is frequently associated with malposition of the superior mesenteric artery and vein and the detection of varices, as well as the determination of directional flow within them. The left gastric or coronary vein is the most common portosystemic collateral. Normal flow in the left gastric vein is toward the splenic and portal vein confluence, but in most cases of portal hypertension with esophageal varices, this flow is reversed and oriented cephalad. Doppler flow studies may also be used to evaluate blood flow to the bowel wall in an assessment for ischemia, which precludes necrosis.

- **Esophageal and gastric lesions:** Assessed with endosonography; include varices, typically located in the EG junction, intramural tumors, and peptic ulcers, which typically demonstrate thickening of all the gut wall layers. Endosonography is also useful in generally evaluating the esophagus, stomach, and rectum. The normal thickness of the esophageal wall is approximately 3 mm, visible as 5 identifiable layers (Figures 19-27 and 19-28). Endoscopic ultrasound guidance is being investigated as an adjunct intervention for angiotherapy in the treatment of GI bleeding. Endoscopic sonography can also depict direct extension of GI malignancies into adjacent soft tissues and perivisceral adenopathy. Transrectal endosonography is typically used to identify and stage previously detected cancer. Endorectal ultrasound is considered at least as accurate as computed tomography (CT) for the preoperative staging of rectal carcinoma. In studies comparing CT with endorectal sonography, ultrasound was shown to be superior for the assessment of both depth of invasion and involvement of lymph nodes. In women, transvaginal ultrasound has been considered an important adjunct to endorectal sonography in both staging of rectal cancer and in localization of tumors that are either stenotic or high or low in the rectum.

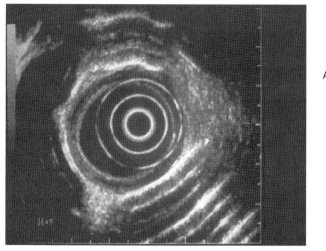

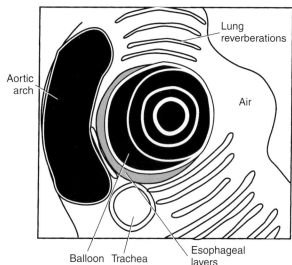

FIGURE 19-27 **Esophagus.** Endoscopic section of the upper esophagus, demonstrating wall layer separation. (Photo courtesy Wui Chong, M.D., Vanderbilt Medical Center.)

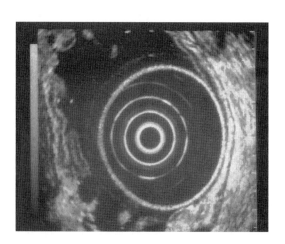

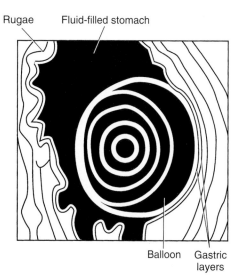

FIGURE 19-28 **Stomach Wall Layers.** Endoscopic section of stomach, demonstrating 5 identifiable wall layers. (Photo courtesy Wui Chong, M.D., Vanderbilt Medical Center.)

NORMAL VARIANTS

- **Meckel's diverticulum:** The remains of the prenatal yolk stalk (vitelline duct) projecting from the side of the ileum. The diverticulum measures between 5 and 25 cm in length and is attached by a peritoneal fold. Some 2% to 3% of the population have Meckel's diverticulum.

REFERENCE CHARTS

■ ■ ■   ASSOCIATED PHYSICIANS

- **Gastroenterologist:** Specializes in treating diseases of the gastrointestinal tract, including the stomach, small and large bowel, gallbladder, and bile ducts.
- **Internist:** Specializes in studying the physiology and pathology of internal organs and diagnosing and treating disorders of those organs.
- **Oncologist:** Specializes in the study and treatment of tumors and malignancies.
- **Pediatrician:** Specializes in guiding the development of children; concerned with the prevention and treatment of childhood diseases.
- **Surgeon:** Utilizes operative procedures to treat diseases, trauma, and organ deformity.
- **Proctologist:** Treats disorders of the colon, rectum, and anus.
- **Otolaryngologist:** Specializes in the diagnosis and treatment of diseases and injuries of the ears, nose, and throat.
- **Radiologist:** Specializes in performing and interpreting radiologic diagnostic studies of the gastrointestinal tract.

■ ■ ■   COMMON DIAGNOSTIC TESTS

- Computed tomography (CT)
  - **Abdomen:** Computed axial tomographic scans using oral and IV contrast demonstrate superior visualization of the small and large bowel.
  - **Enterography:** A multidetector CT (MDCT) scanner is used for visualization of the mucosa of the small bowel. Patients must drink a large volume (1350 mL) of 0.1% barium sulfate before imaging. If GI bleeding, small bowel tumors, or chronic ischemia is suspected, the patient will undergo a biphasic contrast-enhanced multidetector (MDCT) study.
  - **Colonography (virtual colonoscopy):** 2-D and 3-D images of the colon are generated using MDCT and a combination of oral contrast and gas distention of the large bowel. High-resolution 3-D images simulate the appearance of optical endoscopy. This technique requires cleansing the large bowel carefully and distending the colon. Residual stool may cause problems similar to those seen with the barium enema, because they may simulate polyps or masses. Three-dimensional endoluminal images are used to confirm the presence of a mass and increase diagnostic confidence.

- **Abdominal plain film:** This radiograph is used to evaluate bones and soft tissue densities of the intra-abdominal contents. Fluid-filled loops of bowel may be seen as tubular densities. Bowel gas patterns are evaluated and compared with normal gas patterns. Identification of the air-filled stomach, portions of the small intestine, and portions of the colon is possible. The examination is performed by a radiologic technologist and interpreted by a radiologist.
- **Upper GI series (barium swallow):** The upper GI series is a set of fluoroscopic and radiographic examinations used to evaluate the GI tract from the esophagus to the small bowel. Fluoroscopy permits observation of real-time motion of the tract. Contrast media are used to increase the density of the GI tract so that the anatomy and mucosal detail are visualized. Barium sulfate is most commonly used for these procedures. An iodinated contrast medium is another preparation used to opacify the tract for optimum visualization. Compression and palpation are techniques used by radiologists who perform and interpret the fluoroscopic examinations. Radiologic technologists assist the physician by adjusting the equipment controls, maintaining adequate film supplies, preparing media, and providing patient care and positioning. These examinations include the following: barium swallow and small-bowel follow-through.
- **Upper GI endoscopy (EGD):** Upper GI endoscopy is used for diagnostic and therapeutic indications. Following appropriate patient preparation, the endoscope is placed in the throat of the sedated patient. It must be swallowed. The scope is guided through the esophagus and into the stomach and duodenum and provides direct visualization of the upper GI tract. Photography, cytology, and biopsy sampling supplement the procedure, which is usually performed and interpreted by a gastroenterologist.
- **Barium enema:** Similar to the upper GI series, this examination involves the study of the colon. Single- or double-contrast media are used in the fluoroscopic procedure. Barium sulfate is infused into the cleaned rectum and x-ray studies are performed. The procedure is also used therapeutically in children with non-strangulated intussusception. A radiologist performs and interprets the examination. A radiologic technologist assists the physician.
- **Colonoscopy, sigmoidoscopy, anoscopy:** These procedures are done to further evaluate an abnormality previously identified by barium enema. For the colonoscopy, the sedated patient is given a rectal examination, followed by insertion of the colonoscope. Air is infused into the anus and the instrument is moved through the colon to the cecum and terminal ileum. The diagnostic evaluation involves structure visualization, photography, and biopsy or lesion removal. The procedures are similar in sigmoidoscopy, in which the sigmoid colon and rectum are examined, and anoscopy, in which the perianal region and the distal rectum are examined, utilizing smaller probes. The procedures are performed and interpreted by gastroenterologists.

■ ■ ■ LABORATORY VALUES

Test	Normal	Increase	Decrease
LIVER FUNCTION TESTS			
CO_2	A:19 to 24 mM V: 22 to 26 mM		Severe diarrhea
Carcinoembryonic antigen (CEA) (P)	0 to 25 mg/mL	Inflammatory bowel disease	
Cholesterol (S)			
Total	150 to 250 mg/dL		Cancer, fat malabsorption
HDL cholesterol (P)	29 to 77 mg/dL		
LDL cholesterol (P)	62 to 185 mg/dL		
VLDL cholesterol (P)	0 to 40 mg/dL		
Lipids (S)			
Total	400 to 800 mg/dL		Fat malabsorption
Cholesterol	150 to 250 mg/dL		
Triglycerides	10 to 190 mg/dL		
Phospholipids	150 to 380 mg/dL		
Fatty acids	9.0 to 15.0 mM/L		
Chloride (CL^-) (U)	110 to 254 mEq/24 hr		Pyloric obstruction, diarrhea
Potassium (K^+) (U)	25 to 100 mEq/L		Diarrhea, malabsorption
Sodium (NA^+) (U)	75 to 200 mg/24 hr		Diarrhea
Stool			
Fat	<5 g/day in patients on 100-g fat diet		
Nitrogen	<2 g/day		
Urobilinogen	40 to 280 mg/24 h		
Weight	<200 g/day		

A, Arterial; **P,** plasma; **S,** serum; **U,** urine; **V,** venous; **WB,** whole blood.

■ ■ ■ VASCULATURE

Vessel	Branch of	Supplies
ARTERIAL SYSTEM		
Esophageal artery	Descending thoracic aorta	Esophagus
Inferior thyroid esophageal branch	Subclavian artery	Esophagus
Left inferior phrenic esophageal branch	Abdominal aorta	Esophagus
Left gastric artery	Celiac artery	Stomach
Right gastric artery	Hepatic artery	Stomach, duodenum
Short gastric arteries (vasa brevia)	Splenic artery	Stomach
Gastroduodenal artery	Hepatic artery	Stomach, duodenum
Supraduodenal artery	Gastroduodenal artery	Duodenum
Right gastroepiploic artery	Gastroduodenal artery	Stomach, greater omentum
Left gastroepiploic artery	Splenic artery	Stomach, omentum
Superior pancreaticoduodenal artery	Gastroduodenal artery	Pancreas, duodenum
Inferior pancreaticoduodenal artery	Superior mesenteric artery	Pancreas, duodenum
Superior mesenteric artery	Abdominal aorta	Midgut
Inferior mesenteric artery	Abdominal aorta	Hindgut
Right colic artery	Superior mesenteric	Large intestine
Middle colic artery	Superior mesenteric	Transverse colon
Ileocolic artery	Superior mesenteric	Cecum, ascending colon, ileum, appendix
Left colic artery	Inferior mesenteric	Descending colon
Sigmoid artery	Inferior mesenteric	Sigmoid colon
Hemorrhoidal artery	Inferior mesenteric	Rectum, anal canal, anus
Superior rectal artery	Inferior mesenteric	Rectum

Continued

■ ■ ■ VASCULATURE—cont'd

Vessel	Tributary to	Drains
VENOUS SYSTEM		
Esophageal vein	Azygos	Esophagus
Left gastric vein	Splenic vein	Stomach, esophagus
Right gastric vein	Portal vein	Stomach
Superior mesenteric vein	Portal vein	Midgut
Inferior mesenteric vein	Splenic vein	Hindgut
Portal vein	Liver	GI tract
Left gastroepiploic vein	Splenic vein	Stomach, omentum
Right gastroepiploic vein	Superior mesenteric vein	Stomach, pancreas
Pancreaticoduodenal vein	Splenic vein	Pancreas, duodenum
Ileocolic vein	Superior mesenteric vein	Intestine
Right colic vein	Superior mesenteric vein	Colon
Middle colic vein	Superior mesenteric vein	Colon
Left colic vein	Inferior mesenteric vein	Sigmoid
Superior hemorrhoidal veins	Inferior mesenteric vein	Rectum, anal canal, anus
Superior rectal veins	Inferior mesenteric vein	Rectum

■ ■ ■ AFFECTING CHEMICALS

Nonapplicable

■ ## CHAPTER 20
■
■
■ # The Male Pelvis: Prostate Gland and Seminal
■ # Vesicles Sonography
■
■

TIMOTHY L. OWENS, MICHAEL J. KAMMERMEIER, AND ZULFIKARALI H. LALANI

OBJECTIVES

Describe the location of the prostate gland and seminal vesicles.
Describe the size of the prostate gland and seminal vesicles.
Identify the gross anatomy of the prostate gland and seminal vesicles.

Describe the sonographic appearance of the prostate gland and seminal vesicles.
Identify the associated physicians, related diagnostic tests, and laboratory values.

■

KEY WORDS

Central Zone — One of four zones of the glandular prostate; accounts for approximately 20% of the gland; located at the superior edge bordering the bladder and seminal vesicles. The ejaculatory ducts course through this zone.

Denonvilliers' Fascia — Two-layered fascia separating the prostate gland from the rectum.

Ductus (Vas) Deferens — One of 2 muscular tubes, each joining with its corresponding seminal vesicle to form an ejaculatory duct.

Ejaculatory Ducts — Two ducts that course through the prostate gland and empty into the prostatic urethra.

Fibromuscular Region — Anterior and smallest portion of the prostate gland; located anterior to the prostatic urethra.

Glandular Region — Posterior and largest portion of the prostate gland. Includes four zones: peripheral, central, transition, and periurethral.

Levator Ani Muscle — Muscle that supports the prostate gland laterally.

Obturator Internus Muscle — Muscle that supports the prostate gland laterally.

Peripheral Zone — Largest (70%) of four zones or areas that make up the posterior glandular portion of the prostate gland; occupies the area lateral and posterior to the distal prostatic urethra.

Periurethral Glandular Zone — One of 4 zones of the glandular portion of the prostate gland; consists of the tissue that lines the proximal prostatic urethra.

Prostate Gland — Gland surrounding the neck of the urinary bladder and male urethra. Supplies a secretion to semen.

Prostatic Urethra — Portion of the male urethra surrounded by the prostate gland. It is adjacent to the urinary bladder.

Semen — Fluid that contains sperm and secretions of glands associated with the male urogenital tract.

Seminal Vesicles — Paired glands at the base of the urinary bladder that are connected to the prostate gland. They empty into the distal portion of the ductus (vas) deferens to form the ejaculatory ducts. They are convoluted, pouchlike structures that secrete an alkaline, viscous fluid rich in fructose, which contributes to sperm viability.

Transition Zone — One of 4 zones of the prostate gland; accounts for only about 5% of the glandular prostate. It has 2 lobes situated on the lateral aspects of the proximal prostatic urethra superior to the verumontanum. This zone borders the central zone posteriorly and laterally and fibromuscular tissue anteriorly.

Verumontanum — Area close to the center of the prostate gland; near the area where the ejaculatory ducts join the prostatic urethra.

■

■ ■ ■ NORMAL MEASUREMENTS

Anatomy	Measurement
Seminal vesicles	5 cm in length, less than 1 cm in diameter
Prostate	4 cm wide, 3 cm anteroposterior, 3.8 cm in length

This chapter covers the prostate gland and seminal vesicle glands, which are structures located in the male pelvis that help make up the male urogenital system (Table 20-1). Other urogenital structures, such as the penis and scrotum, are discussed in Chapter 29. The ureters, urinary bladder, and related muscles and vasculature are described in Chapter 17. Figure 20-1 shows a cross-section of the male pelvis.

LOCATION
Prostate Gland
The prostate lies inferior to the urinary bladder and surrounds the proximal urethra. It lies behind the symphysis pubis and is separated posteriorly from the rectum by 2 layers of tissue called Denonvilliers' fascia. Laterally, the prostate is supported by the obturator internus and levator ani muscles.

Seminal Vesicles
The seminal vesicles lie posterior to the urinary bladder just superior to the prostate. Each seminal vesicle angles medially toward the apex of the bladder and lies medial to the ureters.

SIZE
Prostate Gland
The prostate weighs approximately 20 g. It normally measures approximately 4 cm (less than 2 inches) wide, 3 cm (1.5 inches) in anteroposterior dimension, and 3.8 cm (1.5 inches) in length. Unlike most other organs that atrophy with age, the prostate sometimes enlarges because of benign changes, infection, malignant tumors, or other causes.

Seminal Vesicles
Each seminal vesicle measures approximately 5 cm (2 inches) in length and less than 1 cm in diameter.

GROSS ANATOMY
Prostate Gland
The prostate gland is shaped like a cone with a central core, the prostatic urethra. The tip of the cone, or apex, is the inferior margin of the prostate and provides an exit for the urethra. The base of the gland is the superior aspect, which is in contact with the urinary bladder. The prostate is perforated by the two ejaculatory ducts, which enter the prostate at its posterior margin and course obliquely and anteriorly to join the prostatic urethra near the verumontanum, an area close to the center of the prostate.

The prostate gland consists of a small anterior fibromuscular region, or stroma, and a much larger posterior glandular region. The anterior fibromuscular stroma is

■ ■ ■ **Table 20-1** Location of Male Pelvis Structures Routinely Visualized with Ultrasound

	Prostate Gland	Seminal Vesicles	Testicles	Epididymis
Anterior to	Rectum			
Posterior to	Peritoneum, symphysis pubis	Urinary bladder	Tunica albuginea, tunica vaginalis, scrotum, skin	Testicle
Superior to		Prostate gland		Testicle
Inferior to	Urinary bladder (at proximal urethra), ejaculatory duct, seminal vesicles			
Medial to	Obturator internus muscle, levator ani muscle	Right and left ureters		
Lt lateral to				
Rt lateral to				

	Corpus Spongiosum	Corpora Cavernosa		Cavernosal Arteries
Anterior to		Cavernosal arteries		
Posterior to	Skin	Corpus spongiosum, cavernosal arteries, skin		
Superior to				
Inferior to				
Medial to	Corpora cavernosa			Corpora cavernosa
Lt lateral to		Cavernosal arteries		
Rt lateral to		Cavernosal arteries		

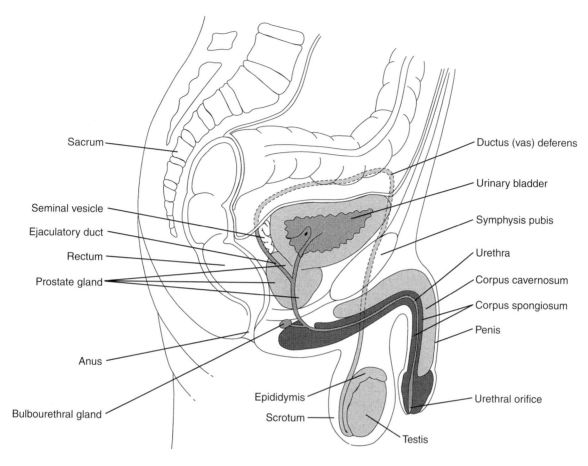

FIGURE 20-1   Male Pelvis. Sagittal cross-section of the male pelvis, illustrating the relationships of genital organs to surrounding structures.

located anterior to the prostatic urethra and is generally of less clinical significance because most pathology occurs in the glandular areas. The posterior glandular portion of the prostate has been described as consisting of zones. Dividing the glandular prostate into zones is probably the most useful representation for imaging. There are 4 zones within the glandular prostate: the peripheral zone, the central zone, the transition zone, and the periurethral glandular zone.

The **peripheral zone** is the largest, making up approximately 70% of the glandular prostate. This zone occupies the area lateral and posterior to the distal prostatic urethra. The **central zone** forms about 20% of the glandular prostate and is located at the superior edge bordering the bladder and seminal vesicles. The ejaculatory ducts course through this zone. The **transition zone** accounts for only about 5% of the glandular prostate and has 2 lobes situated on the lateral aspects of the proximal prostatic urethra superior to the verumontanum. The transition zone borders the central zone posteriorly and laterally and the fibromuscular tissue anteriorly. The tissue that

lines the proximal prostatic urethra forms the **periurethral glandular zone**. Figure 20-2, *A*, depicts the zonal anatomy of the prostate in the coronal plane; Figure 20-2, *B*, illustrates the prostatic anatomy in the sagittal plane. The prostate is surrounded by a thin capsule consisting of dense fibrous tissue and smooth muscle. This capsule connects with the muscle layers of the prostatic urethra. The prostatic urethra is divided by the verumontanum (area near the center of the prostate) into proximal and distal segments. These proximal and distal segments form an angle of approximately 35 degrees at the verumontanum.

Seminal Vesicles

The seminal vesicles are paired glands, each encapsulated by connective tissue. Beneath the connective tissue is a thin layer of smooth muscle that surrounds the submucosa and mucous membrane. The seminal vesicles are convoluted, pouchlike structures emptying into the distal portion of the **ductus (vas) deferens** to form the ejaculatory ducts.

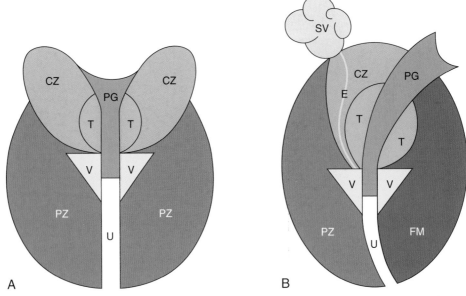

FIGURE 20-2 **A,** Zonal anatomy of the prostate gland in the coronal plane. *CZ,* Central zone; *PG,* periurethral glandular tissue (or zone); *PZ,* peripheral zone; *T,* transition zone; *U,* prostatic urethra; *V,* verumontanum. **B,** Zonal anatomy of prostate gland in the sagittal plane. *CZ,* Central zone; *E,* ejaculatory duct; *FM,* fibromuscular stroma; *PG,* periurethral glandular tissue (or zone); *PZ,* peripheral zone; *SV,* Seminal vesicles; *T,* transitional zone; *U,* prostatic urethra; *V,* verumontanum.

PHYSIOLOGY

The production of sperm, or male germ cells, might be considered the most important function of the male reproductive system, but without the secretions of the accessory organs, the sperm could not survive to complete the process of reproduction. The prostate gland and seminal vesicles secrete alkaline fluids that contribute to sperm viability. The fluid the prostate produces and secretes is believed to neutralize the acid environment of the vagina, uterus, and fallopian tubes, where fertilization of the ovum takes place. It constitutes between 13% and 33% of the volume of semen, the fluid that consists of sperm, the secretions of the prostate and seminal vesicles, and other glands associated with the male urogenital tract. The seminal vesicles secrete a viscous fluid rich in fructose. It constitutes about 60% of the volume of semen. Prostatic and seminal secretions are conveyed through numerous ducts to the prostatic urethra. The fluids are then carried outside the body through the penis via the distal urethra and finally exit through the external urethral orifice.

SONOGRAPHIC APPEARANCE
Prostate Gland and Seminal Vesicles

Ultrasound examination of the seminal vesicles and prostate may be performed either by the transabdominal method through a distended urinary bladder, as seen in Figures 20-3, *A* and *B,* or by the transrectal approach, as shown in Figure 20-4.

The transabdominal method is used only to assess the size of the glands (Figure 20-3, *C*), because most pathology is not well demonstrated with this technique. The transrectal approach is superior for scanning the seminal vesicles and prostate because of the close proximity of the transducer to the area of interest.

Sonographically, the seminal vesicles appear as low-gray structures. In the transverse scanning plane, they are seen in long axis (Figure 20-5). Normal seminal vesicles should appear symmetric in size and shape and display the same echogenicities.

In a sagittal scanning plane, the axial sections of the seminal vesicles are identified as ovoid structures with low-level echoes superior to the prostate gland (Figure 20-6).

The prostate gland is sonographically heterogeneous, with medium-level echoes (Figure 20-7). The normal prostate should always appear symmetric in shape and size.

Transrectally, in the transverse scanning plane the normal prostate gland will appear semilunar in shape near the base (superiorly) and will become more rounded near the apex (inferiorly). It will appear hyperechoic relative to the normal seminal vesicles. An area of low-level echoes situated anteriorly and in the midline of the prostate gland represents the periurethral tissue

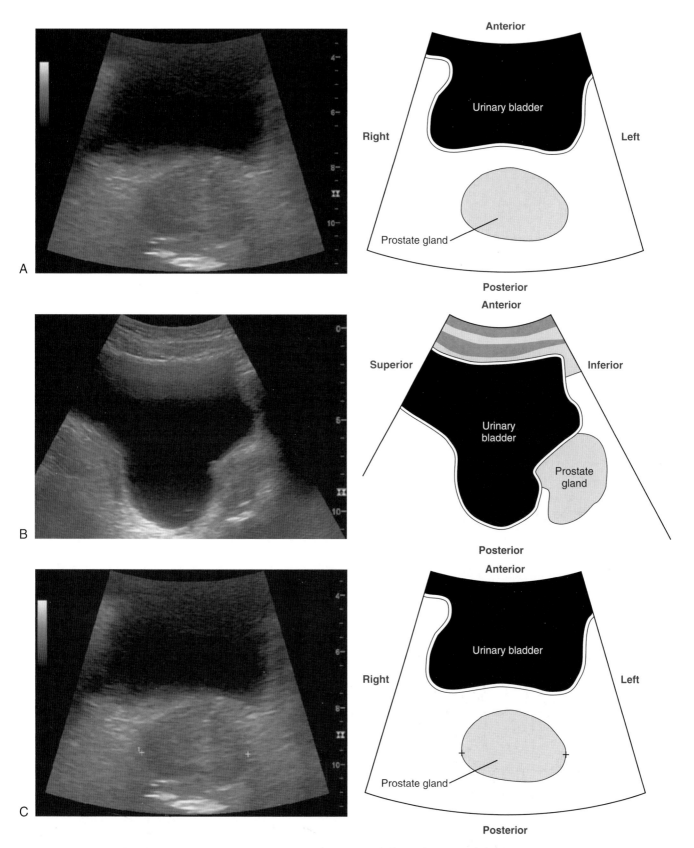

FIGURE 20-3 **A,** Transverse scanning plane; transabdominal image of the prostate gland. **B,** Sagittal scanning plane; midline transabdominal image of the prostate gland. **C,** Transverse scanning plane with width measurement; transabdominal image of the prostate gland.

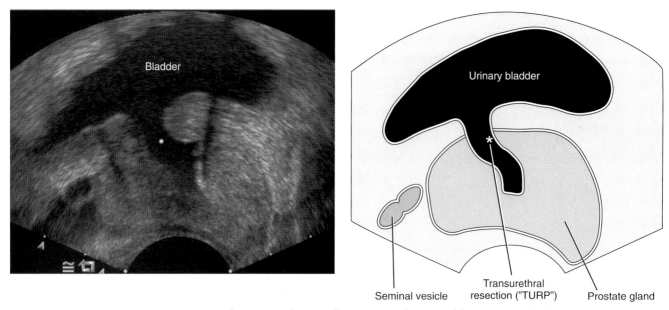

FIGURE 20-4 Sagittal scanning plane; midline transrectal image of the prostate gland.

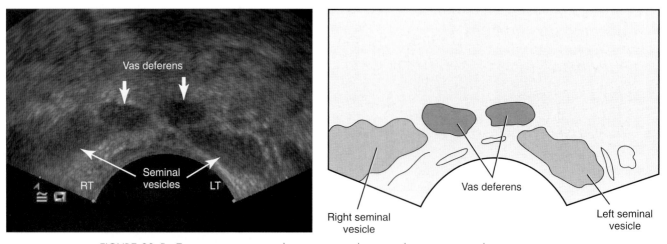

FIGURE 20-5 Transverse scanning plane; transrectal image demonstrating a long axis section of the seminal vesicles.

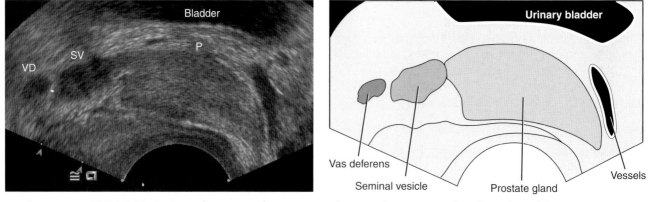

FIGURE 20-6 Sagittal scanning plane; transrectal image demonstrating the relationship of the prostate gland and seminal vesicles.

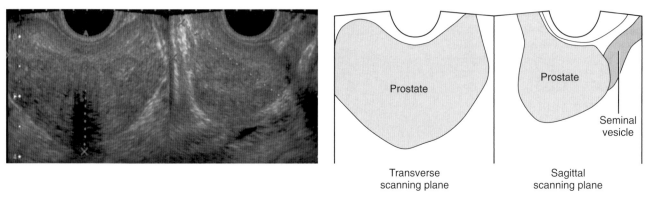

FIGURE 20-7 Transverse and sagittal scanning planes; transrectal images of the heterogeneous, medium-level echoes of the prostate gland. (Courtesy Ultrasoundpaedia.com.)

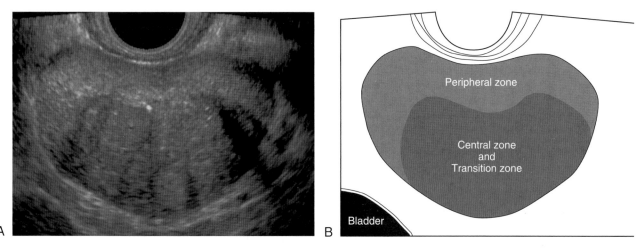

FIGURE 20-8 **A,** Transverse scanning plane; transrectal image of the prostate gland showing zonal anatomy. **B,** Another transverse scanning plane; transrectal image of the prostate gland showing zonal anatomy.

and fibromuscular stroma. In the normal prostate, the central zone and transition zone cannot be individually distinguished, whereas the peripheral zone may appear hyperechoic and homogeneous in comparison. The peripheral zone occupies the posterior and lateral portions of the gland (Figure 20-8).

The periurethral tissues appear hypoechoic relative to the urethra and surrounding structures and may be difficult to differentiate from the fibromuscular stroma, anteriorly, which can also appear hypoechoic when compared with adjacent structures. The peripheral zone should normally be homogeneous and slightly more echogenic.

SONOGRAPHIC APPLICATIONS
Prostate Gland
- Size and echo texture
- Prostatitis (infection)
- Detection of masses
- Evaluation of benign prostatic hypertrophy (BPH)
- Sonographic correlation of findings on a digital rectal examination

- Sonographic correlation of evaluated serum prostatic specific antigen (PSA)
- Evaluation of extracapsular spread of prostatic carcinoma
- Evaluation of postoperative transurethral resection (TURP)
- Ultrasound-guided biopsies of prostatic lesions

Seminal Vesicles
- Evaluation of size, symmetry, and echo texture
- Ruling out presence of cysts or calculi
- Inflammatory processes
- Congenital anomalies

REFERENCE CHARTS
■■■ ASSOCIATED PHYSICIANS

- **Urologist:** Specializes in surgical diseases of the male genitourinary tract and female urinary system.

■ ■ ■ COMMON DIAGNOSTIC TESTS

- **Magnetic resonance imaging (MRI):** A noninvasive imaging modality that is very useful in identifying soft tissue structures. It is performed by a radiologic technologist and interpreted by a radiologist.
- **Sonography:** As a method of evaluating the structures of the male genitourinary system, ultrasonography is second only to direct physical palpation of the prostate by a urologist.

■ ■ ■ LABORATORY VALUES

- **Serum prostatic specific antigen (PSA):** Used to evaluate the function of the prostate. Normal serum PSA is less than 4.0. Elevated serum PSA may indicate presence of disease but is not specific for carcinoma.

■ ■ ■ VASCULATURE

Nonapplicable

■ ■ ■ AFFECTING CHEMICALS

Nonapplicable

- # CHAPTER 21

The Female Pelvis

BETTY BATES TEMPKIN AND MARILYN DICKERSON PRINCE

OBJECTIVES

Describe the anatomy of the female pelvis and its sonographic appearance.

Describe the location of the female pelvic anatomy with relation to adjacent structures.

Describe the muscles of the pelvis and their sonographic presentations.

Describe the physiology of the female reproductive organs.

Describe the variable positions of the uterus and their sonographic presentation.

Describe the localization of bowel segments within the female pelvis.

KEY WORDS

Adnexa — Regions of the true pelvis posterior to the broad ligaments.

Anteflexed Uterus — When the bladder is empty and the cervix and vagina form a 90-degree angle, and the uterine body and fundus are bent at a great anterior angle until the fundus is pointing inferiorly and resting on the cervix.

Anterior Cul-de-sac (Vesicouterine Pouch) — Area between the uterus and pubic bone.

Anteverted Uterus — When the bladder is empty and the cervix and vagina form a 90-degree angle, and the uterine body and fundus are tipped or tilted anteriorly.

Bicornuate Uterus — Most common of the congenital malformations of the female genital tract. Recognized sonographically by the presence of two endometrial canals that usually communicate at the level of the cervix.

Broad Ligaments — Double folds of peritoneum that extend from the uterine cornua to the lateral pelvic walls. They are not true ligaments and only provide minimal support for the uterus.

Cervix — Lower cylindrical portion of the uterus that projects into the vagina.

Corpus — Body and largest part of the uterus; lies between the uterine fundus and cervix.

Endocervical Canal — Cervical canal extending 2 to 4 cm from its internal os, where it joins the endometrial canal to its external os, which projects into the vaginal vault.

Endometrial Canal — Proximal portion of the birth canal that is formed by the uterine

endometrium. It is continuous with the endocervical canal.

Endometrial Stripe — The thin, bright, reflective sonographic appearance of the central, linear, opposing surfaces of the endometrium that form the endometrial canal.

Endometrium — Innermost, mucosal layer of the uterine wall that is continuous with vaginal epithelium inferiorly and uterine tube mucosa superolaterally.

Estrogen — Hormone produced by the ovaries that promotes proliferation or preparation of the uterine endometrium for possible implantation by a zygote.

External Os — Portion of the endocervical canal that projects into the vaginal vault.

False Pelvis (Greater or Major Pelvis) — Descriptive area given to the area superior to the pelvic inlet (linea terminalis) and inferior to the iliac crests.

Follicles — Ovarian encasement containing an immature ovum. Site of ova maturation.

Fundus — Widest and most superior segment of the uterus situated between the insertion of the uterine tubes at the level of the uterine cornua; continuous with the body of the uterus.

Graded Compression — Slow and steady compression of the bowel between the anterior and posterior abdominal walls.

Iliac Crests — Portion of innominate bones that define the most superior, bilateral aspect of the pelvic cavity. They are palpable external landmarks that aid in evaluating the pelvis.

Internal Os — Portion of endocervical canal that joins or opens into the endometrial canal.

Isthmus (Uterine) — Constricted portion of the uterus where the body or corpus meets or is continuous with the uterine cervix.

Linea Terminalis — Imaginary line drawn from the symphysis pubis around to the sacral promontory, marking the dividing plane between the true and false pelves. The circumference of this plane is termed the *pelvic inlet.*

Menarche — Onset of menstruation.

Menses/Menstruation — Monthly sloughing off of the endometrial lining of the non-pregnant uterus.

Mesentery — Double layer of visceral peritoneum that wraps around a bowel segment and attaches it to the posterior abdominal wall.

Multiparous — Multiple viable births.

Myometrium — Muscle layer that forms the bulk of the uterus. Composed of three layers of different muscle fibers: outer longitudinal fibers, intermediate spiral bands, and inner circular and longitudinal fibers, which are responsible for the dramatic enlargement of the uterus during pregnancy and the radial muscle contractions necessary to expel the fetus at parturition.

Nulliparous — No viable births.

Ovulation — Occurs when the ovarian follicle bursts and releases the mature ovum. Approximately 14 days after follicle formation.

Continued

Parametrium — Fat and cellular connective tissue surrounding the two layers of each broad ligament and the structures they contain. (The fallopian tube, round ligament, ovarian ligament, and vascular structures of the uterus and ovaries are positioned between the two layers of each broad ligament.)

Parity — Number of viable offspring.

Parturition — Act of giving birth.

Posterior Cul-de-sac (Rectouterine Pouch or Pouch of Douglas) — Area between the rectum and the uterus.

Psoas Major Muscles — Somewhat triangular in shape; situated vertically in the body.

Prominent paired muscles that originate at the lateral aspects of the lower thoracic vertebrae and course anterolaterally in their descent to the iliac crests.

Pubic/Pubis Symphysis — Anterior fusion of the innominate bones (sacrum and coccyx are the posterior fusion). Palpable external land mark that aids in evaluating the pelvis.

Retroflexed Uterus — When the bladder is empty and the cervix and vagina are linearly oriented, and the uterine body and fundus are bent at a great posterior angle until the fundus is pointing inferiorly, adjacent to the cervix.

Retroverted Uterus — When the bladder is empty and the uterine body and fundus are tipped posteriorly and the angle of the cervix and vagina increases, making them more linearly oriented.

Serosa — Thin membrane that covers the myometrium and forms the outer layer of the uterus.

Space of Retzius — Space that separates the anterior bladder wall from the pubic symphysis and is typically filled with extra peritoneal fat.

True Pelvis (Lesser or Minor Pelvis) — Descriptive term given to the region deep to the pelvic inlet (linea terminalis).

■

In most cases, sonography is the imaging method of choice for evaluating the female pelvis. It is a commonly performed examination that requires knowledge of the normal anatomy in the female pelvis and its sonographic (cross-sectional) presentation.

The organs contained within the female pelvis include the genital tract (uterus, vagina, uterine tubes), ovaries, urinary bladder, and pelvic colon. The pelvic bones form its outer boundaries, while deep to this lie skeletal muscles that form its inner margins.

LOCATION

True pelvis, false pelvis, pelvic skeleton, pelvic musculature, pelvic ligaments, pelvic spaces, genital tract (uterus, vagina, uterine tubes), ovaries, urinary bladder, pelvic colon

The location of the pelvis can be defined as that part of the peritoneal cavity extending from the iliac crests superiorly to the pelvic diaphragm inferiorly. The area encompassing the pelvis is described in regions and compartments.

■ ■ ■ NORMAL MEASUREMENTS

Anatomy	Length	Width	Thickness
Vaginal canal	9 cm		
Cervical canal	2 to 4 cm		
Premenarchal uterus	2.5 cm	2 cm	1 cm
Nulliparous uterus	7 cm	4 cm	3 cm
Multiparous uterus	8.5 cm	5.5 cm	4.5 cm
Uterine tubes	7 to 12 cm		
Adult ovary	2.5 to 5.0 cm	1.0 to 3.0 cm	0.6 to 2.2 cm

Ovarian Volumes*	Mean (mL)
Premenarche (3 to 15 years)	3.0 (±2.3)
Menstruating	9.8 (±5.8)
Premenopausal	6.8
Postmenopausal (1 to 5 years after)	6.2 (±2.7) to 4.0 (±1.8)
Postmenopausal (10 to 15 years after)	2.8 (±2.1) to 2.2 (±1.4)

*Length × width × thickness (height) × 0.523.

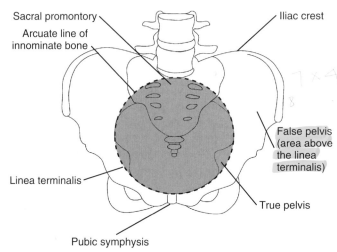

FIGURE 21-1 **True and False Pelves.** The linea terminalis extends from the sacral promontory, along the arcuate lines of the innominate bones, to the pubic symphysis. The true pelvis is the region deep to the linea terminalis. The false pelvis is the region of the abdominopelvic cavity that is superior to the linea terminalis and inferior to the iliac crests.

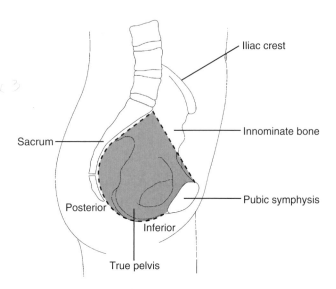

FIGURE 21-2 **True Pelvis.** The true pelvis is a bowl-shaped cavity that tilts inferoposteriorly.

There are three descriptive regions of the pelvis: *right iliac, hypogastric,* and *left iliac* (see Chapter 7, Figure 7-1). The pelvis is also described in terms of two structurally continuous compartments that make up the pelvic cavity area: the *true pelvis* and the *false pelvis.* An arbitrary division defined by the sacral promontory and linea terminalis designates the true and false pelves. The **linea terminalis** is an imaginary arcuate line drawn along the inner surface of the pelvic bone—from the pubic or pubis symphysis anteriorly to the sacral promontory posteriorly—that marks the plane separating the false from the true pelvis (Figure 21-1).

- **True pelvis location.** The **true pelvis (minor or lesser pelvis)** extends from the linea terminalis to the pelvic diaphragm inferiorly. It is a bowl-shaped cavity aligned posteriorly and inferiorly within the skeletal framework (Figure 21-2). The urinary bladder, various loops of small bowel, the genital tract, and the ovaries are situated within the true pelvis.
- **False pelvis location.** The **false pelvis (major or greater pelvis)** is defined as the more superior aspect of the pelvic cavity, extending from the iliac crests superiorly to the linea terminalis inferiorly.
- **Pelvic skeleton location.** *Sacrum, coccyx, innominate bones (ilium, ischium, pubis)*
  - ○ **Sacrum and coccyx.** The sacrum and coccyx constitute the distal segment of the vertebral spine and form the posterior border of the pelvic cavity (Figure 21-3).

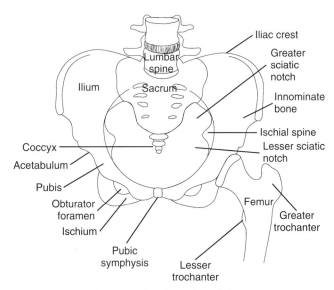

FIGURE 21-3 The Pelvic Skeleton.

- ○ **Innominate bones.** The innominate bones encircle most of the pelvic cavity, forming its lateral and anterior margins. Each innominate bone is composed of the ilium, ischium, and pubis. The innominate bones join posteriorly at the sacrum and coccyx and fuse anteriorly at the pubis or pubic symphysis. The iliac crests of the innominate bones define the most superior aspect of the pelvic cavity. The two **iliac crests** and the **pubic symphysis** are palpable external landmarks that aid in evaluating the pelvis (see Figure 21-3).

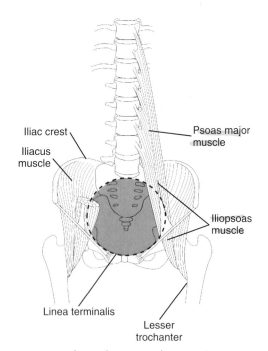

FIGURE 21-4 False Pelvis Musculature. The psoas major muscles and the iliacus muscles join at the level of the iliac crests to form the iliopsoas muscles of the false pelvis. The iliopsoas muscles pass over the pelvic brim, exiting the false pelvis to reach the lesser trochanter of the femurs.

- **Pelvic musculature locations**. *Psoas, false pelvis (iliopsoas, rectus abdominis, transverse abdominis), true pelvis (obturator internus, piriformis, pelvic diaphragm muscles [pubococcygeus, iliococcygeus, coccygeus])*
  - **Psoas muscles.** The **psoas major muscles** are prominent paired muscles extending across the posterior wall of the abdominopelvic cavity. These muscles originate at the lateral aspects of the lower thoracic vertebrae and course anterolaterally in their descent to the iliac crests.
  - **False pelvis muscles.** *Iliopsoas, rectus abdominis, transverse abdominis*
    - (i) **Iliopsoas muscles.** The psoas major muscles join the iliacus muscles at the level of the iliac crests to form the iliopsoas bundles of the false pelvis. Each iliopsoas muscle courses anteriorly along the linea terminalis, to travel over the pelvic brim and insert into the lesser trochanter of the femur (Figure 21-4).
    - (ii) **Rectus abdominis muscles.** Much of the anterior wall of the abdominopelvic cavity is formed by the rectus abdominis muscles, which extend from the sixth ribs and the xiphoid process down to the pubic symphysis (Figure 21-5, *A*). These paired muscles are

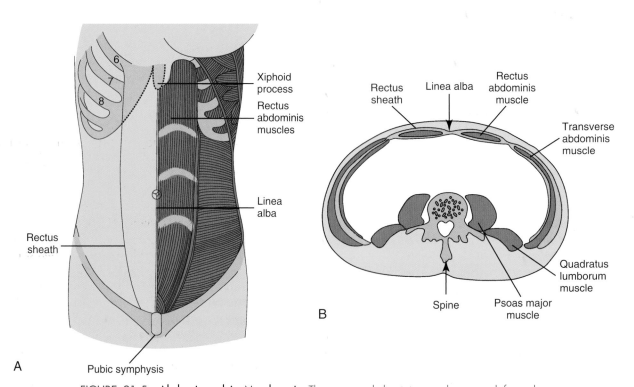

FIGURE 21-5 Abdominopelvic Muscles. A, The rectus abdominis muscles extend from the xiphoid process to the pubic symphysis along the anterior abdominal wall. The muscular rectus sheath surrounding the rectus abdominis muscles fuses midline at the linea alba. **B,** Axial section through the midabdomen. The skeletal muscles lining the abdominopelvic cavity include the rectus abdominis muscles anteriorly, the transverse abdominis muscles laterally, and the psoas major and quadratus lumborum muscles posteriorly.

Pelvic diaphragm

intersected by transverse tendinous bands and are wrapped in a muscular sheath. The rectus sheath fuses with the transversus abdominis muscles to form the linea alba, at the midline of the body.

(iii) **Transverse abdominis muscles.** The transverse abdominis muscles form the antero-lateral borders of the abdominopelvic cavity. This muscle group lies deep to the internal and external oblique muscles (Figure 21-5, *B*).

○ **True pelvis muscles.** *Obturator internus, piriformis, pelvic diaphragm (pubococcygeus, iliococcygeus [levator ani], coccygeus)*

(i) **Obturator internus muscles.** The obturator internus muscles originate along the arcuate line of the innominate bones and course parallel to the lateral walls of the true pelvis. These triangular muscles narrow inferiorly to pass through the lesser sciatic notch. The obturator internus is secured to the medial aspect of the greater trochanter. The internal surface of this muscle is covered by a tough membranous layer called the obturator fascia (Figure 21-6).

(ii) **Piriformis muscles.** The piriformis muscles originate in the most posterior aspect of the true pelvis, along the lower portion of the sacrum, posterior to the uterus. These muscles travel anterolaterally, narrowing to pass through the greater sciatic notch. The piriformis muscles are attached to the superior aspect of each greater trochanter (see Figure 21-6).

(iii) **Pelvic diaphragm muscles.** The pelvic diaphragm is a group of skeletal muscles lining the floor of the true pelvis and supporting the pelvic organs (Figure 21-7). This muscular

floor is composed of three paired muscles: the *pubococcygeus, iliococcygeus,* and *coccygeus muscles.*

- The pubococcygeus muscles are the most medial and anterior muscle pair of the pelvic diaphragm muscles. These muscles extend from the pubic bones to the coccyx, encircling the urethra, vagina, and rectum.
- The iliococcygeus muscles are located lateral to the pubococcygeus muscles. This pair extends from the obturator fascia and ischial spine anteriorly to the coccyx posteriorly. Together, the pubococcygeus and iliococcygeus muscles form a hammock across the floor of the true pelvis and are termed the *levator ani muscles.* These muscles provide primary support to the pelvic viscera and aid in the contraction of the vagina and rectum.
- The coccygeus muscles are the most posterior muscle pair of the pelvic diaphragm. These muscles extend from the ischial spine to the sacrum and coccyx.

• **Pelvic ligaments location.** *Broad, round, cardinal, uterosacral, infundibulopelvic, ovarian, pubovesical, lateral*

○ **Broad ligaments.** The anterior and posterior peritoneal reflections covering the uterus extend anterolaterally to the walls of the true pelvis (Figures 21-8 and 21-9). These double folds of peritoneum extend from the uterine cornua to the lateral pelvic walls to form the **broad ligaments**. The broad ligaments are not true ligaments, and they provide minimal support for the uterus.

The fallopian tube, round ligament, ovarian ligament, and vascular structures of the uterus and ovaries are positioned between the two layers of each broad ligament. These structures are surrounded by fat and cellular connective tissue, called the **parametrium**. The spaces within the peritoneal cavity located posterior to the broad ligaments are referred to as the **adnexa** (see Figure 21-8).

○ **Round ligaments.** Three paired ligaments provide structural support to the uterus: the round ligaments, the cardinal ligaments, and the uterosacral ligaments. Each round ligament originates at the uterine cornu and courses within the broad ligaments to the anterolateral pelvic wall (see Figure 21-9). The round ligament passes over the pelvic brim, through the inguinal canal, and is secured at the labia majora. The round ligaments maintain the forward bend of the uterine fundus.

○ **Cardinal ligaments and uterosacral ligaments.** The cardinal and uterosacral ligaments provide

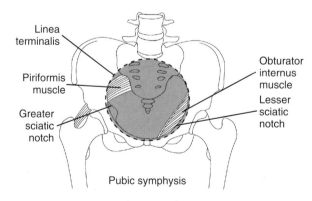

FIGURE 21-6 True Pelvis Muscles. The obturator internus muscles line the lateral walls of the true pelvis. The piriformis muscles are situated in the posterior region of the true pelvis and course cross-grain to the obturator internus muscles.

Linea terminalis

Piriformis muscle

Greater sciatic notch

Pubic symphysis

Obturator internus muscle

Lesser sciatic notch

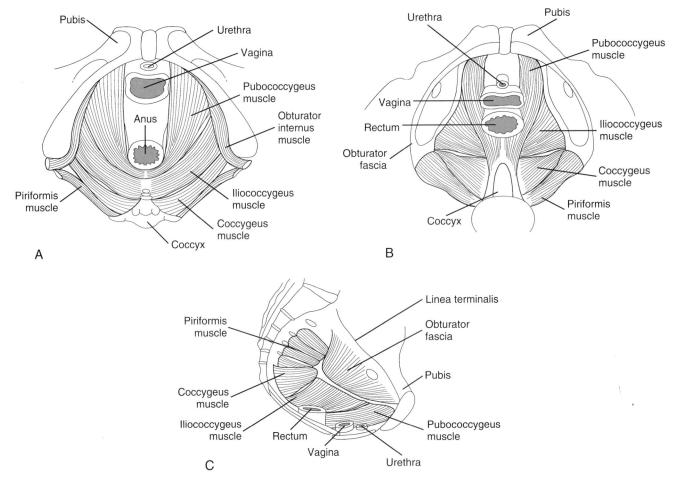

FIGURE 21-7 **The Pelvic Diaphragm.** Three muscle pairs, the pubococcygeus, iliococcygeus, and coccygeus, form the floor of the true pelvis and provide support for the pelvic organs. **A,** Viewed from below. **B,** Viewed from above. **C,** Viewed laterally.

Cardinal + Uretrosacral lig.

more rigid support for the cervix. These ligaments maintain the normal axis of the cervix, roughly perpendicular to the vaginal canal. The cardinal ligaments extend from the upper cervix and isthmus to the obturator fascia at the lateral walls of the pelvis (see Figure 21-9). The uterosacral ligaments extend from the posterior aspect of the cervix around the lateral walls of the rectum to the sacrum (see Figure 21-9).

○ **Infundibulopelvic ligaments and ovarian ligaments.** There are two paired ligaments supporting the ovaries and maintaining their relative positions in the adnexal regions. The infundibulopelvic ligament extends from the infundibulum and the lateral aspect of the ovary to the lateral pelvic wall. The ovarian ligament supports the medial aspect of the ovary to the uterine cornu. This ligament lies within the peritoneal folds of the broad ligament. The mesovarium is a short, double fold of peritoneum extending from the posterior aspect

of the broad ligament to the ovarian hilum (Figure 21-10 on p. 349).

○ **Pubovesical ligaments and lateral ligaments.** The pubovesical ligaments extend anteriorly from the bladder neck and attach to the pubic bones. The lateral ligaments extend to fuse with the tendinous arch of the obturator internus muscles.

• **Pelvic spaces locations.** *Anterior cul-de-sac, posterior cul-de-sac, space of Retzius*

○ **Anterior cul-de-sac.** Area between the uterus and pubic bone that is formed by the peritoneum, which expands over the urinary bladder and covers the anterior wall of the uterus. This peritoneal reflection creates a shallow space within the peritoneal cavity, known as the **anterior cul-de-sac** or vesicouterine pouch (Figure 21-11 on p. 350). This space is usually empty but may contain loops of small bowel.

○ **Posterior cul-de-sac.** The rectouterine reflection of the peritoneum creates a larger potential space

Endo
75° ≤ 5mm
w/tamaxofin ≤ 8mm

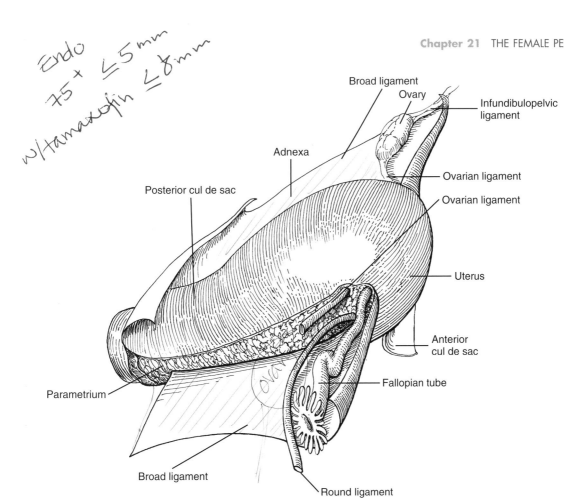

FIGURE 21-8   Broad Ligaments, Ovaries, and Uterine Tubes Locations. The ovaries are situated in the adnexa, the regions of the true pelvis posterior to the broad ligaments. The broad ligaments are double folds of peritoneum extending from the lateral aspects of the uterus to the pelvic wall. The uterine (fallopian) tubes, round ligaments, and ovarian ligaments are all located within the double folds of the broad ligaments.

between the posterior wall of the uterus (particularly the cervix) and the anterior wall of the rectum. This space is known as the posterior cul-de-sac, rectouterine pouch, or pouch of Douglas. The posterior cul-de-sac is the most dependent space in the abdominopelvic cavity. Any fluid collecting within the peritoneal cavity often drains into this space (see Figure 21-11).

○ **Space of Retzius.** The space of Retzius separates the anterior bladder wall from the pubic symphysis; it is filled with extraperitoneal fat (see Figure 21-11).

- **Genital tract location.** *Vagina, uterus, uterine tubes*

○ **Vagina location.** The vagina sits in the hypogastric portion of the peritoneal cavity (or midregion of the true pelvis) between the urinary bladder and urethra (anteriorly) and the rectum (posteriorly) (see Figure 21-11 and Table 21-1 on p. 351). It extends superior to inferior, from the external os of the uterine cervix to the external genitalia. The external orifice of the vagina is located posterior to the urethral orifice between the labia minora.

○ **Uterus location.** The nonpregnant uterus is also located in the hypogastric portion of the peritoneal cavity, between the urinary bladder (anteriorly) and rectum (posteriorly) (see Figure 21-11). The cervical portion of the uterus enters the vagina and lies at right angles to it.

Congenital uterine malformations result in anatomic variations of the uterus, cervix, and vagina resulting from the incomplete fusion or agenesis of the müllerian ducts (Figure 21-12 on p. 352). The bicornuate uterus is the most common of the congenital malformations of the female genital tract. It is recognized sonographically by the presence of 2 endometrial canals that usually communicate at the level of the cervix. Bicornuate uterus is best appreciated in axial or short axis sections, as seen in Figure 21-13 on p. 352. Note the gestational sac in the right horn of the uterus and myometrial tissue separating the 2 endometrial canals.

○ **Uterine tubes location.** The uterine, or fallopian, tubes extend laterally from the uterus to the

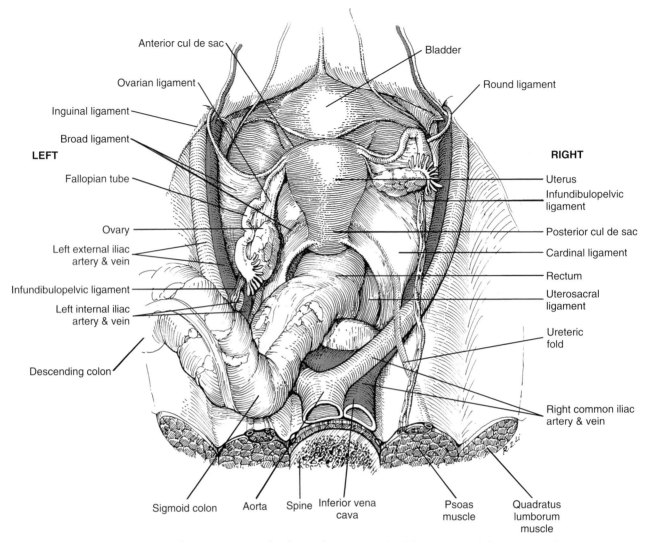

FIGURE 21-9 **Pelvic Ligaments and Pelvic Colon.** The cardinal ligaments and the uterosacral ligaments provide rigid support for the uterine cervix. The round ligaments extend from the cornua to the anterior wall of the pelvis. These ligaments pass through the inguinal canal and are secured to the external genitalia. The round ligaments maintain the anterior bend of the normal anteverted uterus. The rectosigmoid colon lies within the true pelvis and is continuous with the descending colon in the left lower quadrant of the abdominopelvic cavity.

ovaries, within the true pelvis. The tubes course within the peritoneal folds of the broad ligaments. They are lateral to the uterus, anteromedial to the ovaries, and posterior to the urinary bladder (see Figures 21-8 and 21-9).

- **Ovaries location.** The ovaries typically lie posterolateral to the uterus within the adnexa (see Figure 21-8). Ovaries are quite mobile and influenced by the condition of surrounding structures. Even though their position is variable, the ovaries never move anterior to the uterus or broad ligaments (see pelvic ligament anatomy).

During a first pregnancy, it is common for the ovaries to become displaced and never return

to their original position. The ovaries in nulliparous (no viable births) women lie in a craniocaudal long axis direction on the iliopsoas muscles of the lateral pelvic walls between the external iliac vessels anteriorly and the internal iliac vessels and ureters posteriorly.

- **Urinary bladder location.** The urinary bladder is fixed inferiorly at its base in the true pelvis, posterior to the pubic symphysis and anterior to the uterus and vagina. It is anchored to the pelvis by pubovesical and lateral ligaments.

Location of the superior portion is variable depending on the amount of urine in the bladder. As the bladder fills with urine, the dome can extend into

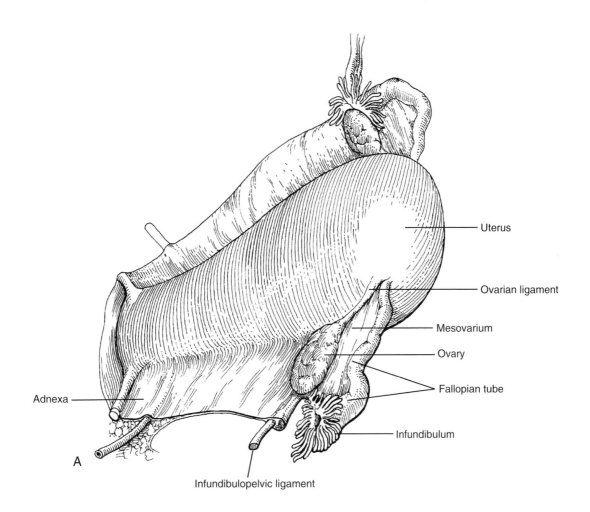

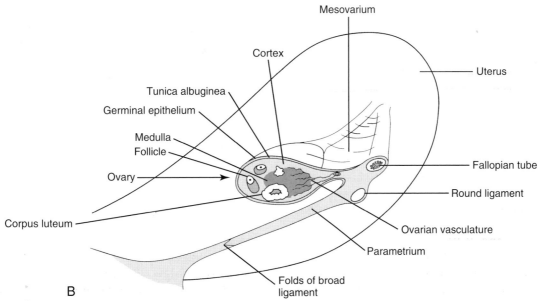

FIGURE 21-10 **The Ovaries and Associated Ligaments. A,** Each ovary is located on the posterior surface of each broad ligament and is anchored in this position by the ovarian and infundibulopelvic ligaments and the mesovarium. The ovaries are the only organs located within the peritoneal cavity that are not covered by peritoneum. **B,** The innermost ovarian tissue is the medulla, composed of ovarian vessels, nerves, and connective tissue. Follicular development takes place in the cortex of the ovary, which surrounds the medulla. The cortex is enclosed by a fibrous capsule called the tunica albuginea. The germinal epithelium is the outermost cellular layer.

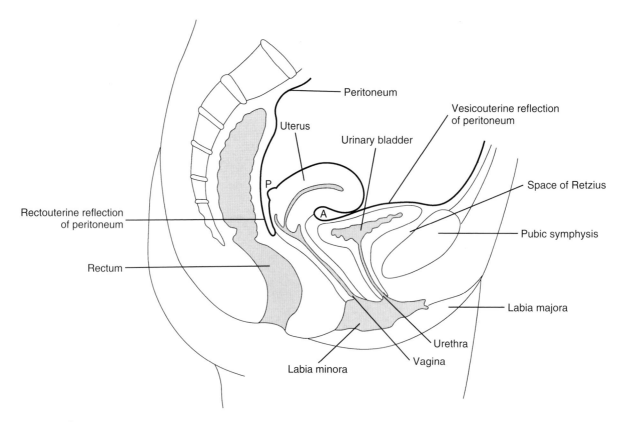

(P) Posterior cul de sac

(A) Anterior cul de sac

FIGURE 21-11   Female Pelvis, Sagittal Plane Cross-Section. The peritoneal lining of the abdominopelvic cavity is seen covering the superior aspect of the urinary bladder, the uterus, and the anterior region of the rectum. The anterior and posterior cul-de-sacs are potential peritoneal spaces created by folds in the peritoneum.

the false pelvis, displacing movable pelvic organs and loops of small bowel. Only the dome is covered by an extension of peritoneum (see Figure 21-9).
- **Pelvic colon location**. *Sigmoid colon, rectum*
  - **Sigmoid colon.** The sigmoid colon lies within the true pelvis and is somewhat variable in length and position. It is continuous with the descending colon in the left lower quadrant of the abdominopelvic cavity and is loosely secured to the posterior pelvic wall by the mesocolon (see Figure 21-9). The sigmoid colon descends toward the rectum in the inferoposterior aspect of the pelvis at the level of the third sacral vertebra.
  - **Rectum.** The rectum is situated posterior to the vagina (see Figure 21-11). It is fixed in its position and is largely retroperitoneal.

SIZE
The size of pertinent female pelvic structures is included with the gross anatomy of female pelvic structures and

can also be found in the Normal Measurements box shown earlier in this chapter.

GROSS ANATOMY
Pelvic Organs
- **Pelvic organs anatomy**. *Genital tract (vagina, uterus, uterine tubes), ovaries, urinary bladder*
  - **Genital tract anatomy.** *Vagina, uterus, uterine tubes*
    The genital tract (vagina, uterus, and uterine tubes) and ovaries make up the primary reproductive organs of the female. The vagina, uterus, and uterine tubes all have the same basic structure: cavities or canals enclosed by an inner mucosal lining, a smooth muscle wall, and an outer layer of connective tissue. Together, these communicating cavities are known as the genital tract. Variations in the mucosa and muscular walls of the genital tract are dictated by the location and function of each segment:

■ ■ ■   **Table 21-1**   Location of Female Pelvis Structures Routinely Visualized With Ultrasound

	Vagina	Uterus	Rt and Lt Uterine Tubes	Rt and Lt Ovaries
Anterior to	Rectum	Posterior cul-de-sac (primarily the cervix), rectum, sigmoid colon, piriformis muscles	Rt and lt ovaries	Rt and lt ovarian fossa, rt and lt ureter, rt and lt internal iliac vessels
Posterior to	Urinary bladder, urethra, parametrium, peritoneum, terminal portions, right and left ureters	Anterior cul-de-sac, rectus abdominis muscle, symphysis pubis, space of Retzius, urinary bladder, peritoneum, some small intestine (fundus)	Urinary bladder	Rt and lt uterine tubes, uterus, rt and lt external iliac vessels, rt and lt broad ligaments
Superior to		Vagina		
Inferior to	Cervix			
Medial to	Rt and lt levator ani muscles	Uterine tubes, rt and lt ovaries, rt and lt broad ligaments, rt and lt obturator internus muscles, rt and lt iliopsoas muscles, external iliac vessels	Rt and lt ovaries, rt and lt iliopsoas muscles	
Lt lateral to			Uterine fundus (left ovary)	
Rt lateral to			Uterine fundus (right ovary)	

(i) **Vaginal anatomy.** The vagina extends from the external genitalia to the uterine cervix. The vaginal canal is approximately 9 cm in length and receives the penis during coitus. The canal also forms the distal portion of the birth canal. The uterine cervix protrudes through the anterior vaginal wall into the upper portion of the vaginal canal. The space within the vaginal canal encircling the cervix forms the anterior, posterior, and lateral fornices of the vagina (Figures 21-14 and 21-15).

The walls of the vagina conform to the general structure of the genital tract. They are composed of a mucosal lining of epithelial cells, a thin smooth muscle wall, and an outer adventitia. The vagina is highly elastic, permitting gross distention during parturition. In the relaxed state the vaginal walls collapse together, and the epithelial lining folds into transverse ridges, or rugae (see Figure 21-15).

(ii) **Uterine anatomy.** As previously mentioned, the uterus lies in the true pelvis between the bladder and the rectum. Uterine walls are composed of 3 tissue layers: endometrium, myometrium, and serosa (see Figure 21-15).

The innermost layer of the uterine wall, the endometrium, is a mucosal layer that is continuous with vaginal epithelium inferiorly and uterine tube mucosa superolaterally. It forms the walls of the endometrial canal, the proximal portion of the birth canal. The endometrium consists of 2 layers: superficial (functional) and deep (basal). The superficial layer is referred to as the functional layer or functional zone because it increases in size during the menstrual cycle and partially sloughs off at the time of menses. The deep, or basal, layer of the endometrium is composed of dense cellular stroma and mucosal glands; it is not significantly influenced by the menstrual cycle.

The myometrium, or muscle layer, forms the bulk of the uterus. It is composed of 3 distinct layers of different muscle fibers: outer longitudinal fibers, intermediate spiral bands, and inner circular and longitudinal fibers. This combination of fibers is responsible for the myometrium dramatically enlarging during pregnancy and producing the radial muscle contractions necessary to expel the fetus at parturition (the act of giving birth).

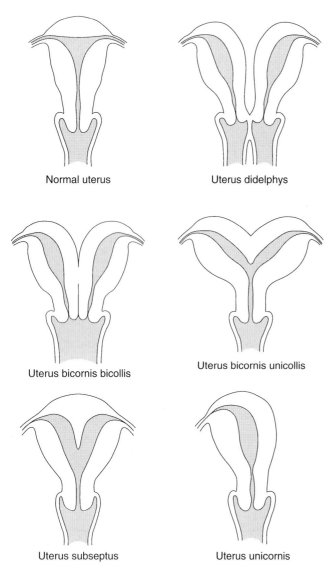

Normal uterus

Uterus didelphys

Uterus bicornis bicollis

Uterus bicornis unicollis

Uterus subseptus

Uterus unicornis

FIGURE 21-12 Congenital Uterine Malformations. This figure illustrates different congenital uterine malformations with anatomic variations of the uterus, cervix, and vagina resulting from the incomplete fusion or agenesis of the müllerian ducts. Complete duplication of the vagina, cervix, and uterine horns is seen in *uterus didelphys*. The *bicornuate uterus* has 2 uterine horns that are fused at 1 cervix (uterus bicornis unicollis) or at 2 cervices (uterus bicornis bicollis). *Uterus subseptus* is a milder anomaly marked by a midline myometrial septum within the endometrial canal. In some cases, only 1 müllerian duct develops, forming a single uterine horn and a uterine tube continuous with 1 cervix and vagina (*uterus unicornis*).

The **serosa** is the thin membrane that covers the myometrium and forms the outer layer of the uterus. The uterus is descriptively divided into 4 parts: fundus, corpus, isthmus, and cervix (see Figures 21-14 and 21-15):

The **fundus** is the widest and most superior segment of the uterus situated between the

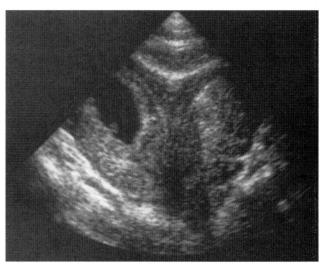

FIGURE 21-13 Bicornuate Uterus. This transabdominal, transverse scanning plane image of the pelvis demonstrates a bicornuate uterus containing a gestational sac within the right endometrial cavity. The gestational sac appears anechoic and is surrounded by the bright decidual reaction of the endometrial lining. Notice how the homogeneous, midgray myometrial tissue separates the endometrial canals of the right and left uterine horns.

insertion of the uterine tubes at the level of the uterine cornua. It is continuous with the body and largest part of the uterus, called the corpus.

The **corpus** is continuous with the uterine cervix at a point marked by a constriction of the uterus called the **isthmus**. During late pregnancy the isthmus is taken up into the corpus to form the lower uterine segment.

The **cervix** is the lower cylindrical portion of the uterus that projects into the vagina. The **endocervical canal** extends 2 to 4 cm (1.6 in) from its **internal os** (or opening), at approximately the same level as the isthmus, where it joins the endometrial canal (uterine canal) to its **external os**, which projects into the vaginal vault. The endometrial, endocervical, and endovaginal canals form a continuous channel through which the fetus passes at birth.

Although the cervix is part of the uterus, the walls of the cervix are structurally unique compared with the rest of the uterus. The smooth muscle fibers are interlaced with collagen fibers, creating a more rigid framework.

Furthermore, a histologic difference has been noted between the endometrial and endocervical mucosa in the internal os. The mucosal lining of the vaginal portion of the

hCG : 36000 T/A

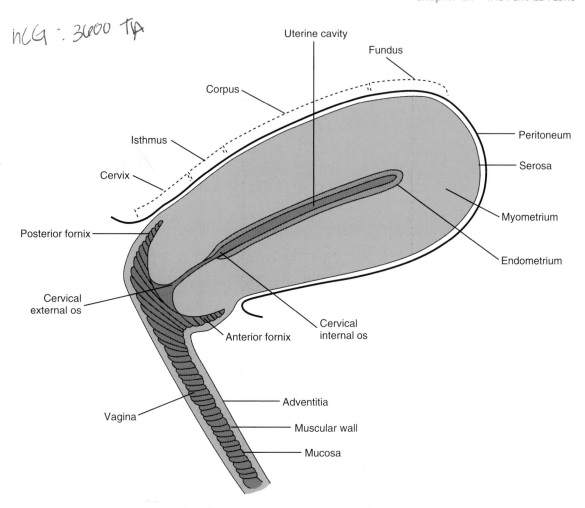

FIGURE 21-14 **Vaginal and Uterine Anatomy.** The wall of the vagina comprises an inner mucosa, a middle smooth muscle layer, and an outer adventitia. The anterior and posterior fornices of the vagina are seen as spaces between the vaginal walls and the portion of the cervix protruding into the vaginal canal. The uterine wall comprises an inner mucosa, called the endometrium; a thick, smooth muscle wall, called the myometrium; and an outer serosa. The regions of the uterus include the cervix, isthmus, corpus, and fundus. Note the narrow anteroposterior dimension of the uterine cavity.

cervix is identical to the epithelial lining of the vagina.

In a female child the uterus is approximately 2.5 cm long, 2 cm wide, and 1 cm thick. The mean dimension of the adult **nulliparous** (no births) uterus is approximately 7 cm long and 4 cm wide. **Multiparous** (multiple viable births) uterine mean dimensions are generally 8.5 cm long and 5.5 cm wide. After menopause, uterine size reduces significantly and the uterus assumes a prepubertal shape. Examples of sonographic measurements of the uterus are shown in Figure 21-16 on p. 355.

Age and **parity** (number of viable offspring) are obviously 2 important factors influencing uterine size and shape. The corpus and fundus of the uterus show considerably more variation in size than the more rigid cervix. Before puberty, the cervix accounts for a significantly greater proportion of the organ than it does during adulthood. During puberty the dimensions of the uterus and endometrial thickness markedly increase. The corpus and fundus portions of the uterus enlarge, changing the uterus from tubular to pear shaped. After **menarche** (menstrual function), the uterus continues to grow for several years. Uterine size is directly related to the number of years post menarche.

As previously mentioned, the uterus normally tilts forward, resting on the dome of

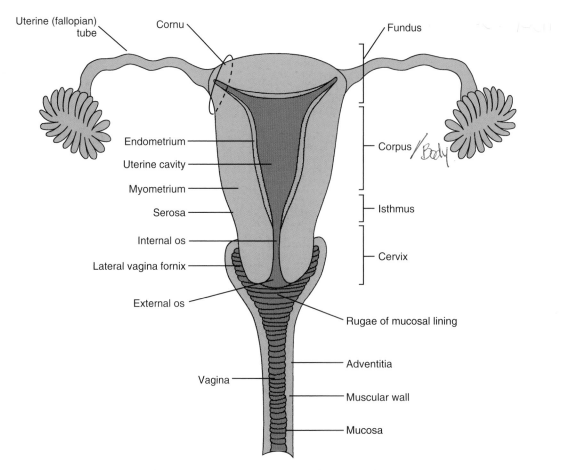

FIGURE 21-15   **Genital Tract.** In this coronal diagram of the genital tract, notice the 3 tissue layers that make up the uterine wall: endometrium, myometrium, and serosa. Note the uterine (fallopian) tubes adjoining the uterus at the cornua. The lateral fornices of the vagina are also evident.

the bladder. The ligaments and peritoneal connections of this organ allow considerable mobility within the true pelvis. This mobility affords subtle displacements of the uterus with filling of the urinary bladder or the rectum, as well as marked displacement of this organ during pregnancy.

The support structures of the uterus give it considerable flexibility. This flexibility affords variations in normal uterine position *(anteversion, anteflexion, retroversion, retroflexion)* (Figure 21-17 on p. 356). When the bladder is empty, the uterus is in an **anteverted** position, in which the cervix and vagina form a 90-degree angle, and the body and fundus are tipped or tilted anteriorly. If the body and fundus are bent at a greater anterior angle until the fundus is pointing inferiorly and resting on the cervix, the uterine position is described as **anteflexed**. Inversely, the uterus can also be retroverted and retroflexed. In a **retroverted** position, the

body and fundus are tipped posteriorly and the angle of the cervix and vagina increases, making them more linearly oriented. If the body and fundus are bent at a greater posterior angle until the fundus is pointing inferiorly adjacent to the cervix, the uterine position is described as **retroflexed**.

(iii) **Uterine tubes** anatomy. The uterine tubes ("fallopian tubes," "oviducts") are coiled, muscular, bilateral tubes emerging from the cone-shaped cornua of the uterus, which are located at the junction of the superior and lateral uterine margins.

The uterine tubes vary in length from 7 to 12 cm as they course within the peritoneum along the superior free margin of the broad ligaments, until they reach the ovaries.

These tubes conduct mature ovum (egg cell) from the ovaries to the uterus through gentle peristalsis of their smooth muscle walls (Figure 21-18, *B*). The mucosal lining of

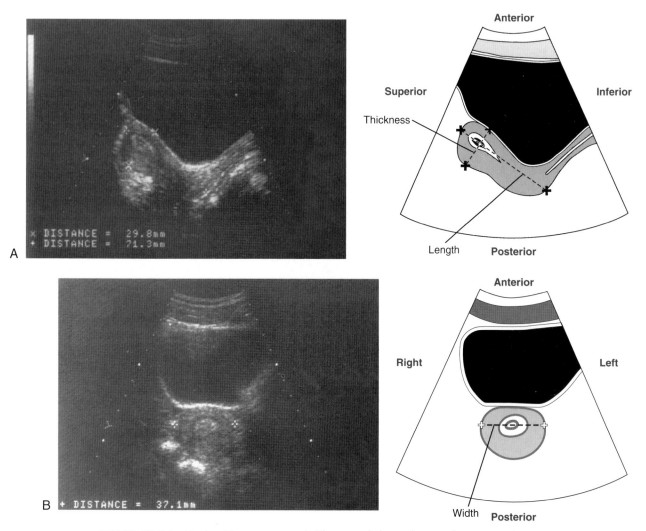

FIGURE 21-16 **Uterine Measurements. A,** This transabdominal, sagittal scanning plane image shows the correct caliper placement for measuring the long axis and greatest anteroposterior measurements of the uterus. The length of the uterus is measured from the fundus to the inferior cervical region. The anteroposterior thickness is measured perpendicular to the length at the widest point of the uterine corpus. **B,** This transabdominal, transverse scanning plane image demonstrates the correct caliper placement for measuring the width of the uterus, which is taken at the widest point of the uterine corpus (or body) in a short axis section.

the tubes consists of ciliated epithelial cells and secretory cells. The cilia propel a gentle current of secreted fluid, which aids in the transport of the ovum.

Uterine tubes are descriptively divided into 4 segments: *interstitial* or *intramural*, *isthmus*, *ampulla*, and *infundibulum* (Figure 21-18, *A*). The interstitial, or intramural, segment of the uterine tube is the narrowest portion and is enclosed within the muscular wall of the uterus. The isthmus is immediately adjacent to the uterine wall, connected to the interstitial segment. It is a short, straight, narrow portion of the tube. The tube widens laterally, forming the ampullary and infundibular sections.

The longest and most coiled portion of the uterine tube is the ampulla. Fertilization most often occurs in the ampulla. The mucosal lining of the ampulla folds into complex matrices, filling much of the tubular lumen.

The infundibulum is the funnel-shaped end portion of the uterine tube. The tube terminates at the fimbriated end of the infundibulum and opens into the peritoneal cavity adjacent to the ovary. The peritoneal ostium of the uterine tube is approximately 3 mm in diameter.

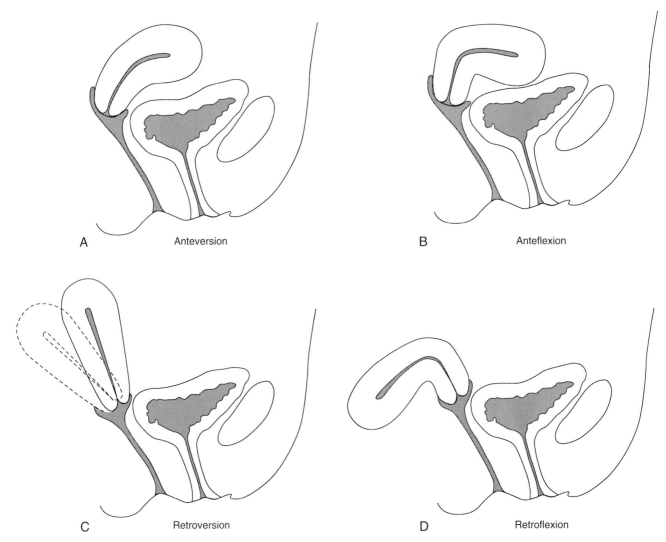

FIGURE 21-17 **Uterine Position Variations. A,** Anteversion. **B,** Anteflexion. **C,** Retroversion. **D,** Retroversion with retroflexion.

Specifically, the infundibulum passes through the posterior aspect of the broad ligament to reach the ovary. The uterine tube and the ovary are not intimately connected; thus the genital tract creates a channel between the outside and the peritoneal cavity. The fimbriae of the uterine tube are fringe-like extensions of the infundibulum, which overlie the ovary and direct the released ovum into the tube.

○ **Ovarian Anatomy.** The ovaries are paired, almond-shaped organs lying on the posterior surface of the broad ligaments. They are the only organs within the abdominopelvic cavity not lined by visceral peritoneum. The germinal epithelium is a single layer of epithelial cells lining the outer surface of the ovary. (This name arose from the mistaken belief that the germ cells originated from this tissue layer.)

The tunica albuginea is a fibrous connective tissue capsule found beneath the epithelial layer. The ovarian stroma, or the body of the ovary, consists of the peripheral cortex and the central medulla. The cortex constitutes the bulk of ovarian tissue and is the site of oogenesis, the production of female gametes (egg cells). The medulla contains the ovarian vasculature, lymphatics, and nerves supported by fibrous connective tissue. This highly vascular core communicates with the parametrium of the broad ligament at the ovarian hilum. The hilum is located along the superoanterior aspect of the ovary.

As previously mentioned, the infundibulopelvic and ovarian ligaments support and maintain

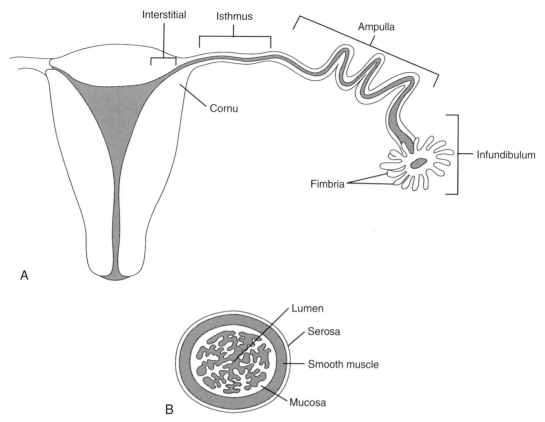

FIGURE 21-18 **Uterine (Fallopian) Tubes Anatomy.** The uterine (fallopian) tubes or oviducts are continuous with the endometrial cavity at the uterine cornua. The 4 regions of the oviduct include the interstitial segment, isthmus, ampulla, and infundibulum. **A,** The regions of the uterine tube. **B,** Cross-section through the ampulla of the tube. This section demonstrates the intricate folds of the mucosal lining. The wall of the oviduct comprises the inner mucosa, middle muscular, and outer serosal layers.

the relative position of the ovaries in their adnexal location. In most cases the ovaries are situated posterolateral to the broad ligaments; however, they are quite mobile and may be located anywhere within the adnexa, except anterior to the uterus or anterior to the broad ligaments (see Figures 21-8 and 21-9).

Ovarian size varies during the life span depending on age, menstrual status, pregnancy status, body habitus, and menstrual cycle phase. At birth, the ovaries are relatively large as a result of maternal hormone stimulus. There is little change in ovarian size until age 5 or 6, after which age-related growth is seen, associated with an increase in cystic functional changes. Normal measurements during reproductive years range from 2.5 to 5 cm in length, 0.6 to 2.2 cm in anteroposterior (AP) thickness (or height), and 1.5 to 3 cm in width.

Ovarian volume may also be used as a measure of normal size and is calculated as follows:

Volume = length × height (AP thickness) × width × 0.523

In women between 15 and 55 years of age, normal ovarian volume is 6.8 mL. Ovarian volume parameters can be influenced by the presence of a large follicle(s) or pathology. Ovarian volume is only marginally affected by cyclic changes. The lowest volumes can be observed during the luteal phase and highest volumes during the preovulatory phase.

○ **Urinary Bladder Anatomy.** The urinary bladder is a muscular sac that receives and stores urine produced by the kidneys. It consists of 4 layers of tissue: an *inner mucosa*, a *submucosa layer*, the *muscularis*, and the outer *serosa*. The *mucosa* folds when the bladder is empty, and it distends and becomes

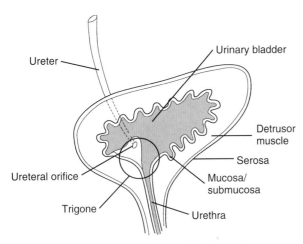

Ureter

Urinary bladder

Detrusor muscle

Serosa

Ureteral orifice

Mucosa/ submucosa

Trigone

Urethra

FIGURE 21-19 **Urinary Bladder.** The bladder wall is composed of an innermost mucosa; followed by a submucosal layer; a thick, middle muscular layer; and an outer serosal lining. The trigone is the region of the urinary bladder at which the ureters enter and the urethra exits this cavity.

smooth when the bladder is full. The *muscularis* layer is composed of 3 layers of smooth muscle, called the detrusor muscle. The outermost layer, the *serosa*, is located at the superior portion of the bladder. It is an extension of pelvic peritoneum (Figure 21-19).

The inferior portion of the urinary bladder is composed of a posterior base (or trigone area) and the neck, which communicate with the ureters and urethra. The external urethral orifice is located between the labia minora of the external genitalia. The inferolateral surfaces of the bladder meet anteriorly and are in contact with the pelvic floor muscles.

The superior and posterior walls of the bladder are lined by visceral peritoneum, which is continuous with the peritoneal lining of the abdominopelvic space. As previously discussed, the peritoneum covering the bladder walls and extending over the uterine fundus creates a potential space between the bladder and the uterus, known as the anterior cul-de-sac. The space of Retzius, also discussed earlier, separates the anterior bladder wall from the pubic symphysis and is typically filled with extraperitoneal fat (see Figure 21-11).

The urinary bladder is a hollow, symmetric organ whose size depends on the quantity of contained urine. The wall of a distended bladder normally measures 3 to 6 mm, depending on the degree of bladder distention.

When the bladder is empty, loops of small bowel rest in the anterior region of the abdominopelvic cavity. A distended urinary bladder pushes the small intestine superiorly, out of the true pelvis.

BLOOD SUPPLY

Internal iliac artery, uterine artery, arcuate arteries, radial arteries, straight arteries, spiral arteries, ovarian artery, gluteal arteries, vaginal artery, azygos arteries, vascular arch, lymph nodes

- **Uterine blood supply.** *Internal iliac artery, uterine artery, arcuate arteries, radial arteries, straight arteries, spiral arteries*
  - **Internal iliac artery.** Continuation of the common iliac artery. Multiple branches that include the uterine artery.
  - **Uterine artery.** Branch of the internal iliac artery that supplies blood to the reproductive organs of the pelvis (Figure 21-20, A). At the level of the cervix the uterine artery gives rise to the vaginal artery, which courses inferiorly. The uterine artery continues superiorly toward its termination at the fundus of the uterus, giving off small branches of itself and the ovarian and uterine tube arterial branches along the way.
  - **Arcuate arteries.** Small uterine artery branches give rise to the arcuate arteries. These arteries loop around and encircle the periphery of the uterus and branch into the radial arteries (Figure 21-20, B).
  - **Radial arteries.** Radial arteries penetrate the uterine myometrium and give rise to the straight arteries (see Figure 21-20, B).
  - **Straight arteries.** The straight arteries supply the uterine endometrium, except for its first layer of tissue, which receives its blood supply from small branches of the straight arteries, called spiral arteries (see Figure 21-20, B).
  - **Spiral arteries.** Spiral arteries perfuse the proliferating uterine endometrium (see Figure 21-20, B). Blood flow in the spiral arteries is responsive to hormonal changes of the menstrual cycle.
- **Vaginal blood supply.** *Internal iliac artery, uterine artery, vaginal artery, azygos arteries*
  - **Internal iliac artery.** Continuation of the common iliac artery. Multiple branches that include the uterine artery.
  - **Uterine artery.** Branch of the internal iliac artery that supplies blood to the reproductive organs of the pelvis. At the level of the cervix the uterine artery gives rise to the vaginal artery, which courses inferiorly (see Figure 21-20, A).
  - **Vaginal artery.** The vaginal artery branches inferiorly from the uterine artery to supply blood to the vagina as well as the fundus of the bladder. Branches of the uterine artery that supply blood

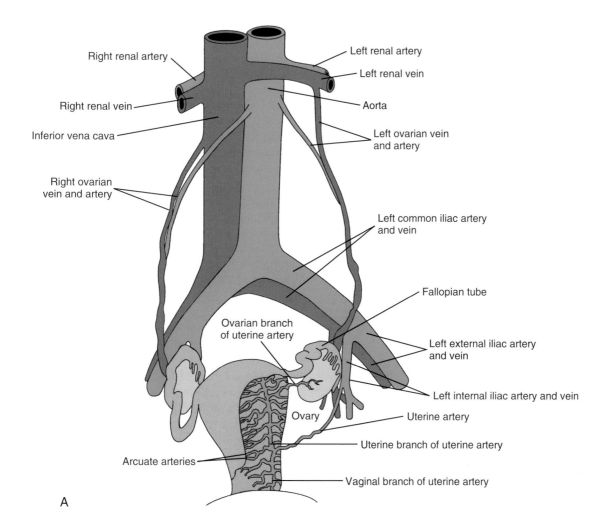

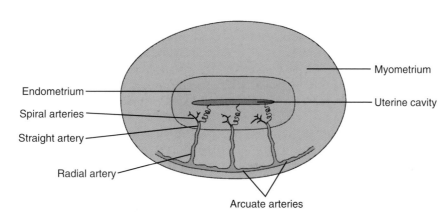

FIGURE 21-20 **Genital Tract and Ovarian Vasculature. A,** The uterine artery is a branch of the internal iliac artery. The uterus, vagina, and ovaries receive blood from branches of this artery, such as the vaginal artery branch, which supplies the vagina and fundus of the urinary bladder. The ovaries also receive blood from the ovarian arteries arising from the abdominal aorta. **B,** The arcuate arteries encircle the outer tissue of the uterus. The myometrium is penetrated by the radial arteries. The endometrium receives blood from the straight and spiral arteries. The spiral arteries become more dilated during the secretory phase of the menstrual cycle. During menses, the spiral arteries are shed along with much of the endometrial lining.

to the cervical portion of the uterus anastomose (join with) branches of the vaginal artery to form the anterior and posterior azygos arteries of the vagina.

- **Azygos arteries.** Formed by anastomosed uterine and vaginal arteries to supply blood to the anterior and posterior portions of the vagina.
- **Uterine tubes blood supply.** *Vascular arch*
  - **Vascular arch.** Formed by anastomosed uterine and ovarian arteries to pass through the mesosalpinx of the broad ligament, to meet the uterine tubes.
- **Ovarian blood supply.** *Uterine artery, ovarian arteries*
  - **Uterine artery.** Branch of the internal iliac artery that supplies blood to the reproductive organs of the pelvis. The uterine artery is 1 of 2 separate vascular pathways that maintain the blood supply to each ovary. At the level of the uterine cornu the ovarian branches of the uterine artery travel laterally within the broad ligament to reach the ovarian hilum.
  - **Ovarian artery.** Right and left ovarian arteries branch off the abdominal aorta at a level inferior to the renal artery branches. Each ovarian artery courses anterior to the psoas and iliopsoas muscles within the retroperitoneum. They travel medially along the infundibulopelvic ligaments to reach the ovarian hilum (see Figure 21-20, *A*).
- **Urinary bladder blood supply.** *Vesicular arteries, vaginal artery*
  - **Vesicular arteries.** Blood is supplied to the urinary bladder by the superior and inferior vesicular arteries, tributaries of the internal iliac arteries.
  - **Vaginal artery.** The vaginal artery branches inferiorly from the uterine artery to supply blood to the vagina as well as the fundus of the bladder.
- **Pelvic lymph nodes blood supply.** *External iliac artery, internal iliac artery, common iliac artery*
  - **External iliac artery.** Supplies blood to the external iliac lymph nodes.
  - **Internal iliac artery.** Supplies blood to the internal iliac lymph nodes.
  - **Common iliac artery.** Supplies blood to the common iliac lymph nodes.

PHYSIOLOGY

Between puberty and menopause, the female reproductive system normally undergoes monthly cyclical changes referred to as the menstrual cycle. The menstrual cycle usually follows a 28-day course, during which a single ovum (egg cell) reaches maturity and is released into the genital tract. Hormones secreted by the anterior pituitary gland and the ovaries control changes in the ovaries and the uterine endometrium throughout this cycle.

The Ovarian Cycle

At menarche the ovaries contain thousands of primordial **follicles**, each composed of a single primary oocyte (immature egg cell or ovum) and surrounding follicular cells that form an encasement. During the follicular phase of the ovarian cycle (days 1 to 14 of the menstrual cycle), 10 to 20 primordial follicles begin to mature. Follicle-stimulating hormone (FSH) is a gonadotropin produced by the anterior pituitary gland, which initiates follicular development. This initial maturation process results in the development of several primary follicles.

A primary follicle contains a primary oocyte surrounded by a membranous protein layer, called the zona pellucida. Proliferating follicular cells, collectively called the zona granulosa, encircle this layer. Outer connective tissue layers of a primary follicle include the theca interna and the theca externa (Figure 21-21).

As a primary follicle grows, the oocyte reaches a mature size. The follicular antrum is a fluid-filled cavity that forms between the cellular layers of the zona granulosa. The developing oocyte rests along the wall of the follicular antrum and is surrounded by the cumulus oophorus, a layer of follicular cells continuous with the zona granulosa. At this stage of development the oocyte and its surrounding structures are called secondary follicles. The theca interna cells of multiple secondary follicles fulfill an endocrine function as they differentiate into estrogen-secreting cells. The hormone **estrogen** promotes proliferation or preparation of the uterine endometrium for possible implantation by a zygote.

Although many follicles develop in the ovaries in response to FSH, only one follicle matures completely and ruptures to release an ovum (egg cell) at **ovulation** (see Figure 21-21). Most of the follicles undergo follicular atresia beyond the stage of the secondary follicle. One secondary follicle continues to mature to become a graafian or dominant follicle before ovulation (see Figure 21-21). The ovum continues to mature through meiotic division, forming the secondary oocyte. Now the oocyte floats freely within the enlarged follicular antrum of the graafian follicle. The follicular cells of the cumulus oophorus now completely surround the zona pellucida and the secondary oocyte, and are called the corona radiata.

The theca interna cells of the graafian follicle continue to produce estrogen. The graafian follicle migrates to the surface of the ovary, while the remaining secondary follicles undergo atresia. At approximately day 14 of the ovarian cycle, ovulation occurs when the mature ovum is expelled into the genital tract. The fimbria of the uterine tube draws the released egg into the infundibulum.

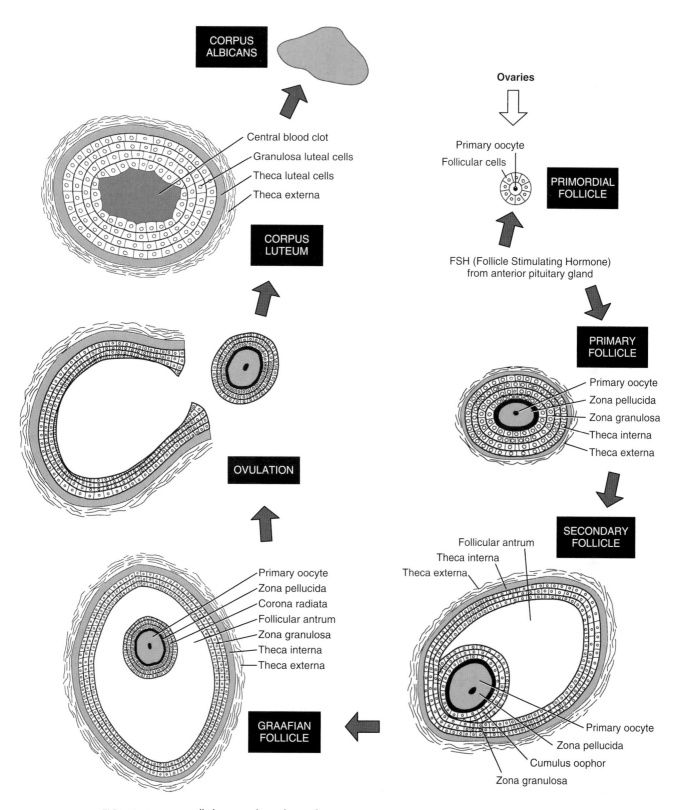

FIGURE 21-21 **Follicle Growth and Development.** Maturation of a follicle during the normal menstrual cycle.

At ovulation, 5 to 10 mL of follicular fluid are released into the peritoneal cavity, settling into the posterior cul-de-sac, a space between the uterus and rectum. The ruptured follicle collapses, fills with blood, and is transformed into a temporary endocrine gland. This begins the luteal phase of the ovarian cycle (days 15 to 28). The remaining follicular structure is now called the corpus luteum and contains a central blood clot surrounded by granulosa luteal cells, theca luteal cells, and the theca externa.

The granulosa luteal cells enlarge and secrete progesterone, which promotes glandular secretions of the endometrium. The theca luteal cells continue the estrogen secretion of their precursors (theca interna), maintaining the proliferated endometrial lining of the uterus. The outer theca externa cells support the rich vascular network characteristic of an endocrine gland.

Luteinizing hormone (LH) is produced throughout the ovarian cycle by the anterior pituitary gland. This hormone promotes secretion of estrogen and progesterone by the ovary. Both estrogen and LH peak immediately before ovulation. Although the corpus luteum depends on LH, progesterone negatively inhibits the production of LH. Consequently, the corpus luteum eventually regresses because of LH stimulation, and only a fibrous tissue mass, called the corpus albicans, remains in the ovary (see Figure 21-21). When the levels of estrogen and progesterone diminish, the thickened endometrial lining of the uterus is shed through menstruation (Figure 21-22).

Pregnancy interrupts the normal menstrual cycle. The developing placenta secretes human chorionic gonadotropin (hCG) after implantation of the fertilized ovum. This hormone has an analogous function to LH, maintaining the corpus luteum. Thus, during pregnancy the corpus luteum continues to secrete estrogen and progesterone throughout the first trimester. The placenta ultimately takes over this endocrine function and the corpus luteum regresses, forming the corpus albicans.

The Endometrial Cycle
The days of the endometrial or menstrual cycle are numbered according to changes in the endometrial lining of the uterus. Days 1 through 5 generally correspond to menses, when the thickened superficial layer of the endometrium is shed in the form of blood through the vagina (see Figure 21-22).

Proliferation is the next phase of the endometrial cycle, occurring between menses and ovulation (see Figure 21-22). The endometrium thickens under the influence of estrogen, preparing the uterine cavity to receive the fertilized egg.

Ovulation usually occurs near day 14 of the menstrual cycle, marking the beginning of the secretory phase (see Figure 21-22). The continued production of

estrogen and now progesterone by the corpus luteum promotes continued thickening and swelling of the endometrium. Exocrine glands of the endometrial lining secrete a glycogen-rich mucus, preparing a suitable environment for implantation.

In the absence of fertilization, the production of LH, estrogen, and progesterone diminishes, and a new cycle begins on day 1 with menses. The timing of menses and proliferation in the endometrial cycle correspond to the follicular phase of the ovarian cycle (days 1 to 14). The secretory phase of the endometrial cycle corresponds to the luteal phase of the ovarian cycle (days 15 to 28).

SONOGRAPHIC APPEARANCE
Pelvic: skeleton, musculature, ligaments, spaces, organs, colon, vasculature
Standard ultrasound examination of the female pelvis is composed of transabdominal (TA) sonography combined with endovaginal or transvaginal (TV) sonography (Figures 21-23 to 21-27). In some cases, standard TA and TV studies may be supplemented by either TA or TV color-flow Doppler or hysterosonography (HS).

TA sonography is performed from the anterior skin surface of the abdominopelvic cavity. When imaging the female pelvis, the urine-filled bladder serves as a "sonic window" because the urine does not obstruct passage of the sound waves. This provides a large field of view, especially when compared with TV imaging. TV sonography provides better anatomic detail than TA imaging because the high-frequency transducer is placed inside the vagina and thus closer to pelvic anatomy. Ideally, TA sonography may show the size and location of a mass, which can then be better characterized with TV sonography.

TA or TV color-flow Doppler is often used as a supplemental study to better differentiate vascular structures in the pelvis or to distinguish the blood supply to a mass. In some cases, HS is necessary. This involves the slow infusion of sterile saline solution into the uterus to delineate the shape, size, and lining of the uterine cavity.

- **Pelvic skeleton sonographic appearance.** *Sacrum, coccyx, innominate bones (ilium, ischium, pubis)*

   Sonography is not the modality of choice for evaluating osseous or bony structures because sound waves cannot penetrate their density; thus bones cast shadows. On the other hand, the distinctive sonographic appearance of the pelvic skeleton creates useful landmarks. The highly echogenic vertebrae of the lower spine form the posterior boundary of the true pelvis (Figure 21-28 on p. 368). The iliac crests of the innominate bones can be identified as hyperechoic linear structures casting posterior shadows. These crests can be visualized extending from the near field to the far field on a TA image when the

Text continued on p. 369

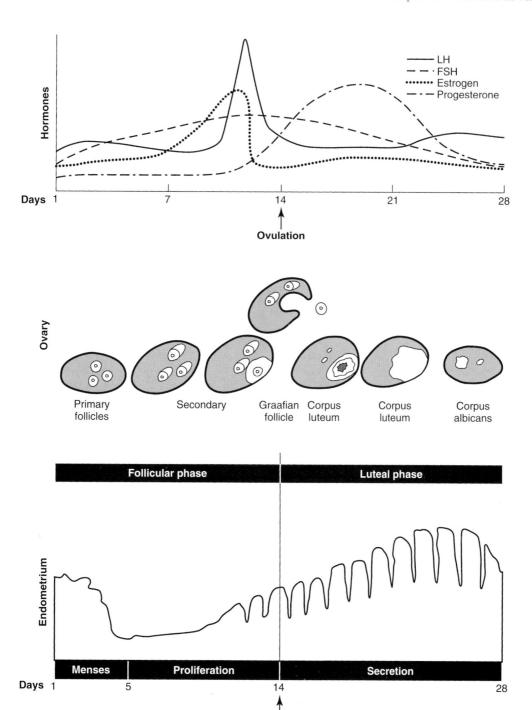

FIGURE 21-22 **Menstrual Cycle.** The first day of bleeding corresponds to the first day of the female menstrual cycle. The thickened endometrial lining of the uterus is shed during menses. At this point the production of follicle-stimulating hormone (FSH) promotes the follicular phase of the ovarian cycle. Developing follicles within the ovaries begin to produce estrogen, which in turn causes proliferation of the endometrial lining. At approximately day 14 of the menstrual cycle, luteinizing hormone (LH) peaks; at this point, ovulation occurs and the graafian follicle releases a mature ovum. The latter half of the menstrual cycle corresponds to the luteal phase of the ovary, during which the corpus luteum produces estrogen and progesterone. These hormones promote the secretory phase of the endometrial cycle, during which the endometrium continues to thicken. Inhibited production of LH at the end of the menstrual cycle leads to a breakdown of the corpus luteum and the shedding of the endometrium with the onset of menses.

Sagittal Scanning Plane/Transabdominal (TA)
Anterior Sound Wave Approach

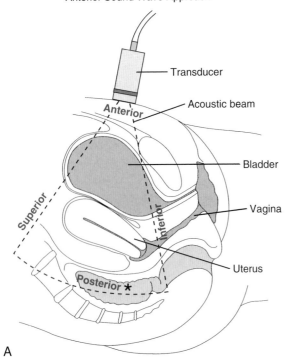

— Transducer

— Acoustic beam

— Bladder

— Vagina

— Uterus

A

IMAGE DISPLAY MONITOR
TA Sagittal Scanning Plane Image Orientation

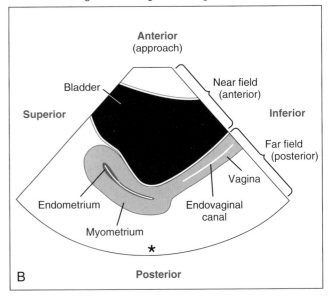

B

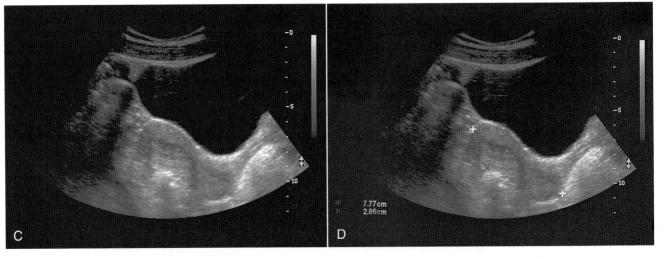

FIGURE 21-23   **Transabdominal (TA), Sagittal Scanning Plane Pelvic Imaging. A,** Illustrates how TA pelvic sonography is performed from an anterior approach using the fully distended urinary bladder as an acoustic window. **B,** Image orientation of the sagittal scanning plane on the image display monitor. The anterior portion of the pelvis is displayed in the near field of the image, and the posterior region of the pelvis is displayed in the far field of the image. In a TA sagittal scanning plane image, the left and right sides of the image correspond to the superior and inferior regions of the pelvis, respectively. **C,** TA sonogram from a midsagittal scanning plane. The fully distended urinary bladder is the large anechoic structure with bright walls in the near field of the image, anterior to the uterus. Notice the smooth contour and medium-gray echo texture of the uterine myometrium and vaginal walls. Note how the uterus is pushed superoposteriorly by the distended bladder and is roughly perpendicular to the ultrasound beam. **D,** Represents the caliper placement for measuring the long axis section of the uterus. *Denotes corresponding location.* (C and D, Images courtesy the University of Virginia Health System, Department of Radiology, Division of Ultrasound, Charlottesville, Virginia.)

Transverse Scanning Plane/Transabdominal (TA)
Anterior Sound Wave Approach

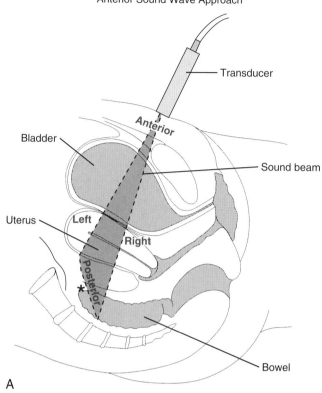

IMAGE DISPLAY MONITOR
TA Transverse Scanning Plane Image Orientation

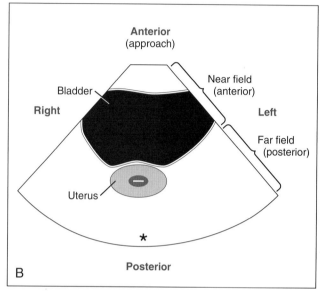

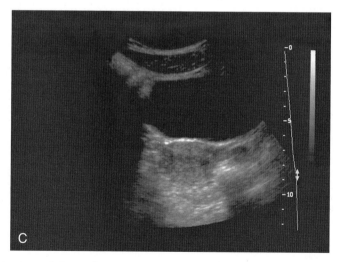

FIGURE 21-24   **Transabdominal (TA), Transverse Scanning Plane Pelvic Imaging. A,** Illustrates the anterior transducer position for TA imaging of the pelvis in the transverse scanning plane. **B,** Image orientation of the transverse scanning plane on the image display monitor. The near and far fields of the image correspond to the anterior and posterior regions of the pelvis, respectively. The left and right sides of the image correspond to the right and left sides of the pelvis, respectively. **C,** TA transverse scanning plane sonogram of a short axis section of the uterus. Note the anechoic urinary bladder in the near field of the image, anterior to the medium-gray uterus. *Denotes corresponding location.

Sagittal Scanning Plane/Transvaginal (TV)
Inferior Sound Wave Approach

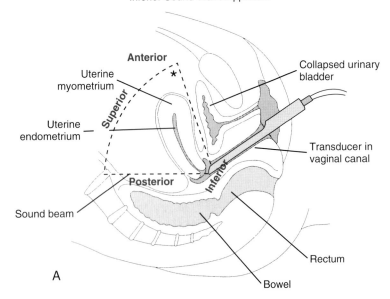

TV Sagittal Scanning Plane Image Orientation

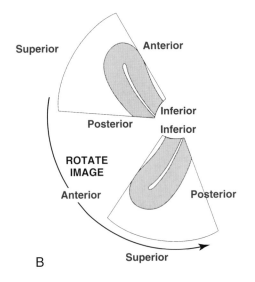

IMAGE DISPLAY MONITOR
TV Sagittal Scanning Plane Orientation

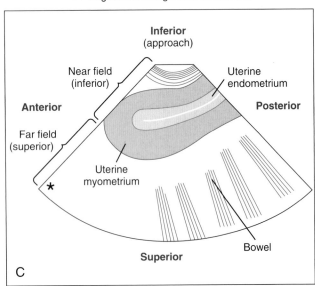

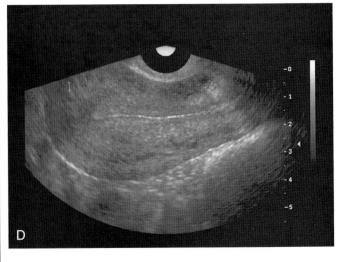

FIGURE 21-25 Transvaginal (TV), Sagittal Scanning Plane Pelvic Imaging. **A,** The transvaginal transducer position for TV imaging of the pelvis; **B** and **C,** The TV sagittal scanning plane image orientation and the rotation of the image on the display monitor. The apex of the TV image corresponds to anatomic structures that are closest to the face of the transducer. In the sagittal scanning plane, the near field of the TV image generally corresponds to the inferior region of the true pelvis. The far field of the TV image generally corresponds to the superior region of the true pelvis. The left and right sides of the display monitor correspond to anterior and posterior regions of the pelvis, respectively. **D,** Longitudinal section of the uterus from a midsagittal scanning plane in TV pelvic imaging. Note the limited field of view (compared with TA imaging) but the increase in anatomic detail. *Denotes corresponding location.

Coronal Scanning Plane/Transvaginal (TV)
Inferior Sound Wave Approach

TV Coronal Scanning Plane
Image Orientation

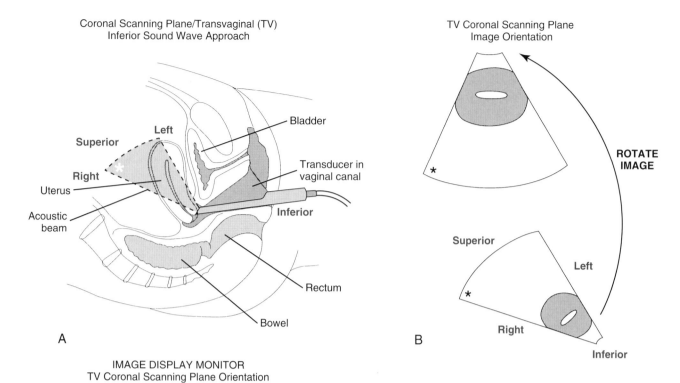

A

B

IMAGE DISPLAY MONITOR
TV Coronal Scanning Plane Orientation

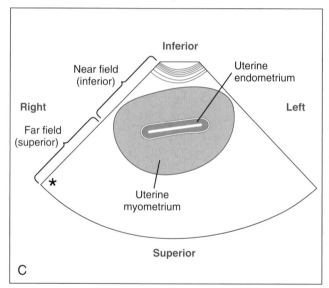

C

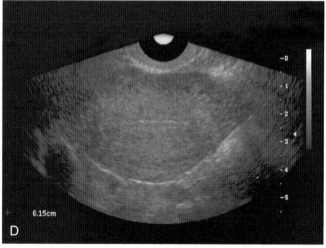

D

FIGURE 21-26 **Transvaginal (TV), Coronal Scanning Plane, Pelvic Imaging. A,** Illustrates the endovaginal transducer position for TV imaging of the pelvis. With an empty urinary bladder, the fundus of the anteverted uterus is tilted forward toward the anterior abdominal wall. Consequently, the TV coronal imaging plane demonstrates a short axis section of the anteverted or anteflexed uterus. **B** and **C,** Illustrate the TV coronal scanning plane image orientation and the rotation of the image on the display monitor. The near and far fields of the TV coronal scanning plane image correspond to inferior and superior regions of the pelvis, respectively. The left and right sides of the display monitor correspond to the right and left sides of the pelvis, respectively. **D,** Short axis section of the uterus from TV coronal scanning plane pelvic imaging. As mentioned previously, note the limited field of view, compared with TA imaging, but the increase in anatomic detail. *Denotes corresponding location.* (**D,** Image courtesy the University of Virginia Health System, Department of Radiology, Division of Ultrasound, Charlottesville, Virginia.)

Sagittal Scanning Plane/Transvaginal
(TV)
Anteroinferior Sound Wave Approach

IMAGE DISPLAY MONITOR
TV Sagittal Scanning Plane Orientation

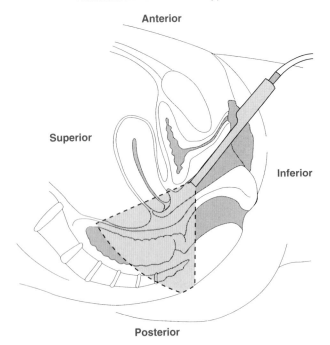

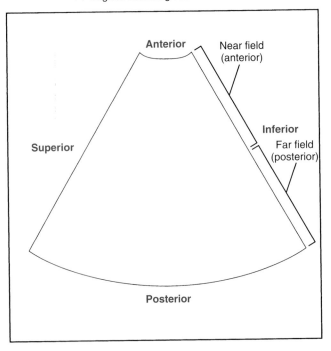

FIGURE 21-27 Transvaginal (TV) Imaging: Anteroinferior Approach. Most TV imaging is performed from a standard inferior approach, as demonstrated in Figures 21-25 and 21-26. However, manipulation of the TV transducer causes variation from the standard TV image orientation previously described. For example, when the transducer handle is lifted anteriorly (toward the pubic symphysis), the sound beam is directed more posteriorly. In this case, the near and far fields of the sagittal image correspond to anterior and posterior regions of the pelvis, respectively, and the left and right sides of the image display monitor more closely correspond to superior and inferior regions of the pelvis. A posteroinferior TV approach would also cause significant variation in image orientation. Thus, image orientation for TV sonography may vary between authors and ultrasound texts.

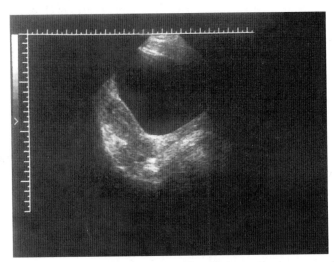

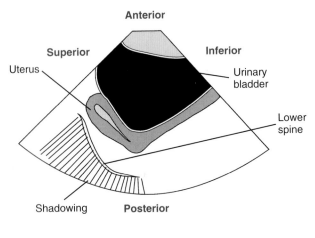

FIGURE 21-28 Pelvic Skeleton. The lower vertebral spine forms the posterior boundary of the true pelvis. The vertebral bodies appear highly echogenic and cast posterior shadows.

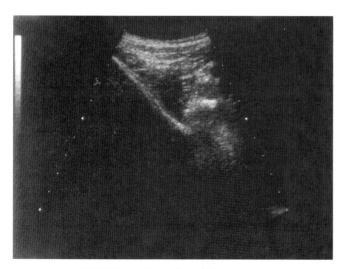 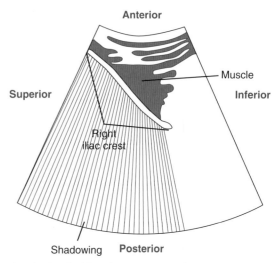

FIGURE 21-29 **Pelvic Skeleton.** The iliac crest is easily identified as highly echogenic, extending superiorly on this longitudinal view. As with the spine, the iliac crest is reflective and casts shadows so that structures behind the crest cannot be visualized in this view.

approach is along the superolateral aspect of the pelvis (Figure 21-29).

- **Pelvic musculature sonographic appearance.** *Iliopsoas, obturator internus, pelvic diaphragm, (pubococcygeus, iliococcygeus, coccygeus), piriformis, rectus abdominis*

  The muscles most commonly visualized in TA pelvic sonography include the iliopsoas muscle bundles, obturator internus muscles, pelvic diaphragm muscles, piriformis muscles, and rectus abdominis muscles. The skeletal muscles of the pelvis exhibit the same characteristic low-gray sonographic muscular pattern seen from other muscles throughout the rest of the body. The pelvic muscles typically appear hypoechoic relative to the pelvic organs. Linear striations in the muscles can be visualized when imaged in a plane longitudinal to the muscle fibers. The skeletal muscles define the external borders of the abdominopelvic cavity.

  ○ **Iliopsoas muscles.** The iliopsoas muscle bundle formed by the psoas major and iliacus muscles exhibits low-gray echoes with a distinct, fairly central, bright focus from the iliopsoas fascia that lies between the psoas major and iliacus muscle. The paired iliopsoas muscles can be identified on each side of the lateral walls of the urinary bladder, in the anterior portion of the pelvis. The anechoic external iliac vessels and homogeneous, low-gray rectus abdominis muscle can be identified anterior to the iliopsoas.

    In short axis the iliopsoas can be identified on each side of the urinary bladder as rounded low-level echoes surrounding the centrally located

echogenic femoral nerve sheath (Figure 21-30). In longitudinal sections the low-gray iliopsoas muscle bundle is ovoid and divided by the femoral nerve sheath, which appears thick, horizontal, and hyperechoic relative to the muscle's appearance (Figure 21-31).

○ **Obturator internus muscles.** The obturator internus muscles appear posterior and medial to the iliopsoas muscles. They present sonographically as thin, bilateral, linear, low-level echoes abutting the lateral walls of the urinary bladder (Figure 21-32). The obturator internus muscles are best seen in TA transverse scanning plane images of the true pelvis.

○ **Pelvic diaphragm muscles.** The muscles of the pelvic diaphragm (*pubococcygeus, iliococcygeus [levator ani muscles], coccygeus*) are easiest to visualize in longitudinal sections in TA, transverse scanning plane images of the most inferior portions of the true pelvis (Figure 21-33, see Figure 21-32). They can be identified as the bilateral, low-gray echoes meeting posterior to the vagina and cervix.

○ **Piriformis muscles.** The bilateral piriformis muscles appear as low-level echoes visualized posterior to the uterus and anterior to the sacrum (Figure 21-34).

○ **Rectus abdominis.** The paired, paramedian rectus abdominis muscles are easiest to identify in transverse scanning plane images of the pelvis. They appear low-gray in the most anterior portion of the abdominopelvic wall. Thin, bright lines representing the rectus sheath delineate the anterior and posterior borders (see Figure 21-32).

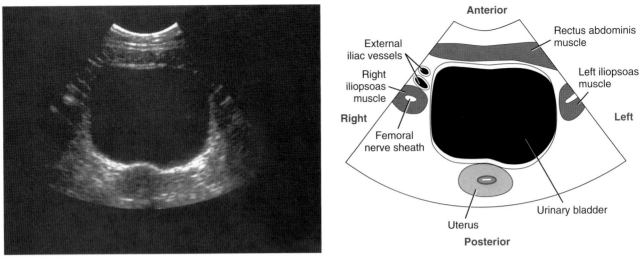

FIGURE 21-30 **Iliopsoas Muscles.** This transabdominal, transverse scanning plane image of the pelvis demonstrates short axis sections of the iliopsoas muscles seen bilateral to the urinary bladder. These skeletal muscles have low-level echoes and appear hypoechoic relative to the echogenic appearance of the centrally located femoral nerve sheath.

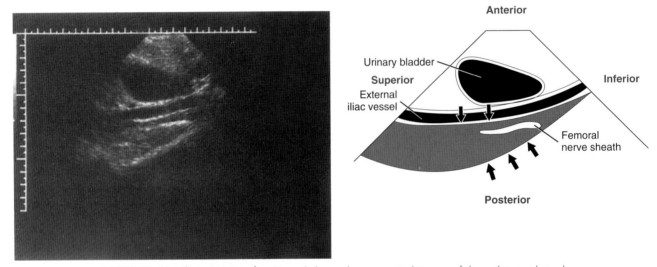

FIGURE 21-31 **Iliopsoas Muscles.** Transabdominal, parasagittal image of the pelvis just lateral to the right ovary. This image demonstrates longitudinal sections of the iliopsoas muscle (shown by arrows), femoral nerve sheath, and external iliac vein.

- **Pelvic ligaments sonographic appearance.** Unless they are outlined by free intraperitoneal fluid, the ligaments of the female pelvis, with the exception of the broad ligaments (Figure 21-35), are not routinely identified sonographically.
- **Pelvic spaces sonographic appearance.** *Posterior cul de sac, anterior cul de sac, space of Retzius*
  - **Posterior cul-de-sac.** It is not uncommon or abnormal to visualize a small amount of free fluid between the cervix and the rectum, in the posterior cul-de-sac, especially after ovulation. Identifica-

tion of a large amount of fluid in the posterior cul-de-sac suggests an abnormality.
  - **Anterior cul-de-sac.** Normally, this space is empty, but loops of small bowel may be visualized in the anterior cul-de-sac, the shallow peritoneal area between the uterus and pubic bone.
  - **Space of Retzius.** The space of Retzius is generally not sonographically significant unless the urinary bladder appears to be displaced posteriorly. This is a characteristic feature of a mass or multiple masses in the space of Retzius, which

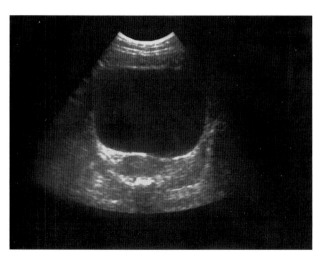

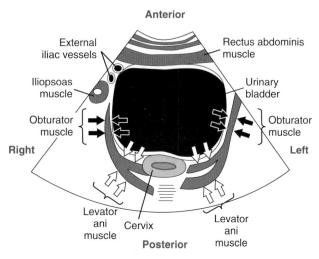

FIGURE 21-32 **Pelvic Musculature.** Transabdominal, transverse scanning plane image of the pelvis demonstrating longitudinal sections of the obturator internus muscles located on each side of the urinary bladder *(black arrows)*. Long sections of the bilateral levator ani muscles of the pelvic diaphragm are seen hammocking across the pelvic floor to meet posterior to the cervix *(white arrows)*. Axial sections of the right iliopsoas muscle and right external iliac artery and vein are seen anterior to the right obturator internus muscle. The rectus abdominis muscle is seen lining the anterior abdominal wall, anterior to the urinary bladder.

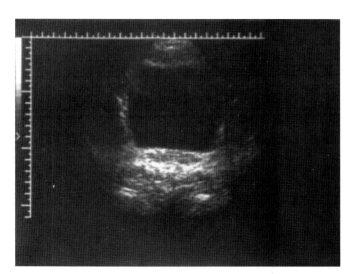

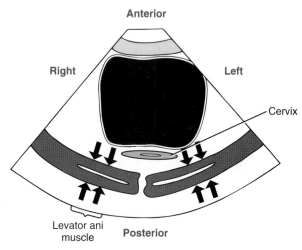

FIGURE 21-33 **Levator Ani Muscles.** Transabdominal, transverse scanning plane image of the lower portion of the true pelvis demonstrating longitudinal sections of the bilateral levator ani muscles of the pelvic diaphragm meeting just posterior to the axial section of the cervix.

separates the anterior bladder wall from the pubic symphysis.

- **Pelvic organs sonographic appearance.** *Genital tract (vagina, uterus, uterine tubes), ovaries, urinary bladder*
  - ○ **Genital tract**. *Vagina, uterus, uterine tubes*

    The sonographic presentations of the vagina, uterus, and uterine tubes are very similar because they share the same basic structure: cavities enclosed by an inner mucosal lining, a smooth muscle wall, and an outer layer of connective tissue. Variations in the sonographic appearance of the mucosa and muscular walls of the genital tract are dictated by size, location, and function of each segment.

    (i) **Vagina sonographic appearance.** The vagina can be identified in the inferior portion of the pelvis between the urinary bladder (anteriorly) and rectum (posteriorly). In transabdominal, sagittal scanning plane images, longitudinal sections of the vagina appear as

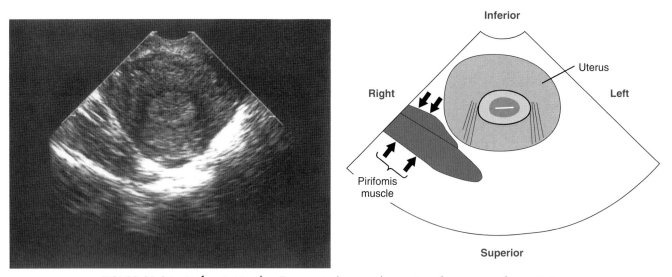

FIGURE 21-34 **Piriformis Muscles.** Transvaginal, coronal scanning plane image demonstrating a longitudinal section of the right piriformis muscle posterolateral to the uterus *(arrows)*. The corresponding piriformis muscle on the left side is obscured by overlying bowel gas.

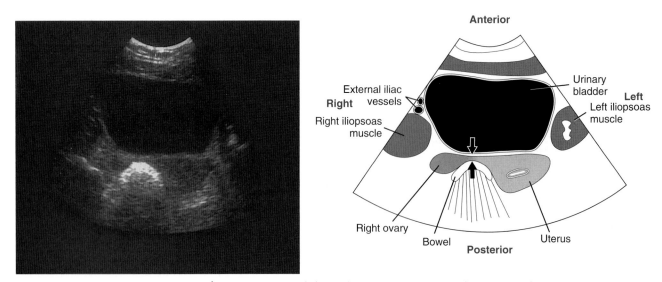

FIGURE 21-35 **Broad Ligaments.** Transabdominal, transverse scanning plane image showing a longitudinal section of the right broad ligament *(between arrows)*, which appears as the region of medium- to low-level echoes extending between the uterine cornu and right ovary.

a tubular, inferior extension of the uterus (posterior to the bladder and anterior to the rectum). In transabdominal, transverse scanning plane images, short axis sections of the vagina have a flattened, oval shape.

The muscular vaginal walls appear low-gray and homogeneous with smooth contours. The central mucosal lining of the normally collapsed vaginal canal walls appears thin, linear, and bright (Figures 21-36 and 21-37). The muscles of the pelvic diaphragm can be visualized posterior to the vagina.

(ii) **Uterus sonographic appearance.** The uterus is well visualized sonographically, using either transabdominal sonography or transvaginal sonography. Size and sonographic pattern of the uterus are described according to corresponding cyclical changes.

As mentioned earlier, the endometrial layer of the uterus is composed of a deep basal layer and superficial layer (or functional zone). Sonographically, the basal layer appears highly echogenic due to the reflective mucosal glands that compose the layer. The

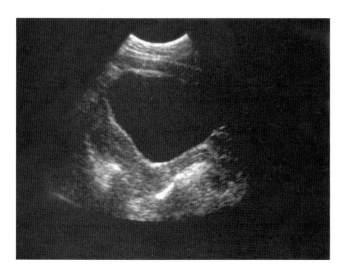
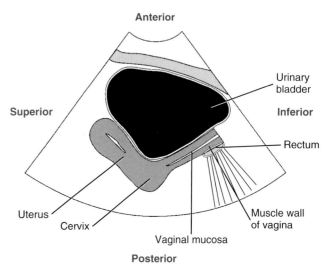

FIGURE 21-36 **Vagina.** This transabdominal, sagittal scanning plane image demonstrates a longitudinal section of the vagina, seen posteroinferior to the distended, anechoic urinary bladder and anterior to the rectum. Notice how the muscular walls of the vagina exhibit low- to mid-level echoes and are hypoechoic relative to the bright appearance of the mucosal lining of the centrally located vaginal canal.

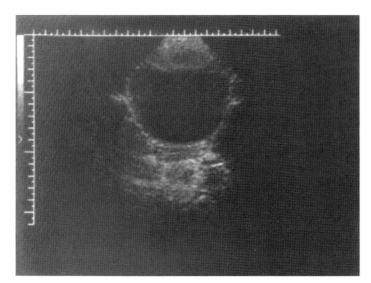
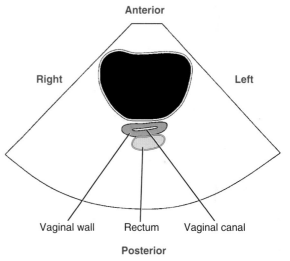

FIGURE 21-37 **Vagina.** Transabdominal, transverse scanning plane image of the pelvis showing an axial section of the vagina, seen posterior to the urinary bladder and anterior to the rectum. The centrally located vaginal canal appears thin and hyperechoic relative to the vaginal walls.

superficial layer generally appears hypoechoic compared with the bright basal layer. The central, linear, opposing surfaces of the endometrium that form the endometrial canal present sonographically as a bright, reflective, thin, midline strip, called the **endometrial stripe**.

The width of the endometrium is greatest near the uterine fundus and narrows toward the cervix (Figure 21-38). Measurement of endometrial thickness is most accurate on a longitudinal section of the uterus and should include the endometrial layers anterior and posterior to the bright endometrial canal (Figure 21-39). Some refer to this as "double-layer" thickness. The darker halo from the inner myometrial layer should not be part of the measurement.

As the thickness of the endometrium changes cyclically with the menstrual cycle, so does its sonographic appearance:

- During the menstrual phase the endometrium appears thin and bright as the superficial layer is shed.

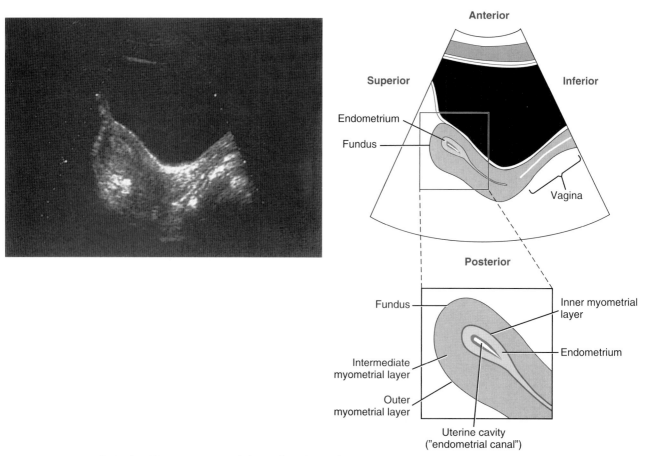

FIGURE 21-38 **Uterus.** Transabdominal, midsagittal scanning plane image of the pelvis showing longitudinal sections of the uterus and vagina just posterior to the urinary bladder. Notice how the width of the uterine endometrium is greatest near the fundus and narrows toward the cervix. Remember that as the thickness of the endometrium changes cyclically with the menstrual cycle, so does its sonographic appearance. Note that the thick walls of the uterus normally compress together, collapsing the centrally located uterine cavity (endometrial canal), giving it a bright, single-stripe appearance.

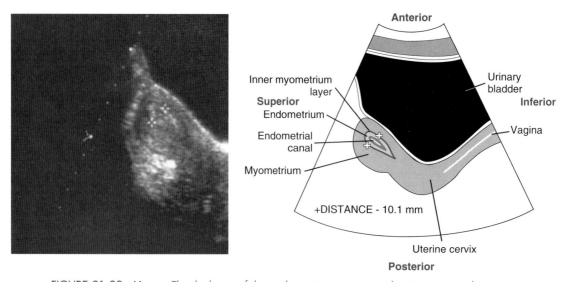

FIGURE 21-39 **Uterus.** The thickness of the endometrium is measured at its greatest dimension in a longitudinal section of the uterus.

- In the early proliferative phase (days 5 to 9), the endometrium measures 4 to 8 mm thick and appears hyperechoic relative to surrounding structures.
- Later in the proliferative phase (days 10 to 14), the functional zone of the endometrium thickens under the influence of estrogen and appears hypoechoic relative to the bright, echogenic basal layer.
- Just before ovulation, near the 14th day of the menstrual cycle, the endometrium measures from 6 to 10 mm and takes on a multilayered appearance (Figure 21-40). The bright endometrial stripe is surrounded by the thickened, darker functional zone. The functional zone is separated from the inner layer of the myometrium by the fairly thin basal layer, which appears hyperechoic in comparison.
- This layered appearance continues during the early secretory phase when the endometrium achieves its maximum echogenicity and thickness from 7 to 14 mm (Figure 21-41). During the secretory phase (days 15 to 28), the functional zone is even thicker and edematous from the influence of progesterone and becomes isoechoic to the basal layer (see Figure 21-41).
- The endometrium normally measures less than 8 mm in postmenopausal women.

The myometrium is isoechoic to and continuous with the muscular walls of the vagina. As mentioned earlier, the uterine myometrium accounts for the bulk of uterine tissue and consists of 3 sonographically distinguishable muscle fiber layers. The outer longitudinal fiber layer appears hypoechoic relative to the intermediate layer and is separated from the intermediate layer by anechoic arcuate vessels. The spiral fiber bands of the intermediate layer constitute the thickest and most echo-dense layer, which exhibits a midgray to low-gray, homogeneous echo texture. The inner circular and longitudinal fibers are significantly less echogenic than the intermediate layer and give the appearance of a thin hypoechoic halo surrounding the endometrium (Figure 21-42).

During periovulatory and menstrual phases, myometrial contractions have been identified sonographically as a rippling effect along the endometrium, extending from the cervix to the fundus. These muscular contractions are thought to play a role in sperm transport.

The only notable sonographic characteristic of the outer serosa layer of the uterus is its smooth contour. It is otherwise indistinguishable.

The sonographic pattern of the uterine cervix is similar to that of the rest of the uterus (Figure 21-43). The muscular walls are homogeneous, with midgray to low-gray echoes that surround the thin, bright mucosal lining of the cervical cavity or canal (Figure 21-44). The endocervical canal is a continuation of the endometrial canal and appears as a fairly thin, bright stripe. It is normal to occasionally see anechoic fluid in the endocervical canal, particularly during the preovulatory phase. In some cases, shadows are cast by air visualized in the vaginal fornices surrounding the external os of the cervix (Figure 21-45, see Figure 21-44, *B*).

The internal os of the cervix is difficult to visualize except during pregnancy, when it is identified as the point where the cervical canal and the amniotic membrane or presenting parts meet.

The external os is recognized as the point where the anterior and posterior lips of the cervix meet. In most cases, TV sonography provides a clear image of the cervix. In situations where TV sonography is contraindicated and TA sonography does not provide enough detailed information of the cervix, translabial (transperineal) sonography provides another scanning option. In translabial imaging the cervical canal is generally oriented at a right angle from the distal vagina.

On TAS when the urinary bladder is full, the uterus appears "straightened out" rather than anteflexed. If the uterus is retroverted, with the fundus pointing posteriorly, it can be difficult to image the fundus with TA sonography as a result of attenuation of sound by the anterior portion of the uterus. This echo-poor appearance is referred to as the "dropout" phenomenon. Usually the dropout in the fundus of a retroverted uterus is not a problem for TV sonography.

(iii) **Uterine tubes appearance.** Unless there is free fluid in the lateral pelvic recesses or tubal pathology, the infundibulum, ampulla, and isthmus cannot be identified sonographically. The interstitial portion of the oviduct,

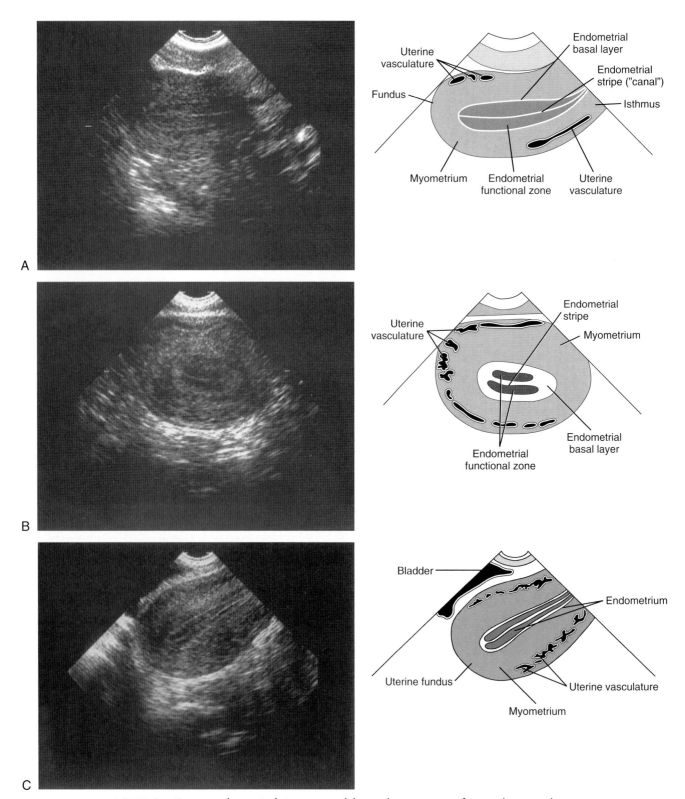

FIGURE 21-40   **Preovulatory Endometrium. Multilayered appearance of preovulatory endome-trium. A,** Transvaginal image showing a longitudinal section of the uterus. Notice the thickness of the endometrium. The bright, single stripe of the endometrial canal is hyperechoic relative to the surrounding low-gray appearance of the functional zone, the thickest portion of the endome-trium. The functional zone is separated from the dark inner myometrial layer by the thin, bright basal layer of the endometrium. **B,** Transvaginal, coronal scanning plane image demonstrating a short axis of the uterus. The myometrium exhibits low- to mid-level gray echoes; the endometrium presents with a multilayered preovulatory appearance. **C,** Another longitudinal section of the uterus prior to ovulation. The multilayered appearance of the endometrium presents as a central bright stripe surrounded by a thicker, darker layer, which is surrounded by a thin, bright border.

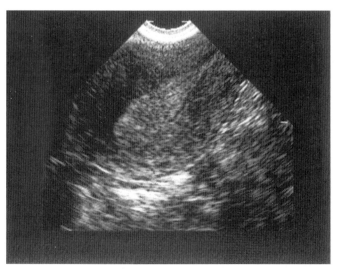

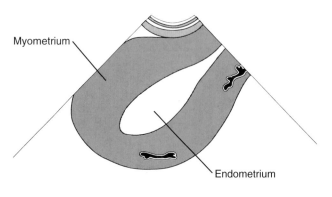

FIGURE 21-41 **Endometrial Secretory Phase.** Transvaginal, sagittal scanning plane image showing a longitudinal section of the uterus and the appearance of the endometrium during the secretory phase. In addition to an increased overall thickness, the endometrial basal layer, functional zone, and canal become isoechoic.

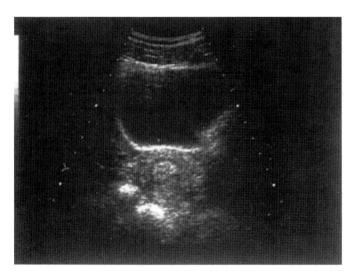

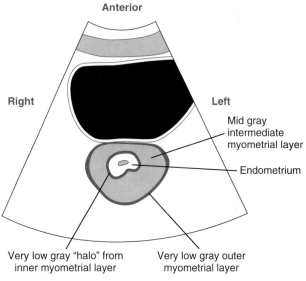

FIGURE 21-42 **Myometrium.** The muscle fiber layers of the myometrium are well distinguished on this axial section of the uterus. The inner and outer layers appear hypoechoic compared with the mid-gray appearance of the intermediate layer.

however, can be imaged with TV sonography. It appears as a 1-cm long, tenuous, echogenic line arising from the endometrial canal and extending through the uterine wall.

○ **Ovarian appearance.** The bilateral, almond-shaped ovaries are most commonly identified lateral to the uterine fundus, usually with the long axis vertically orientated (Figure 21-46 on p. 380).

Normal ovarian echo texture is homogeneous unless otherwise interrupted by anechoic ovarian follicles, a common finding during reproductive years. Generally, the ovary presents sonographically with a periphery representing the tunica that appears hypoechoic compared with the low-gray appearance of the central core that represents the stroma. The ovaries usually appear hypoechoic relative to the uterine myometrium. Sonographic landmarks that help locate the ovaries include the bilateral iliopsoas muscles, which appear low-gray and posterolateral to the ovaries, the anechoic

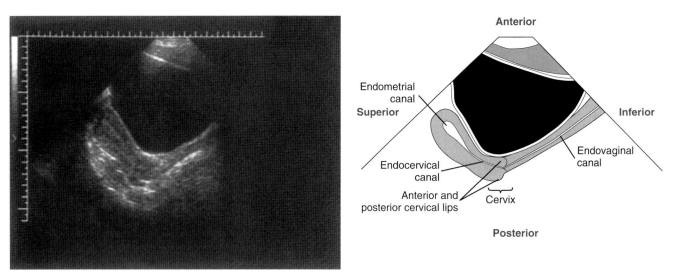

FIGURE 21-43 **Cervix.** Transabdominal, sagittal scanning plane image of the pelvis showing a longitudinal section of the cervix at the most inferior aspect of the uterus, closest to the vagina. Notice how the anterior and posterior lips of the cervix can be distinguished as the cervix protrudes into the vagina.

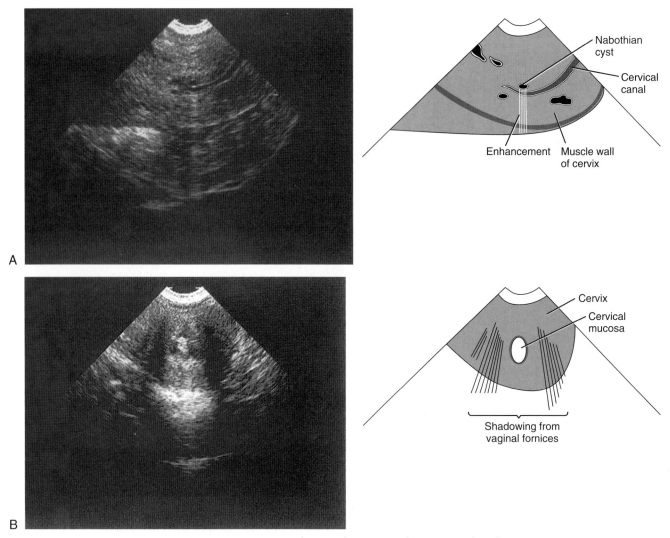

FIGURE 21-44 **Cervix. A,** Transvaginal, sagittal scanning plane image that demonstrates a longitudinal section of the cervix. A slight quantity of anechoic fluid is seen within the cervical canal. A small nabothian cyst is seen within the wall of the cervix exhibiting posterior enhancement. **B,** Transvaginal, coronal scanning plane image showing an axial section of the cervix. Note the shadowing from the vaginal fornices.

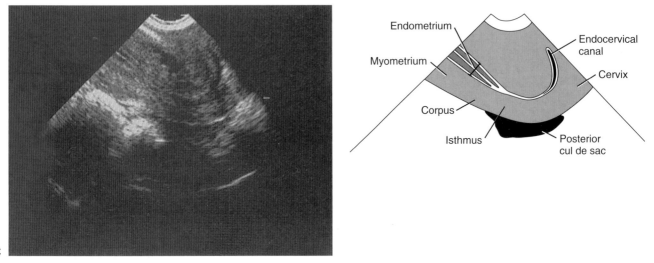

C

FIGURE 21-44, cont'd **Cervix. C,** Transvaginal, sagittal scanning plane image of a longitudinal section of the uterus in an anteflexed uterus. A small quantity of anechoic fluid is seen in the endocervical canal and the posterior cul de sac.

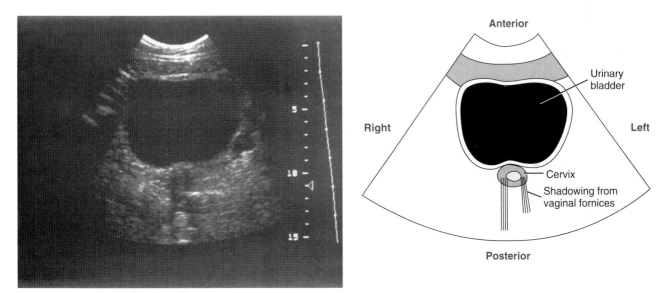

FIGURE 21-45 **Cervix.** Transabdominal, transverse scanning plane image demonstrating shadowing from the vaginal fornices, which confirms that the axial section posterior to the urinary bladder is the cervix.

external iliac vessels anterolateral to the ovaries, and the anechoic internal iliac vessels posterior to the ovaries. TA sonography and, especially, TV sonography provide excellent definition of the ovaries and follicular structures.

As mentioned earlier, ovarian volume is marginally affected by cyclical changes. The lowest volumes are seen during the luteal phase and highest volumes during the preovulatory phase.

Developing follicles within the ovary vary in both size and number. The anechoic appearance of a follicle accompanied by bright, posterior enhancement is due to the fluid-filled follicular antrum (Figure 21-47). The oocyte and cellular layers of the developing follicle cannot be identified sonographically. However, just before ovulation, the granulosa layer separates from the theca layer, resulting in a low-gray ring. Also at

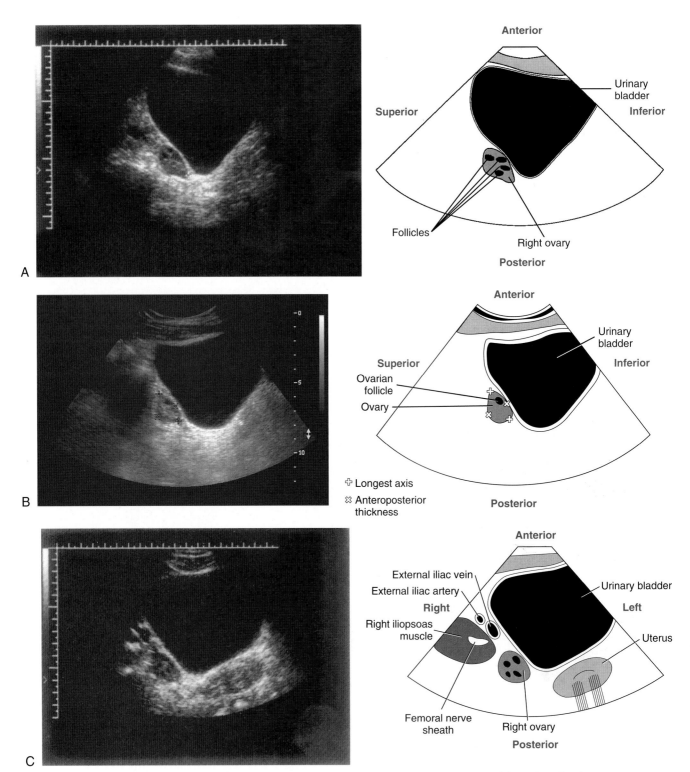

FIGURE 21-46 **Ovaries. A,** Transabdominal, sagittal scanning plane image of the right side of the pelvis. Note the typical almond shape of the ovary. The ovaries appear medium- to low-gray and homogeneous unless otherwise interrupted by anechoic, fluid-filled follicles, as seen in this image. **B,** The length and thickness of the ovary are measured on a long axis section. Since the position of the ovaries is not fixed, the long axis may be viewed in either transabdominal a sagittal or transverse scanning plane. The length is calculated from the longest longitudinal dimension of the ovary. The anteroposterior thickness is measured perpendicular to the length; width is measured on the largest axial section. **C,** This transabdominal, transverse scanning plane image demonstrates the anatomic position of the ovary relative to its surrounding structures. The iliopsoas muscle and external iliac vessels are seen anterior to the right ovary. Typically the uterus is medial to the ovaries as seen in this image.

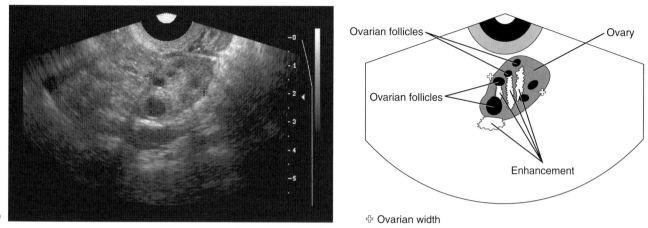

⊹ Ovarian width

FIGURE 21-46, cont'd   **Ovaries. D,** Transvaginal imaging provides detailed anatomy of the ovaries as seen in this image. (**B** and **D,** Images courtesy the University of Virginia Health System, Department of Radiology, Division of Ultrasound, Charlottesville, Virginia.)

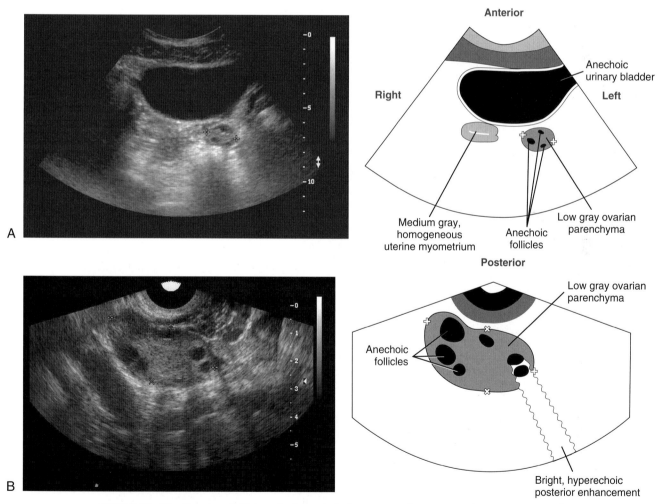

FIGURE 21-47   **Ovarian Follicles. A, B,** and **C** demonstrate the sonographic appearance of normal ovarian parenchyma and developing follicles. Notice the detail afforded by transvaginal imaging in **B** and **C** (on the following page). (Images courtesy the University of Virginia Health System, Department of Radiology, Division of Ultrasound, Charlottesville, Virginia.)

Continued

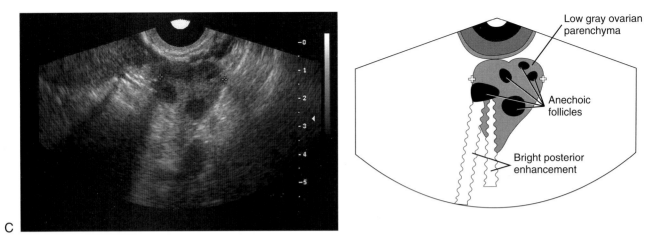

C

FIGURE 21-47, cont'd Ovarian Follicles. C, Sonographic appearance of normal ovarian parenchyma and developing follicles. Notice the detail afforded by transvaginal imaging. (Images courtesy the University of Virginia Health System, Department of Radiology, Division of Ultrasound, Charlottesville, Virginia.)

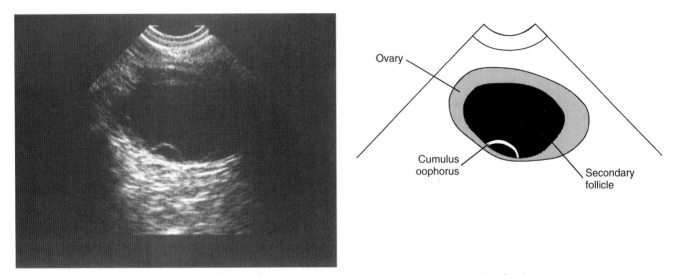

FIGURE 21-48 Cumulus Oophorus. The cumulus oophorus appears as a thin, bright crescent along the wall of the mature follicle. The secondary oocyte is contained within the cumulus oophorus.

this time, the cumulus oophorus of the secondary follicle can occasionally be seen as a thin, bright crescent along the wall of the anechoic follicular antrum (Figure 21-48). A mature graafian or dominant follicle presents as anechoic, with smooth bright walls, and measures approximately 20 mm (within a range of 16 to 28 mm) (Figure 21-49).

As mentioned, after ovulation, the anechoic fluid of the ruptured graafian follicle can be identified in the posterior cul-de-sac, molding to the shape of surrounding structures (Figure 21-50). Also after ovulation, the corpus luteum appears irregular in shape and contains internal echoes as a result of hemorrhage and blood clot. The internal echoes vary in appearance from multiple, fine, bright septations to diffuse, low-level echoes (Figure 21-51). This blood clot may become completely anechoic over time, at which point the corpus luteum resembles the sonographic appearance of a mature follicle. Eventually the corpus luteum regresses, leaving a small amount of scar tissue in the ovary, called the corpus albicans, which appears as a bright focus within the ovarian stroma (Figure 21-52).

○ **Urinary bladder appearance**. It is important to note that the size and shape of the bladder can vary depending on the quantity of urine being stored at any given time. Nevertheless, the distended bladder should appear symmetric on ultrasound.

The fully distended urinary bladder presents as a large, anterior, anechoic structure in the

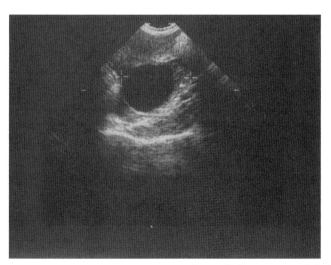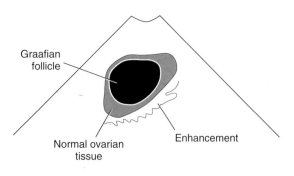

FIGURE 21-49 Graafian Follicle. Dominant follicles appear anechoic with smooth, thin, bright walls, and are round or oval in shape. Mature follicles are usually 18 to 22 mm in size and exhibit posterior enhancement.

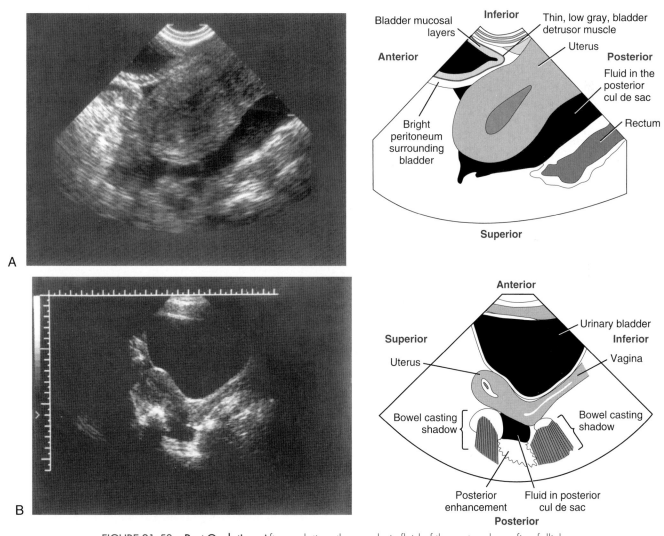

A

B

FIGURE 21-50 Post Ovulation. After ovulation, the anechoic fluid of the ruptured graafian follicle can be identified in the posterior cul-de-sac, molding to the shape of surrounding structures. **A,** The posterior cul-de-sac is well delineated when fluid filled. Note the partially filled urinary bladder in the upper left corner, which correlates to an anteroinferior orientation in this transvaginal, sagittal scanning plane image. Notice how the inner mucosa of the bladder wall is less visible and the relaxed detrusor muscle and the peritoneal lining surrounding the bladder are clearly visualized. **B,** Obvious anechoic collection of fluid in the posterior cul-de-sac located posterior to the uterus.

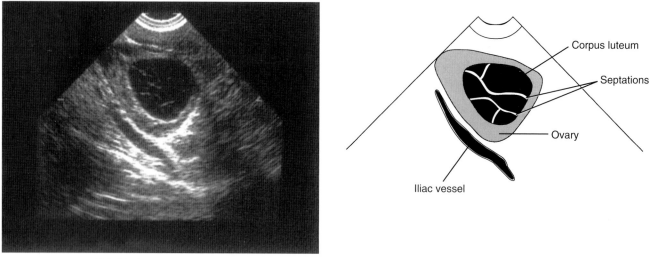

FIGURE 21-51 **Corpus Luteum.** The internal echoes of a corpus luteum vary in appearance from multiple, fine, bright septations to diffuse, low-level echoes. This corpus luteum is visualized with multiple, fine septations.

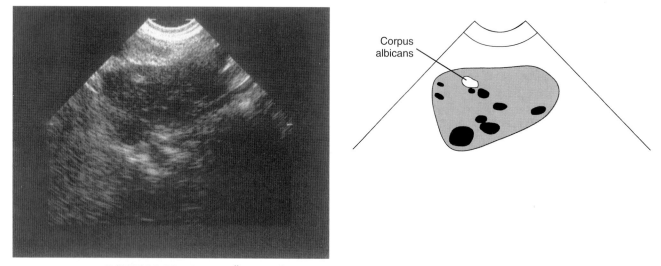

FIGURE 21-52 **Corpus Albicans.** The corpus albicans is the remaining scar tissue in the ovary after regression of the corpus luteum. This transvaginal image shows the corpus albicans, which appears as a highly echogenic foci within the ovary.

midregion of the true pelvis surrounded by smooth, bright, uniformly thick walls.

On superior short axis sections the distended bladder has a rounded appearance. Inferiorly, the short axis bladder sections appear square, shaped by the pelvic musculature and bones.

In longitudinal sections the contour of the posterior surface of the bladder can normally appear somewhat indented by an anteverted uterus.

As previously discussed, the bladder is composed of 4 layers of tissue: an inner mucosa, a submucosa layer, the muscularis, and the outer serosa. The thin inner layers of mucosa appear as narrow bright lines along the circumference of the bladder (Figure 21-53). The middle muscularis, or muscular, layer of the bladder wall stretches thin with bladder distention and is not well visualized sonographically. When the bladder is only slightly distended, the relaxed detrusor muscle can be visualized as a low-gray layer surrounding the mucosa (Figure 21-54, see Figure 21-50, *A*, noting how the detrusor muscle is better appreciated with TV sonography). The thin outer serosal layer of the bladder is sonographically indistinct.

Normally, the ureters are not sonographically appreciated as they enter the bladder. Yet the effect

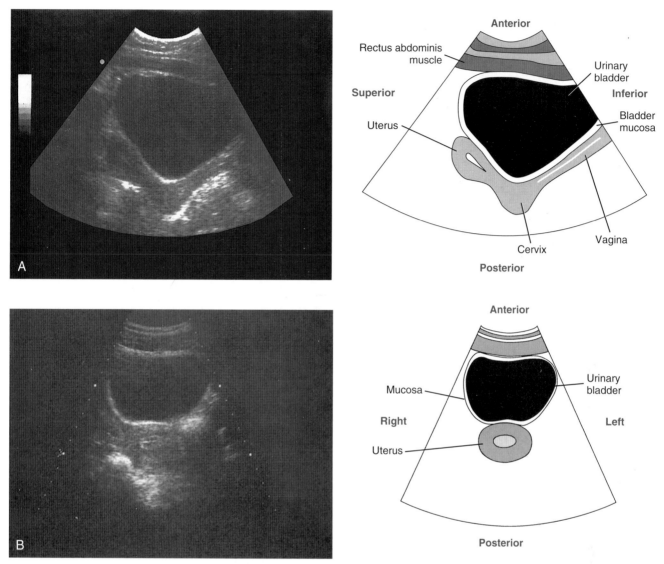

FIGURE 21-53 **Urinary Bladder. A,** Longitudinal section. **B,** Axial section. The bright mucosal lining of the distended anechoic bladder is seen along its circumference. The muscular wall of the bladder is stretched thin due to distention; thus the detrusor muscle is not visible. Notice how the bladder appears square-shaped in a short axis section. The uterus can be identified in both images, posterior to the bladder.

of the ureters ejecting urine into the bladder can be routinely observed on real-time examination. As discussed in Chapter 17, bright "ureteral jets," or squirts of urine, can be visualized in the trigone portion of the bladder.

- **Pelvic colon appearance.** An understanding of TA and TV sonography of the pelvic colon is rapidly becoming essential in performing a complete pelvic evaluation of premenopausal women presenting with pelvic pain. Within the pelvis, the colon is the most commonly visualized segment of the gastrointestinal tract and may be fairly easy to identify by the localization of stratified bowel segments. Loops of bowel within the pelvic cavity may appear heterogeneous, homogeneous, or fluid filled. It may or may not be visualized because of content. Bowel can present as bright and reflective, anechoic, or a combination of both.

The ascending and descending colon as well as the sigmoid colon, the cecum, appendix, and the rectum may be identified by the location of the bowel segment within the pelvic field of view and by internal components that may be distinguishable using TA or TV scanning.

Small bowel is displaced superiorly when the urinary bladder is full for TA sonography. During TV sonography, peristalsis can be observed in the loops of small bowel around the uterus and ovaries. The

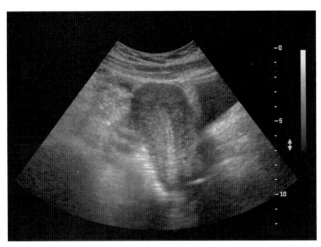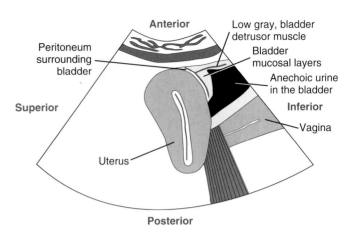

FIGURE 21-54 **Urinary Bladder.** Transabdominal, sagittal scanning plane image of midline of the pelvis with a partially filled urinary bladder. In this case the detrusor muscle is relaxed and is seen as a low-gray layer of the bladder wall.

lack of peristalsis is a sonographic clue to disease that has affected the colon. In some cases, gas in the intestine can obscure visualization of the ovaries and adnexa; however, diseased segments are often gasless. *Graded compression* and moving a patient into variable positions can displace gas from the field of view. Graded compression also may be used to improve visibility of a bowel segment and to minimize tenderness and discomfort. **Graded compression** means to slowly and steadily compress the bowel between the anterior and posterior abdominal walls.

The knowledge of which bowel segments are fixed and which are mobile aids in localizing a segment of interest. The free edge of small bowel mesentery is essentially the entire length of the small bowel, thus making it mobile. Therefore it is difficult to be precise about location along the small bowel. A **mesentery** is a double layer of visceral peritoneum that wraps around a bowel segment and attaches it to the posterior abdominal wall.

Appendicitis is the most common cause for emergent surgery in the United States. For female premenarchal patients and children, ultrasound is the safest and often the initial imaging modality to use in efforts to localize the cause of right lower quadrant (RLQ) pain.

The ileocecal valve connecting the ileum of the small bowel to the cecum of the large bowel is a landmark on US ultrasound images when trying to localize the terminal ileum, the cecum, and the appendix. The cecum does not have a mesentery and so has a variable attachment to the posterior abdominal wall. The appendix arises approximately 2.5 cm inferior to the cecum and posteromedial to the ileocecal valve. This relationship is fixed although the

appendix has a variable length (normally < 5 cm) and tip. Once the ileocecal valve and terminal ileum are identified, the appendix may be seen arising from the cecum without a valve. The mesentery of the appendix, the mesoappendix, attaches to the edge of the small bowel mesentery.

The right colon is fixed and retroperitoneal. The sigmoid is a suspended segment of bowel with a superior attachment to the descending colon along the medial side of the left iliac vessels. The inferior part is rooted along the third sacral vertebra, causing the sigmoid mesentery to attach to the pelvic sidewall in the shape of an inverted V and enabling mobility such that the sigmoid can extend to the RLQ and cause pain in that area.

As with the small bowel, the sonographic appearance of the rectosigmoid colon is variable, depending largely on content. Typically, the sigmoid colon and the rectum contain gas and fecal material, giving them an echogenic appearance with posterior shadowing (Figure 21-55).

- **Pelvic vasculature appearance.** *Uterine, ovarian*
  - **Uterine vasculature appearance.** The high resolution of TV sonography provides visualization of much of the uterine vasculature. Vessels coursing within the peripheral myometrium appear as anechoic structures (see Figure 21-40).

    As a rule, the uterine arteries and veins can be identified with color-flow Doppler (TA sonography or TV sonography) lateral to the cervix and ascending lateral to the uterus in the broad ligament to the junction of the uterine tubes and uterus.

    During the periovulatory period the spiral arteries can be identified in the functional zone of the

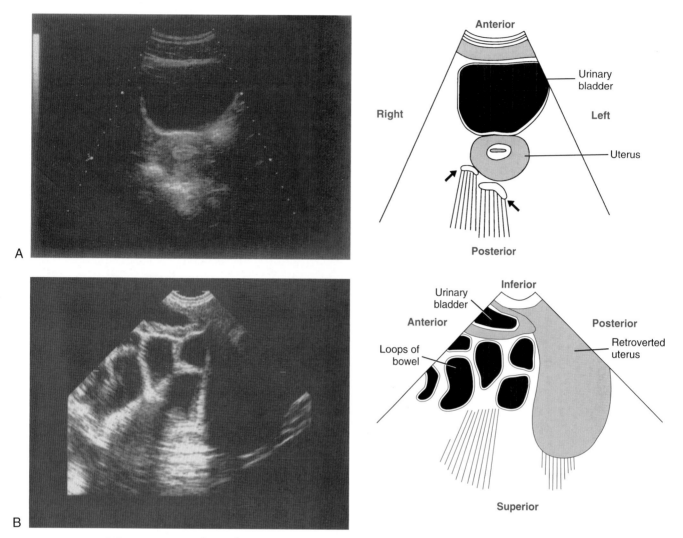

FIGURE 21-55   **Pelvic Colon. A,** This transabdominal, transverse scanning plane image shows a reflective portion of the sigmoid colon *(arrows)* posterior to the uterus. **B,** Detailed peristaltic loops of small bowel are often visualized during transvaginal imaging. Fluid-filled loops of bowel are seen resting in the anterior cul-de-sac in this sagittal scanning plane image. (Images courtesy the University of Virginia Health System, Department of Radiology, Division of Ultrasound, Charlottesville, Virginia.)

endometrium with TV color-flow Doppler. In cases of infertility, the spiral arteries cannot be imaged.

○ **Ovarian vasculature appearance.** Color-flow and spectral Doppler are valuable tools in assessing blood flow to the ovaries and to ovarian masses. During the normal ovulatory cycle the functional ovary receives greater vascular perfusion between days 9 and 28 of the menstrual cycle. This is reflected in a lower-resistance Doppler waveform in the ovary producing the dominant follicle. A low-resistance waveform has a high amount of diastolic flow. The luteal phase is the best time to observe blood flow within the ovary using power Doppler and TV color-flow Doppler. In postmenopausal women, ovarian flow cannot be detected.

• **Pelvic lymph nodes appearance.** Normal pelvic lymph nodes are not appreciated sonographically. Abnormally large nodes appear hypoechoic relative to surrounding structures or even anechoic with indistinct bright walls. Typically, they appear in multiples and are closely related in groups. Pathologically enlarged lymph nodes in the pelvis would be visualized in the areas surrounding the common iliac artery, external iliac artery and vein, pelvic sidewalls, and in the area of the false pelvis.

SONOGRAPHIC APPLICATIONS

- Ruling out the presence of a mass: if a mass is found, sonography can provide the site of origin, size, and composition. Sonography is limited, however, in providing definitive diagnoses of the benignity or malignancy of such masses. Clinical studies suggest great potential in the future for differentiating benign from malignant tumors utilizing TV color-flow Doppler and spectral Doppler.
- Diagnosing congenital uterine anomalies

- Evaluating pelvic inflammatory processes
- Ruling out ectopic pregnancy
- Diagnosing and managing infertility: This includes the sonographic assessment of contributing causes of infertility such as:
  - ○ Endometriosis
  - ○ Congenital anomalies
  - ○ Myomas
  - ○ Pelvic inflammatory disease
- Follicle monitoring: For infertility cases, particularly in patients undergoing hormone therapy.
- Ultrasound-guided ovum retrieval: For in vitro fertilization.
- Detecting intrauterine contraceptive devices (IUDs, IUCDs): Figure 21-56 demonstrates four common types of IUDs. These devices generally appear highly reflective on ultrasound images with varying degrees of posterior acoustic shadowing. Figures 21-57 and 21-58 demonstrate the typical sonographic patterns of IUDs.
- Evaluating ovaries in posthysterectomy patients: In the absence of the uterus, the ovaries typically rest within the posterior cul de sac. Figure 21-59 illustrates a TA midsagittal scanning plane image posthysterectomy.
- Hysterosonography (HS): This technique was developed to better evaluate the endometrium. HS has provided a more accurate distinction between endometrial abnormalities such as hyperplasia, polyp, fibroid, or carcinoma.

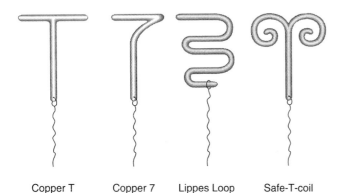

Copper T   Copper 7   Lippes Loop   Safe-T-coil

FIGURE 21-56 Intrauterine devices (IUDs), which provide contraception.

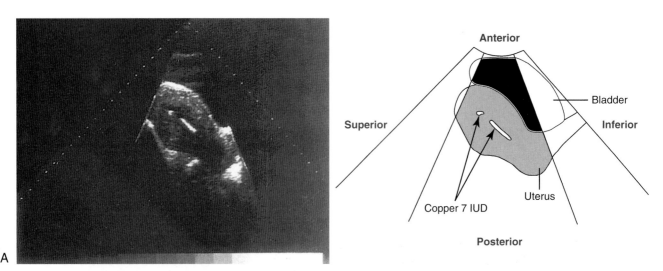

A

FIGURE 21-57 **Copper Seven IUD. A,** The Copper Seven IUD is easily visualized in a longitudinal section of the uterus. This contraceptive device is highly echogenic and rests within the endometrial cavity.

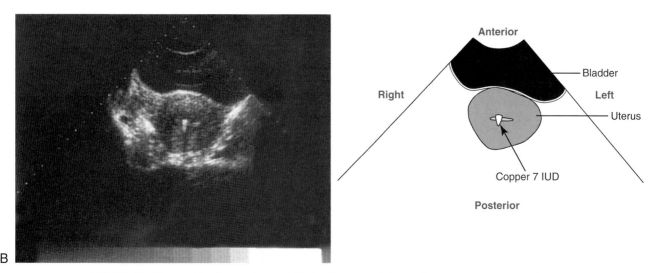

FIGURE 21-57, cont'd **Copper Seven IUD. B,** This transabdominal, transverse scanning plane image of the pelvis demonstrates the appearance of the Copper Seven IUD within the endometrial canal in this axial section of the uterus.

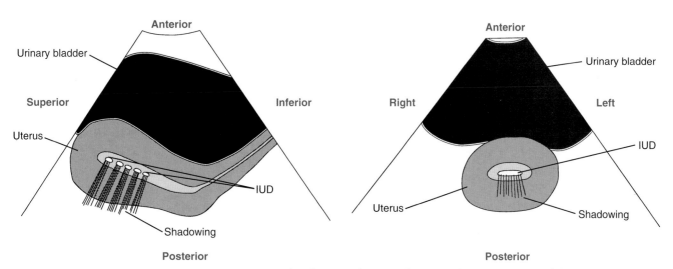

FIGURE 21-58 **Lippes Loop IUD.** This illustrates the typical sonographic appearance of the Lippes Loop IUD within the endometrial canal. Posterior shadowing is frequently associated with IUDs.

NORMAL VARIANTS

- **Uterine normal variations:** Consists of specific uterine positions identifiable with ultrasound that include tilting of the uterus to the right or left, tilting of the uterine fundus and body posteriorly (retroversion) (Figure 21-60), and bending of the uterine fundus and body posteroinferiorly (retroflexion). It should be noted that these posi-

tion variations are considered to be normal standard deviations unless the uterus is displaced by pathology.

- **Ovarian normal variations:** A congenital ovarian malformation identifiable with ultrasound is alteration of the typical shape of the ovary, giving it a distinctive L-shape. The ovary appears normal in all other respects.

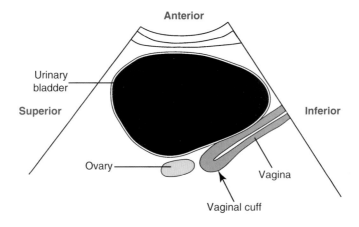

FIGURE 21-59   Post Hysterectomy Pelvis. This illustrates the typical appearance of the pelvis post hysterectomy. The vaginal cuff can be identified, and with the absence of the uterus, the ovary moves into the posterior cul-de-sac.

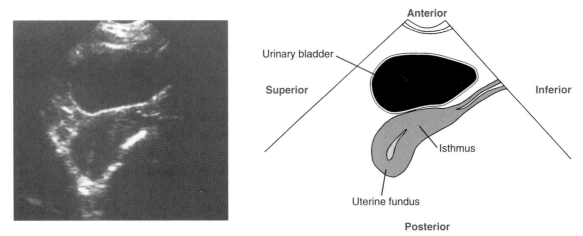

FIGURE 21-60   Retroverted Uterus. This transabdominal, sagittal scanning plane image demonstrates the typical appearance of a longitudinal section of a retroverted uterus. Notice how the fundus is tilted posteriorly. A retroverted uterus is considered to be a normal variation in uterine position.

REFERENCE CHARTS

▪ ▪ ▪   ASSOCIATED PHYSICIANS

- **Gynecologist:** A physician specializing in female reproduction, including physiology, endocrinology, and diseases of the genital tract.
- **Obstetrician:** A physician specializing in the medical care of pregnant women.
- **Radiologist:** A physician specializing in the administration and interpretation of diagnostic medical imaging.
- **Endocrinologist:** A physician specializing in the physiologic and pathologic association of hormonal secretions of the body.

▪ ▪ ▪   COMMON DIAGNOSTIC TESTS

- **Computed tomography and magnetic resonance imaging:** Computed tomography (CT) and magnetic resonance imaging (MRI) are both extremely important diagnostic tools in evaluating the female pelvis. Improvements in contrast agents continue to enhance the superior tissue characterization of these modalities. These tests are performed by trained technologists and interpreted by radiologists.
- **Laparoscopy:** An endoscopic procedure performed under local or general anesthesia in which a telescopic instrument is inserted into the abdominal cavity from the area of the navel. The laparoscope can be manipulated in order to visualize the abdominal or pelvic organs. This test is performed and interpreted by a gynecologist.
- **Hysteroscopy/salpingoscopy:** An endoscopic procedure in which a telescopic instrument is inserted through the vagina and into the uterus. This test allows visualization of the interior uterine walls. This technique can also be used to visualize the fallopian tubes. These tests are performed and interpreted by a gynecologist or a similarly trained physician.
- **Hysterosalpingography:** A radiologic examination of the uterus and fallopian tubes after dye (contrast agent) administration. Tubal blockage and structural abnormalities of the uterus can be diagnosed. This procedure is performed and interpreted by a radiologist.
- **Hysterosonography:** A sonographic procedure used to examine the endometrium and uterine cavity. The procedure provides enough detail to differentiate endometrial pathologies that are otherwise not distinguishable with standard TA or TV sonography. Radiologists perform the procedure and interpret the results.

▪ ▪ ▪   LABORATORY VALUES

- **Estrogen/progesterone:** These hormones are produced by the ovary during the normal menstrual cycle. Serum concentrations of these hormones can be useful in evaluating ovulatory function.
- **Human chorionic gonadotropin (hCG):** A highly accurate blood pregnancy test. This hormone is produced by placental trophoblastic cells and plays an important role during the first trimester of pregnancy.
- **Leukocytosis:** An abnormally high serum white blood cell count (exceeding 10,000 per mm³). This condition is indicative of an infectious process (such as pelvic inflammatory disease).

▪ ▪ ▪   VASCULATURE

UTERINE VASCULATURE

Aorta → common iliac artery → uterine → internal iliac artery → uterine artery → arcuate arteries → radial arteries → straight arteries → spiral arteries → spiral veins → straight veins → radial veins → arcuate veins → uterine vein → internal iliac vein → common iliac vein → inferior vena cava

OVARIAN VASCULATURE

Pathway One

Aorta → common iliac artery → internal iliac artery → uterine artery → ovarian branch of uterine artery → ovarian branch of uterine vein → uterine vein → internal iliac vein → common iliac vein → inferior vena cava

Pathway Two

Aorta → right ovarian artery → right ovarian vein → inferior vena cava or aorta → left ovarian artery → left ovarian vein → left renal vein → inferior vena cava

▪ ▪ ▪   AFFECTING CHEMICALS

- **Birth control pills:** Estrogen and progestin provide a highly effective form of birth control. These medications mimic the hormonal conditions of pregnancy, resulting in an ovulatory state.
- **Diethylstilbestrol (DES):** A synthetic estrogen commonly administered to pregnant women from the late 1940s to the early 1970s. This medication was thought to reduce the risks for spontaneous abortion. DES was taken off the market after it was discovered to cause multiple problems involving the reproductive organs of offspring exposed to the drug in utero. A small, irregular, T-shaped uterus is a common malformation associated with DES exposure.
- **Menotropins (Pergonal), urofollitropin (Metrodin), clomiphene citrate (Clomid):** Medications commonly prescribed in infertility to stimulate follicular maturation and induce ovulation.

■ **CHAPTER 22**

First Trimester Obstetrics (0 to 12 Weeks)

BETTY BATES TEMPKIN AND ROBBI R. KING

OBJECTIVES

Describe the role of the female reproductive system in creating and supporting a developing embryo.

Describe the sonographic appearance of the gestational sac and early embryo.

Describe the sonographic appearance of embryologic development.

Describe the sonographic appearance of the placenta during the 1st trimester.

Describe how gestational age is determined sonographically during the 1st trimester.

Identify related tests performed during the 1st trimester.

KEY WORDS

Amnion — Innermost membrane of the developing embryo; eventually fuses with the chorion.

Amniotic Cavity/Sac — Enclosure containing the developing embryo and fetus; filled with amniotic fluid to cushion and protect the embryo/fetus.

Amniotic Fluid — Liquid enclosed by the amnion that surrounds and bathes the embryo/fetus. Permits symmetric growth of the embryo/fetus; prevents adhesions from forming in the fetal membranes; cushions the embryo/fetus and acts as a shock absorber; helps to maintain proper temperature of the embryo; allows normal development of the respiratory, gastrointestinal, and musculoskeletal systems; helps to prevent infection; and may be a source of nutrients for the developing embryo.

Amniotic Fluid Volume (AFV) — Amount of amniotic fluid in the amniotic cavity. Reflects the state of gestational well-being. Many abnormalities are associated with marked increases (polyhydramnios) or decreases (oligohydramnios). Determined by a variety of methods.

Aneuploidy — Abnormal chromosome number.

Chorion — Outermost tissues of the developing embryo. Eventually fuses with the amnion.

Chorionic Cavity — Part of early development that surrounds the amniotic cavity and contains the yolk sac. Eventually obliterated by the amniotic cavity that increases in size to accommodate the developing embryo.

Chorionic Villi — Fetal portions of the placenta that are finger-like projections of the trophoblast layer (outer cell layer of the blastocyst) that extend into the deciduate endometrium. They are surrounded by lacunae, pools of maternal blood. Contact of the villi of the embryonic circulatory system with the maternal lacunae facilitates the transfer of oxygen and metabolites and the transfer of carbon dioxide and waste products.

Corpus Luteum — What remains of the ovarian follicle following ovulation. Produces progesterone and a small amount of estrogen to prepare the uterus for pregnancy. May become enlarged and fluid filled during pregnancy and thereafter, gradually diminishing without complication.

Crown Rump Length (CRL) — Age-determining measurement of the length of the embryo/fetus from the top of the head (crown) to the middle of the buttocks (rump), during the 1st trimester of pregnancy. Commonly accepted as the most accurate assessment of GA.

Decidua — Term applied to the gravid endometrium. Functional reaction of the endometrial lining to pregnancy. The endometrium becomes thick and edematous from vascular and structural changes to accommodate embryo implantation and development.

Decidua Basalis — Section of decidualized uterine endometrium where the blastocyst implants.

Decidua Capsularis — Thin portion of endometrium that overlies the section of gestational sac facing the uterine cavity.

Decidua Parietalis — Remaining endometrium, or peripheral portion, that is unoccupied by the implanted ovum.

Double Bleb Sign — Description of the distinctive sonographic appearance of the embryonic disk situated between the newly developed amniotic cavity and secondary yolk sac within the chorionic cavity at 4 to 5 weeks' gestational age.

Double Sac Sign — Sonographic identification of the decidua capsularis, decidua parietalis, and decidua basalis to differentiate a "pseudo sac" associated with ectopic pregnancies from a gestational sac.

Estrogen — Hormone produced by the ovarian corpus luteum to help prepare the uterus for pregnancy. Regularly produced by the ovaries as a "feminizing" hormone.

Fetal Vernix — Flakes of fetal skin that are sonographically distinguishable in amniotic fluid.

Follicle-Stimulating Hormone (FSH) — Hormone produced by the anterior pituitary gland in the brain to promote ovarian follicular growth.

Gestational Age (GA) — Synonymous with menstrual age; used to date the age of a pregnancy.

Gestational Sac — Term used by sonologists to describe the fluid-filled cavity of an intrauterine pregnancy during the 1st trimester. First fundamental sonographic finding in early pregnancy.

Gravid — Pregnant.

Human Chorionic Gonadotropin (hCG) — Hormone secreted by the developing placenta to communicate to the rest of the body that a gestation is present within the uterus.

Intradecidual Sign — Description of the sonographic appearance of the normal location of a very early intrauterine pregnancy when the gestational sac is visualized right next to the centrally located endometrial cavity at the level of the fundus or body of the uterus.

Lacunae — Small pools of maternal blood that surround the chorionic villi in the placenta.

Luteinizing Hormone (LH) — Hormone that, when increased, causes ovulation to occur.

Mean Sac Diameter (MSD) — Age-determining measurement of the mean diameter of the gestational sac during the early 1st trimester of pregnancy.

Nuchal Translucency (NT) Measurement — Measurement of the fluid that normally collects at the back of the fetus' neck between 11.3 and 13.6 weeks of gestation to determine the fetal risk estimate for aneuploidy (abnormal number of chromosomes; example is Down syndrome). An increase in the amount of fluid is indication of possible abnormality.

Ovulation — Release of the ovum (egg cell) into the genital tract from a mature ovarian follicle.

Placenta — Temporary maternal-fetal organ that provides nutrition, waste removal, gas exchange, and immune and endocrine support required for the developing embryo/fetus. It is delivered with the fetus at birth.

Progesterone — Hormone produced by the corpus luteum that helps prepare the uterus for pregnancy.

Pseudo Sac — Associated with pregnancies outside the uterus (ectopic pregnancy).

Rhombencephalon — Normal cystic hindbrain that is sonographically distinguishable in the developing embryo during the eighth week of gestation.

Umbilical Cord — Connection between the embryo/fetus and placenta. Consists of two arteries and one vein through which embryonic/fetal blood passes to and from the placenta.

Vitelline (Omphalomesenteric) Duct — Connection between the yolk sac and early developing embryo. It eventually becomes part of the umbilical cord. Also known as the "yolk stalk."

Yolk Sac — Nutrient-filled sac formed by and adjacent to the outer layer of the early developing embryo.

Zygote — Product of fertilization when the egg and sperm fuse together.

■■■ NORMAL MEASUREMENTS

Mean Sac Diameter (MSD):
Length + Depth + Width ÷ 3

Gestational Sac
- Visible with transvaginal sonography when MSD is 2 to 3 mm, which corresponds to 4 weeks' gestational age (GA)
- Visible transabdominally when MSD is 5 mm, which corresponds to 5 gestational weeks

Gestational Age (GA) in Days
- MSD (in millimeters) + 30 = GA (in days)
- MSD of 6 mm corresponds to 36 gestational days

Crown Rump Length (CRL)
- Long axis measurement of the embryo
- CRL increases by approximately 1 mm/day

Yolk Sac
- Maximum diameter is 5 to 6 mm, which corresponds to a CRL of 30 to 45 mm

Nuchal Translucency (NT) 11.3 – 13.6 wks
- First trimester, anteroposterior (AP) measurement of the fluid collection at the back of the fetus' neck
- Normal measurement: 2.5 to 3.0 mm

This chapter and Chapter 23 describe the anatomy, physiology, embryology, and ultrasound appearance of the embryo/fetus and its support structures at various stages of pregnancy. Chapter 24 discusses high-risk pregnancies and associated ultrasound studies and associated ultrasound-guided procedures.

Based on a 28-day menstrual cycle, the 1st trimester of pregnancy is defined as 12 weeks after the 1st day of the last menstrual period. Typically, the term **gestational age (GA)** is synonymous with menstrual age and is used to date the age of a pregnancy.

...a remarkable
...embryonic, and
...g the normal
...in early preg-
...interpretable

...of the female
...nancy begins
...2nd weeks of
...enstrual cycle.
...matures, and
usually on the fourteenth day, ovulation, the release of
an ovum (egg cell) into the genital tract, occurs when
the follicle ruptures (Figure 22-1). This *ovarian phase*, or
cycle, depends on follicle-stimulating hormone (FSH) to
promote follicular maturity and a rise in luteinizing
hormone (LH) to cause ovulation. After ovulation, the
follicle transforms into the corpus luteum, which produces the hormones progesterone and a small amount
of estrogen to prepare the uterus for pregnancy. During
pregnancy the corpus luteum may become enlarged
and fluid filled (Figure 22-2). It can reach greater than
6 cm in diameter by 7 weeks. Thereafter, it gradually
diminishes without complication.

Fertilization usually takes place within 1 day of ovulation, day 15, at the ampulla of the uterine ("fallopian") tube, and is considered complete when the egg
and sperm fuse to form a zygote. The zygote repeatedly
divides and eventually forms a cluster of 16 or more
cells, the morula. The morula exits the fallopian tube
on the 18th or 19th day and enters the uterine cavity.
Endometrial fluid penetrates the cell mass, creating a
blastocyst. The blastocyst consists of an inner cell mass
(or embryoblast) that develops into the embryo and
an outer shell of cells, or trophoblast, that later forms
the placenta. The placenta is a temporary maternal-
fetal organ that provides nutrition, waste removal, gas
exchange, and immune and endocrine support required
for the developing embryo/fetus. It is delivered with the
fetus at birth.

The blastocyst's inner embryoblast layer will also
develop into the secondary yolk sac, the amnion, and
umbilical cord. The outer trophoblast layer eventually
creates the chorionic membranes of the fetal portion of
the placenta. The blastocyst cavity converts the inner cell
mass into an embryonic disk, a flattened inner cell mass
from which the embryo begins to differentiate. A primary
yolk sac filled with nutrients forms on the anterior
aspect of the embryonic disk. It provides nourishment
for the early embryo and serves as the developmental
circulatory system before internal circulation.

By day 20 or 21, the blastocyst begins to implant into
the decidualized endometrium. Decidua is the term
applied to the gravid, or pregnant, endometrium. It is
the functional reaction of the endometrial lining to
pregnancy. The endometrium becomes thick and edematous from vascular and structural changes to accommodate embryo implantation (Figure 22-3). By the 28th
day, the blastocyst has become fully embedded within
the myometrium of the uterus and implantation is
complete.

Weeks 4 to 5
During week 4, initiation of placental development
occurs, resulting in a primitive uteroplacental circulation. The primary yolk sac regresses as the secondary
yolk sac forms between the amnion (innermost membrane of the embryo) and the chorion (outermost tissues
of the embryo). A bilaminar embryonic disk distinguishes itself from the embryoblast layer. It lies between
the secondary yolk sac and developing amniotic cavity.
Sonographers refer to this anatomic relationship as the
double bleb sign (Figure 22-4).

Also during week 4, as the embryo grows and elongates, a long, hollow tube is formed on the anterior
surface of the embryo that develops into the alimentary
canal. The canal is the rudimentary gastrointestinal
system and divides into the foregut (the most superior
end), midgut, and hindgut (the most inferior end). The
foregut will eventually give rise to the pharynx, esophagus, stomach, and proximal duodenum. It will also give
rise through outpouching to the liver and pancreas. The
midgut gives rise to the small intestine and a portion of
the colon. The hindgut eventually develops into the
distal colon, rectum, and portions of the bladder.

The neuroplate, the most primitive component of the
neurologic axis, develops after 4 to 5 weeks. This plate
forms the neurotube, which eventually forms the brain
and spinal cord.

The fetal lungs begin development as small paired
buds arising from the anterior surface of the most superior portion of the tube that becomes the alimentary
canal. The fetal lung buds are present at about 5 weeks
GA and form numerous branching buds, which grow
and increase in number until 17 weeks of gestation.

Toward the end of week 5, the bilaminar embryonic
disk changes into a trilaminar structure (3 layers: endoderm, mesoderm, ectoderm).

Weeks 6 to 10: Embryonic Phase
The *embryonic phase*, weeks 6 to 10, is considered a critical phase of human development. Major structures
begin to form, and although organ function is minimal,
the primitive heart starts to beat at the beginning of
the 6th week. Between approximately 5 to 7 weeks'
gestation (embryonic disk length of 2 to 10 mm) the

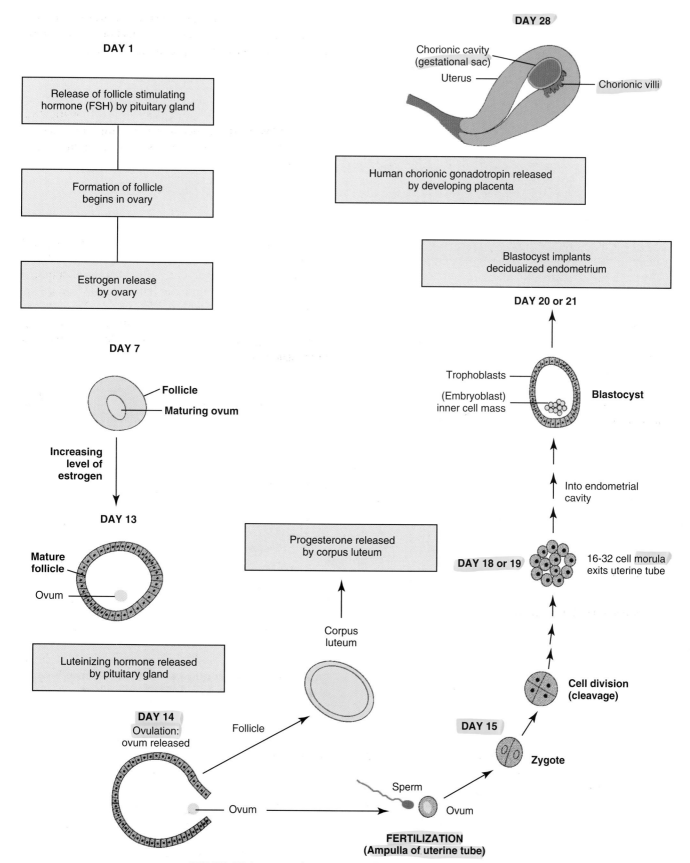

FIGURE 22-1 Normal events in the first 4 weeks of gestation.

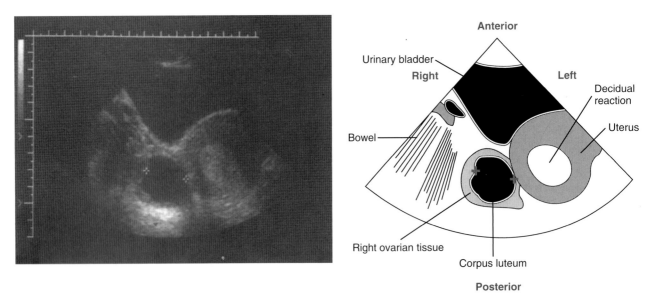

FIGURE 22-2 **Corpus Luteum.** During pregnancy, the corpus luteum may become enlarged and cystic, as seen in this image.

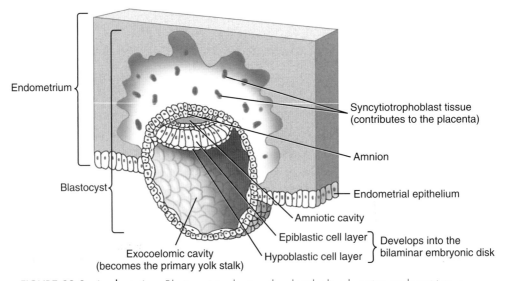

FIGURE 22-3 **Implantation.** Blastocyst implanting the decidualized uterine endometrium.

heartbeat can be visualized by ultrasound. The embryonic heart begins as two tubes that eventually fuse along their midlines to form a very primitive tubular heart. Later in the 1st trimester, the four-chambered heart is formed by a series of folds and fusions of tissues in the tubular pump. Initially, the heart is required only to move blood across the circulatory system of the yolk sac. After development of the four chambers, internal circulation begins and the heart pumps fetal blood throughout the growing embryo/fetus and its placenta.

Week 6
By week 6 the neurotube has developed into the primitive embryonic brain, which consists of 3 segments:

forebrain (the *prosencephalon*), midbrain (the *mesencephalon*), and hindbrain (the *rhombencephalon*). The forebrain develops into the cerebrum, lateral ventricle, and thalamus. The midbrain becomes the adult midbrain and forms the aqueduct of Sylvius. The hindbrain grows into the adult pons, medulla, and cerebellum and forms the fourth ventricle.

Weeks 7 to 8
While it is growing, the embryo folds on itself along its different surfaces to differentiate anatomy. Two lateral folds lead to the formation of the anterior and lateral abdominal walls. At the same time, the midgut forms from the roof of the yolk sac, thereby reducing the

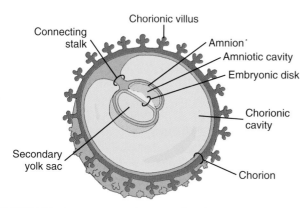

FIGURE 22-4 **4 to 5 Weeks' GA.** The chorionic cavity (gestational sac) measures 5 mm in diameter and is well visualized sonographically. The bilaminar embryonic disk is situated between the newly formed amniotic cavity and secondary yolk sac. This anatomic relationship is described in sonography as the "double bleb sign."

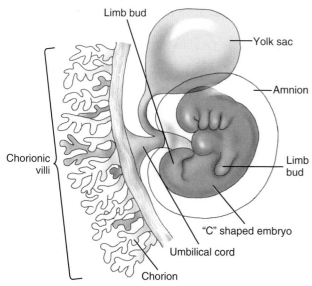

FIGURE 22-5 **7 to 8 Weeks' GA.** The umbilical cord resolves, and the embryo changes from flat to C-shaped.

connection between them to a narrow yolk stalk. At approximately 7 or 8 weeks, the yolk stalk fuses with the omphalomesenteric duct (vitelline duct) to become the umbilical cord. The **umbilical cord** is the connection between the embryo/fetus and the placenta. It consists of two arteries and one vein through which embryonic/fetal blood passes to and from the placenta. With development the amnion expands to form an external covering for the umbilical cord and embryo. At this point the appearance of the embryo changes from flat and trilaminar to a C-shaped embryo with limb buds (Figure 22-5). The heart comes to lie ventrally and the brain cranially.

Week 8
Mineralization of the fetal skeleton begins at 8 weeks. During weeks 8 to 11 the small bowel usually herniates out of the embryo at the base of the umbilical cord. This is a normal event, and the bowel retracts into the embryo by 12 weeks of development.

Week 10
Functional fetal kidney tissue appears at approximately 10 weeks. The production of fetal urine does not occur until early in the 2nd trimester. (The fetal kidneys and bladder are discussed in Chapter 23.) By the end of week 10, major organ systems are established and the embryo demonstrates human features.

Weeks 11 to 12: Fetal Phase
Weeks 11 and 12, the final 2 weeks of the 1st trimester, begin the *fetal phase*. Growth is rapid, and organ development continues. Fetal intestinal activity begins the eleventh week of development; fetal swallowing usually starts in week 12. The skull and femur are adequately mineralized by 11.5 to 12 weeks. The fetal head is disproportionately large compared to the body and constitutes half the length. As development continues, the head and body subsequently become more proportional.

DEVELOPMENT OF THE PLACENTA
As discussed, the decidualized endometrium becomes thick and edematous from vascular and structural changes to accommodate embryo implantation and development of the embryo. During these changes, the decidualized endometrium differentiates into 3 distinct areas: *decidua basalis, capsularis,* and *parietalis,* all of which, except the deepest, are shed at parturition (birth) (Figure 22-6).
- The **decidua basalis** is the portion of thick decidua at the implantation site, which makes it the maternal portion and deepest layer of the placenta.
- The **decidua capsularis** is a thin portion of endometrium that overlies the section of gestational sac facing the uterine cavity.
- The **decidua parietalis** (or decidua vera) is the remaining endometrium, or peripheral portion, which is unoccupied by the implanted ovum.

The fetal components of the placenta are the **chorionic villi**, or finger-like projections of the trophoblast layer (outer cell layer of the blastocyst), which extend into the deciduate endometrium (Figure 22-7). Some of these villi degenerate to form a membrane-like structure, the smooth chorion (chorion laeve, or chorionic membrane). The remaining villi comprise the chorion frondosum, the portion of chorion at the implantation site that actively invades the decidua basalis to establish nutrition for the embryo. The chorion frondosum villi

At 12wks placenta: thickness 1-2cm
full term: 2.5-4cm (20cm diameter)

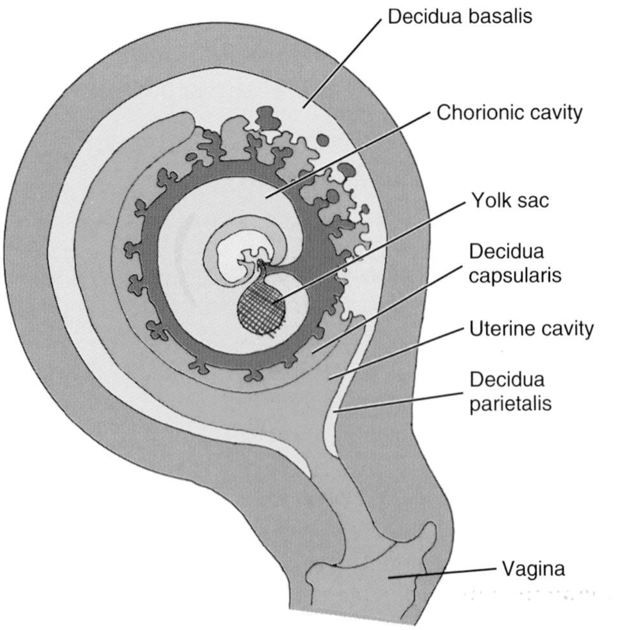

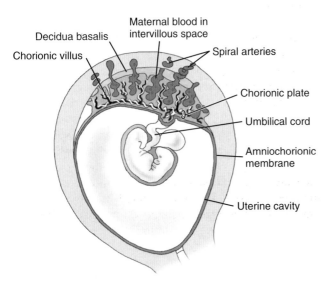

FIGURE 22-6 **Decidualized Endometrium.** Differentiation of the gravid endometrium into decidua basalis (implantation site), capsularis (overlies sac facing uterine cavity), and parietalis (remainder of endometrium).

FIGURE 22-7 **Placenta Development.** Chorionic villi invade the decidua basalis, forming embryo-maternal circulation. Resulting intervillous spaces receive maternal blood from the spiral arteries that surround and perfuse villi containing fetal blood.

are surrounded by maternal tissue called the lacunar network. The lacunar network is a tissue extremely rich in small blood vessels; after contact with the villi, this tissue breaks down and forms small pools of maternal blood, or lacunae. It is the contact of the villi of the embryonic circulatory system with the maternal lacunae

that facilitates the transfer of oxygen and metabolites and the transfer of carbon dioxide and waste products.

Each chorionic villus branches to form groups of villi. Large groups of villi are known as cotyledons, and groups of cotyledons form between one and five lobules. As the gestation increases in size, so do its requirements for nutrition and waste product removal. The placenta also increases in size to keep up with this increasing demand. At 12 weeks, the placenta is between 1 and 2 cm in thickness. By 40 weeks of gestation, the placenta may be between 2.5 and 4 cm in thickness. The diameter of a term placenta can be as much as 20 cm.

The placenta may be divided into 3 basic areas: the *chorionic plate*, the *base plate*, and the *placental substance*.

1. The *chorionic plate* is the portion toward the inside of the sac that touches the amniotic membrane.
2. The *base plate*, or basal layer, is the portion on the outside that touches the uterus.
3. The *placental substance* is the placental material between the basal layer and the chorionic plate.

Functional circulatory groups separate the lobes of the placenta. Small venules course through the substance of the placenta, becoming progressively larger as they converge, eventually forming a single umbilical vein. Conversely, the maternal blood, which supplies the oxygen and nutrients and removes waste products and carbon dioxide, arrives at the placenta via two umbilical arteries that enter the substance of the placenta and progressively divide with the villi to form even smaller spiral arterioles that coil their way up to the base of the placenta from the endometrial layer of the uterus. As previously discussed, the single umbilical vein and the two umbilical arteries form the umbilical cord that connects the fetus to the placenta.

The placenta also functions as an endocrine gland. It produces **human chorionic gonadotropin (hCG)**, which communicates to the rest of the body that a gestation is present within the uterus. It also produces estrogen and progesterone throughout the pregnancy.

DEVELOPMENT OF FETAL MEMBRANES

Prior discussion included that two fetal membranes surround the embryo, the amnion and the chorion. The amnion or amniotic membrane develops from the inner blastocyst layer and enlarges to enclose the **amniotic cavity/sac**, which is separated from the secondary yolk sac by the small bilaminar embryonic disk (see Figure 22-4). Figure 22-8 illustrates how the amnion and amniotic cavity enlarge to accommodate the developing embryo. The amniotic membrane remains attached to the embryo at the cord insertion site and ultimately covers the umbilical cord. The yolk sac, within the shrinking chorionic cavity, moves away from the embryo. The amnion and its cavity grow rapidly,

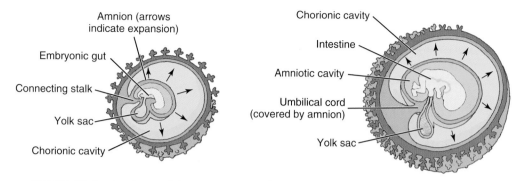

FIGURE 22-8 **Amnion and Amniotic Cavity.** The amnion or amniotic membrane enlarges to enclose the amniotic cavity.

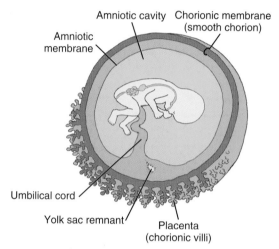

FIGURE 22-9 **Chorion and Chorionic Cavity.** During development, the chorionic membrane and chorionic cavity shrink while the amniotic membrane and amniotic cavity enlarge to accommodate the developing embryo.

containing the developing embryo and the amniotic fluid that "bathes" the embryo/fetus throughout its course of development and protects it from injury. The amnion consists of four connective layers and one epithelial layer; it is not a vascular membrane.

As mentioned, the chorionic membrane (smooth chorion, or chorion laeve) develops from the outer blastocyst layer. This vascular structure encloses the **chorionic cavity**, which surrounds the amnion, yolk sac, and embryo. Figure 22-9 shows that as development continues, the chorionic membrane and cavity shrink; the amniotic membrane and cavity enlarge. Eventually, the membranes fuse, usually after 16 weeks. Complete fusion of the amniotic and chorionic membranes occurs with obliteration of the chorionic cavity.

DEVELOPMENT OF AMNIOTIC FLUID

Amniotic fluid is the liquid enclosed by the amnion. As it surrounds and bathes the embryo/fetus, amniotic fluid has several important functions:

- Permits symmetric growth of the embryo/fetus
- Prevents adhesions from forming in the fetal membranes
- Cushions the embryo/fetus and acts as a shock absorber
- Helps to maintain proper temperature of the embryo
- Allows normal development of the respiratory, gastrointestinal, and musculoskeletal systems
- Helps to prevent infection
- Possibly serves as a source of nutrients for the developing embryo

The amount of fluid present in the amniotic cavity is calculated as the **amniotic fluid volume (AFV)**, which depends on the balance between amniotic fluid production and its removal or absorption. The AFV reflects the state of gestational well-being. In fact, many abnormalities are associated with marked increases (polyhydramnios) or decreases (oligohydramnios) in the AFV. (Various methods of calculating AFV are discussed in Chapter 23.)

During pregnancy, the structures responsible for production and passage of fluid into the amniotic cavity are the chorion frondosum, chorionic and amniotic membranes, skin, and respiratory and urinary tracts. Structures involved in the reduction of amniotic fluid are the gastrointestinal system and the amniotic-chorionic interface. Intramembranous and transmembranous pathways are also involved with the exchange, across membranes, of amniotic fluid and fetal blood (intramembranous) and amniotic fluid and maternal blood (transmembranous).

The 1st trimester contributes very little in the production of amniotic fluid. Electrolytes, water, urea, and creatinine pass freely through the membranes and into the cavity. Later, amniotic fluid is produced primarily by the lungs and kidneys. Fetal lung fluid leaves the trachea during breathing, becoming part of the amniotic fluid. The exact amount is unknown. Urine production also becomes part of amniotic fluid. Urine contribution is estimated at approximately 30% of fetal body weight daily.

The quantity of amniotic fluid increases until about 30 weeks of gestation. At that point the volume of fluid begins to decrease considerably until delivery. The reduction of amniotic fluid is due primarily to gastrointestinal activity (swallowing amniotic fluid) and absorption of amniotic fluid into fetal blood perfusing the surface of the placenta. Fetal swallowing removes about half of the daily urine produced. At term, the fetus may swallow up to 50% of the AFV. It should be noted that at one time the respiratory system was considered part of AFV reduction; however, the current theory is that the lungs do not provide a pathway for the absorption of fluid in the normal fetus.

SONOGRAPHIC APPEARANCE OF FIRST TRIMESTER ANATOMY

Transvaginal sonography has made it possible to routinely image early embryonic/fetal structures. A sonographer needs to be familiar with embryology and how it presents sonographically to be able to distinguish normal and abnormal development. Early identification of anomalies influences decisions about pregnancy termination or fetal therapy.

Gestational sac is the term used by sonologists to describe the fluid-filled cavity of an intrauterine pregnancy during the 1st trimester.

Gestational Sac Appearance

The gestational sac is the first fundamental sonographic finding in early pregnancy. Transvaginal transducers can visualize the gestational sac as early as 3 to 5 weeks. Normally, it is located within the fundus or body of the uterus and appears as a very small, round or oval, anechoic, fluid-filled collection enclosed by echogenic walls (the bright choriodecidual reaction) right next to the centrally located, bright, linear endometrial cavity. There should be no displacement or change in size of the endometrial cavity at this early stage. This sonographic finding is referred to by some as the intradecidual sign.

Double Sac Sign

As the normal gestational sac enlarges, it has a distinct sonographic appearance known as the double sac sign, when the fluid-filled gestational sac and the fluid-filled uterine cavity are identified together. This sign distinguishes a pseudo sac, associated with pregnancies outside the uterus (ectopic pregnancy), from a gestational sac. Figure 22-10 demonstrates the double sac sign. Two bright concentric lines are seen surrounding a portion of the gestational sac. The line closest to the sac is the decidua capsularis (DC)—smooth chorion. The peripheral line is the decidua parietalis (DP). The uterine cavity is the anechoic, fluid-filled space between these two lines. The uterine cavity is always a potential anechoic space containing a small amount of fluid visualized between the DC and DP. The decidua basalis (DB) combines with the chorion frondosum at the gestational sac-endometrium interface; it appears hyperechoic relative to adjacent structures and thick due to developing placental tissue.

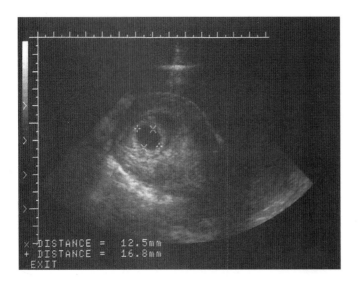

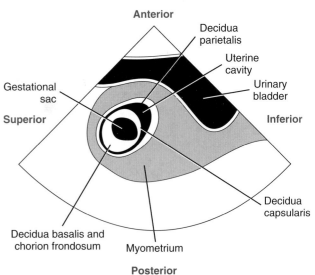

FIGURE 22-10 **Double Sac Sign.** When the fluid-filled gestational sac and the fluid-filled uterine cavity are identified together it is termed the *double sac sign*, a sign that distinguishes a pseudo sac from a gestational sac.

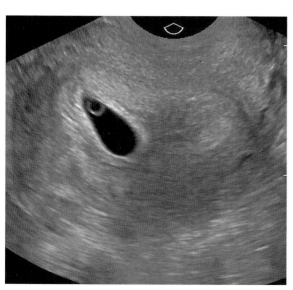
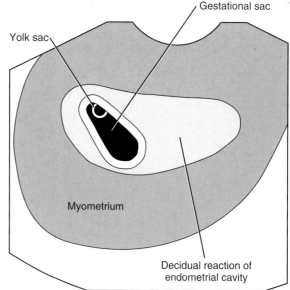

FIGURE 22-11 **Yolk Sac.** The secondary yolk sac is the first structure identified within the gestational sac. Sonographic identification of the yolk sac confirms pregnancy.

Yolk Sac Appearance

The secondary yolk sac is the first structure identified within the gestational sac. As seen in Figure 22-11, the yolk sac appears small and round with bright, well-defined walls and an anechoic fluid-filled center. Normally, it measures less than 6 mm. Transvaginally, the yolk sac can be identified as early as the 5th week. Using a transabdominal approach, the yolk sac should be visible by the 7th week.

Sonographic visualization of the yolk sac confirms pregnancy and, like the double sac sign, rules out a pseudo sac. The yolk sac also serves as a landmark for locating the embryonic disk and cardiac activity. A faint, flickering motion visualized adjacent to the yolk sac represents neurologically active heart tissue. It is often seen before the embryo can be sonographically distinguished.

As previously discussed, the yolk sac and embryo retreat from one another as the amnion and its cavity enlarge and the chorionic cavity obliterates. When a distinguishable area is seen on the periphery of the yolk sac, the embryonic disk has differentiated itself from the embryoblast layer. Occasionally, during the later portion of the 5th week the embryonic disk can be seen lying between the yolk sac and developing amniotic membrane. When these structures are visualized together, they are described as the *"double bleb"* or *"double bleb sign."* With developmental changes, the double bleb is not detectable after the 7th week. When the yolk sac comes to lie outside the amniotic cavity, it remains attached to the embryo by the **vitelline (omphalomesenteric) duct.** Although small, the duct can be sonographically identified as the bright, linear connection between the embryo and yolk sac, surrounded by anechoic fluid.

Embryo Appearance

At 5 to 6 gestational weeks the early developing embryo is evident with transvaginal scanning. At this point, it is approximately 1 to 2 mm in length, ovoid or shapeless, and hugs the wall of the gestational sac.

As seen in Figure 22-12, the embryo appears as a small, highly echogenic, focal thickening along the bright outside edge of the yolk sac, surrounded by anechoic chorionic fluid.

At 6 gestational weeks, it is not possible to distinguish the embryo crown (cephalic end/cephalic pole) from the rump (caudal end/caudal pole), but by the 7th week, as seen in Figure 22-13, the embryo begins to assume a shape that reveals the head at one end and rump at the other.

Fetal limb buds should start to be visible by 8 weeks as the embryo develops a C-shaped configuration (see Figure 22-5). The crown becomes prominent and contains the anechoic developing **rhombencephalon** (cystic hindbrain), as seen in Figure 22-14. In some cases, a normal tail-like appendage that eventually regresses is identifiable at the rump.

Figure 22-15 shows a 9.5-week-old embryo. All four developing limbs can be seen, as well as the previously mentioned normal protruding caudate pole referred to as the *embryonic tail* that resolves with further development.

Figure 22-16 shows a 10.6-week-old gestation with normal gut herniation into the base of the umbilical cord. Also, at this stage of development the head

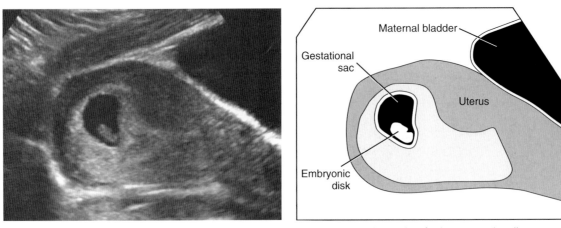

FIGURE 22-12   **The Embryo.** The early embryo (embryonic disk) is identified sonographically as a small, bright, focal thickening along the highly echogenic outside edge of the yolk sac.

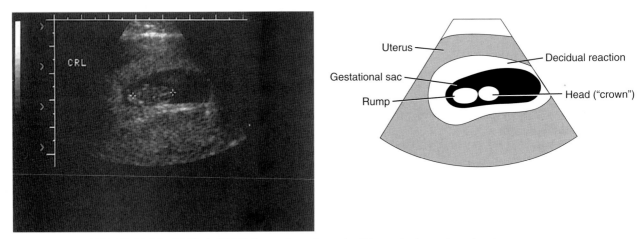

FIGURE 22-13   **7-Week-Old Embryo.** As early as the 7th week, the embryo begins to assume a shape that reveals the head or crown at one end and rump at the other.

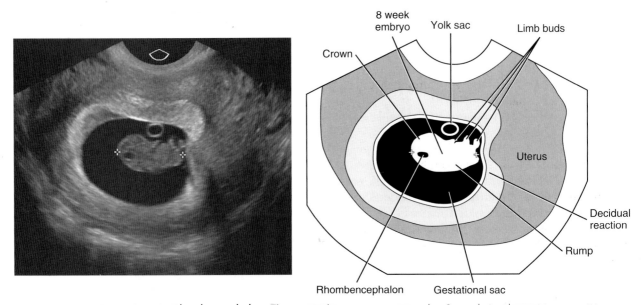

FIGURE 22-14   **Rhombencephalon.** The crown becomes prominent by 8 weeks and contains the developing rhombencephalon.

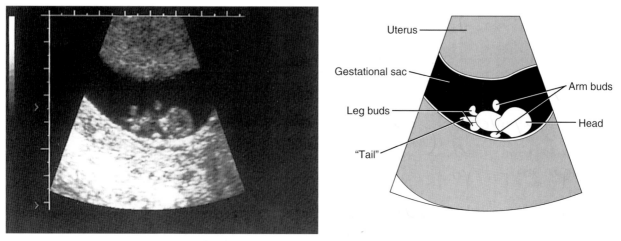

FIGURE 22-15 **9.5-Week-Old Gestation.** Note how the 4 developing limbs are seen and normal protruding caudate pole ("tail") are observed at this stage of development.

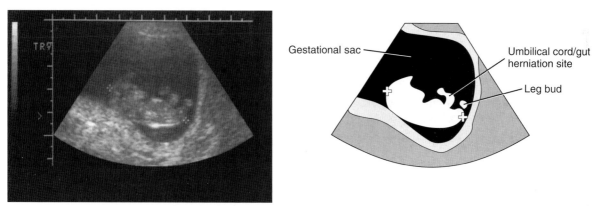

FIGURE 22-16 **Normal Gut Herniation in a 10.6-Week-Old Gestation.** Note how the head becomes disproportionately larger than the body at this stage of development.

becomes disproportionately large compared to the body and constitutes half the length. As growth continues, the head and body subsequently become more proportional.

During week 10, the fluid-filled anechoic stomach and homogeneous embryonic liver can be seen, and the brain may appear anechoic. By 12 weeks, echogenic brain structures can be visualized within the fetal skull.

Individual fingers and toes are usually identified by 11 weeks. The anechoic, urine-filled bladder might be seen by this time and should always be visualized by week 13.

Umbilical Cord Appearance

The umbilical cord is well visualized at 8 weeks. Figure 22-17 illustrates how the cord appears thick and about

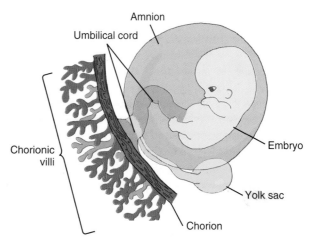

FIGURE 22-17 Week 8 of development.

Umbilical Cord diameter ✗ 2 cm

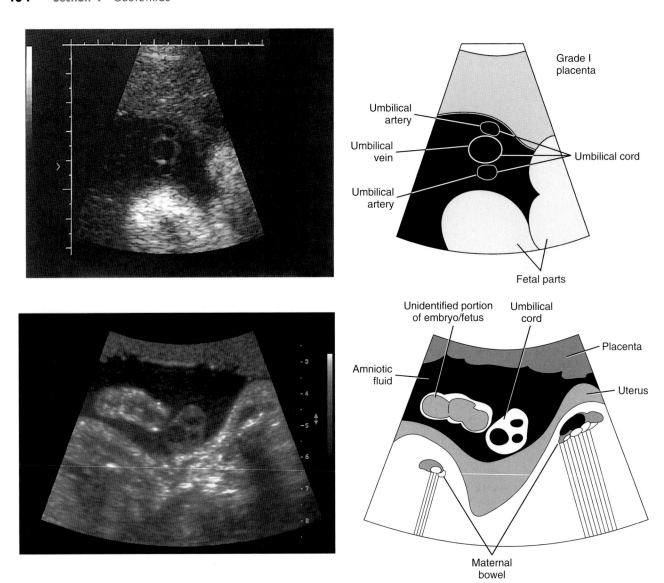

FIGURE 22-18 **Umbilical Cord.** Short axis umbilical cord views. (Bottom image, Scan courtesy the University of Virginia Health System, Department of Radiology, Division of Ultrasound, Charlottesville, Virginia.)

Vein Runs Sup.
Arteries Run Inf

as long as the embryo. The cord grows at a rate similar to that of the embryo. As it increases in length, the cord develops multiple spiral turns thought to be caused by helic arterial muscle layers.

As mentioned, the cord is composed of two umbilical arteries and one umbilical vein that appear anechoic with walls that are thick and bright. The normal diameter of the cord is less than 2 cm. The two images in Figure 22-18 are the cord viewed in short axis. The cord presents as one large anechoic circle with thick hyperechoic walls (the vein), flanked by two small anechoic circles with thick hyperechoic walls (the arteries).

Umbilical cord blood vessels enter the embryo/fetus at the umbilicus and immediately diverge there.

The umbilical vein runs superiorly to join embryo/fetal portal circulation. The umbilical arteries course inferiorly along both sides of the urinary bladder and can be differentiated from dilated ureters with color Doppler.

Placenta Appearance

What begins as a diffusely thick echogenic ring surrounding the early gestational sac changes to a bright focal area of thickening, the chorionic frondosum, which eventually becomes the placenta. Figure 22-19 clearly shows the differentiated deciduas, including the decidua basalis, which combines with the chorionic frondosum to become the placenta.

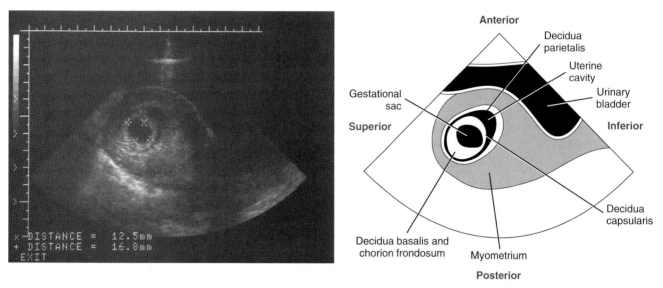

FIGURE 22-19 **Early Placenta Development.** The deciduas are clearly differentiated including the decidua basalis that combines with the chorion frondosum to become the placenta.

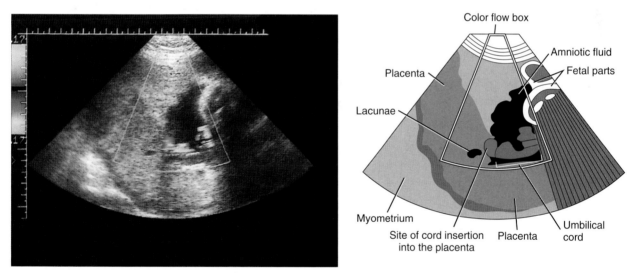

FIGURE 22-20 Color-flow image demonstrating the placental cord insertion site.

The placenta appears homogeneous to heterogeneous. It is primarily medium-level, homogeneous echoes that are interrupted by the retroplacental complex early in the 2nd trimester of pregnancy and later by retroplacental and intraplacental arteries. The homogeneous substance of the placenta is further interrupted by "insertion" of the umbilical cord shown in the color-flow image in Figure 22-20. Ultrasound identification of the cord insertion into the placenta is important for certain invasive obstetric procedures, such as fetal blood sampling. The area is considered optimal because the cord is fixed at this location, making the needle approach more accurate.

Membrane Appearance

Sonographic identification of the amnion and its cavity confirms the presence of an intrauterine gestational sac. Its size and appearance determine whether an early pregnancy is progressing normally. The amniotic membrane is very thin and, as a rule, is not visualized before 7 gestational weeks. Once in a while, however, as previously stated, it is identifiable during the later portion of the 5th week as a small, round, echogenic ring containing anechoic fluid; it is contiguous with the embryonic disk but on the opposite side of the yolk sac (see Figure 22-4). The yolk sac is easily distinguishable from the amniotic membrane because it is thicker and more

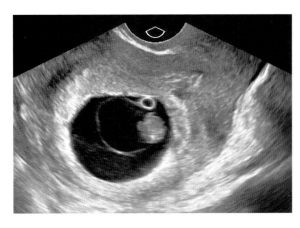
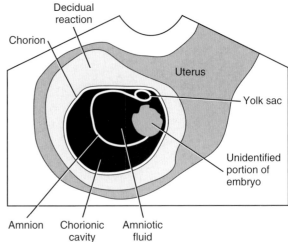

FIGURE 22-21 Sonographic identification of the amnion and its cavity confirms the presence of an intrauterine gestational sac.

echogenic. As mentioned, the term *double bleb sign* has been used to describe the sonographic appearance of this early anatomic relationship.

By 7 weeks the amniotic membrane has developed beyond the double bleb sign. The amnion is best visualized with transvaginal transducers and high gain settings and, as seen in Figure 22-21, it appears as a thin, bright, outline of the anechoic, fluid-filled amniotic cavity. Before fusion of the amnion and chorion, the chorionic cavity can be appreciated sonographically only when the amniotic membrane is visible. Another sonographic marker of the chorionic cavity is the distinctive chorionic fluid, which is very slightly hyperechoic relative to the appearance of amniotic fluid. Figure 22-21 also shows the low-level echoes in chorionic fluid that are probably from increased concentrations of protein and albumin within the chorionic cavity. When the amnion is not visualized, it does not indicate an abnormality, and when the amnion completely fuses with the chorion, between 12 and 16 weeks, the amnion is no longer visible.

Amniotic Fluid Appearance

Amniotic fluid appears anechoic; however, it is not unusual to view free-floating particles in the fluid. In most cases this occurs early or midway into the second trimester of pregnancy. The particles are believed to be fetal vernix (flakes of skin) with no pathologic significance.

As mentioned, the amniotic fluid volume is a sonographic marker for fetal well-being. In the past, sonographic assessment of amniotic fluid amounts was subjective. Extremes of too little fluid (oligohydramnios) or too much fluid (polyhydramnios) were fairly easy for experienced sonologists and sonographers

to recognize; yet there were no criteria for use by less-experienced examiners. The importance of amniotic fluid in fetal development brought about the development of methods to accurately assess the AFV throughout pregnancy. (Because these assessments are more applicable to 2nd and 3rd trimester gestations, they will be discussed in Chapter 23.)

SONOGRAPHIC DETERMINATION OF GESTATIONAL AGE

Every gestation begins as a single cell, but eventually individual differences in growth rate give rise to a range of sizes and biologic variations, all of which are normal for a given GA. Early in the pregnancy these individual differences are much less pronounced than they are later. Therefore the most accurate time to date a pregnancy is during the 1st trimester, when variations are relatively minimal.

Measurement guidelines for dating pregnancy during the 1st trimester are:
- Gestational sac (no yolk sac, embryo, or heartbeat) at 5 weeks
- Gestational sac with yolk sac (no embryo, no heartbeat) at 5.5 weeks
- Gestational sac with yolk sac (living embryo too small to measure) at 6 weeks
- Crown rump length (CRL) measurement of the embryo from 6 weeks + days to 12 weeks

Several methods, such as *sac volumes* and *mean diameters*, have been developed to determine gestational sac size to calculate GA:
- **Mean sac diameter (MSD).** Many institutions use the MSD method (Figure 22-22). Three measurements of the gestational sac—length, depth, and width—are obtained, summed, and then divided by

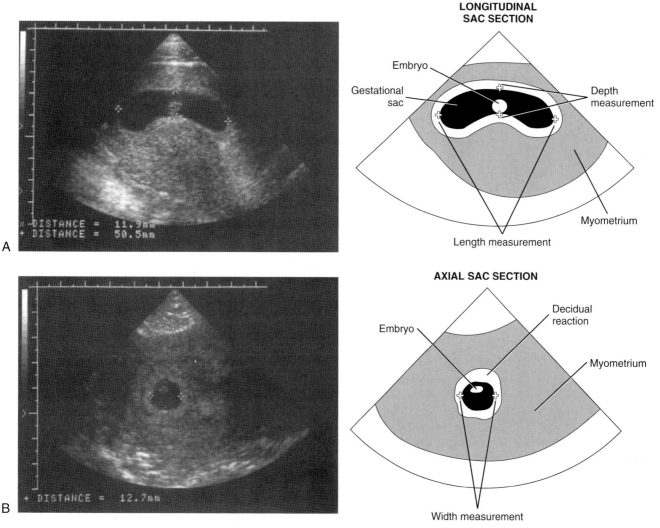

FIGURE 22-22 **Mean Sac Diameter (MSD).** Three measurements of the gestational sac (length, depth, and width) are obtained, summed, and then divided by 3 to determine the MSD. Gestational age (GA) (in days) is calculated by adding 30 to the MSD (in millimeters): MSD + 30 = GA (in days). **A,** How to correctly measure the length and depth of the gestational sac on a longitudinal section. **B,** How to correctly measure the width of the gestational sac on an axial section.

3 to determine the MSD. Length and depth are measured on a longitudinal section of the gestational sac as demonstrated in the top image below. GA (in days) is calculated by adding 30 to the MSD (in millimeters): **MSD + 30 = GA (in days)**

- **Mean internal diameter**. To accurately obtain the mean internal diameter of the gestational sac, measurement calipers are placed at the fluid-tissue interface; the wall (the bright choriodecidual reaction) is not included in the measurement.
- **Crown rump length**. CRL is commonly accepted as the most accurate assessment of GA. As development continues in the 1st trimester, the CRL and amniotic sac diameter increase 1 mm per day; it is interesting to note that these measurements are equal throughout the 1st trimester. *Measurement guidelines for CRL are:*

○ *Embryonic disk length:* (not possible to distinguish the crown from the rump) at 6+ weeks not to exceed 8 gestational weeks
○ *Neck rump measurement:* (prominent head flexion causing C shape of embryo makes longest axis from neck to rump) at 6+ to 8 gestational weeks
○ *CRL:* (head extends, making true crown rump long axis) at 8+ to 12 gestational weeks

The CRL measurement is reported to be accurate to within ±4.7 days for dating pregnancies. CRL of the embryo/fetus is measured from the top of the head (crown) to the middle of the buttocks (rump). Figure 22-23 demonstrates correct caliper placement for CRL measurement. The CRL measured 36.9 mm, which correlates to a 10.7-week GA. Several methodology tables are available that convert CRL (in millimeters) to GA.

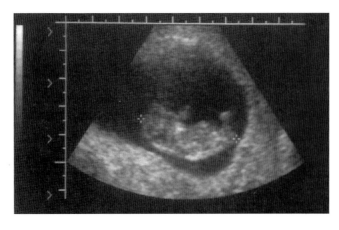
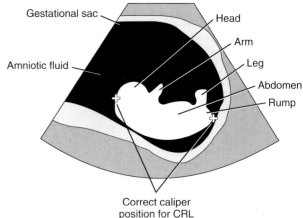

FIGURE 22-23 **Crown Rump Length (CRL).** The CRL measurement is said to be the most accurate measurement for dating pregnancies. Note that correct caliper placement is from the top of the head or crown to the middle of the buttocks or rump.

As development continues into the second trimester, CRL measurements are replaced by biparietal measurements of the fetal head and femur length measurements to determine GA.

SONOGRAPHIC APPLICATIONS

Ultrasound can be used to confirm or rule out a variety of things during the 1st trimester. The most common indications for a 1st trimester ultrasound are:

- **Gestational age (GA):** To confirm GA for patients who require invasive studies such as chorionic villi sampling, elective repeat cesarean delivery, or elective termination of pregnancy.
- **Vaginal spotting or bleeding:** To rule out ectopic pregnancy, threatened abortion, abortion in progress, or incomplete or complete abortion.
- **Large for dates:** To rule out a mass, a multiple gestation, a fetal anomaly, or an incorrect menstrual history.
- **Small for dates:** To rule out embryonic/fetal death, blighted ovum, ectopic pregnancy, fetal anomaly, or incorrect menstrual history.
- **Pelvic pain:** To rule out a mass, a placental abruption, or an ectopic pregnancy.
- **Fetal growth:** To determine cases of severe preeclampsia, diabetes mellitus, renal disease, chronic hypertension, or fetal malnutrition.
- **Substance abuse or prescription drugs early in pregnancy:** To rule out embryonic/fetal anomalies and determine fetal growth rate.
- **Fetal presentation:** To determine when presenting part cannot be established in labor.
- **Trauma:** To determine embryonic/fetal well-being.
- **History of miscarriage:** To determine the status and well-being of an early gestation.
- **History of multiple gestations or fertility drug treatment:** To determine the number of gestations.

- **Fetal risk for aneuploidy:** The nuchal translucency (NT) measurement is used in a combination with a maternal serum screen and maternal age to determine the fetal risk for aneuploidy, an abnormal chromosome number. The NT measurement is of the fluid that normally collects at the back of the fetus' neck during the 1st trimester between 11.3 and 13.6 weeks of gestation. A magnified image of the fetal head, neck, and upper thorax in a midsagittal plane should be used to obtain the NT measurement. The head should not be flexed or extended, and the spinal column should face the bottom of the imaging screen. Calipers must be placed on the inner borders of the widest portion of the NT. Figure 22-24 demonstrates the correct caliper placement for the NT measurement.

NORMAL VARIATIONS

- **Uterine synechia (amniotic sheets):** Synechiae are membranes formed from scarring or adhesions secondary to surgery or infection. They extend from the uterus with amnion and chorion growing around them. The membrane is 4 layers thick (2 layers of amnion and 2 of chorion) and highly echogenic. Synechiae do not attach to the embryo/fetus and are not associated with gestational abnormalities. They should not be confused with amniotic bands. Figure 22-25 shows the bright, membranous appearance of synechiae.
- **Myometrial contraction:** Contractions of the myometrium of the uterus are frequently seen on sonograms and should not be confused with a myoma (uterine mass). Contractions are distinguishable by their inward bulge without disturbing uterine contour and their temporary nature.

NT (inner to inner at widest portion)
11.3 – 13.6 wks.

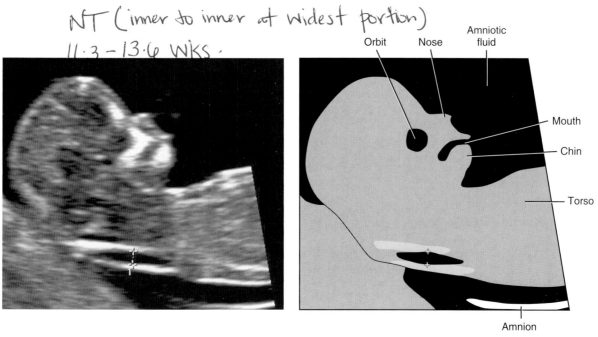

FIGURE 22-24 Nuchal Translucency (NT). Correct caliper placement for the NT measurement.

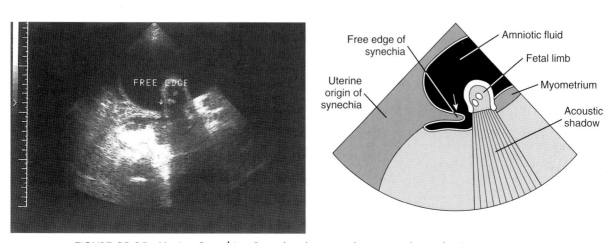

FIGURE 22-25 Uterine Synechia. Considered a normal variation during the 1st trimester, synechiae are membranes formed from scarring or adhesions secondary to surgery or infection. They do not attach to the embryo/fetus and are not associated with gestational abnormalities.

REFERENCE CHARTS

■ ■ ■ ASSOCIATED PHYSICIANS

- **Obstetrician/Gynecologist:** Manages preterm obstetric care and delivers the fetus. This physician is also responsible for the care of the infant immediately following delivery.
- **High-risk obstetrician:** Specializes in the preterm management of women whose pregnancies are at risk due to various medical conditions. This physician delivers the fetus and is responsible for the care of the infant immediately following delivery.
- **Fertility specialist:** Typically, this physician is an obstetrician/gynecologist who specializes in treating disorders of the female reproductive system associated with fertility and pregnancy.
- **Radiologist/Sonologist:** Specializes in the administration and diagnostic interpretation of ultrasound and other imaging modalities.

COMMON DIAGNOSTIC TESTS

- **Pregnancy test:** Detects human chorionic gonadotropin (hCG) levels in urine or blood when pregnancy exists. A lab technician usually runs the test, which is interpreted by a pathologist or obstetrician/gynecologist.
- **Beta-hCG test:** Blood is tested to quantitate the serum level of hCG to estimate gestational age. A lab technician usually runs the test, which is interpreted by a pathologist or obstetrician/gynecologist.
- **Maternal/paternal blood typing:** Determines blood type and whether Rh factor is positive or negative. The Rh factor is a group of autoantibodies that react with a person's own immunoglobulin.
- **Chorionic villus sampling (CVS):** Transabdominal or transcervical penetration of the uterus and amniotic sac for a sample of the chorion covered by villi, which is used for obtaining pertinent genetic information regarding the embryo/fetus.
- **Computed tomography (CT):** Evaluation of fetal and maternal anatomy when sonographic evaluation is indeterminate. CT is generally used as a "last resort" because of the radiation exposure and in most cases is limited to assessment of the acute maternal abdomen.
- **Magnetic resonance imaging (MRI):** Traditionally used to evaluate maternal anatomy during pregnancy and abnormalities such as adnexal masses, which require further characterization beyond the ultrasound findings. Typically, MRI evaluation of the fetus is hindered by fetal motion.

LABORATORY VALUES

- **hCG:** An hCG of 2000 is the level at which a sac will be seen in most normal early pregnancies.
- **Alpha-fetoprotein (AFP):** Found in maternal blood and amniotic fluid. Elevated levels indicate fetal abnormalities or defects.
- **Triple marker screening (AFP, uE3, hCG):** Abnormal levels of alpha-fetoprotein (AFP), unconjugated estriol (uE3), and human chorionic gonadotropin (hCG) are indicators of certain embryonic/fetal abnormalities, possible multifetal gestations, and when combined with maternal age, screening markers for Down syndrome (the most common cause of malformation and mental retardation in newborns).

VASCULATURE

Internal iliac artery—Paired uterine arteries—Multiple arcuate arteries—Arcuate branches enter the endometrium—Spiral arteries located within decidua basalis invade trophoblastic chorionic villi—Trophoblastic chorionic villi plug the spiral arteries and erode small portions of the decidua, which enlarges to form intervillous spaces—Intervillous spaces receive maternal blood from spiral arteries.

AFFECTING CHEMICALS

- **Menotropins (Pergonal), urofollitropin (Metrodin), clomiphene citrate (Clomid):** Medications prescribed for infertility to stimulate follicular maturation and induce ovulation. In some cases, these medications have been associated with multifetal gestations.

CHAPTER 23

Second and Third Trimester Obstetrics (13 to 42 Weeks)

BETTY BATES TEMPKIN AND ROBBI R. KING

OBJECTIVES

Describe the sonographic appearance of the placenta and its role in supporting gestation.

Describe the significance of the location of the placenta in relation to the internal cervical os.

Describe the fetal effect on the amniotic fluid volume (AFV).

Describe the sonographic appearance of the development of the fetus from the second to third trimester.

Describe how the placenta functions as an organ of respiration for the fetus.

Describe the sonographic markers used to properly orient the transducer planes for the biparietal diameter (BPD), head circumference (HC), and abdominal circumference (AC).

Be familiar with related tests performed during the second and third trimester.

KEY WORDS

Amniocentesis — Percutaneous penetration of the uterus and amniotic sac for aspiration of a sample of amniotic fluid.

Amniotic Fluid Index (AFI) — In each of four equal quadrants of the gravid uterus, the anteroposterior diameter of the deepest amniotic fluid pocket free of cord and extremities is measured. These four measurements are added together to determine the AFI. A sum of 8 cm is considered normal.

Amniotic Fluid Volume (AFV) — Amount of amniotic fluid in the amniotic cavity. Determined by various methods.

Cerebrospinal Fluid (CSF) — Acts as a protective cushion encasing the brain and spinal cord, and regulates the pressure within the spaces that it fills.

Ductus Arteriosus — Connects the pulmonary artery and the aorta. Closes at (or shortly after) birth.

Foramen Ovale — Opening between the atria of the fetal heart allowing blood to move from right to left in the atrial chambers. May remain patent after birth but is held closed by the normal pressure gradient between left and right atria.

Lacunae — Small pools of maternal blood that surround the chorionic villi in the placenta.

Lecithin-to-Sphingomyelin Ratio (L-S ratio) — Ratio of the chemicals lecithin and sphingomyelin, found in amniotic fluid, which measures the degree of fetal lung development.

Low-Lying Placenta — Also known as "potential placenta," occurs when the placenta's lower edge lies within 0.5–5 cm from the internal cervical os.

Marginal Placenta Previa — Exists when the placenta extends up to, but not above, the internal cervical os.

Meconium — Fetal waste material that accumulates in the bowel during the middle to late second trimester. Consists of swallowed amniotic fluid, glandular secretions, vernix, and bile.

Nuchal Fold (NF) Measurement — Measurement of skin thickness at the back of the fetus' neck between 15 and 22 weeks of gestation to determine the fetal risk estimate for aneuploidy (abnormal number of chromosomes; example is Down syndrome). Increased thickness is indication of increased fetal risk for abnormalities.

Partial ("Incomplete") Placenta Previa — Occurs when a portion of the cervical os is obstructed by overlying placenta.

Placenta — Temporary maternal-fetal organ that provides nutrition, waste removal, gas exchange, and immune and endocrine support required for the developing embryo/fetus. Delivered with the fetus at birth.

Placenta Previa — Condition that occurs when the cervical os is obstructed by an overlying placenta. Placenta previa usually requires cesarean delivery.

Placental Grading — Method of classifying placental maturation according to sonographic appearance.

Placental Volume — Second-trimester predictor for abnormal fetal outcome. Placenta should be approximately equal in thickness (in millimeters) to the gestational age in weeks + 10 mm.

Total ("Complete") Placenta Previa — Occurs when the entire cervical os is obstructed by an overlying placenta.

Vernix — Free-floating particles visualized in amniotic fluid; believed to be flakes of skin and hair with no pathologic significance.

The 2nd and 3rd trimesters of a pregnancy are a progressive period when the organs and organ systems formed during the 1st trimester become fully developed. By the 12th week the majority of organs formed during the 1st trimester are located in their final anatomic positions. Thus the 1st trimester can be referred to as "a trimester of differentiation and development," and the 2nd and 3rd trimesters may be referred to collectively as "trimesters of growth and maturation."

This chapter addresses the fetal organs, organ systems, and associated structures that can be examined with sonography during the 2nd and 3rd trimesters of pregnancy, and the measurements used to determine gestational age (GA) during this time.

THE PLACENTA

The tremendous amount of growth that occurs during the second and third trimesters is highly dependent on the ability of the fetus to acquire nutrients and oxygen. It is also dependent on fetal ability to remove the waste products of metabolism. The organ that accomplishes these tasks is the **placenta**.

The enormous circulatory surface provided by the many fetal and maternal blood vessels allows nutrients and metabolic waste products to be exchanged in the placenta. Carbon dioxide is at a much higher concentration in the fetal blood and thus tends to move into the maternal blood. Oxygen is at a much higher level in the maternal bloodstream and thus moves into the fetal blood. The placenta thus functions as an organ of respiration for the fetus.

The placenta may be sonographically visible by 10 weeks. As discussed in Chapter 22, it appears as the thickened, bright portion of the rim of tissue surrounding the gestational sac. At 12 to 13 GA weeks, the early placenta appears homogeneous and hyperechoic relative to adjacent structures. Intervillous blood flow can be demonstrated with color or power Doppler sonography. During the second and third trimesters the placenta's appearance becomes slightly darker. In some cases, small anechoic areas representing maternal venous lakes, or **lacunae**, may interrupt the placenta's otherwise homogeneous appearance. It is often possible to see a swirl-like motion within these pools of venous blood. This presumably represents very slow circulation of maternal blood. A prominent venous lake is shown in Figure 23-1. Anechoic tubular structures on the uterine surface of the placenta representing maternal marginal veins may also be visualized, as seen in Figure 23-2.

Between 14 and 15 GA weeks the placenta is well established and the retroplacental complex can be observed. It presents as an area of low-level, mixed echoes composed of the uterine decidua (gravid endometrium), myometrium, and uterine blood vessels. At 16 to 18 weeks, color power Doppler may be able to demonstrate small intraplacental arteries. By the third trimester the mature placenta becomes extremely vascular. Both retroplacental and intraplacental arteries are readily identified and appear as anechoic structures with bright, thin walls.

Some experts believe that **placental volume** in the second trimester can be used as an accurate predictor for abnormal fetal outcome. In most normal cases the placenta should be *approximately equal in thickness (in millimeters) to the gestational age in weeks +10 mm.*

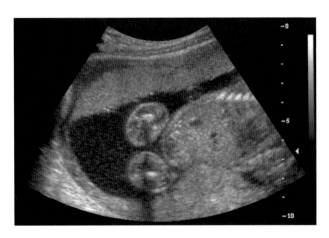 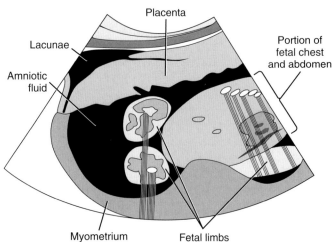

FIGURE 23-1 **Lacunae.** Lacunae are normal, small, anechoic pools of maternal venous blood that may visualized throughout the placenta during the second and third trimesters of pregnancy. (Scan courtesy the University of Virginia Health System, Department of Radiology, Division of Ultrasound, Charlottesville, Virginia.)

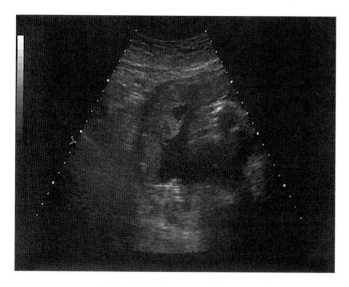
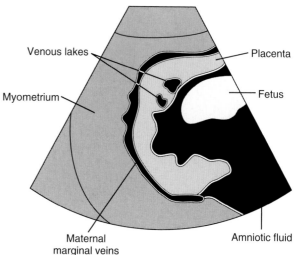

FIGURE 23-2 **Maternal Marginal Veins.** Anechoic areas visualized along the uterine surface of the placenta represent maternal marginal veins.

Measuring the placenta is not standard practice, but most experts agree that it should not exceed 4.0 cm. With experience, a sonographer will probably recognize a placenta that appears too thick or too thin secondary to a primary pathology.

Throughout pregnancy, the placenta matures and calcifies (the sonographic sign of "aging") at a fairly reproducible rate. During the 1970s, Grannum and colleagues developed **placental grading**, a method that classifies placental maturation according to sonographic appearance (Figure 23-3). The categories of placental classification are *Grades 0, I, II, and III*:

- *Grade 0.* Represents the normal placenta. It has a smooth chorionic plate (sac border), a substance that is devoid of focal bright areas, and a basal layer (uterine border) that is free of bright, reflective densities as well. The placental substance (between borders) appears homogeneous, with medium- to low-level echoes; it may be interrupted by anechoic lacunae.
- *Grade I.* The chorionic plate shows some subtle indentation. The homogeneous placental substance exhibits a few scattered, punctate densities ("calcifications") that appear hyperechoic relative to the placental substance. The basal layer of a Grade I placenta appears hypoechoic to anechoic compared to the placental substance. These placental findings are considered as normal changes at any time after 34 weeks of development.
- *Grade II.* The placenta exhibits mild or medium-sized indentations in the chorionic plate. The homogeneous substance of the placenta contains scattered, "comma-like" densities (calcifications) that are hyperechoic relative to the placental substance. The basal plate in a Grade II placenta contains a few small,

bright, linear densities. Grade II placental findings are considered normal at any time after 36 weeks of development.

- *Grade III.* The placenta contains obvious indentations in the chorionic plate that extend as far as the basal layer, dividing the placenta into segments. The otherwise homogeneous substance of the placenta may contain both bright, highly echogenic areas and anechoic areas. Bright, scattered calcifications appear significantly larger and may exhibit acoustic shadowing. The basal layer of a Grade III placenta has very long, highly echogenic, linear echoes and may, in advanced stages, appear as an unbroken line. Grade III placental findings are considered normal at any time after 38 weeks of development.

Initially it was believed that the placental grading system, which essentially measures amounts of calcification within the aging placenta, could be used as a means to date a gestation. Experts attempted to correlate placental maturity with lung maturity. It is now known that dating the gestation by placental grading techniques is highly inaccurate. However, there is a distinct relationship between the age of the gestation and the grade of the placenta. Normally, a Grade I placenta should not appear before 34 weeks, a Grade II placenta should not appear before 36 weeks, and a Grade III placenta should not appear before 38 weeks. Appearance of these grades before the stated times may indicate an abnormality. When the placenta exhibits premature aging or accelerated calcification, it is usually due to maternal cigarette smoking or to thrombotic disorders and the medicines used to treat them.

Sonographic evaluation of the placenta also includes noting its position within the uterus relative to the

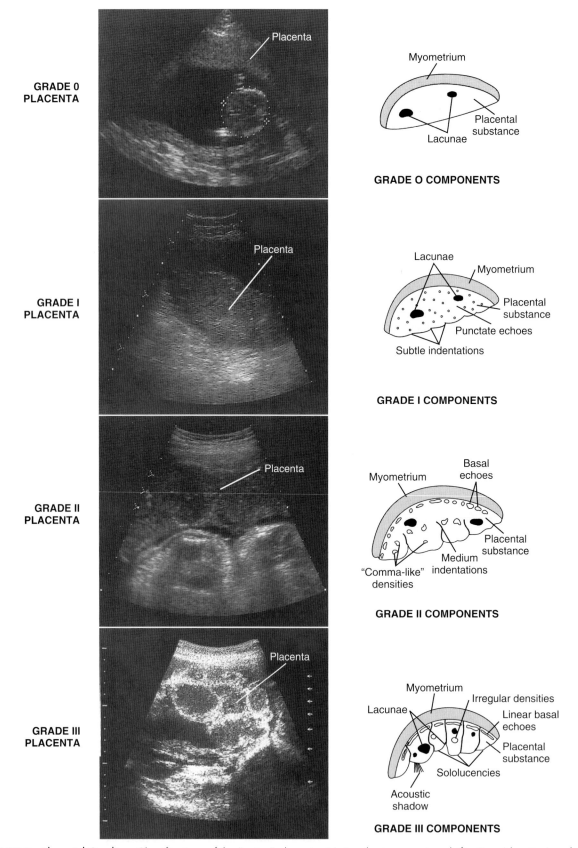

FIGURE 23-3 Placental Grading. Classifications of the "aging" placenta. Notice the increase in calcifications (densities) and changes in contour from Grades 0 to III. **Grade 0.** Represents the *normal placenta*. The placental substance appears homogeneous, with medium- to low-level echoes that may be interrupted by anechoic lacunae. No densities are evident and contours are smooth. **Grade I.** The chorionic plate begins to show some signs of subtle indentations, a few scattered densities are present, and the basal layer appears anechoic. **Grade II.** Medium-sized indentations are evident in the chorionic plate, "comma-like" densities are prevalent throughout the placental substance, and a few small linear densities appear in the basal plate. **Grade III.** The chorionic plate contains indentations extending to the basal layer, dividing the placenta into segments. The placental substance appears complex, with both anechoic areas and bright focal areas representing large calcifications that may cast shadows. Long, linear densities are evident in the basal plate. In advanced stages they may appear as an unbroken line.

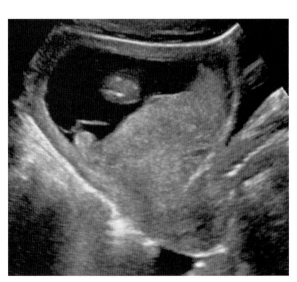

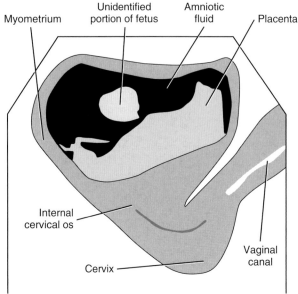

FIGURE 23-4 Total ("Complete") Placenta Previa. Note how the placenta entirely covers the internal cervical os.

internal os of the cervix to rule out placenta previa. **Placenta previa** occurs when any portion of the internal cervical os is covered by part of the placenta. There are 4 types of placenta previa: *total, partial, marginal* and *low-lying*.

1. **Total ("complete") placenta previa.** Occurs when the entire cervical os is obstructed by an overlying placenta, as seen in Figure 23-4. Generally indicated by vaginal bleeding during the second or third trimesters. The patient usually requires cesarean delivery because vaginal delivery would be dangerous for the fetus and mother.
2. **Partial ("incomplete") placenta previa.** Occurs when a portion of the cervical os is obstructed by overlying placenta. This condition is associated with vaginal bleeding and necessitates cesarean delivery.
3. **Marginal placenta previa.** Exists when the placenta extends up to, but not above, the internal cervical os. These patients have follow-up examinations during the final weeks of their pregnancy to see whether the position of the placenta has changed as the uterus enlarges to accommodate the growing fetus.
4. **Low-lying placenta.** Occurs when the placenta's lower edge lies within 0.5 to 5 cm from the internal cervical os. Occasionally, the term "potential placenta" is also used to describe a placenta that stops within a few centimeters of the internal cervical os. In follow-up ultrasound exams, the placenta frequently appears to move upward and away from the internal os when, in fact, it is the stretched lower uterine segment that has moved as a result of the growing fetus pushing the uterus upward.

There are multiple *risk factors* for placenta previa, including history of placenta previa, history of cesarean section, increased maternal age, increased parity, enlarged placenta, and maternal history of smoking. There are 3 *causes* of placenta previa: (1) a low-lying placenta in a normal uterus, (2) a low-lying placenta resulting from the presence of a benign fibroid tumor, and (3) a vascular malformation that causes placental formation only in the lower portion of the uterus.

AMNIOTIC FLUID

The fetal effect on **amniotic fluid volume (AFV)** increases with the pregnancy. During the third trimester, fetal kidneys may produce between 600 and 800 mL of fluid per day; near term, the fetus may swallow up to 450 mL of fluid per day. As discussed in Chapter 22, the volume of amniotic fluid reflects the state of gestational well-being. For that reason, various methods of calculating amniotic fluid volumes have been developed. One method assesses the AFV by totaling the individual pockets of amniotic fluid. The maximum vertical pocket (MVP) method to assess the AFV was developed to determine oligohydramnios (deficiency in the amount of amniotic fluid). It uses the greatest vertical dimension of the single deepest pocket of amniotic fluid free of umbilical cord and extremities. Most institutions use 2 cm as the minimum normal amount; less than 2 cm usually indicates oligohydramnios. An alternative method, the 4-quadrant analysis, assesses AFV by finding the **amniotic fluid index (AFI)**. The following illustration shows how this measurement is based on the division of the gravid uterus into 4 equal quadrants using the umbilicus and linea nigra.

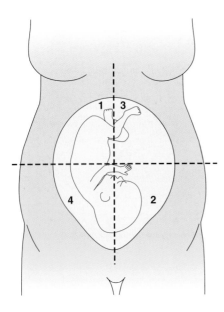

The anteroposterior diameter of the deepest amniotic fluid pocket free of cord and extremities in each quadrant is measured. These four measurements are added together to determine the AFI. A sum of 8 to 25 cm is considered normal.

In the early to middle portion of the second trimester of pregnancy, it is not unusual to view free-floating bright particles in the otherwise anechoic amniotic fluid. The particles as mentioned in Chapter 22, are believed to be fetal **vernix** (flakes of skin and hair) with no pathologic significance.

FETAL ORGAN SYSTEMS

Musculoskeletal System

The fetal skeleton is visualized earlier and more consistently than any other organ system. The *axial skeleton* begins to form between the 6th and 8th menstrual weeks, beginning with the vertebrae and ribs, followed by the skull and sternum. The *appendicular skeleton* also begins to form during the 6th menstrual week when the upper and lower limbs first appear as small buds on the lateral body wall. This is followed by formation of the pectoral and pelvic girdles. The soft tissues of the skeleton develop in a similar sequence to that of the skeletal structures. The bones continue to grow and accumulate minerals (ossify) throughout the second and third trimesters.

As early as the latter half of the first trimester, ultrasound is able to demonstrate how ossified or bony portions of the fetal skeleton appear highly echogenic or hyperechoic compared to the low-gray appearance of adjacent cartilaginous structures.

The bright reflection of the fetal skeleton is an indication of the degree of mineralization that has taken place within the developing bones. The density of bone attenuates the sound waves, preventing through transmission. The sound waves are reflected from the surface of the bones, causing a highly echogenic appearance with a shadow cast behind it. As discussed in earlier chapters, the degree of echogenicity depends on the density of the bone, its distance from the sound beam, and the angle at which the beam strikes the bone. The brightest reflections occur at normal (perpendicular) incidence.

Axial Skeleton

Spine

During the second and third trimesters the majority of bones or components of bones of the axial skeleton can routinely be visualized. This includes the fetal spine, and even though it matures at varying degrees and levels, the vertebrae have a highly reflective appearance, making them easy to recognize. Three primary ossification centers of each vertebra are sonographically distinguishable (Figure 23-5). They are the anterior centrum of the body and one on each side of the posterior neural arch. As ossification continues, the transverse processes, pedicles, and laminae can be differentiated.

The anterior ossification center of the vertebrae is equidistant from the two posterior ossification centers. In axial or "short axis" sections, these bright echoes are parallel, or actually converge toward each other (Figure 23-6). Normal vertebral laminae angle inward, the opposite of the outward splaying of the laminae observed with spina bifida, a bony anomaly.

Several vertebrae imaged at once in a longitudinal section appear as two rows of closely spaced reflectors on each side of spinal cord, which appears hypoechoic in comparison. These two rows are roughly parallel, but wider in the cervical and lumbar regions and narrower in the sacral region (Figure 23-7).

Rib Cage

In the region of the thorax, the bright, echogenic appearance of the fetal rib cage is easily identified and serves as an excellent anatomic landmark. The reflective ribs found between the spine and the sternum stand out against the midgray to low-gray background of the lungs and heart muscle.

Skull

In the skull region a number of vivid, echogenic bones can be identified. The calvaria—composed of the frontal, temporal, parietal, and occipital bones—is easily distinguishable. Similarly, the cartilaginous portions of these bones, the cranial sutures, are commonly seen

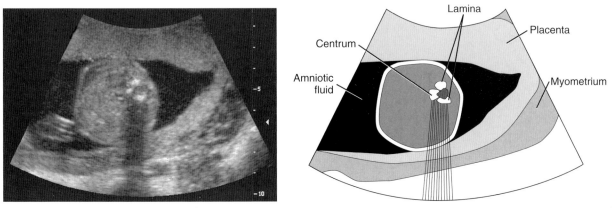

FIGURE 23-5 **Axial Skeleton.** Short axis section of the fetal lumbar spine. Note how the anterior ossification center (centrum) of the vertebrae is equidistant from the 2 posterior ossification centers (lamina). (Scan courtesy the University of Virginia Health System, Department of Radiology, Division of Ultrasound, Charlottesville, Virginia.)

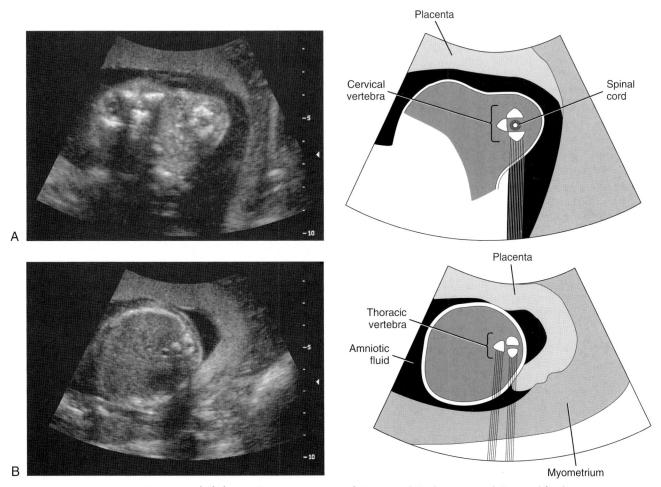

FIGURE 23-6 **Axial Skeleton.** Short axis sections of **A,** cervical; **B,** thoracic; and **C,** sacral fetal vertebrae. In axial or "short axis" sections, these bright echoes are parallel, or actually converge toward each other. Normal vertebral laminae angle inward, the opposite of the outward splaying of the laminae observed with spina bifida, a bony anomaly. *Continued*

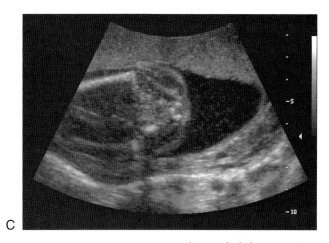

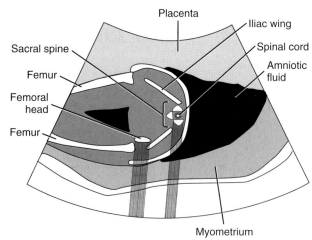

FIGURE 23-6, cont'd **Axial Skeleton. C,** The distinctive appearance of the pelvic iliac bones serve as an excellent landmark for confirming the lower portion of the fetal spine. (Scan courtesy the University of Virginia Health System, Department of Radiology, Division of Ultrasound, Charlottesville, Virginia.)

(Figure 23-8), as well as the fontanelles or "bone-free windows" to the fetal brain. The petrous ridge and greater wing of the sphenoid bone are visualized without difficulty as they delineate the anechoic anterior, middle, and posterior cranial fossae.

In almost all normal cases the mandible, bony nasal ridge, and orbits can be visualized. Usually, in older fetuses, the orbital contents can be assessed. The globe and lens appear very low-gray and hypoechoic to adjacent structures. The bright retrobulbar fat and bony orbital walls appear hyperechoic compared to the midgray appearance of the rectus muscles, optic nerve, and eyelid.

Appendicular Skeleton
Extremities
During the early-to-mid second trimester the majority of bones of the appendicular skeleton can be visualized. In most cases the upper extremity phalanges, metacarpals, radius, ulna, humerus, clavicle, and scapula can be identified. Because the metacarpals and metatarsals are ossified at 16 weeks, they are easier to distinguish than the carpals and tarsals (except for the tarsal talus and calcaneus), which remain cartilaginous throughout pregnancy. Figure 23-9, *A*, shows all five digits of a 33-week fetal hand. The lower extremity phalanges, metatarsals, tibia, fibula, and femur can also be imaged in the first half of the second trimester, as can the hip and knee joints. Figure 23-9, *B*, shows all five metatarsals and phalanges of a 22-week fetal foot.

In axial sections the long bones of the forearms and lower legs appear as two bright, echogenic foci surrounded by soft tissue, which appears low-gray and hypoechoic in comparison. Normally, these bones end at the same level distally. Proximally, the ulna is

longer than the radius. In the lower leg the tibia is the medial bone; the fibula, the lateral. In long axis and longitudinal sections the long bones appear "long" and highly echogenic with posterior acoustic shadowing (Figure 23-10 on pp. 421-422).

Muscles
Normal fetal muscles appear very low-gray on ultrasound. In fact, some muscles may appear anechoic, especially in the abdominal wall where they can mimic the appearance of ascites (abnormal fluid). High-resolution ultrasound equipment makes it possible to differentiate the individual layers of the transversus abdominus and the internal and external oblique muscles. These muscles can be identified as the anechoic areas between the bright subcutaneous and peritoneal fat (Figure 23-11 on p. 422).

Cardiovascular System
This discussion will concentrate on the sonographic presentation of uterine and fetal blood vessels, as well as the fetal heart. Given that the anatomy of the heart and great vessels is the focus of Chapters 25, 30, and 31, this discussion will concentrate on the features unique to the fetal heart and their sonographic presentation.

The fetal vascular system has some unique features that do not exist after birth. As discussed in Chapter 22, the umbilical cord contains one vein and two arteries. The umbilical vein carries oxygenated blood from the placenta to the fetus, where it connects with the left portal vein in the liver. After birth, the umbilical vein closes off, and eventually becomes the ligamentum teres. Specifically, the umbilical vein courses from the midline of the fetal abdominal wall posteriorly and slightly cephalad into the liver along the free margin of

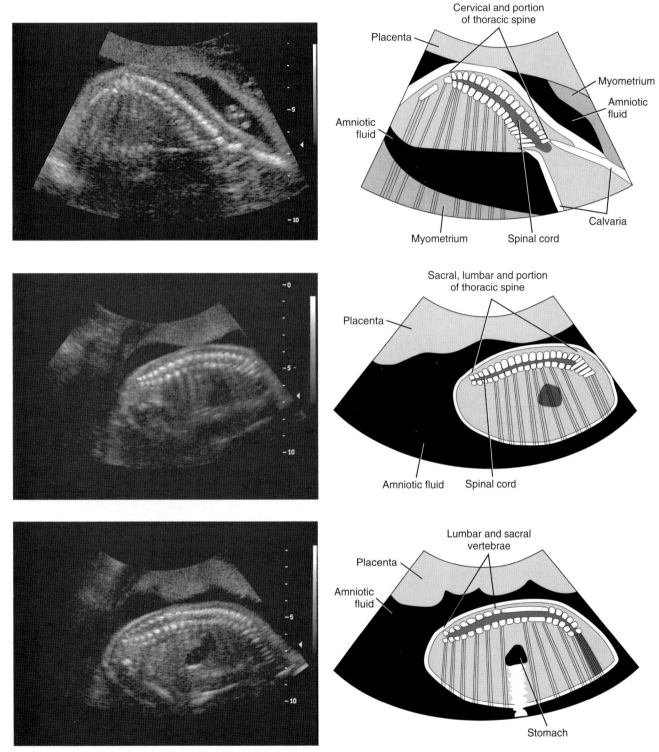

FIGURE 23-7 **Axial Skeleton.** Observe in these images of longitudinal fetal spine sections how much wider the cervical spine is compared to the normal tapering of the vertebrae in the sacrum. Gaps between vertebral bodies are composed of the nonossified margins of adjoining vertebral bodies and the intervertebral disks. Spinal cord neural tissue appears hypoechoic compared with the bright appearance of the meninges and vertebral bodies. (Scans courtesy the University of Virginia Health System, Department of Radiology, Division of Ultrasound, Charlottesville, Virginia.)

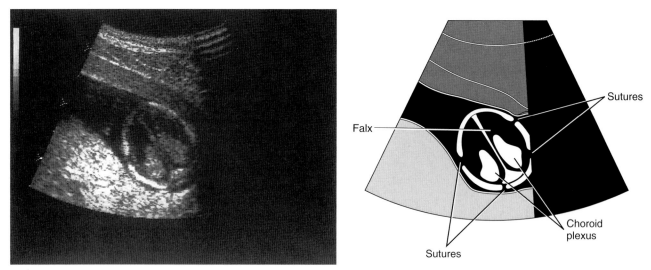

FIGURE 23-8 **Axial Skeleton.** Observe how the cartilaginous fetal skull sutures appear hypoechoic relative to the bright reflection from the bones that make up the calvarium or "skull." The sutures along with the fontanelles serve as the windows for sonographic brain imaging. These nonossified "gaps" between the bones of the skull allow the sound waves to pass through, making brain imaging possible.

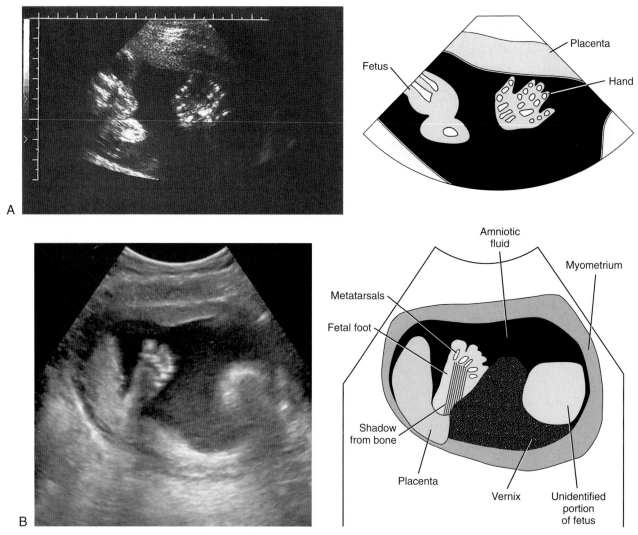

FIGURE 23-9 **Appendicular Skeleton. A,** All 5 highly echogenic digits of this 33-week fetal hand are visualized. The areas between the pieces of bone are cartilages that assist hand movement. Note that the cartilages appear hypoechoic relative to the bright appearance of the bones. **B,** All 5 metatarsals and phalanges of a 22-week fetal foot.

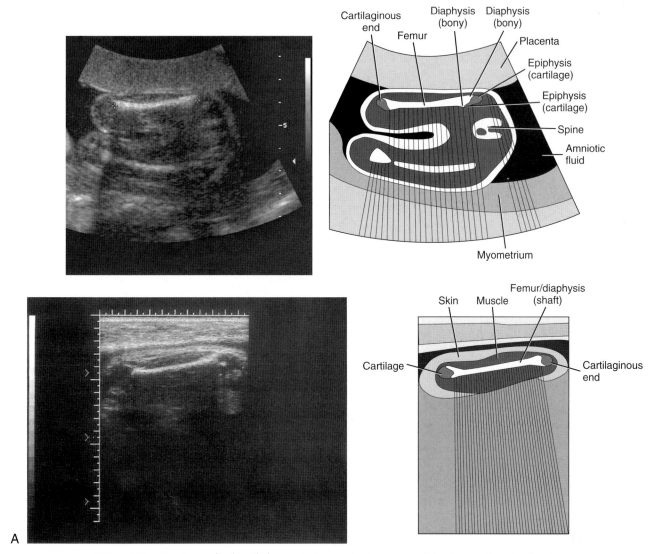

FIGURE 23-10 **Appendicular Skeleton. A,** Longitudinal sections of the femur. Note the bright, reflective appearance of the bone. The low-gray areas immediately adjacent to each bony end of the femur are the cartilaginous ends of the bone. Shadowing prevents the full thickness of the ossified diaphysis of long bones from being visualized. Therefore the width of the cartilaginous epiphysis can appear greater than the width of the bony diaphysis. When both femurs are visualized, the shadowing can also give the appearance that the femur in the far field of the image is bowed. The posterior shadow cast by the femur becomes more apparent as ossification increases with advancing gestational age. *Continued*

the falciform ligament. It joins the umbilical segment of the left portal vein, which courses superiorly and to the right, forming the transverse portion, or pars transversa, of the left portal vein, where it joins the right portal vein (Figure 23-12).

The ductus venosus, which shunts oxygenated blood into the inferior vena cava, originates from the pars transversa, or in some cases more rightward. It courses unbranched to join the left, or middle, hepatic vein and ultimately the inferior vena cava (Figure 23-13). Shortly before birth, the ductus venosum closes and becomes

the fibrous ligamentum venosum, marking the left anterolateral border of the caudate lobe of the liver.

Figure 23-14 shows examples of the umbilical cord insertion into the placenta and into the fetus. As discussed in Chapter 22, ultrasound identification of the cord insertion into the placenta is important for invasive obstetric procedures such as fetal blood sampling. The area is considered optimal because this is the only location where the cord is fixed, making needle approach more accurate. At the cord insertion site into the fetus, the umbilical vein courses superiorly and to the right to

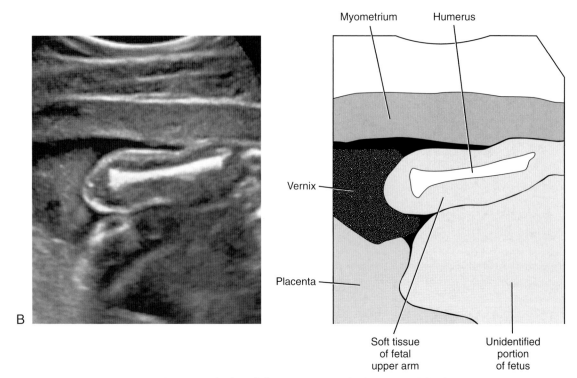

FIGURE 23-10, cont'd   **Appendicular Skeleton. B,** Longitudinal section of the humerus. Notice its hyperechoic appearance compared to adjacent structures. Observe the shadow posteriorly. (**A,** Scans courtesy the University of Virginia Health System, Department of Radiology, Division of Ultrasound, Charlottesville, Virginia.)

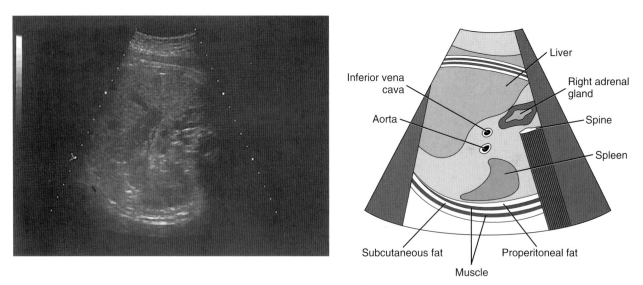

FIGURE 23-11   **Muscles.** High-resolution ultrasound equipment makes it possible to differentiate the individual layers of the transversus abdominus muscles and the internal and external oblique muscles. These muscles can be identified as the anechoic areas between the bright subcutaneous and peritoneal fat.

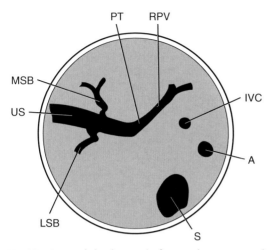

FIGURE 23-12 **Umbilical Vein/Left Portal Vein Circulation.** *A,* Aorta; *IVC,* inferior vena cava; *LPV,* umbilical segment of left portal vein; *LSB,* lateral segment branch; *MSB,* medial segment branch; *PT,* pars transversa of left portal vein; *RPV,* right portal vein; *S,* stomach.

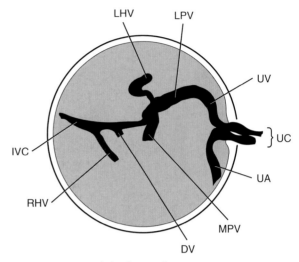

FIGURE 23-13 **Umbilical Circulation.** *DV,* Ductus venosus; *IVC,* inferior vena cava; *LPV,* umbilical segment of left portal vein; *RHV,* right hepatic vein; *UA,* umbilical artery; *UC,* umbilical cord; *UV,* umbilical vein.

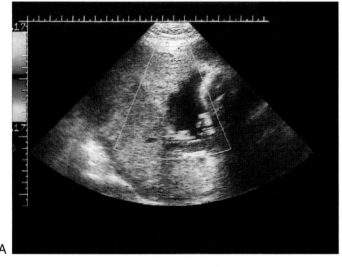

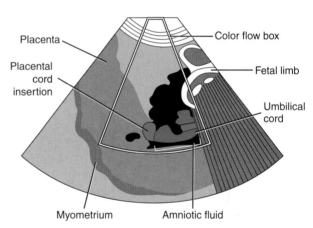

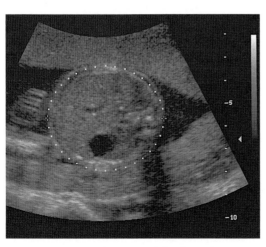

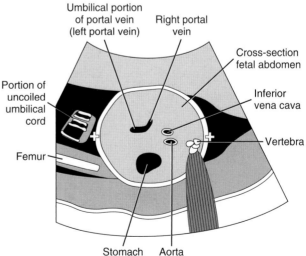

FIGURE 23-14 **Umbilical Cord Insertion.** (B and C, Scans courtesy the University of Virginia Health System, Department of Radiology, Division of Ultrasound, Charlottesville, Virginia.)

Continued

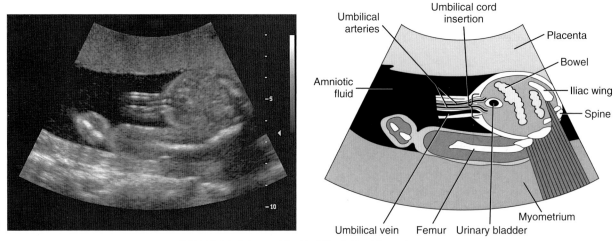

FIGURE 23-14, cont'd   Umbilical Cord Insertion.

enter the liver and become part of portal circulation; the umbilical arteries run inferiorly along the margin of the urinary bladder and ultimately carry blood from the fetus back to the placenta. Some of the blood, however, does bypass the umbilical arteries at the internal iliac arteries to oxygenate and nourish the lower extremities of the fetus.

Before birth, the anatomy of the fetal heart and great vessels is the same as that in the pediatric and adult heart, with two exceptions. The basic anatomy includes four chambers consisting of two atria and two ventricles, atrioventricular connections (valves), and inflows and outflows (great vessels). The two unique features of the fetal heart are the foramen ovale and ductus arteriosus. As illustrated in Figure 23-15, the fetal heart allows blood to move from right to left in the atrial chambers via the **foramen ovale**. This opening between the atria may remain patent after birth, but it is held closed by the normal pressure gradient between left and right atria. The pulmonary artery and the aorta are connected by the **ductus arteriosus**. This duct allows blood to move from the pulmonary artery to the aorta. Because the fetal lungs do not have a respiratory function, they do not require large quantities of blood. The ductus arteriosus closes at (or shortly after) birth.

Heart Chambers and Septa
As early as 15 weeks, and certainly by 20 weeks, the fetal heart presents sonographically as a four-chambered structure (Figure 23-16). Chamber walls appear hyperechoic relative to the anechoic appearance of the blood within them. Chambers should appear relatively symmetric, divided by the bright atrioventricular septa, which should be "broken" only at the foramen ovale. Normally, the heart should be visualized on the left side of the thorax. The axis of the heart should be tilted

approximately 45 degrees to the anteroposterior axis of the fetal thorax and pointed to the left (Figure 23-17). Sometimes it is necessary to image the ventricles and atria separately because of fetal position (Figure 23-18).

Cava, Aorta, and Pulmonary Artery
Figure 23-19 shows examples of how sonography also provides information regarding the position and size of the great vessels. Blood vessels in the fetus appear as they do after birth: bright walls with anechoic, blood-filled lumens. Identification of the great arteries and outflow tracts in their usual positions confirms normal ventriculoarterial connections. Notice how the left atrium lies closest to the spine and the right ventricle lies closest to the anterior chest wall. Both atria and both ventricles are approximately the same size.

During the second trimester the superior vena cava, thoracic aorta, and pulmonary artery appear in the upper mediastinum, just superior to the heart. In older fetuses, the transverse aorta branches (brachiocephalic, left common carotid, left subclavian), right common carotid, and jugular veins are frequently seen with ultrasound. The posterior position of the abdominal aorta and inferior vena cava in the abdomen makes them easy to identify as well. The iliac arteries and veins are also frequently observed. Color Doppler is useful for identifying smaller branches of the abdominal aorta, such as the celiac axis, superior mesenteric artery, and renal arteries and veins.

Respiratory System
The lungs begin development as small-paired buds branching off the primitive alimentary canal during the fifth menstrual week. These buds increase in size, and multiple diverticula (outpouchings) form until about 17 weeks of gestation. The surfaces for gas exchange

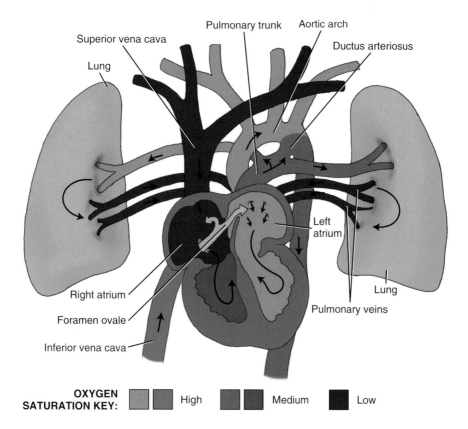

FIGURE 23-15 **Fetal Heart.** Two features unique to the fetal heart are the foramen ovale and ductus arteriosus. The foramen ovale is an opening between the atria of the heart; allowing blood to move from right to left in the atrial chambers. The foramen ovale may remain patent after birth, but it is held closed by the normal pressure gradient between left and right atria. The ductus arteriosus connects the pulmonary artery and the aorta. This duct allows blood to move from the pulmonary artery to the aorta. Because the fetal lungs do not have a respiratory function, they do not require large quantities of blood. The ductus arteriosus closes at (or shortly after) birth.

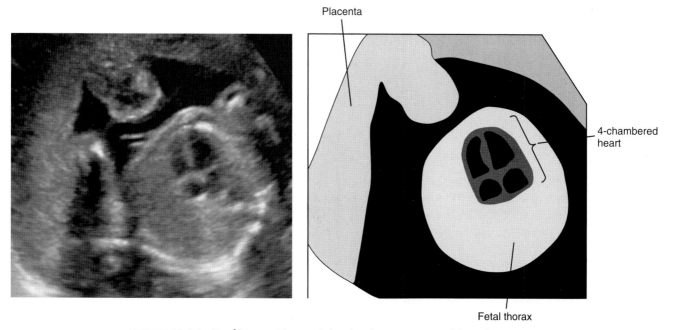

FIGURE 23-16 **Fetal Heart.** Classic 4-chamber heart view in a 26-week gestation.

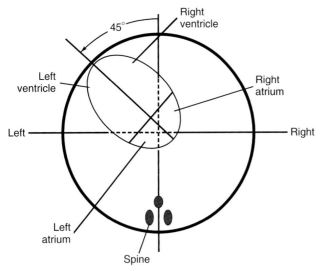

FIGURE 23-17 **Fetal Heart.** Short axis section of the fetal thorax, illustrating the normal position of the heart.

are not developed during this period. Therefore respiration is not possible, and fetuses born during this period are unable to survive. The primitive lungs mature and become capable of functioning sometime after 25 weeks' gestation. Some fetuses born at this stage will survive if given intensive care. During the last weeks of gestation, the final stage of development of the lungs begins. The lungs grow until they nearly fill the thoracic cavity. Lung growth continues into early childhood. The ability of the lungs to function can be measured in utero by monitoring the **lecithin-to-sphingomyelin ratio (LS ratio)**. During the 16th GA week, amniotic fluid is tested to detect the chemicals lecithin and sphingomyelin. The ratio of the amount of lecithin to the amount of sphingomyelin, the LS ratio, measures the degree of fetal lung development. Depending on the LS ratio, elective delivery may be delayed to allow time for the lungs to develop, and in required preterm deliveries, prenatal

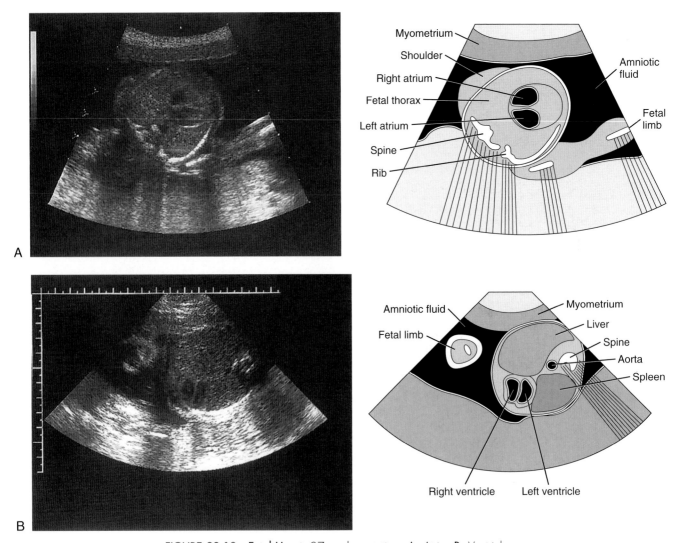

FIGURE 23-18 **Fetal Heart.** 27-week gestation. **A,** Atria. **B,** Ventricles.

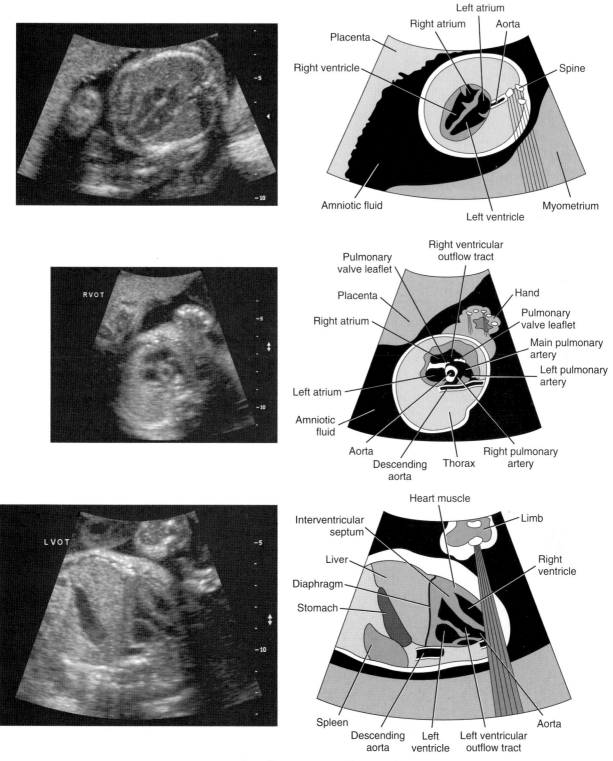

FIGURE 23-19 **Great Arteries and Outflow Tracts.** Identification of the great arteries and outflow tracts in their usual positions confirms normal ventriculoarterial connections. Notice how the left atrium lies closest to the spine and the right ventricle lies closest to the anterior chest wall. Both atria and both ventricles are approximately the same size. (Scans courtesy the University of Virginia Health System, Department of Radiology, Division of Ultrasound, Charlottesville, Virginia.)

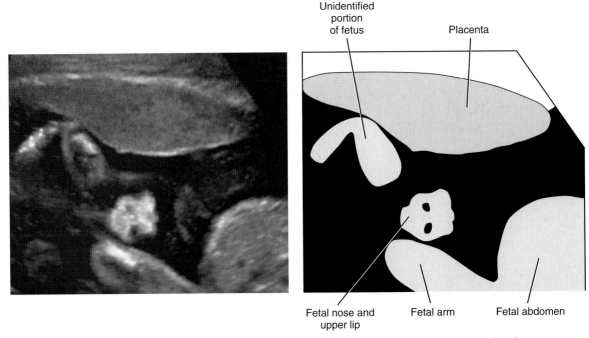

FIGURE 23-20 **Upper Respiratory Tract.** The fetal nose, naval cavity and septum, and palate are visualized. This image demonstrates a normal fetal palate, there is no cleft present between the nose and upper lip.

medications are administered to prevent or decrease the severity of respiratory distress.

Upper Respiratory Tract

The portions of the fetal upper respiratory tract visible with sonography include the nose, nasal cavity and septum, and the palate (Figure 23-20). The presence of anechoic amniotic fluid in portions of the tract makes structures such as the pharynx, hypopharynx, piriform sinuses, and the epiglottis (in older fetuses) commonly visible. When the hypopharynx is fluid filled, the larynx is usually detectable. Generally, the fluid-filled trachea can be traced from its distal end, passing posterior to the aortic arch.

Lungs, Ribs, and Diaphragm

Early in pregnancy, identification of the lungs is derived more from the structures adjacent to them such as the heart (medially), ribs (superolaterally), diaphragm (inferiorly), and liver (inferiorly). The homogeneous lung tissue contrasts with the anechoic blood in the heart chambers. The ribs are easily recognized by their bright, reflective appearance. Figure 23-21 shows the sonographic appearance of the fetal diaphragm. Unlike the bright appearance of the adult diaphragm, the fetal diaphragm typically appears hypoechoic compared to adjacent structures. Further, it should appear slightly concave, with the cuplike portion opening toward the abdomen and the arched position pointing toward the thorax. It is not unusual

to see the diaphragm move with fetal respiration, especially during the latter half of the third trimester. During most of the second trimester, the liver and lungs appear homogeneous, mid-gray, and isoechoic. The lungs become more echogenic as the pregnancy progresses.

Gastrointestinal System

During gestational week 4, the foregut and hindgut develop from embryonic folds. The midgut is connected to the yolk sac. The foregut divides into the esophagus, stomach, and duodenum in week 5. The liver, gallbladder, pancreas, and spleen arise as diverticula from the primitive alimentary tube. The midgut splits into the remainder of small bowel, ascending colon, and a portion of transverse colon. The hindgut differentiates into the remainder of transverse colon, descending colon, and rectum. In the second trimester, bidirectional bowel peristalsis occurs. By the third trimester, peristalsis is unidirectional from the esophagus to the anus.

During the mid-to-late second trimester, fetal **meconium** ("waste") will accumulate in the bowel. It consists of swallowed amniotic fluid, glandular secretions, vernix, and bile. The cecum acts as an accumulation point for this fetal waste material.

As early as the end of the first trimester, several components of the fetal gastrointestinal system, such as the tongue, along with the stomach, gallbladder, liver, and bowel, can be identified sonographically.

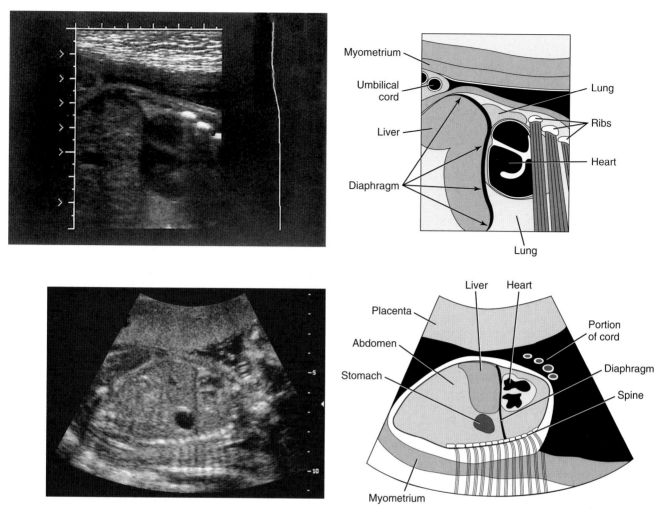

FIGURE 23-21 Fetal Diaphragm. The fetal diaphragm appears as a smooth, hypoechoic muscular boundary between the thorax and the abdomen. (Bottom scan courtesy the University of Virginia Health System, Department of Radiology, Division of Ultrasound, Charlottesville, Virginia.)

Oral Cavity and Esophagus

The oral cavity, including the hard and soft palates and the tongue, is visualized fairly consistently with sonography. On the other hand, the proximal portion of the esophagus is nearly impossible to see; however, the mid and distal portions may occasionally be visualized anterior to the descending thoracic aorta as five parallel lines. The line appearance is created by the contrast between the low-gray muscular wall and brighter serosa and lumen.

Stomach and Gallbladder

Because they are the only subdiaphragmatic fetal gastrointestinal system structures normally filled with fluid, the stomach and gallbladder are consistently easy to identify. The fluid-filled stomach appears as an anechoic structure on the left side of the fetal abdomen (Figure 23-22). The size of the stomach is variable and depends on the amount of amniotic fluid swallowed

by the fetus. The fluid (before bile production) or bile-filled gallbladder appears as an anechoic structure on the right side of the fetal abdomen (Figure 23-23). The gallbladder may be difficult to visualize after 32 weeks' gestation. It is thought that it contracts, releasing bile, as a result of the initiation of gallbladder function.

Liver

By the second trimester the homogeneous, midgray liver is routinely visualized occupying the right side and much of the rest of the fetal abdomen (see Figure 23-23). The fetal liver is the largest parenchymal organ of the gastrointestinal system and of the abdomen. It is the site of production of red blood cells and is proportionately much greater in size in the fetus than in the adult; the left lobe extends as far as the left abdominal wall. It is the large size of the fetal liver that forces the diaphragm upward into the thorax and causes the fetal heart to be in a nearly horizontal plane.

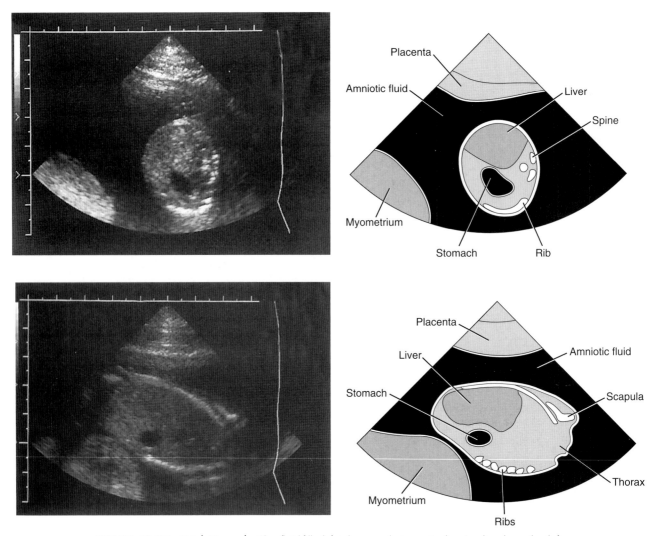

FIGURE 23-22 **Fetal Stomach.** The fluid-filled fetal stomach is routinely visualized on the left side of the abdominal cavity. It appears anechoic with relatively smooth walls. Stomach size and shape are determined by the amount of fluid it contains.

The anechoic umbilical vein courses through the liver, interrupting its otherwise homogeneous appearance. The vein's course is nearly perpendicular to the axis of the fetus as it nears its bifurcation point within the liver. Because of this, it is possible to see a fairly lengthy segment of the umbilical vein, in an axial section of the fetal abdomen, taken at a level of the fetal stomach (Figure 23-24). Also at this level, the umbilical vein, stomach, spine, and liver are important landmarks for measurement of the fetal abdominal diameter or abdominal circumference (described in more detail later in this chapter). The cord insertion into the fetal abdomen is shown in Figure 23-25.

Pancreas

The pancreas is the other major parenchymal organ of the gastrointestinal system; it is rarely seen. In some instances the fetal pancreas may appear hyperechoic

relative to adjacent structures and is visualized lying between the anechoic fluid-filled stomach (posterior wall) and anechoic splenic vein.

Spleen

Even though the spleen is not a gastrointestinal organ, it is associated with the liver by virtue of portal-splenic circulation (see Chapter 18). Between 12 and 24 weeks' gestation, the spleen functions as a hematopoietic organ; lymphocyte and monocyte production continue throughout adult life. Like the fetal liver, the fetal spleen is routinely visualized from the second trimester onward. It occupies the left upper quadrant of the fetal abdomen; it is bounded laterally by the ribs, posteromedially by the spine, anteromedially by the stomach, posteriorly by the kidney, and superiorly by the diaphragm; inferiorly its margin is variable. As seen in Figure 23-23, the sonographic appearance of the fetal

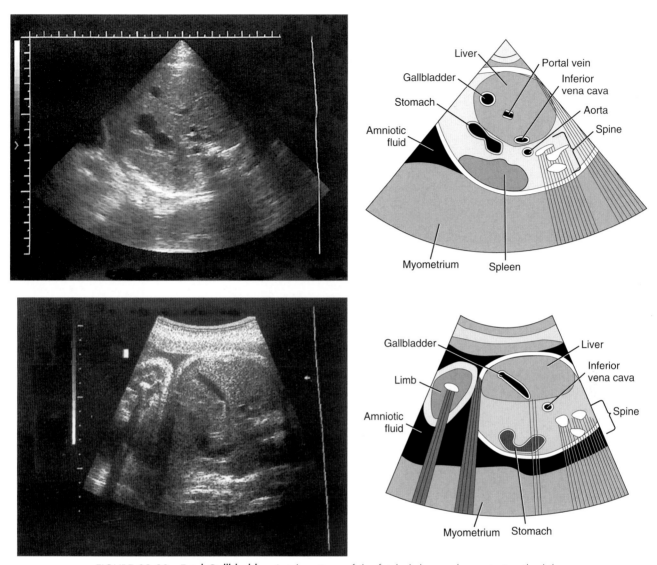

FIGURE 23-23   **Fetal Gallbladder.** Axial sections of the fetal abdomen demonstrating the bile-filled gallbladder. It appears anechoic with smooth walls. Gallbladder lie is variable; therefore, the long axis can be imaged in any scanning plane. The size and shape of the gallbladder depend on the amount of fluid (before bile production) or bile it contains. Note how the liver fills the majority of the abdominal cavity. In the early phases of pregnancy the liver margins may appear ill defined. Also, notice how the fetal spleen is isosonic to the fetal liver (also with indistinct margins during early development).

spleen is comparable to the fetal liver—that is, midgray and homogeneous with indistinct margins during early development. Comparatively, the adult spleen appears slightly hypoechoic compared to the liver.

Small and Large Bowel

Through the second and third trimesters, the small bowel gradually becomes more noticeable. Most ultrasound equipment is able to distinguish small bowel loops and the bowel wall. The muscle layers of the bowel wall appear hypoechoic compared with the remarkably echogenic serosa and subserosa.

When the pregnancy nears term, the small bowel is readily imaged in virtually all fetuses. It is thought that mesenteric fat deposits delineate individual bowel loops, which facilitate identification. By late pregnancy it is normal to see a small amount of anechoic fluid within the small bowel and brighter areas of meconium (fetal waste).

The fetal colon is in the same anatomic position as in the adult. The colon ascends from the right flank to the liver, where it bends (at the "hepatic flexure") and traverses the abdomen inferior to the stomach and the spleen, where it bends ("splenic flexure") and then

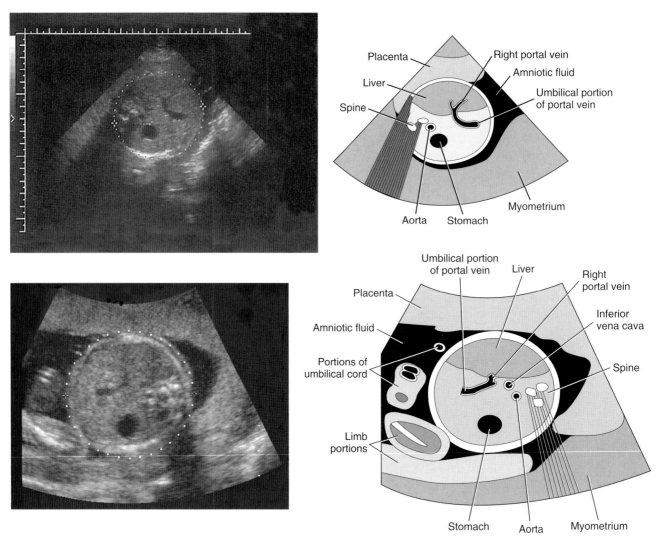

FIGURE 23-24 **Umbilical Portion of the Portal Vein.** Axial sections of the fetal abdomen. Note how the umbilical portion of the portal vein originates in the midline of the abdomen then curves toward the liver as the right branch of the portal vein becomes visible. (Bottom scan courtesy the University of Virginia Health System, Department of Radiology, Division of Ultrasound, Charlottesville, Virginia.)

descends toward the left flank, meeting the sigmoid colon and rectum. Figure 23-26 shows amniotic, fluid-filled portions of the ascending and transverse colon. Collapsed, the fetal colon typically appears hypoechoic relative to adjacent structures.

Genitourinary System
The fetal genitourinary system consists of the kidneys, ureters, urinary bladder, urethra, and genitalia. The kidneys, which form in association with urethral buds, develop between 7 and 9 weeks of gestation and become functional at approximately 10 weeks. The bladder and ureters are formed at approximately 6 weeks of development.

After the 16th week of gestation, the majority of amniotic fluid arises from fetal urination. Assessment of the quantity of amniotic fluid therefore constitutes the initial step in the evaluation of the fetal genitourinary system. A normal amount of amniotic fluid implies the presence of at least one functioning kidney.

Kidneys
Even though fetal kidney position is variable and the sonographic appearance of the kidneys is difficult to differentiate from adjacent structures, they may in some cases be identified sonographically as early as 15 to 16 weeks. Typically, consistent recognition of fetal kidneys begins during the 20th week. Later in pregnancy, the

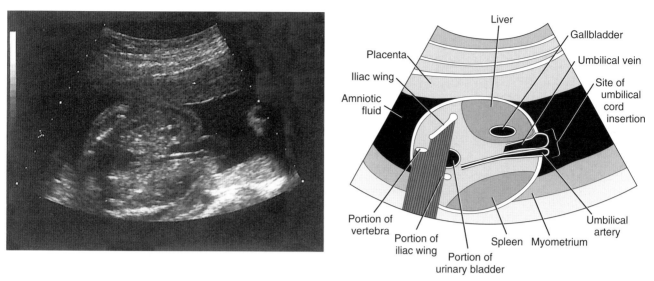

FIGURE 23-25 Umbilical Cord Insertion. Longitudinal sections of the umbilical vein and one umbilical artery as they enter the fetal abdominopelvic cavity.

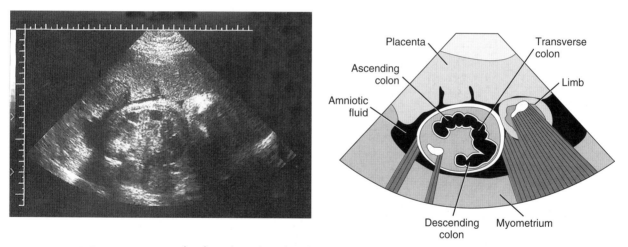

FIGURE 23-26 Fetal Colon. The colon's fluid-filled lumen appears anechoic and distinctly delineates portions of the ascending, transverse, and descending colon.

bright, hyperechoic, retroperitoneal fat surrounding the kidneys makes them easier to visualize.

The fetal kidneys grow at a rate that keeps them proportionately equal to the other developing fetal structures. In general, the length of the fetal kidneys may be represented by the length of 4 to 5 vertebrae of the fetus. The ratio of kidney diameter to the diameter of the fetal abdomen should remain between 0.27 and 0.23 throughout the gestation.

Cortex, Medulla, and Sinus

The normal fetal renal cortex appears homogeneous and moderate to low in echogenicity. As in the adult kidney, columns of Bertin (cortical extensions) separate the medullary pyramids from each other. The pyramids are only sonographically distinguishable when filled with urine, and then their anechoic appearance is easily identified because it is in such contrast to the appearance of the renal cortex. Unlike adult kidneys, the fetal renal sinus has very little fat, making it virtually indistinguishable or slightly hyperechoic relative to the renal cortex. Because of this, it is common to visualize urine-filled, intrarenal collecting structures that are otherwise not appreciated sonographically; the infundibula and renal pelvis appear anechoic.

Normal fetal kidneys can be identified in their paraspinous location; longitudinal sections appear elliptical; axial sections appear round (Figure 23-27).

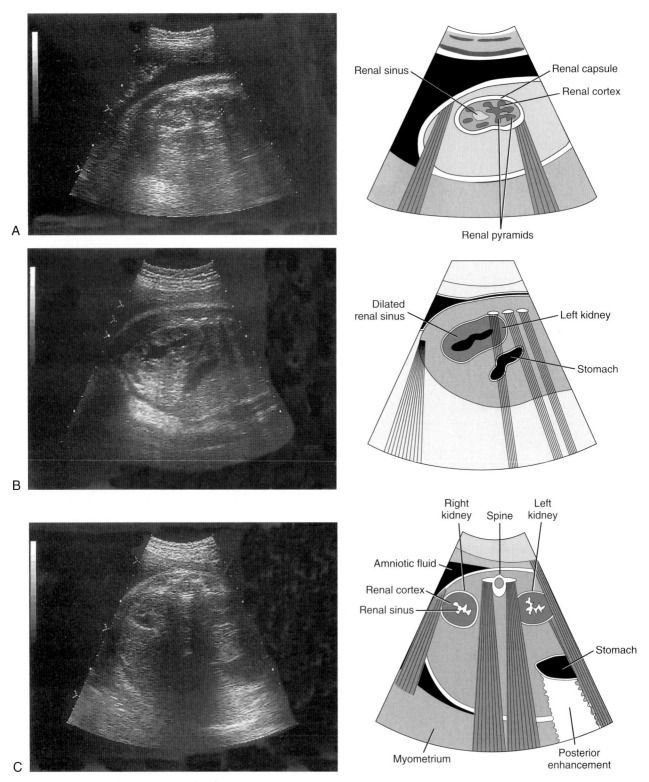

FIGURE 23-27 Fetal Kidneys. A, Longitudinal section of the fetal kidney (between measurement calipers). The distinctive elliptical shape and bright appearance of the renal capsule assist sonographic identification of the kidneys. Later in the trimester, the highly echogenic appearance of the retroperitoneal fat surrounding the kidneys also makes visualization easier. **B,** In this longitudinal section of fetal kidney the centrally located area of the renal sinus appears anechoic because the collecting system is marginally dilated with urine/fluid. **C,** In axial sections the fetal kidneys appear round. Notice how closely they lie to the bilateral lumbar spinal ossification centers.

Ureters

As a rule, normal fetal ureters are not visualized sonographically. In almost all cases, identification of a fetal ureter is an indication of abnormal dilatation.

Urinary Bladder

By 15 weeks' menstrual age, over 90% of all normal fetal urinary bladders can be visualized. Figure 23-28 demonstrates the ultrasound appearance of the fluid-filled fetal urinary bladder. Note how the bladder is located at the midline of the fetal pelvis. Also notice the thin, hyperechoic bladder wall surrounding the anechoic fluid. With normal fetal renal function, the size of the fetal bladder will often be seen to increase and decrease in size during an ultrasound examination. Identification of the urine-filled fetal urinary bladder is *necessary* to establish renal function. If the bladder is not seen, the fetus can be examined in 30-minute to 45-minute intervals when the fetus normally fills and empties its bladder. If the bladder still cannot be visualized, follow-up studies are usually mandatory. The fetal bladder grows in proportion to the rest of the fetus during the remainder of pregnancy, and its visualized size depends on the degree of filling.

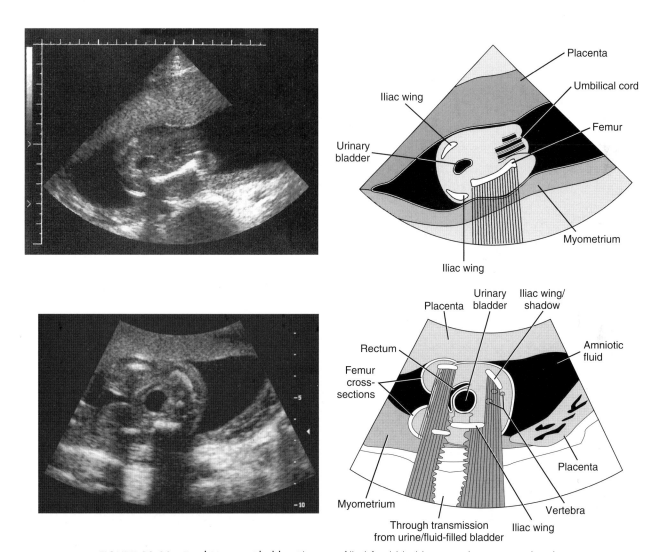

FIGURE 23-28 **Fetal Urinary Bladder.** The urine-filled fetal bladder is easily recognized in the fetal pelvis because of its characteristic anechoic appearance and midline position. Another distinction is the thin, bright appearance of the bladder wall that virtually disappears when the bladder is fully distended. Note the difference in size between these bladders. Changes in the volume of the urinary bladder not only confirms fetal urine production but also, with time, differentiates the bladder from pathologic structures in the pelvis, such as cysts, that have a similar sonographic appearance. (Bottom scan courtesy the University of Virginia Health System, Department of Radiology, Division of Ultrasound, Charlottesville, Virginia.)

Urethra

Occasionally, the urethra may be identified in male fetuses. If the penis is erect, the urethra presents as a bright, reflective line running along the length; otherwise, it is not identifiable.

Genitalia

From the early second trimester, fetal gender can be established sonographically. Determination of fetal gender depends on the visualization of either the male scrotum or the female labia. Assignment of gender should not be made on the basis of the presence or absence of a fetal penis. The penis may be quite small and not visualized, suggesting the presence of a female fetus, or a female clitoris may suggest the presence of a small penis. Thus if the gender of the fetus is to be determined, the labia must be distinguished from the scrotum. Figure 23-29 demonstrates the ultrasound appearance of male and female external genitalia in utero.

Fetal male genitalia are easier to identify than female genitalia. The midgray to low-gray homogeneous penis and scrotum are most apparent. In some cases the testes have been differentiated within the scrotum as early as the third trimester. It is not unusual for small, anechoic testicular hydroceles (fluid collections) to be visualized bilaterally. Details of the penis, including the glans, urethra, and corpora cavernosa, may also be identified; in some cases even the foreskin is visible. The prostate cannot be distinguished.

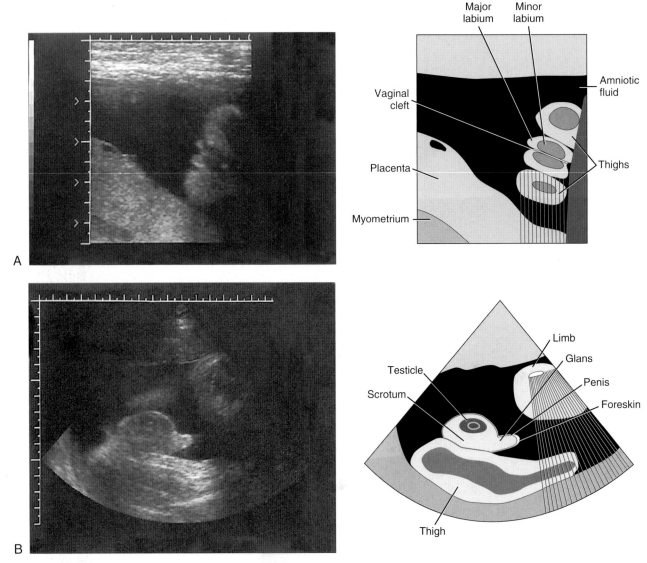

FIGURE 23-29 **Fetal Genitalia. A,** Female genitalia in a 32-week gestation. Female gender is confirmed only when the major and minor labia have been identified. **B,** Male genitalia in a 30-week gestation. Male gender is confirmed only when the scrotum has been identified.

In the fetal female the bilateral major and minor labia may be detectable as early as 17 or 18 menstrual weeks. The major labia flank the minor labia; they appear more echogenic than the hypoechoic minor labia. The bright, linear vaginal cleft lies at the midline, between the minor labia. Typically, the fetal uterus and ovaries cannot be visualized.

Adrenal Glands

Although the fetal adrenal glands are not part of the genitourinary system, their close proximity to the kidneys and relatively conspicuous appearance make them a significant sonographic marker. The triangular-shaped adrenals appear to "cap" the upper renal poles. High-resolution scanning reveals a low-gray organ that is predominantly hypoechoic relative to the liver, spleen, and renal cortex (Figure 23-30).

Central Nervous System

The central nervous system consists of the brain and the spinal cord. It arises from the posterior surface of the embryo (ectoderm). A linear depression is formed along the midline of the early embryo. The borders of the depression fold over to form the neurotube that gives rise to the spinal cord and the brain. Closure of this tube begins in mid-embryo and continues in both cephalad and caudad directions, completing the cephalad first. The brain is composed of 3 elements: the brain stem, the cerebrum, and the cerebellum. Membranes known as the meninges, which also surround the spinal cord, surround these elements. The brain and spinal cord have an elaborate system of circulation composed of ventricles, cisterns, and sinuses.

The Brain
Brain Stem

The brain stem is composed of the *medulla oblongata, pons, midbrain, thalamus,* and *hypothalamus.* It is a continuation of the spinal cord and is the base of the brain. The *medulla oblongata* is closest to the spinal cord and is responsible for control of respiration, heart rate, blood pressure, and certain involuntary reflexes (sneezing, coughing, etc.). The *pons* is located between the medulla and the cerebellum and helps to regulate respiration. The pons also transmits signals from the spinal cord to the cerebellum and cerebrum. The *midbrain* sits between the pons and the thalamus. It relays signals from one part of the brain to another and controls head and eye movements. The *thalamus* and *hypothalamus* are superior to the midbrain. The thalamus is a relay system for cerebral impulses. The hypothalamus is the communication relay between the nervous system and the endocrine system.

Cerebrum

The cerebrum is the center of higher mental faculties. It is concerned with the interpretation of impulses and voluntary muscular activities; it is the largest component of the brain and is composed of 5 lobes: parietal, temporal, occipital, frontal, and insula. The cerebral (or callosal) fissure that extends anteriorly to posteriorly almost completely divides the cerebrum into two lateral hemispheres; the corpus callosum keeps them connected. A fold of dura mater in the cerebral fissure, called the falx cerebri, is a significant sonographic marker because it is an extremely bright reflection. The falx is seen at right angles to the sound beam in axial

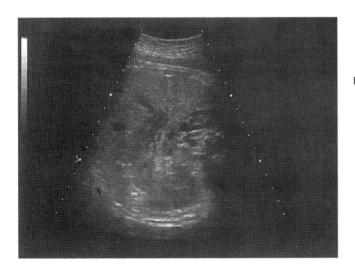
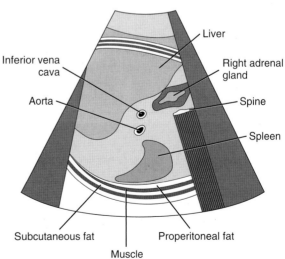

FIGURE 23-30 **Fetal Adrenal Gland.** The prominent size and low-gray sonographic appearance of the fetal adrenal glands make them distinguishable from surrounding structures.

sections of the brain as a bright line dividing the homogeneous, midgray to low-gray cerebrum into equal right and left halves.

Cerebellum

The cerebellum helps to coordinate movements, balance, and posture; it is located just below the cerebrum and superoposterior to most of the brain stem. The cerebellum is composed of two lateral hemispheres (Figure 23-31). A small central lobe, the vermis, relays information between the two hemispheres. On ultrasound the cerebellar vermis often appears strikingly echogenic due to its intertwined meninges covering; it is the bright, reflective line dividing the homogeneous, low-gray cerebellum.

Meninges

The meninges are composed of 3 layers: *dura mater, arachnoid,* and *pia mater.* The *dura mater* is the outermost layer and functions as a tough protective cover for the brain and spinal cord. The *arachnoid layer* is a fibrous, cobweb-like structure and is the thin middle layer. The *pia mater* is a delicate and highly vascularized inner layer that closely follows the contours of the brain and

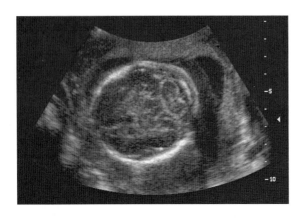
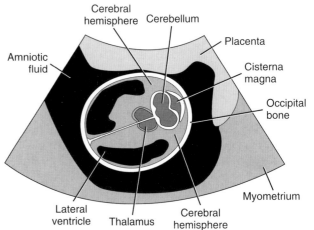
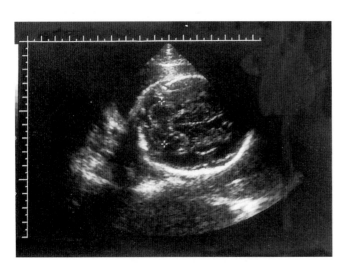
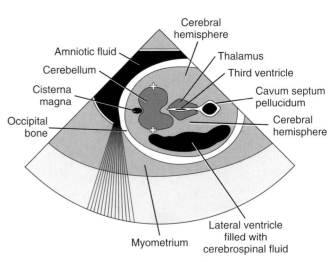

FIGURE 23-31 **Intracranial Anatomy.** The *cerebellum* helps to coordinate movements, balance, and posture; it is located just below the cerebrum and appears low-gray, homogeneous, and symmetric. The anechoic *cisterna magna,* located at the base of the cerebellum, is the largest cerebrospinal fluid (CSF)–filled cistern in the brain. The *cerebrum* is the center of higher mental faculties and accounts for the largest part of the brain; its hemispheres appear midgray to low-gray on ultrasound. Peripheral to the edges of the cerebrum are *subarachnoid spaces* that range in appearance from anechoic to varying levels of echogenicity; some are filled with anechoic CSF, some with echogenic mater, and some with areas of both. The *ventricles* appear anechoic because they are filled with cerebrospinal fluid; their walls appear bright. (Top scan courtesy the University of Virginia Health System, Department of Radiology, Division of Ultrasound, Charlottesville, Virginia.)

spinal cord. The layers have the sonographic distinction of appearing very bright and hyperechoic compared to adjacent structures.

The meninges not only provide protection for the central nervous system, but also facilitate cerebrospinal fluid movement from the subarachnoid space to the dural sinuses. The dura mater is actually two layers. The thicker outer layer firmly adheres to the bones of the skull. The thin inner layer follows the basic curvature of the brain, and together with the arachnoid and pia mater layers, serves to separate the structures of the brain. At the area where the outer and inner layers first separate, there are small spaces. Collectively, these spaces are known as the dural sinuses.

Cerebrospinal fluid (CSF) is similar to plasma in chemical composition except for the concentration of sodium ions, which is much higher in CSF. CSF appears anechoic on ultrasound and is seen filling the central canal of the spinal cord, the ventricles of the brain (see Figure 23-31), and the subarachnoid space. It also is present within the cisterns of the brain (discussed later in this chapter). CSF acts as a protective cushion encasing the brain and spinal cord, and regulates the pressure within the spaces that it fills. CSF may also have a metabolic role; however, this role is not clearly defined.

Ventricles

Ventricles of the brain are part of a system that helps manufacture and distribute CSF. Four ventricles constitute this system: *two lateral ventricles; the third ventricle;* and the *fourth ventricle.*

The *lateral ventricles* are considered the first and second ventricles. They are composed of 5 regions: (1) frontal horns (most anterior), (2) lateral bodies (most superior), (3) occipital horns (most posterior), (4) temporal (most lateral), and (5) atria (the juncture of the temporal and occipital horns with the body of the lateral ventricle). Occipital and temporal horns are the last to fully develop. They can be identified by the 18th or 20th gestational week. At this stage all of the components of the lateral ventricles have developed. Nevertheless, their shape and proportion will change as they and adjacent neural tissue continue to grow. Between 24 weeks and term, the increase in brain volume causes the slow-growing lateral ventricles to gradually become less prominent.

A lateral ventricle is located in each cerebral hemisphere (see Figure 23-31). Each lateral ventricle is connected to the third ventricle by the foramen of Monro, which runs from the juncture of the frontal horn and body of the lateral ventricle to the roof of the third ventricle.

The *third ventricle* is found in the midline of the brain and is located centrally in the thalamus (see Figure 23-31). The *fourth ventricle* is also found in the

midline in a more posterior location. The third and fourth ventricles are connected by a long tubular structure known as the aqueduct of Sylvius, and the fourth ventricle is also connected to the central canal of the spinal cord by two lateral ducts, the foramina of Luschka, and a single medial duct, the foramen of Magendie.

Highly echogenic, prominent choroid plexus can be identified with ultrasound within the lateral ventricles (with the exception of the frontal and occipital horns) by the 11th gestational week (Figure 23-32). The choroid plexus is a highly vascularized tissue that develops from the pia mater and secretes CSF. Except for the areas containing choroid plexus, the remaining portions of the lateral ventricles are clearly delineated by anechoic CSF. Ventricle walls appear vivid and hyperechoic relative to the CSF and adjacent brain matter. As mentioned, between 24 weeks and term, the increase in brain volume causes the slow-growing lateral ventricles and choroid plexus to gradually become less prominent.

CSF flows from the lateral ventricles to the third and fourth ventricles, to the subarachnoid space, and then to the dural sinuses, where it is absorbed in the venous bloodstream.

The subarachnoid space (the space between the pia mater and the arachnoid layer) is very small in most areas, but in certain areas it is enlarged, and CSF will pool there. These pools of CSF are called cisterns. The lumbar cistern is the largest of these spaces and is found in the distal end of the spine. Other such cisterns are found in various locations within the brain. The largest of these cisterns is the cisterna magna, which is located at the base of the cerebellum in a posterior location within the skull (see Figure 23-31).

Vasculature

Two internal carotid arteries and two vertebral arteries supply the circulatory system of the brain. The vertebral arteries join in the inferior and posterior portion of the brain to form basilar arteries, which enter the circle of Willis. The internal carotid arteries enter the circle laterally and inferiorly. The middle cerebral arteries arise laterally from the circle of Willis and course medially to the sylvian fissures. Paired anterior and posterior cerebral arteries also arise from this circle. The veins draining the brain are all tributaries of the dural sinuses and drain into the internal jugular veins.

The Spinal Cord

The spine is a continuation of the brain stem. It contains a nerve bundle floating in CSF that is covered by meninges. The CSF in the spinal column freely communicates with the CSF in the cranium. The spinal cord is clearly visible by gestational week 15 or 16. It is seen best in longitudinal sections, as the very low-gray

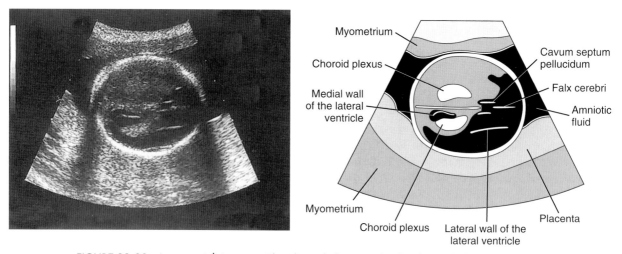

FIGURE 23-32 **Intracranial Anatomy.** The *choroid plexus* are bright, drumstick-shaped structures on either side of the falx cerebri within the lateral ventricles. The *falx cerebri* is the bright, reflective fold of dura mater in the cerebral fissure that separates the cerebral hemispheres. Except for the areas containing choroid plexus, the remaining portions of the *lateral ventricles* are clearly delineated by anechoic cerebrospinal fluid (CSF). Ventricle walls appear hyperechoic relative to CSF and brain matter.

echoes lying between the highly reflective, echogenic vertebrae.

Sonographic Appearance

Intracranial anatomy. By the 11th gestational week, the ovoid appearance of the large *lateral ventricles* filled with highly echogenic choroid plexus is easily identified. The *choroid plexus* are the most prominent intracranial structures seen at this time. They are bright, drumstick-shaped structures on either side of the falx cerebri in the posterior portion of the brain. The *falx* is the bright, reflective fold of dura mater in the cerebral fissure that separates the cerebral hemispheres. The anechoic *frontal horns* are free of the choroids, yet are easily identified because they are filled with CSF. Except for the areas containing choroid plexus, the remaining portions of the lateral ventricles are clearly delineated by anechoic CSF. Ventricle walls appear vivid and hyperechoic to the CSF and midgray to low-gray brain matter. At this point of development only the rudiments of the *occipital* and *temporal horns* are present. Also at this time, the homogeneous, medium-level to low-level gray appearance of the *cerebrum, cerebellum, brain stem,* and highly reflective *third ventricle* is established and will remain fairly consistent, other than developmental enlargement, throughout the gestation. The *brain linings* (dura-arachnoid and pia) are also established and have the distinction of appearing very bright or hyperechoic compared with adjacent structures. The *falx cerebri* is a significant sonographic marker because it is an extremely bright reflection. The falx is seen at right angles to the sound beam in the axial plane as a reflective line dividing the homogeneous, mid-gray to low-gray cerebrum into equal right and left halves. The *cerebellar vermis* often appears strikingly echogenic due to its intertwined meninges covering; it is the reflective line dividing the homogeneous, low-gray cerebellum.

Peripheral to the edges of the brain are *subarachnoid spaces* that range in appearance from anechoic to varying levels of echogenicity; some are filled with anechoic CSF and some with echogenic mater, and some with areas of both.

As development continues, specific portions of brain matter are identifiable as they differentiate sonographically. Nuclei such as the *caudate* and *lentiform* appear as low-level, gray echoes, hypoechoic to surrounding structures with the exception of anechoic CSF. The *tegmentum portion of the brain stem* is also hypoechoic as opposed to the *ventral area of the pons,* which presents as an area of midgray or moderate echogenicity, a little brighter than the nuclei and tegmentum.

Highly reflective brain fissures can be identified before 20 weeks. Two are commonly seen, the small and less important *parieto-occipital fissure* and the larger *lateral fissure* that is often mistaken for the lateral wall of the lateral ventricles, an error that can present as hydrocephalus (over enlargement of the lateral ventricles). By 38 to 42 weeks (term), the lateral fissure closes with progressive growth of the parietal and temporal lobes and eventually becomes the sylvian cistern.

The *thalamus* is a diamond-shaped area visualized in the center of an axial section taken through the temporal lobe of the brain; it appears homogeneous with medium- to low-level echoes and is divided into two equal sections by the *third ventricle*, a bright line, which extends upward into the space between the two halves (see Figure 23-31). At times a very small quantity of fluid, which appears anechoic, can be seen giving the third ventricle a slit-like appearance.

The *cavum septum pellucidum* is another anechoic, fluid-containing structure seen in the midline of the brain (see Figure 23-32). It appears as two small, bright lines separated by CSF, parallel to the falx. This structure contains more fluid than the third ventricle. It is located superoanterior to the thalamus and third ventricle and lies between the frontal horns and bodies of the two lateral ventricles.

An axial section of the brain just above the level of the thalamus should show three bright lines parallel with the long axis of the head. The middle of these three lines is the *falx cerebri*. It should be seen to bisect the head left to right. Lateral to the falx are two bright lines. These represent the *lateral borders of the lateral ventricles*. The distance from the falx to either of the lines should be approximately one third the distance from the falx to one side of the calvarium (skull) or less. Before 18 weeks, the ventricles fill most of the skull, and this rule does not apply, but should hold, beyond 18 weeks of gestation.

Familiarity with the development of fetal intracranial anatomy and its sonographic presentation assists the sonographer in recognizing normal versus abnormal anatomy at different growth stages. For instance, before the 13th gestational week, it is normal to view the choroid plexus filling the lateral ventricle. It assumes a more posterior location between 13 and 15 weeks, and the anterior horns of the lateral ventricles become quite prominent. In some cases the prominent anterior horns have been mistaken for abnormally large ventricles (ventriculomegaly). Similarly, development of the corpus callosum is not complete until the 18th or 20th gestational week. Scans performed before this time have, in some instances, wrongly suggested agenesis of the corpus callosum. In the same way, before 18 to 22 weeks, the undeveloped cerebellar vermis leaves the inferior portion of the fourth ventricle only covered by the thin ventricular roof, giving the appearance of abnormal communication between the fourth ventricle and cisterna magna. Later in gestation, this finding suggests the presence of brain malformation.

DETERMINATION OF GESTATIONAL AGE DURING THE SECOND AND THIRD TRIMESTERS

The transition between first and second trimesters (12 to 13 weeks) is the accepted time to make the transition from crown rump length (CRL) measurements to *biparietal diameter (BPD)*, *head circumference (HC)* and

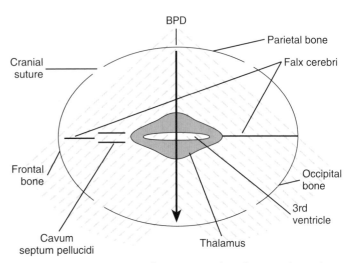

FIGURE 23-33 **Biparietal Diameter.** This illustrates how the sound beam must be perpendicular to the parietal bones and intersect the third ventricle and thalami to obtain an accurate plane for a biparietal diameter (BPD) measurement.

abdominal circumference (AC), and *femur length (FL)* measurements to predict gestational age.

Biparietal Diameter (BPD)

The BPD can be appropriately measured through any plane of section that traverses the third ventricle and thalami. The transducer must be perpendicular to the parietal bones and positioned to intersect the third ventricle and thalami (Figure 23-33). (Refer to the Central Nervous System section to review the sonographic appearance of these brain structures.)

To accurately measure the BPD, the calvaria (cranium) must be symmetric with smooth contours, and measurement cursors may be positioned in 1 of 3 ways: (1) inner edge of near calvarial wall to outer edge of far calvarial wall, (2) outer edge of near calvarial wall to inner edge of far calvarial wall, and (3) middle of near calvarial wall to middle of far calvarial wall. Most institutions use the second method (Figure 23-34, *A*).

The recognizable symmetry of the calvaria and thalami (on either side of the third ventricle) makes it easy to recognize the correct plane of section to obtain accurate and consistent measurements of the BPD. Charts are available that correlate the BPD measurement with gestational age, and most modern ultrasound equipment computes an age while the measurement is obtained.

Cephalic Index (CI)

At times a number of conditions such as multiple gestations and breech presentations can alter the shape of the fetal head; in those cases the cephalic index (CI) should always be determined to assess head shape. The BPD,

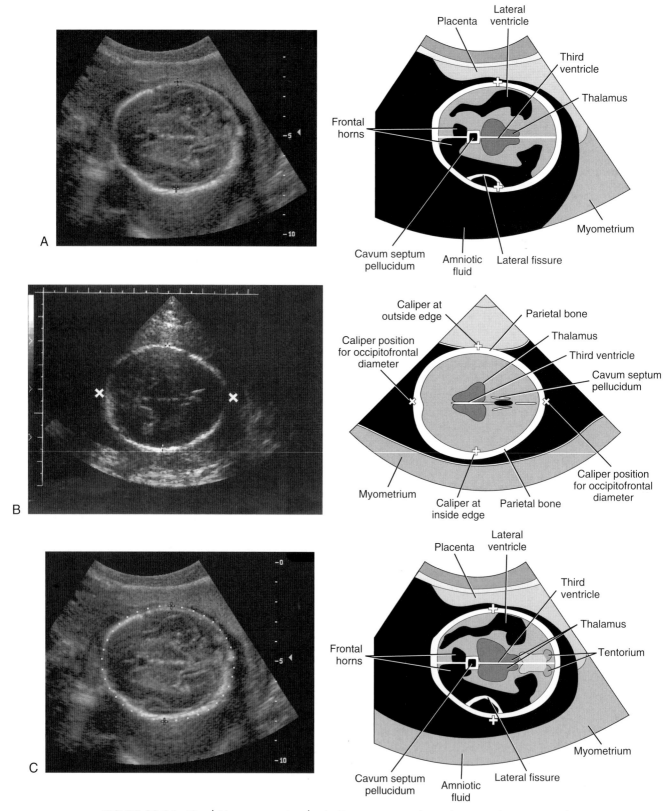

FIGURE 23-34 **Head Measurement Levels. A,** Demonstrates caliper placement (outer to inner) and anatomic level for a *biparietal diameter (BPD)* measurement. **B,** Position of calipers (outer to inner and outer to outer/horizontal) for *BPD* and *fronto-occipital diameter (FOD)* measurements. **C,** Demonstrates caliper placement (outer to outer/vertical) and anatomic level for a *head circumference (HC)* measurement. (**A** and **C,** Scans courtesy the University of Virginia Health System, Department of Radiology, Division of Ultrasound, Charlottesville, Virginia.)

along with a fronto-occipital diameter (FOD), is used to calculate the CI:

$$BPD \div FOD \times 100 = Cephalic \ index$$

The FOD is measured from the outer edge to the outer edge of the calvaria (Figure 23-34, *B*). Today, most ultrasound machines compute the CI using the long and short axes from a head circumference (HC) measurement. The CI should be between 0.72 and 0.86. If the CI is above 0.86, the head is wider than average, or brachiocephalic. If the CI is under 0.72, the head is narrower than average, or dolichocephalic. The HC is usually used for dating the pregnancy when the CI is abnormal.

Head Circumference (HC) *outer to outer*
Unlike the BPD, HC is best obtained through a single plane of section that must be perpendicular to the thalami, the third ventricle (like the BPD), and the cavum septum pellucidum and tentorium.

To accurately measure the head circumference, the calvaria should appear symmetric with smooth contours. In cases where the entire perimeter of the calvaria is not demonstrated, the elliptical measurement cursor on most machines will adequately estimate the portions not imaged. Cursors should be placed at the outer edge of the near calvarial wall to the outer edge of the far calvarial wall (Figure 23-34, *C*). Care should be taken not to fit the ellipse to the surrounding skin edge. Charts are available that correlate the HC measurement with gestational age, and most modern ultrasound equipment computes an age while the measurement is obtained.

As discussed, the BPD can be obtained through multiple planes; the HC, through a single plane of section. Therefore the HC image can be used to obtain the BPD. On the other hand, a BPD image cannot necessarily be used to obtain the HC unless it is at the single level that includes the cavum septum pellucidum and tentorium, along with the thalamus and third ventricle

Abdominal Circumference (AC)
As seen in Figure 23-35, the AC is measured through a single plane of an axial section of the fetal abdomen where the umbilical vein branches, and the right and left portal veins are continuous with one another. At this level the shortest length of the umbilical vein is visualized. Other sonographic markers for the correct AC level include the axial section of the fetal spine that appears as three bright, echogenic reflectors, and the anechoic fluid-filled stomach may be seen on the fetus' left.

The axial section of the fetal abdomen should appear round or nearly round for an accurate AC measurement. The elliptical measurement cursor is fit to the skin edge (Figure 23-36). Charts are available that correlate the

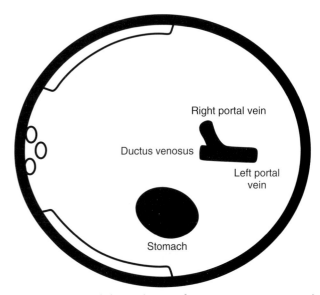

FIGURE 23-35 *Abdominal Circumference Measurement Level.* Illustrated axial fetal abdomen level for accurate abdominal circumference (AC) measurement.

AC measurement with gestational age, and as previously mentioned, most modern ultrasound equipment computes an age while the measurement is obtained.

The AC is considered the most difficult measurement to consistently obtain because of the times when the AC landmarks can be less than optimal to image. In these cases the "roundest" appearance of the abdomen is used. At this level the anteroposterior and transverse diameters of the abdomen should be equal or nearly equal. Because not all ultrasound instruments have the ability to trace or draw ellipses, the AC can be determined by adding the anteroposterior and transverse diameters of the abdomen (measured from skin edge to skin edge) and multiplying the total sum by 1.57:

$$(D1 + D2) \times 1.57 = AC$$

Standard reference tables are used to correlate the AC with predicted age. Other charts use the AC and HC to estimate fetal weight.

Femur Length (FL)
The fetal femur can be measured as early as 12 weeks of development to predict gestational age. The proper plane of section is simply the long axis of the bone. This can be confirmed by showing the highly reflective femoral head and femoral condyle in the same plane. Measurement cursors are placed at the bone-cartilage interface, which are the ossified portions of the metaphysis and diaphysis. The low-gray cartilaginous ends of the femur are not included in the measurement.

Figure 23-37, *A*, demonstrates the measurement of a fetal femur. Both femurs should always be measured. If the femur lengths do not agree with gestational age

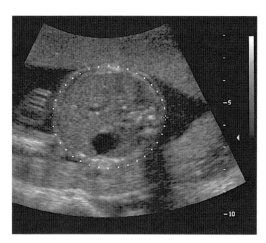

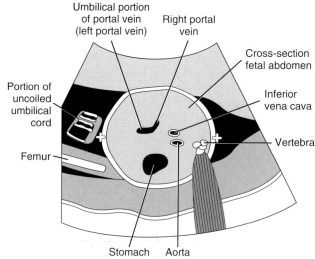

FIGURE 23-36 **Abdominal Circumference Measurement Level.** Demonstrates caliper placement (*outer skin edge to outer skin edge*) and plane of section to obtain the fetal abdominal circumference (AC) measurement. The AC is measured at the position where the short axis diameter of the liver is the greatest. Sonographically, this is identified as the axial section of the fetal abdomen where the anechoic right and left portal veins are continuous with one another. Some refer to this appearance as the "hockey stick." Note that this is also where the shortest length of the umbilical portion of the left portal vein is visualized. (Scan courtesy the University of Virginia Health System, Department of Radiology, Division of Ultrasound, Charlottesville, Virginia.)

head or abdominal measurements, the humeri should also be measured (Figure 23-37, *B*). Charts (often part of ultrasound machine software as mentioned) are available that correlate estimated gestational age with femur and humerus lengths.

In relatively rare cases, when the BPD, HC, or FL is not obtainable, additional measurement parameters (and correlating charts) to estimate fetal age can be used. These include long axis measurements of the fetal tibia, fibula, radius, ulna, clavicle, or foot. Furthermore, interorbital and intraorbital diameters and transverse diameter of the cerebellum are preferred by some experts as supplementary methods for estimating fetal age.

Following the first trimester, fetal age estimates should be based on the multiple measurement parameters discussed in this chapter, preferably before 20 weeks' gestation. Most experts agree that the optimal combination of parameters is based on HC and FL.

Inaccurate measurements can lead to misdiagnoses and serious potential errors in the clinical management of the patient and gestation. Learning the guidelines for obtaining fetal measurements and using them consistently and accurately provide the essential information for correct interpretation.

SONOGRAPHIC APPLICATIONS

Ultrasound can be used to confirm or rule out a variety of things during the second and third trimesters. Some

of the most common indications for a second- and third-trimester ultrasound are:

- **Gestational age (GA):** confirm GA before invasive studies such as **amniocentesis** (percutaneous penetration of the uterus and amniotic sac for aspiration of a sample of amniotic fluid), elective repeat cesarean delivery, discrepancy between size and dates, or evaluation of fetal growth.
- **Fetal growth.**
- **Fetal presentation.**
- **Discrepancy between size and dates:**
    - *Small for dates:* rule out fetal death, fetal anomaly, or incorrect menstrual history.
    - *Large for dates:* rule out a mass, multiple gestation, or fetal anomaly.
- **History of or suspected multiple gestations:** to determine the number of gestations.
- **Vaginal spotting or bleeding:** to rule out placenta previa or placental abruption (partial or complete separation of the placenta from the uterus).
- **Incompetent cervix:** to rule out cervical shortening.
- **Abdominal/Pelvic pain:** to rule out a mass, ectopic pregnancy, placenta previa, or placental abruption.
- **Substance abuse or prescription drugs early in pregnancy:** to rule out fetal anomalies and determine fetal growth rate.
- **Premature labor and/or rupture of membranes.**
- **Trauma:** to determine fetal well-being.

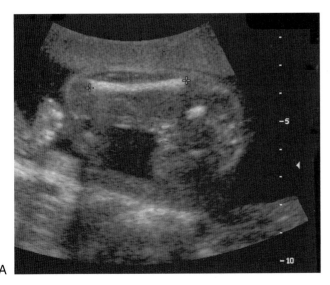

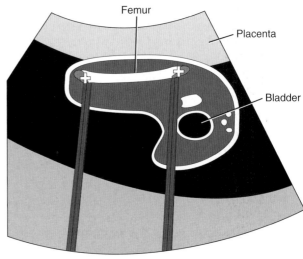

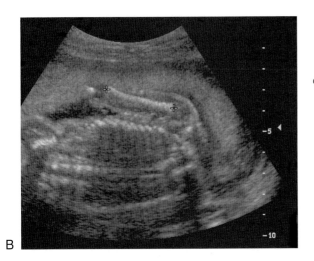

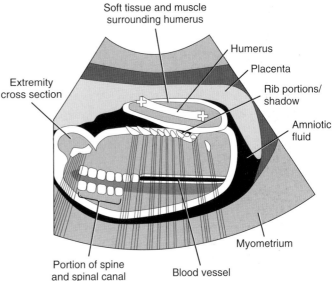

FIGURE 23-37 Long Bone Measurements. The long axis of the *femur* and *humerus* are used for measurements to determine gestational age. If both cartilaginous ends of the long bones are visualized, this guarantees that the plane of section is the long axis. Measurement is confined to the ossified portions. **A,** Femur measurement. **B,** Humerus measurement. (Scans courtesy the University of Virginia Health System, Department of Radiology, Division of Ultrasound, Charlottesville, Virginia.)

- **History of previous congenital anomaly.**
- **Abnormal biochemical markers.**
- **Evaluation of amniotic fluid.**
- **Suspected fetal death.**
- **Fetal risk for aneuploidy:** the **nuchal fold (NF) measurement** is performed during the second trimester and should not be mistaken with the nuchal translucency which is measured in the first trimester. The NF measurement is used to determine the fetal risk for an abnormal chromosome number (aneuploidy). Many believe that a thick nuchal fold (6 mm or greater) detected during the second trimester is a reliable indicator for Down syndrome. Skin thickness at the back of the fetus' neck is measured between 16 and 22 weeks of gestation. An axial section of the fetal head at the level of the cerebellar hemispheres and cavum septum pellucidum is used for the measurement. Calipers are placed on the outer surface of the occipital bone and the outer surface of the skin.

- **Follow-up studies of placenta location or fetal anomaly.**

NORMAL VARIANTS

- **Lemon sign:** Appears as bilateral, frontal, concave scalloping of the calvaria.

- **Prominent cisterna magna:** In the absence of other malformation(s), this is a normal finding.
- **Choroid plexus cyst:** In the absence of other malformation(s), this is a normal finding that usually resolves by 24 to 26 gestational weeks.
- **Cavum vergae:** Normal prominent posterior continuation of the cavum septum pellucidi, which may simulate a dilated third ventricle or arachnoid cyst.
- **Fetal hair:** Commonly seen in the third trimester and should not be mistaken for a calvarial mass or scalp edema.
- **Prominent cardiac moderator band:** Normal enlargement or prominence of the moderator band can simulate a ventricular thrombus or neoplasm.
- **Echogenic Intracardiac Focus (EIF).** Seen as a small, bright, echo focus in the heart on a 4-chamber heart view. If an EIF is seen in isolation in a normal pregnancy it is considered a normal, benign variant. EIFs are seen in 4% to 5 % of normal pregnancies. Figure 23-19 illustrates an EIF in the left ventricle. EIFs normally disappear during the third trimester.

REFERENCE CHARTS

ASSOCIATED PHYSICIANS

- **Obstetrician/Gynecologist:** Manages preterm obstetric care and delivers the fetus. This physician is also responsible for the care of the infant immediately after delivery.
- **High-risk obstetrician:** Specializes in the preterm management of women whose pregnancies are at risk because of various medical conditions. This physician also delivers the fetus and is responsible for the care of the infant immediately after delivery.
- **Fertility specialist:** Typically, this physician is an obstetrician/gynecologist who specializes in treating disorders of the female reproductive system associated with fertility and pregnancy.
- **Radiologist/Sonologist:** Specializes in the administration and diagnostic interpretation of ultrasound and other imaging modalities.

COMMON DIAGNOSTIC TESTS

- **Pregnancy test:** Detects human chorionic gonadotropin (hCG) levels in urine or blood when pregnancy exists. A lab technician usually runs the test, which is interpreted by a pathologist or obstetrician/gynecologist.
- **Beta-hCG test:** Blood is tested to quantitate the serum level of hCG to estimate gestational age. A lab technician usually runs the test, which is interpreted by a pathologist or obstetrician/gynecologist.
- **Maternal/paternal blood typing:** Determines blood type and whether Rh factor is positive or negative.
- **Antibody screen:** Blood test for Rh factor, which is a group of autoantibodies that react with a person's own immunoglobulin.
- **Glucose screen:** Blood test for diabetes between 24 and 28 weeks' gestation.

- **Doppler ultrasound:** Various Doppler ultrasound applications can be used evaluate maternal and fetal blood flow, including the blood vessels of the placenta.
- **Amniocentesis:** Transabdominal or transcervical penetration of the uterus and amniotic sac for aspiration of a sample of amniotic fluid used for obtaining pertinent genetic information regarding the fetus.
- **Computed tomography (CT):** Evaluation of fetal and maternal anatomy when sonographic evaluation is indeterminate. CT is generally used as a "last resort" because of the radiation exposure; in most cases, its use is limited to assessment of the acute maternal abdomen.
- **Magnetic resonance imaging (MRI):** Traditionally used to evaluate maternal anatomy during pregnancy and abnormalities, such as adnexal masses, which require further characterization beyond the ultrasound findings. Typically, MRI evaluation of the fetus is hindered by fetal motion.

LABORATORY VALUES

- **Alpha-fetoprotein (AFP):** Found in maternal blood and amniotic fluid. Elevated levels indicate fetal abnormalities or defects.
- **Lecithin-to-sphingomyelin ratio (LS ratio):** Found in amniotic fluid. Measures the degree of fetal lung development.
- **Triple marker screening (AFP, uE3, hCG):** Abnormal levels of alpha-fetoprotein (AFP), unconjugated estriol (uE3), and human chorionic gonadotropin (hCG) are indicators of certain embryonic/fetal abnormalities, possible multifetal gestations, and combined with maternal age, screening markers for Down syndrome.

ROUTINE MEASUREMENTS

- **Biparietal diameter (BPD):** Easily obtained, reproducible measurement of the fetal head used to calculate an estimated age. An accurate BPD can be obtained through any plane of section that intersects the thalami and third ventricle. Generally, measurement cursors are placed from the outer edge of the near calvarial wall to the inner edge of the far calvarial wall. Experts believe the BPD to be most accurate before 20 menstrual weeks. Standard reference tables are used to correlate the BPD with predicted age.
- **Head circumference (HC):** Elliptical measurement along the calvarial margins that is used to calculate an estimated age. The HC is best obtained through a single plane of section that must be perpendicular to the thalami, third ventricle, cavum septum pellucidum, and tentorium. Measurement cursors should be placed at the outer edge of the near calvarial wall to the outer edge of the far calvarial wall. Standard reference tables are used to correlate the HC with predicted age.
- **Abdominal circumference (AC):** Elliptical measurement along the abdominal skin margin used to calculate an estimated age. The AC is best obtained at the short axis level of the abdomen where the right and left

portal veins are continuous with one another. Elliptical measurement cursors should be placed at the skin edge. Standard reference tables are used to correlate the AC with predicted age. Additional charts use the AC and HC to estimate fetal weight.

- **Femur length (FL):** Long axis measurement of the ossified portions of the fetal femur used to calculate an estimated age. An accurate FL is obtained when the cartilaginous femoral condyle and femoral head are visualized simultaneously. They are not included in the femoral measurement; cursors are placed at the ossified ends of the metaphysis and diaphysis. Standard reference tables are used to correlate the FL with predicted age.
- **Cephalic index (CI):** Calculated measurement to assess fetal head shape. The BPD, along with the FOD (fronto-occipital diameter measured from the outer edge to the outer edge of the calvaria), is used to calculate the CI as follows:

$$BPD \div FOD \times 100 = \text{Cephalic index}$$

A normal CI is between 0.72 and 0.86.

- **Nuchal fold (NF) measurement:** Measurement of the thickness of the skin at the back of the fetus' neck to assess fetal risk of aneuploidy. One caliper is placed on the outer surface of the occipital bone and the other is placed on the outer skin surface on a transcerebellar image that includes the cavum septum pellucidum.
- **Amniotic fluid index (AFI):** Calculated measurement to determine the amniotic fluid volume (AFV). Anteroposterior fluid measurements from four equal, gravid uterine quadrants are added together to total the AFI. An 8-cm AFI is considered normal.

■ ■ ■ AFFECTING CHEMICALS

- **Menotropins (Pergonal), urofollitropin (Metrodin), clomiphene citrate (Clomid):** Medications prescribed for infertility to stimulate follicular maturation and induce ovulation. In some cases, these medications have been associated with multifetal gestations.

■ ■ ■ VASCULATURE

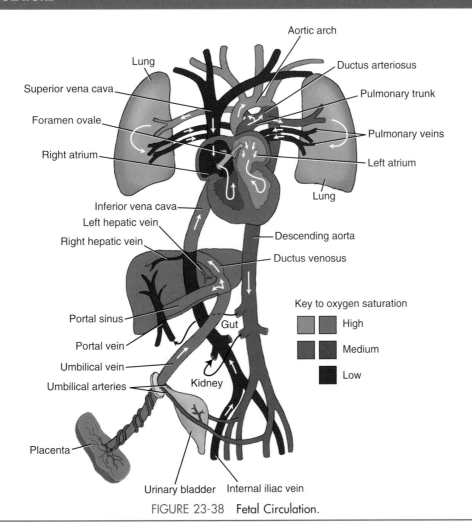

FIGURE 23-38 Fetal Circulation.

CHAPTER 24

High-Risk Obstetric Sonography

BETTY BATES TEMPKIN

OBJECTIVES

Describe the indications for a biophysical profile.
Describe how biophysical profiles are scored.
Describe an amniocentesis and its purpose.
Describe chorionic villus sampling (CVS) and its purpose.

Describe the indications for fetal blood sampling.
Describe the difference between dizygotic and monozygotic twin gestations.

KEY WORDS

Alpha-Fetoprotein (AFP) — Found in maternal blood and amniotic fluid. Elevated levels indicate fetal abnormalities or defects.

Amniocentesis — Transabdominal or transcervical penetration of the uterus and amniotic sac for aspiration of a sample of amniotic fluid used for obtaining pertinent genetic information regarding the fetus.

Biophysical Profile — Test to measure fetal well-being. Several fetal biophysical variables are observed to predict perinatal outcome.

Chorionic Villus Sampling (CVS) — Transabdominal or transcervical penetration of the uterus and amniotic sac for a sample of the chorion covered by villi, which is used for obtaining pertinent genetic information regarding the embryo/fetus.

Dizygotic Twins — Twins that develop embryologically from two separate ova, similar to a single gestation. Commonly called fraternal (not identical) twins.

Lecithin-to-Sphingomyelin Ratio (L-S ratio) — Ratio of lecithin to sphingomyelin, which measures the degree of fetal lung development.

Monozygotic Twins — Twins that develop embryologically from a single ovum. Commonly called identical twins. The number of chorions (placentas) and amnions is variable.

HIGH-RISK PREGNANCIES

High-risk pregnancies include those in which:

- There was a previous child with an abnormality such as a neural tube defect, chromosomal disorder, developmental defect, or malformation syndrome.
- There is a preexisting or existing maternal condition that may jeopardize the pregnancy.
- The biochemical screening results are abnormal.
- There is a suspected or detected abnormality.
- There is a condition such as multifetal gestation, advanced maternal age, intrauterine growth retardation (also known as intrauterine growth restriction), maternal diabetes mellitus, or post-date gestation.

In most high-risk cases, ultrasound evaluation or ultrasound-guided procedures are recommended. This chapter addresses the ultrasound studies used for those higher-risk pregnancies.

FETAL SONOGRAPHIC BIOPHYSICAL PROFILE

In some pregnancies it is necessary to determine whether the fetus is in distress. To assess the status of the fetus, a **biophysical profile** may be performed. Biophysical profiles, which measure fetal well-being, are usually reserved for ultrasound cases with abnormal or ambiguous findings. Several fetal biophysical variables are observed to predict perinatal outcome: fetal heart rate, fetal body movements, fetal tone, fetal breathing movements, amniotic fluid volume, and placental grading. Evaluations begin with a nonstress, electronic fetal heart rate monitoring, followed by real-time ultrasound assessment of the other biophysical components. The examination ends when each of the biophysical components meets normal criteria or when 30 minutes of real-time ultrasonography have elapsed. A scoring system is used in which each biophysical activity or component

■ ■ ■ **Table 24-1** Biophysical Profile Scoring

	Criterion	Score (PTS)
Part I: Nonstress test	Two accelerations of 15 beats per min in 30-min test	2
Part II: Ultrasound examination		
Gross movement	Three separate flexions and extensions in 30-min examination	2
Tone	One episode of fetal opening and closing of hand or clenching of foot in 30-min examination	2
Respiration	At least 60 sec of fetal breathing in 30-min examination	2
Fluid	At least one pocket of amniotic fluid of at least 1 cm in two dimensions	2
	Unqualified pass	8 or more
	Maximum total	10

Data from Manning EA, Platt LD, Sipos L: Antenatal fetal evaluation: development of a fetal biophysical profile, *Am J Obstet Gynecol* 136:787-795, 1980.

is scored as either 0 (when abnormal) or 2 (when normal). Scores of 8 or higher are associated with good perinatal outcome. Scores lower than 8 are generally followed up with additional testing or induced delivery (Table 24-1).

The criteria for scoring biophysical profiles may vary among institutions, but generally the normal fetal biophysical profiles are based on the following observations within 30 minutes: (1) the presence of two or more fetal heart rate accelerations of at least 15 beats per minute in amplitude and at least 15 seconds in duration associated with fetal movement in a 20-minute period and (2) fetal body movement consisting of three or more gross body movements that may include arching of the back or neck or twisting of the trunk. Simultaneous limb and trunk movements are counted as a single movement. Fetal tone consists of at least one incident of limb motion from a position of flexion to extension and rapid return to flexion. Fetal breathing movement is noted in the presence of at least one 60-second episode. Amniotic fluid volume consists of the presence of fluid throughout the uterus and a pocket measuring at least 2 cm or more in vertical diameter. Placental grading (discussed in Chapter 23) is noted as 0, II, or III.

An alternative method for assessing the amount of amniotic fluid or determining the amniotic fluid index (AFI) is the four-quadrant analysis. This measurement is based on the division of the gravid uterus into four equal quadrants using the umbilicus and linea nigra. The anteroposterior diameter of the deepest amniotic fluid pocket in each quadrant is measured. These four measurements are added together to determine the AFI. A sum of 8 cm is considered normal. In most cases, sonographers include only the pockets that are free of extremities and the umbilical cord.

Biophysical profiling is recognized as a reliable method of assessing fetal well-being to predict perinatal outcome in high-risk pregnancies.

DOPPLER ULTRASOUND EVALUATION

Doppler studies of placental and fetal circulation can provide significant data concerning fetal well-being, making it possible to improve fetal outcome.

Umbilical cord Doppler is an examination technique that measures the resistance of blood flow within the placenta. The Doppler signal from the two umbilical arteries is obtained with continuous-wave, or in some cases pulse-wave, Doppler. The spectrum of the signal is analyzed to determine the diastolic flow. The extent of diastolic flow is directly related to the flow resistance of the placenta. There is good correlation between the absence of effective diastolic flow and a poor outcome. In some institutions a poor high-resistance flow pattern will increase the likelihood of an induced delivery. It is believed that damage to the fetus may be minimized by its removal from an inadequate environment.

Doppler measurements may also be used to assess maternal circulation to the uterus. During pregnancy the uterine arteries have very low pulsatility and may appear almost as venous signals when the Doppler waveform is examined. However, a modest cardiac pattern should be obtained. Examples of umbilical artery and maternal uterine artery Doppler waveforms are presented in Figures 24-1 and 24-2.

Fetal responses and adaptation to changes in the intrauterine environment can be evaluated by observing fetal blood circulation. This discussion will focus on applicable blood circulation excluding the fetal heart, since it was discussed in Chapter 23.

Absence of the end-diastolic fetal aortic velocity can easily be determined and is a good predictor of fetal well-being. In fetuses with absent end-diastolic velocity of the thoracic or abdominal aorta, perinatal outcome is poor. Furthermore, abnormal fetal aortic flow velocity waveforms have been associated with neurologic dysfunctions such as lower verbal and global IQ.

Doppler velocity of the renal arteries is clinically applicable for assessing the fetal behavioral state. High renal vascular impedance is an indicator of a fetus

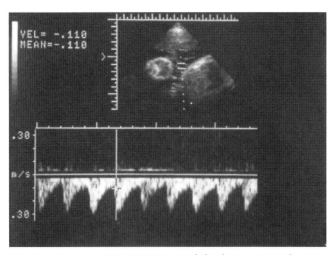

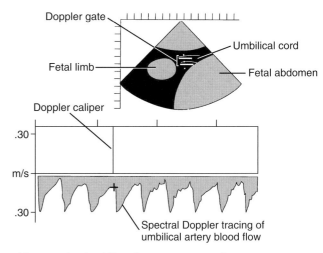

FIGURE 24-1 **Umbilical Artery Doppler Waveform.** Ultrasound-pulsed Doppler interrogation of the umbilical artery. This is a normal low-resistance waveform.

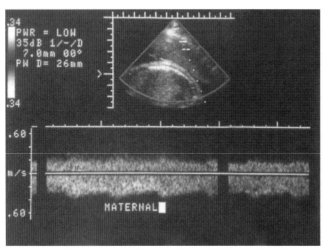

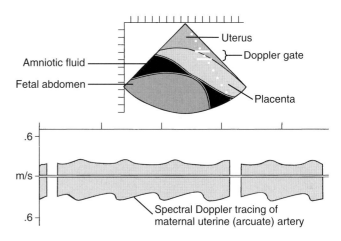

FIGURE 24-2 **Uterine Artery Doppler Waveform.** Ultrasound-pulsed Doppler interrogation of uterine circulation during the third trimester. The waveform on top of the line is a venous signal. The waveform under the line is that of a uterine artery. Note their similarity. The artery has a very low pulsatility.

that is too small for its gestational age. This becomes more obvious with the presence of oligohydramnios. Additionally, there seems to be a significant correlation between the AFI and the renal artery systolic/diastolic ratio.

Normally, the fetal splenic artery has a lower pulsatility than the renal artery. Abnormal splenic artery velocity may be used in predicting fetal hypoxia. In addition, some fetuses that are small for their gestational age demonstrate a decrease in resistance in the splenic artery.

In severe cases of intrauterine growth retardation or restriction, the fetal hepatic artery can usually be detected. The flow velocity waveform displays a low-impedance, high-velocity blood flow, suggesting

redistribution of the hepatic artery, as well as the cerebral, adrenal, and coronary arteries.

Doppler investigation of the umbilical vein is another gauge of fetal well-being. Extraabdominal umbilical venous flow displays regular pulsations up to 15 weeks of gestation; beyond that, the venous pulsations gradually disappear. Occurrence of venous pulsations later in pregnancy is an ominous sign that indicates congestive heart failure in compromised fetuses.

Doppler velocimetry of the ductus venosus plays a valuable role in prenatal fetal assessment. It is easy to distinguish from surrounding vessels and has an acceptable reproducibility with little variation. Abnormal ductus venosus velocity may be useful in determining fetal cardiac disease, severe growth retardation or restriction, fetal anemia, and various chromosomal abnormalities.

Abnormal flow velocity waveform of the inferior vena cava (IVC) is another key sign of fetal compromise. In fetal hypoxia the pulsatility of blood flow in the IVC increases.

With high-risk pregnancies the improvement in outcome of the compromised fetus depends on early identification. Doppler velocimetry studies can provide early data that are critical in the detection and management of fetal abnormalities.

ULTRASOUND-GUIDED PROCEDURES

Amniocentesis

Certain invasive obstetric procedures are routinely assisted by ultrasound for a safer and more accurate study. One of these is transabdominal **amniocentesis**, the percutaneous penetration of the uterus and amniotic sac for aspiration of a sample of amniotic fluid. The fluid contains desquamated fetal cells that can be grown in tissue culture and used for a variety of metabolic assays or DNA extraction. Ideally, amniocentesis is performed at approximately 16 weeks' gestation. Performing amniocentesis any earlier than this increases the risk for possible complications.

As a rule, amniocentesis performed with ultrasound guidance is a safe procedure, but it has the potential to cause serious complications such as premature rupture of membranes, premature labor, and premature separation of the placenta. Additional complications may include injury to the fetus from the needle, fetal or maternal bleeding, placental hemorrhage (if a transplacental approach is used), and even fetal death. Considering the possible complications, each case is evaluated individually, weighing the benefits of the information provided from an amniocentesis against the risks.

When the amniotic fluid is analyzed to determine its biochemical components, the concentration of one component, **alpha-fetoprotein (AFP)**, increases beyond normal limits when certain defects are present. Of particular interest is the karyotype (a chromosomal map) to detect Down syndrome. Many other genetic abnormalities can be detected by this procedure, and the list is growing as research continues. Additionally, through research in molecular biology, molecular probes have been devised that can detect a great number of genetic disorders and can provide test results quicker than other conventional cell culture and chromosomal banding techniques.

Ultrasound plays several roles during the amniocentesis procedure. First, ultrasound is used to assess gestational age, viability, anatomy, number of gestations, and placenta location. Second, the position of the desired pocket of amniotic fluid is determined. The abdomen is then prepped with sterile washes, and the physician anesthetizes the skin and subcutaneous tissues. A sterile cover is positioned over the transducer, and sterile gel is used as the scanning couplant. Next, the position of the amniotic fluid pocket is reconfirmed. In some institutions a sterile needle will be affixed to the ultrasound transducer. In others the transducer is positioned to visualize the amniocentesis needle as it is inserted "freehand" into the amniotic sac. During the procedure, ultrasound provides confirmation that the fetus is not in the needle's path and that the needle is in the correct position for fluid aspiration. After the procedure, ultrasound assesses fetal viability.

As mentioned in Chapter 23, amniotic fluid markers of fetal lung maturity often influence perinatal management. The amniotic fluid is tested to detect two chemicals: lecithin and sphingomyelin. The ratio of lecithin to sphingomyelin, the **Lecithin-to-Sphingomyelin Ratio (L-S ratio)**, measures the degree of fetal lung development. Depending on the L-S ratio, elective delivery may be delayed to allow time for the lungs to develop, and in mandated preterm deliveries, prenatal medications are administered to prevent or decrease the severity of respiratory distress.

Chorionic Villus Sampling

Chorionic villus sampling (CVS) was developed as an early first-trimester means of collecting tissue for genetic analysis, using placental tissue buds or chorionic villi. Because this test can be performed as early as 10 to 12 menstrual weeks, it offers a greater advantage to a woman who is at high risk for giving birth to an abnormal infant. If an affected fetus is diagnosed and the decision is made to terminate the pregnancy, the medical and psychologic risks are fewer with a first-trimester termination compared to a second-trimester termination.

As in amniocentesis, ultrasound is used before the procedure to determine viability, number, trophoblast location, and sampling path. There are two commonly used approaches to CVS: transcervical and transabdominal. The placental implantation site and the position of the uterus dictate the choice of method. Either the abdomen or cervix is prepped with sterile washes, and the physician anesthetizes the site. A sterile cover is positioned over the transducer, and sterile gel is used as the scanning couplant. In both cases, ultrasound guidance informs the clinician when an area rich in chorionic villi has been reached and the collecting device is in place for sampling.

CVS does carry certain risks. After the procedure, spontaneous bleeding or even spontaneous abortion can occur. Generally, procedure-related fetal loss rate due to CVS is extremely low; however, spontaneous abortion has been estimated to occur in approximately 1% of cases.

Fetal Blood Sampling and Fetal Intravascular Transfusion

Ultrasound is essential for safe and reliable access to fetal circulation. The most common indications for the sampling of fetal blood are the confirmation of abnormal findings found on amniocentesis or CVS and the need for rapid chromosomal diagnosis. Analysis of fetal blood requires 48 to 72 hours as compared to 2 to 3 weeks for amniocentesis. Additional indications that require the sampling of fetal blood include diagnosis of a structural anomaly on ultrasound, assessment of fetal anemia, hemophilia and other clotting disorders, and immunodeficiencies and other white cell disorders.

Therapy by intrauterine transfusion of red cells into the umbilical vein is recommended in fetuses with severe hydrops and anemia. Red cells or platelets are routinely transfused for fetal isoimmunization. A transfusion of thrombocytes may be considered in fetuses with severe thrombocytopenia.

The method of choice for fetal blood sampling and fetal intravascular transfusion is as follows. Before the procedure, the area of the umbilical cord insertion into the placenta is established with ultrasound. This area is considered optimal because the cord is fixed at this location. In some cases a free loop of cord may be used; however, this approach is more difficult because of cord movement. The mother is sedated for her own comfort and to reduce movement of the fetus. The abdomen is prepped with sterile washes, and a sterile cover is positioned over the transducer. Sterile gel is used as the scanning couplant. While the physician anesthetizes the skin and subcutaneous tissues, ultrasound is used to check the angle of the needle insertion. Next, under ultrasound guidance, a spinal or transfusion needle is advanced into the umbilical circulation.

The complication rate after fetal blood sampling and fetal intravascular transfusion procedures depends on the indication for the procedure. Fetuses with intrauterine growth retardation and/or structural anomalies are at the highest risk for fetal distress.

Clearly, ultrasound is essential for establishing accuracy during invasive obstetric procedures, making it a valuable asset for prenatal diagnosis and therapy.

MULTIFETAL GESTATIONS

The increase in multiple births since 1980 has been attributed to increased fertility treatments and older maternal populations. Multifetal gestations are considered high-risk pregnancies, both for the fetus and the mother. Complications in multifetal gestations, which parallel those of single gestations but occur with higher frequency, include preterm birth, intrauterine growth retardation or restriction, and fetal anomalies. Complications unique to multifetal gestations include conjoined twins, acardiac twins, twin embolization with co-twin demise, and twin-to-twin transfusion syndrome. Maternal complications associated with multifetal gestations compared with single gestations include higher incidences of preeclampsia, hypertension, placenta abruption, placenta previa, and prepartum and postpartum hemorrhage. The complications and anomalies described for twins are generally applicable to each additional gestation; the risk and severity are usually accentuated.

Sonography is of great value in determining the type of twinning and in accurately identifying fetal complications and anomalies associated with multiple gestations, thus significantly contributing to perinatal management.

Embryology of Multifetal Gestations

Twin gestations result from fertilization of either *two separate ova* or a *single ovum*:

- *Two separate ova* = "*fraternal*" or **dizygotic twins**. Each dizygotic twin develops embryologically similarly to a single gestation. All dizygotic twins form their own blastocyst, resulting in separate amnions (diamniotic) and separate placentas (dichorionic).
- *Single ovum* = "*identical*" or **monozygotic twins**. Monozygotic twins occur after fertilization of a single ovum. The number of chorions (placentas) and amnions is variable and depends on when the zygote (fertilized ovum) divides relative to differentiation of the chorion and amnion. Three types of monozygotic twins are as follows: *dichorionic-diamniotic*, *monochorionic-diamniotic*, and *monochorionic-monoamniotic* (Figure 24-3).
  - **Dichorionic-diamniotic.** Division of the zygote before day 4 (before blastocyst formation) results in a dichorionic-diamniotic gestation. Each embryo will have an individual placenta and amniotic sac.
  - **Monochorionic-diamniotic.** Division between days 4 and 8 (after blastocyst formation but before amnion differentiation) results in a monochorionic-diamniotic gestation. This is the most common type of monozygotic twin gestation. The embryos will share a common placenta but have their own amniotic sac.
  - **Monochorionic-monoamniotic.** Division beyond 8 days postfertilization (after amnion formation) results in a monochorionic-monoamniotic gestation. The embryos will share a common placenta and share a single amniotic sac. In rare cases, division can occur to the embryonic disk more than 13 days postfertilization, resulting in conjoined, or "Siamese," twins. The later the division, the greater the number of shared organs. All conjoined twins are monozygotic, monochorionic-monoamniotic gestations.

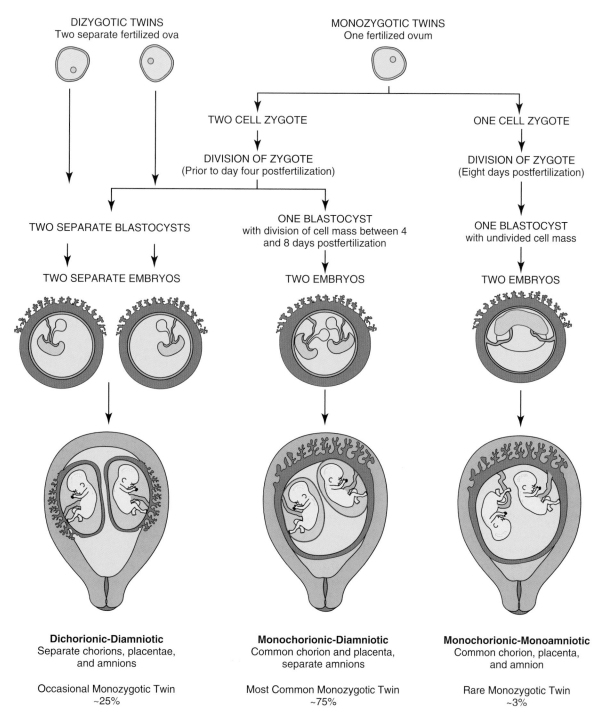

FIGURE 24-3 Development of monozygotic and dizygotic twins, including placentation.

Understanding the embryologic sequence for chorion and amnion formation is essential to the sonographic assessment of multifetal gestations. With twin gestations:

- All dichorionic twins are diamniotic.
- All monoamniotic twins are monochorionic. Monochorionic gestations (because the amnion forms after the chorion) can be either:
  - Diamniotic
    or
  - Monoamniotic

Sonographic Assessment of Multifetal Gestations

There are special considerations in the ultrasound examination of multifetal gestations. All twins should be carefully evaluated with ultrasound to verify the number of chorions and amnions. It should be determined (1) whether the developing embryos (or fetuses) reside in a single amniotic sac, are separated by a membrane(s), or reside in multiple amniotic sacs and (2) whether the chorion/placenta is single and shared or individual and multiple. These determinations can be challenging, particularly beyond the first trimester when, in fact, it may not be possible. For example, a monozygotic dichorionic-diamniotic gestation is identical in appearance to that of a dizygotic gestation. Both involve two complete embryos, two complete sacs, and two separate placentas. Quite often, later in pregnancy, the borders of the placentas will move close to each other and may finally fuse, making differentiation between a monochorionic or dichorionic pregnancy difficult, if not impossible.

From 6 to 10 weeks of gestation, sonographic identification of the number of gestational sacs is an accurate method for predicting chorionicity. An early gestational sac appears as a 2- to 5-mm round, fluid-filled structure surrounded by a rim of high-amplitude echoes that corresponds to the chorion. Early in development, the amniotic membrane is closely applied to the forming embryo, and the fluid-filled gestational sac, as identified on ultrasound, is predominantly chorionic fluid and representative of the chorionic cavity. Therefore counting the number of gestational sacs (chorionic cavities) accurately predicts chorionicity (number of placentas). Two sacs imply dichorionicity, three sacs trichorionicity, and so on. At approximately 10 weeks of gestation the amniotic cavity enlarges until it obliterates the chorionic cavity, and in twin gestations the amnions become opposed and form an intertwin or interfetal membrane.

During the second and third trimesters, the sonographic criteria for determining chorionicity shift to fetal gender, appearance of the interfetal membrane, and number of placentas. If twin fetuses are of opposite gender (dizygotic/fraternal), they are always dichorionic and diamniotic. If, however, the twins are the same gender (identical or fraternal) or the gender is not identified, chorionicity cannot be established, and only genetic analysis can determine the type before delivery.

In a diamniotic twin gestation, whether placentas are shared or not, a membrane should be seen sonographically, separating the fetuses. The thickness of this interfetal membrane can predict chorionicity, whether the pregnancy is monochorionic or dichorionic. The membrane in a diamniotic-monochorionic twin gestation is two layers thick, consisting of two amnions only, one from each fetus. The membrane in a diamniotic-dichorionic twin gestation is the thickest: four layers thick, with two amnions plus two chorions.

Sonographic identification of separate placentas in multifetal gestations depends on the proximity of implantation of the blastocysts. The further apart the implantation, the less likely the placentas are to become fused along their borders, making differentiation easier and the number count accurate. Identification of a single placenta with sonography does not differentiate between a monochorionic gestation and a dichorionic gestation with two continuous fused placentas. However, sonographic identification of two separate placentas in a twin pregnancy does determine dichorionicity.

Utilizing transvaginal sonography, the amnion is visible by 7 or 8 weeks of gestation, when the crown rump length is 8 to 12 mm. Diamnionicity is recognizable as two separate gestational sacs. Monoamnionicity is confirmed when a single amniotic sac containing two embryos is identified.

Amnionicity can also be established by identifying the number of yolk sacs. Sonographically, the yolk sac is identified approximately 2 weeks earlier than the amnion. Therefore in a monochorionic twin gestation, identification of two yolk sacs is an accurate method for confirming diamnionicity in the first trimester before visualization of the amniotic membrane. Monochorionic-monoamniotic gestations are associated with a single yolk sac or, in rare cases, a partially divided yolk sac, depending on when the zygote divides.

THE EXPANDING ROLE OF ULTRASOUND IN HIGH-RISK OBSTETRICS

This chapter has presented the role of ultrasound in high-risk pregnancies. In most cases, high-risk pregnancies utilize the ultrasound examinations and ultrasound-guided procedures discussed here. As new clinical management procedures evolve for handling high-risk pregnancies, ultrasound will continue to play a critical role in the development of new approaches to fetal prenatal diagnosis and therapy.

Recently, fetal surgical procedures have been carried out with a high degree of success. These procedures require the use of ultrasound for, first, detecting the anomaly, and second, locating an incision point within the uterus for extracting the fetus for surgery. The post-surgical period also requires ultrasound examination of the surgical site.

The use of ultrasound in managing high-risk pregnancies has the advantage of being a safe procedure offering an abundance of information that directly affects maternal and fetal management and ultimately reduces adverse perinatal outcome.

REFERENCE CHARTS

■ ■ ■ ASSOCIATED PHYSICIANS

- **High-Risk obstetrician:** Specializes in the preterm management of women whose pregnancies are at risk due to various medical conditions. This physician also delivers the fetus and is responsible for the care of the infant immediately after delivery.
- **Obstetrician/Gynecologist:** Manages preterm obstetric care and delivers the fetus. This physician is also responsible for the care of the infant immediately after delivery.
- **Fertility specialist:** Typically, this physician is an obstetrician/gynecologist who specializes in treating disorders of the female reproductive system associated with fertility and pregnancy.
- **Radiologist/Sonologist:** Specializes in the administration and diagnostic interpretation of ultrasound and other imaging modalities.

■ ■ ■ COMMON DIAGNOSTIC TESTS

- **Fetal biophysical profile:** Ultrasound evaluation to assess fetal well-being by evaluating multiple fetal biophysical activities.
- **Doppler ultrasound:** Various Doppler ultrasound applications are used to evaluate maternal and fetal blood flow, including the blood vessels of the placenta.
- **Amniocentesis:** Transabdominal or transcervical penetration of the uterus and amniotic sac for aspiration of a sample of amniotic fluid used for obtaining pertinent genetic information regarding the fetus.
- **Chorionic villus sampling (CVS):** Transabdominal or transcervical penetration of the uterus and amniotic sac for a sample of the chorion covered by villi; used for obtaining pertinent genetic information regarding the embryo/fetus.
- **Fetal blood sampling:** Generally follows confirmation of abnormal findings on amniocentesis or CVS or the need for rapid chromosomal diagnosis. Analysis requires only 48 to 72 hours, much shorter than the time required for amniocentesis or CVS.

- **Fetal blood transfusion:** Fetal therapy involving fetal intravascular transfusion of red cells or platelets for isoimmunization.
- **Computed tomography (CT):** Evaluation of fetal and maternal anatomy when sonographic evaluation is indeterminate. CT is generally used as a "last resort" because of the radiation exposure and in most cases is limited to assessment of the acute maternal abdomen.
- **Magnetic resonance imaging (MRI):** Traditionally used to evaluate maternal anatomy during pregnancy and abnormalities such as adnexal masses, which require further characterization beyond the ultrasound findings. Typically, MRI evaluation of the fetus is hindered by fetal motion.

■ ■ ■ LABORATORY VALUES

- **Alpha-fetoprotein (AFP):** Found in maternal blood and amniotic fluid. Elevated levels indicate fetal abnormalities or defects.
- **Triple marker screening (AFP, uE3, hCG):** Abnormal levels of alpha-fetoprotein (AFP), unconjugated estriol (uE3), and human chorionic gonadotropin (hCG) are indicators of certain fetal abnormalities and possible multifetal gestations and, when combined with maternal age, screening markers for Down syndrome.
- **L-S ratio –** Amniotic fluid is tested to detect the ratio of lecithin to sphingomyelin, which measures the degree of fetal lung development.

■ ■ ■ ROUTINE MEASUREMENTS

- See Chapter 23.

■ ■ ■ VASCULATURE

- See Chapter 23.

■ ■ ■ AFFECTING CHEMICALS

- Menotropins (Pergonal), urofollitropin (Metrodin), clomiphene citrate (Clomid): Medications prescribed for infertility to stimulate follicular maturation and induce ovulation. In some cases, these medications have been associated with multifetal gestations.

CHAPTER 25

Fetal Echocardiography

JILL BEITHON

OBJECTIVES

Describe the location and size of the heart in the fetus.
Identify normal fetal heart anatomy.
Discuss the three fetal vascular shunts and their purpose.
Understand the screening of the fetal heart and the appropriate timing of this test.
List the five views necessary for imaging during the screening of the fetal heart.

Describe how to maximize resolution while imaging the fetal heart.
Explain what constitutes a technically correct four-chamber heart view.
Name three different types of four-chamber views.
Identify associated physicians.

KEY WORDS

Atrioventricular Septal Defect (AVSD) — Refers to a spectrum of cardiac defects that includes abnormalities of both the interventricular and atrial septum and the atrioventricular valves.

Atrioventricular Valves (AV) — The valves (the tricuspid valve on the right; the mitral valve on the left) that control the openings through which the atria and ventricles on each side of the heart communicate.

Cardiac "Crux" — Point where the lower part of the atrial septum meets the upper part of the ventricular septum and where the atrioventricular valves insert.

Complete Transposition of the Great Arteries (TGA) — Also referred to as dextro-Transposition of the great arteries (*d*-Transposition of the great arteries, dextro-TGA, or *d*-TGA), is a birth defect involving the large arteries of the heart. This is a failure of the truncus arteriosus to divide and position normally during cardiogenesis. The aorta, which normally arises from the left ventricle, will arise from the right ventricle in this condition. The pulmonary artery, which normally arises from the right ventricle, will arise from the left ventricle in this condition.

Congenital heart disease (CHD) — Problem with the structure of the heart that is present at birth. Congenital heart defects are the most common type of birth defect.

Coronary Arteries — Arteries that arise from the aortic root which perfuse the heart muscle.

Ductus Arteriosus — A shunt in fetal circulation that connects the main pulmonary artery to the descending aorta.

Ductus Venosus — One of three fetal shunts; enables oxygenated blood from the mother to pass almost directly into the fetal heart, bypassing the liver. Following birth it will fibrose and become the ligamentum venosum.

Eustachian Valve — Also called the valve of the inferior vena cava, the Eustachian valve lies at the junction of the inferior vena cava and right atrium. In fetal life the Eustachian valve helps direct the flow of oxygen-rich blood through the right atrium into the left atrium and away from the right ventricle. Streaming this blood across the atrial septum via the foramen ovale increases the oxygen content of blood in the left atrium. This, in turn, increases the oxygen concentration of blood in the left ventricle, the aorta, the coronary circulation, and the circulation of the developing brain.

Foramen Ovale — Shunt in fetal circulation between the two atrial chambers.

Inferior Vena Cava (IVC) — Large vein that drains the lower half of the body into the right atrium of the heart.

Interatrial Septum (IAS) — Wall separating the upper chambers of the heart, the right and left atria.

Interventricular Septum (IVS) — Wall separating the lower chambers of the heart, the right and left ventricles.

Moderator Band — Septomarginal trabecula (also known as the moderator band) is a muscular band of heart tissue found in the right ventricle. It is seen near the apex and extends from the ventricular septum to the base of the anterior papillary muscle.

Prostaglandin E — Drug used used in maintaining a patent ductus arteriosus in newborns. This is primarily useful when there is threat of premature closure of the ductus arteriosus in an infant with ductal-dependent congenital heart disease, including cyanotic lesions (e.g., pulmonary atresia/stenosis, tricuspid atresia/stenosis, transposition of the great arteries) and acyanotic lesions (e.g., coarctation of the aorta, hypoplastic left heart syndrome, critical aortic stenosis, interrupted aortic arch).

Pulmonary Artery (Main, Right, Left) — Main pulmonary artery that receives blood from the right ventricle and then branches into a right pulmonary artery to the right lung and a left pulmonary artery to the left lung.

Situs Solitus — Normal arrangement of the abdominal and thoracic organs.

Superior Vena Cava (SVC) — One of the two great veins normally connected to the right atrium. The other is the inferior vena cava. The SVC drains the blood from the head and upper extremities.

Total Anomalous Pulmonary Venous Return (TAPVR) — Rare congenital heart defect in which all four pulmonary veins return blood from the lungs to the systemic venous circulation rather than the left atrium, where they normally return blood.

This condition is fatal in the neonate after closure of the foramen ovale and the ductus arteriosus.

Umbilical Arteries — Two umbilical arteries supply deoxygenated blood from the fetus to the placenta. Branches of the internal iliac arteries, the umbilical arteries surround the urinary bladder and then carry deoxygenated blood out of the fetus through the umbilical cord.

Umbilical Vein — Vein that delivers oxygenated blood from the placenta to the fetus.

■

This chapter will discuss the anatomy and physiology of the fetal heart along with the imaging considerations necessary for the evaluation of this intricate and tiny structure. When one considers that **congenital heart disease (CHD)** (problem with the structure of the heart that is present at birth) is the most common human malformation, it becomes apparent why imaging of the fetal heart is an important element of the second-trimester fetal anatomy examination. This is important because prenatal diagnosis of congenital heart defects can significantly reduce morbidity and mortality of the neonate. This is especially true for abnormalities that are dependent on the two shunts in the fetal heart remaining open after birth. Such abnormalities include coarctation of the aorta, hypoplastic heart syndrome, and **complete transposition of the great arteries (TGA)** (birth defect where the aorta, which normally arises from the left ventricle, will arise from the right ventricle; the pulmonary artery, which normally arises from the right ventricle, will arise from the left ventricle).

PRENATAL DEVELOPMENT

The anatomy of the fetal heart before and after birth are similar, except for two unique features: the foramen ovale and the ductus arteriosus. As discussed in Chapter 23, the **foramen ovale** is an opening in the atrial septum that allows some of the blood entering the right atrium to bypass the lungs and flow directly to the left side of the heart. The **ductus arteriosus**, a shunt between the **main pulmonary artery** and the descending aorta, allows most of the blood coming from the pulmonary artery to bypass the lungs (Figure 25-1). In abnormalities that restrict the flow of blood in or out of the left ventricle the direction of blood can move backward from the left atrium to the right atrium across the foramen ovale, thus allowing blood to continue to flow through the heart. In these anomalies blood also can redirect from the ductus arteriosus backward into the aortic arch, the arch vessels, and the **coronary arteries** (arteries that arise from the aortic root that perfuse [supply] the heart muscle). This allows necessary blood to get to the brain and heart muscle even in the presence of a major flow-restricting

abnormality (Figure 25-2). When a right-sided obstruction is present, the ductus arteriosus can also move blood backward, allowing blood to back up the branch pulmonary arteries that bring necessary blood to the lungs for fetal development (Figure 25-3). After birth these shunts close, which no longer allows for the free flow of blood between the right and left circulations. If flow-restricting abnormalities are found prenatally, measures can be taken to assure that these two shunts remain open until surgical intervention can be performed. A drug, **Prostaglandin E**, can be given to the neonate to allow the ductus arteriosus to remain patent.

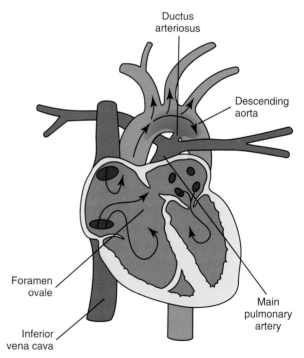

FIGURE 25-1 **Blood Flow in the Normal Fetal Heart.** In this drawing note the opening between the atrial chambers, the foramen ovale, that allows blood to pass from the right atrium to the left atrium. Also note the ductus arteriosus, a shunt between the pulmonary artery and the descending aorta that allows blood to bypass the lungs. The lungs do not have a respiratory function at this time and cannot accept large quantities of blood in fetal life.

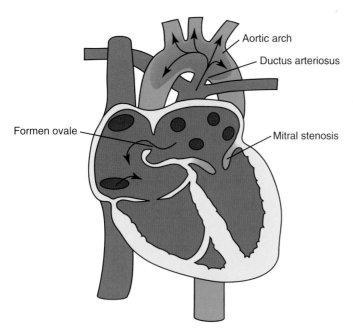

FIGURE 25-2 Blood flow in a left-sided heart abnormality, mitral stenosis, causing hypoplastic left heart syndrome. Blood coming into the right and left atria is redirected backward across the foramen ovale, causing the fossa ovalis flap to move into the right atrium. Blood from the ductus arteriosus is redirected into the aortic arch, supplying blood to the arch vessels and the coronary arteries, allowing blood to get to the brain and heart muscle.

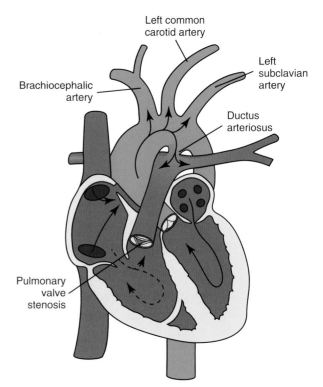

FIGURE 25-3 Blood flow in a right-sided heart anomaly, pulmonary stenosis, causing hypoplastic right heart syndrome. Blood coming into the right atrium is all redirected across the fossa ovalis into the left atrium and ventricle. Blood from the aortic arch is redirected backwards into the ductus arteriosus and into the branch pulmonary arteries supplying necessary blood to the lungs for fetal development.

Refer to Chapter 30, Pediatric Echocardiography, for more in-depth information and diagrams regarding the prenatal development of the heart.

Fetal Circulation

Oxygenation of fetal blood happens within the placenta in the fetus because the lungs are developing and are not ready to perform this function. Normal circulation through the fully developed fetal heart is shown in Figure 25-4. Maternal and fetal blood mix within the small vessels of the placenta, which allows oxygenated blood to return to the fetus via the **umbilical vein**. The umbilical vein delivers blood directly to the liver, where some oxygen is used up. Blood leaves the liver and enters the **inferior vena cava (IVC)** through the hepatic veins. At the entrance of the liver the umbilical vein branches into the **ductus venosus**, which is the first shunt in the fetal circulation. This vessel bypasses the liver and joins the hepatic vein blood entering the IVC. At this suprahepatic portion of the IVC there are three different levels of oxygenated blood. The blood from the ductus venosus is moving faster than the other blood in the IVC at this location and preferentially flows along one edge of the IVC as it enters the right atrium. The **eustachian valve** serves to direct this ductus venosus blood across the second shunt in fetal circulation, the

foramen ovale. Most of the remaining blood in the IVC joins with the blood entering the right atrium from the **superior vena cava (SVC)** and flows across the tricuspid valve into the right ventricle. This mechanism allows the blood with the highest oxygenation level, from the ductus venosus that bypassed the liver, to get to the left ventricle without using up oxygen content (Figure 25-5). The left ventricle gives off the ascending aorta that delivers this highly oxygen concentrated blood to the heart muscle via the coronary arteries, and the brain via the carotid arteries arising from the aorta. The blood that entered the right ventricle leaves via the main pulmonary artery. The main pulmonary bifurcates into the **right** and **left pulmonary arteries**, which allow a small amount of blood to go to the lungs. The rest of the blood from the main pulmonary artery enters the descending aorta via the third shunt in the fetal heart (the ductus arteriosus), mixes with the blood from the aorta, and continues down the descending aorta. There, some of it will perfuse the lower extremities via the iliac arteries and some will return to the placenta for reoxygenation via the **umbilical arteries** (see Figure 25-4).

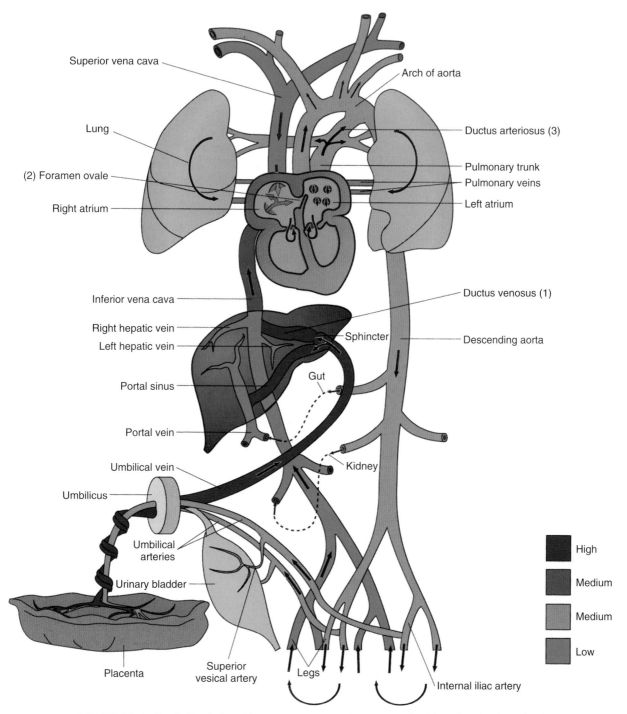

FIGURE 25-4 **Fetal Circulation.** The organs are not drawn to scale. Note that the three fetal shunts permit most of the blood to bypass the liver and the lungs: (1) the ductus venosus, (2) the foramen ovale, and (3) the ductus arteriosus.

LOCATION

The fetal heart is positioned in the anterior half of the chest with the base of the heart, the atria, in the middle of the chest and the apex of the heart, the tip of the ventricles, to the left of the midline. The **interventricular septum (IVS)** and the **interatrial septum (IAS)** divide the heart into right and left sides with a line positioned

along the IVS angled about 45 degrees from a midsagittal plane (Figure 25-6). The fetal heart lies directly transverse in the chest with the lungs occupying the posterior components of the chest. When imaging the fetal heart, it is important to see symmetrical ribs on each side to make sure that a true transverse plane is being obtained. After birth the lungs inflate and push the apex of the

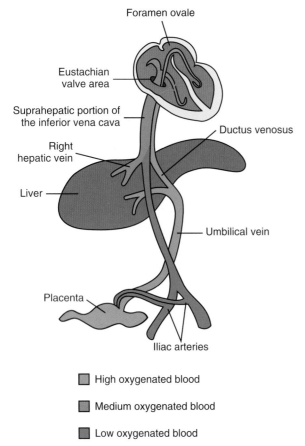

FIGURE 25-5   **Fetal Blood Oxygen Level Concentrations.** The blood from the ductus venosus preferentially shunts along 1 edge of the suprahepatic portion of the IVC, allowing it to enter the right atrium and shunt directly across the foramen ovale, being directed by the Eustachian valve. This allows the blood with the highest oxygen content to get to the cardiac muscle via the coronary arteries, and to the brain via the carotid arteries.

heart inferiorly so the heart then lies at an oblique angle in the chest.

SIZE

The fetal heart is about the size of a quarter at 20 weeks' gestational age. When one considers that it is also beating at a rate of about 150 beats per minute it is not surprising that it is a true imaging challenge. Neonatal dimensions of the heart vary with age and weight.

GROSS ANATOMY

See Chapter 30, Pediatric Echocardiography, for a detailed discussion of cardiac anatomy.

PHYSIOLOGY

The heart is the primary organ of the circulatory system whose mission is to pump oxygenated blood throughout the systemic circulation. In the fetus the placenta provides the method for oxygenating the blood, rather than the lungs, which are not yet ready to take over that function. Three shunts in the fetal circulation, previously described in this chapter, provide the mechanisms to get the oxygenated blood to the tissues while bypassing the lungs.

SONOGRAPHIC APPEARANCE

Screening the fetal heart is typically performed during the second trimester. It differs from a complete fetal echo because the purpose of screening is to determine whether the fetus needs to be referred for further investigation to prepare for delivery. Normal anatomic relationships must be determined, but determining the type of defect an anomaly is, or specifics regarding blood flow, is not necessary. A complete fetal echocardiogram describes a detailed evaluation of all structures of the fetal heart including the use of color Doppler, pulsed-wave Doppler, and when needed, continuous-wave Doppler.

Congenital heart disease is the most common birth defect, affecting 4 to 13 per 1000 births. Half of the cases are minor and may be easily resolved by surgery or resolve on their own. The remainder accounts for over half of the deaths from congenital abnormalities in childhood. Because the majority of fetuses with CHD have no known risk factors, all pregnancies should be screened for CHD. If an anomaly is suspected, or normal anatomy cannot be identified, a complete fetal echocardiogram is recommended.

Five axial views are recommended for the screening examination (Figure 25-7):

1. **Determination of Situs.** **Situs solitus** is the normal arrangement of the abdominal and thoracic organs (Figure 25-8). This means that the organs, which should develop on the right, did so. These are the liver, gallbladder, inferior vena cava, right atrium, and the trilobed right lung. Left-sided structures are normally the spleen, stomach, left atrium, aorta, and the bilobed left lung. With situs solitus there is approximately a 1% chance of a congenital heart defect. The complete reversal of all organs is known as situs inversus and only increases the risk of CHD slightly, as the relationships of all of the organs remain correct. The reversal of some of the organs, but not others, is called situs ambiguous, or heterotaxy, and carries a high risk of CHD.

2. **Four-Chamber View.** The four-chamber view consists of a detailed evaluation of a number of cardiac structures and also the positioning of the fetal heart in an axial view (Figure 25-9). After a technically correct four-chamber view is obtained, the following elements should be evaluated on the image:
   ○ **Cardiac axis.** The normal axis of the heart is 45 degrees to the left of the midline (see Figure 25-6). In an otherwise normal appearing four-chamber

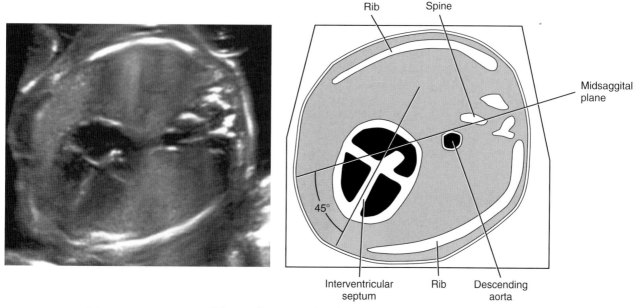

FIGURE 25-6 *Position of the Fetal Heart in the Chest.* The fetal heart lies in a true transverse position in the fetal heart. This can be determined by the ribs seen symmetrically in linear fashion on both sides of the chest. The interventricular septum forms a 45-degree angle with a midsagittal plane.

view, an abnormal cardiac axis should raise a high degree of suspicion for an outflow tract anomaly.

○ **Cardiac position.** The heart should lie anterior in the chest with the heart axis tipped to the left (see Figure 25-9). The heart may be displaced from its normal position by extrinsic factors such as space-occupying lesions of the lungs, or fetal lung hypoplasia or agenesis. A diaphragmatic hernia may displace the heart, or the heart may be displaced to the left in the presence of a gastroschisis or omphalocele.

○ **Cardiac size.** The heart should occupy approximately a third of the thoracic area (see Figure 25-9).

○ **Four chambers.** The presence of four distinct chambers should be seen (see Figure 25-9).

○ **Ventricular chamber size.** The ventricular chambers should be similar in size. Size can be estimated by visualizing the width of the ventricular chambers, inner-to-inner dimensions, just anterior to the **atrioventricular valves (AV)** (the valves that control the openings through which the atria and ventricles on each side of the heart communicate; tricuspid valve on the right; mitral valve on the left.) in end-diastole, immediately after the AV valves close (Figure 25-10). In mid-gestation the chambers should be similar in size. With increasing gestational age the right ventricle normally may be up to 20% larger than the left ventricle. If the right ventricle is disproportionally larger than the left ventricle, careful evaluation of left heart

obstructive lesions should be performed. Likely causes of this disparity include evolving hypoplastic left heart syndrome or coarctation of the aorta. If the left ventricle is disproportionally larger than the right ventricle, lesions that obstruct the flow of blood to the right heart should be carefully evaluated for evolving hypoplastic right heart syndrome.

○ **Atrial chamber size.** The atrial chambers should be approximately equal in size (see Figure 25-9).

○ **Fossa ovalis flap.** The flap of the fossa ovalis should be seen in the left atrium (see Figure 25-9). The flap is very thin and may be best visualized with real time.

○ **Moderator band.** The septomarginal trabecula (also known as the moderator band) is a muscular band of heart tissue found in the right ventricle. It is seen near the apex and extends from the ventricular septum to the base of the anterior papillary muscle (Figure 25-11). The moderator band is important because it carries part of the right bundle branch of the atrioventricular bundle of the conduction system of the heart to the anterior papillary muscle. This shortcut across the chamber of the ventricle seems to facilitate conduction time, allowing coordinated contraction of the anterior papillary muscle. The moderator band is often used to identify the morphologic right ventricle in prenatal ultrasound. The left ventricle does not have a moderator band; the right ventricle can be identified by this structure. It is possible for the morphologic right ventricle to be

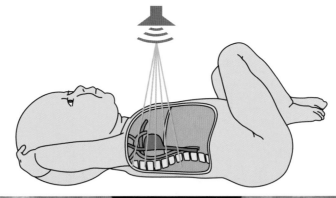

View #1 – Determination of situs

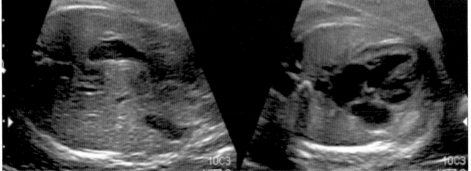

View #2 – Four-chamber view   View #3 – LVOT view

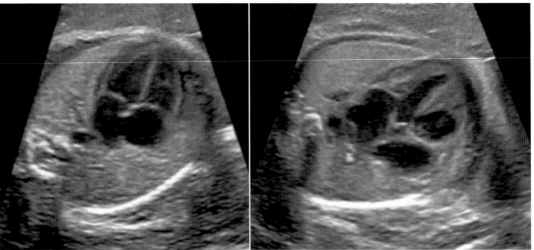

View #4 – RVOT view   View #5 – 3VT view

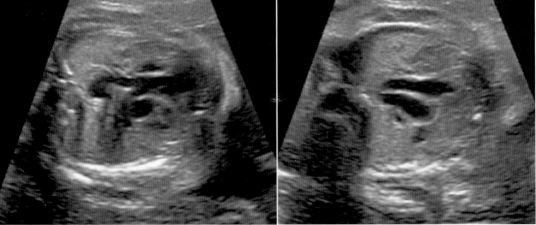

FIGURE 25-7 **Five Axial Views for Fetal Heart Screening.** View #1: Determination of situs; view #2: Four-chamber view; view #3: LVOT view; view #4: RVOT view; view #5: 3VT view.

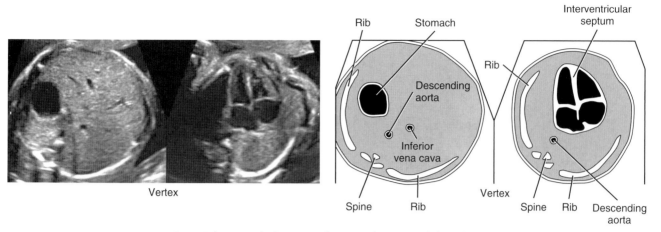

FIGURE 25-8 **Situs Solitus.** A dual image of an axial section of the abdomen and thorax showing the left-sided position of the stomach and apex of the heart proving situs solitus (when the fetal lie is annotated on the image).

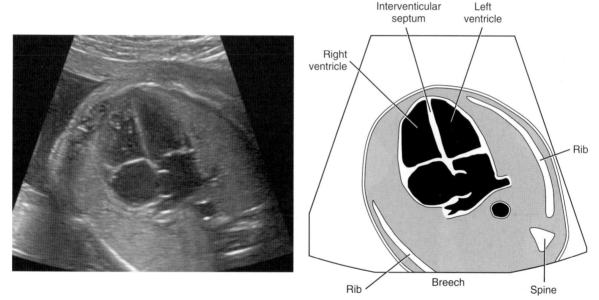

FIGURE 25-9 **Technically Correct Four-Chamber View.** A technically correct four-chamber view should have the following features as shown in this image. One complete rib should be seen on each side of the thorax. The fetal spine should be visible on the image. The interventricular septum should be clearly seen. The ventricles should appear elongated in comparison to the atria. Fetal position should be labeled on the image.

positioned on the left side of the heart in a condition called corrected transposition of the great vessels. It is important to check the lie of the fetus to make sure that the ventricle seen on the right side of the fetus has a moderator band and thus is the morphologic right ventricle.

○ **Intact ventricular septum.** The IVS should be evaluated for any apparent ventricular septal defects (VSDs). VSDs are the most common congenital heart defect in children, with an incidence

that is 20 times more common than the next most frequently found congenital heart defect. This being said it is only about the fifth most-common cardiac defect to be identified prenatally. IVS defects are classified depending on their location and are divided into two basic regions, the muscular septal region and the membranous septal region. The muscular septum has 3 subregions; the inlet, outlet, and trabecular regions (Figure 25-12). The membranous septum is an area just below the

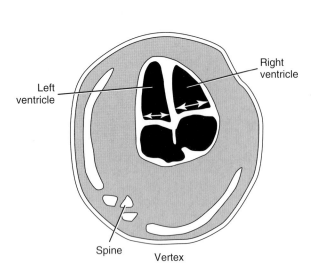

FIGURE 25-10 **Ventricular Size Estimation.** Ventricular size can be estimated by visualizing the width of the ventricular chambers, inner-to-inner dimensions *(arrows)*, just anterior to the atrioventricular valves (AV) in end-diastole, immediately after the AV valves close.

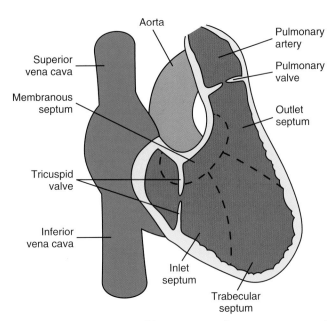

FIGURE 25-12 Regions of the interventricular septum as viewed from the right ventricular side of the heart.

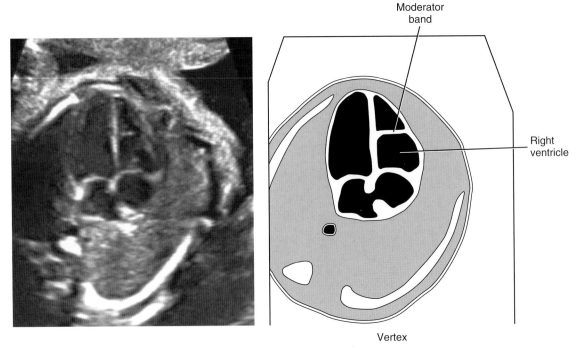

FIGURE 25-11 **Moderator Band in Right Ventricle.** The septomarginal trabecula (also known as the moderator band) is a muscular band of heart tissue found in the right ventricle. It is seen near the apex and extends from the ventricular septum to the base of the anterior papillary muscle on the lateral wall.

aortic valve. Because many membranous septal defects also involve areas of the muscular septum, they are commonly called perimembranous defects. Perimembranous VSDs are the most common and are often associated with outflow and great vessel anomalies. Membranous defects are best seen in the left ventricular outflow tract view and are detected by the interruption of the continuity between the ventricular septum and the ascending aorta. This will be discussed more

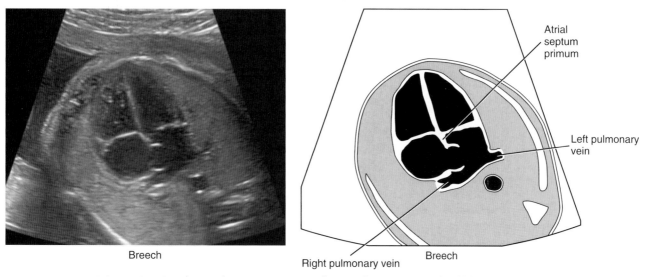

Breech

Right pulmonary vein   Breech

Atrial septum primum

Left pulmonary vein

FIGURE 25-13 The atrial septum primum and two pulmonary veins should be documented.

in the section regarding the left ventricular outflow tract. Muscular septal defects are generally not detected unless they are 2 to 3 mm in size. Because the ventricular septum is a curvilinear structure, several different angles and views are necessary to evaluate all portions of the IVS. Muscular defects are best seen in a view that puts the IVS at a perpendicular angle to the beam. The use of color Doppler may increase the ability to detect in utero defects. However, limitations including axial, lateral, and temporal resolution, along with the variability of fetal movement, continue to make it a very difficult diagnosis. In most cases, however, muscular defects are of limited clinical significance and many will undergo spontaneous closure in utero.

○ **Atrial septum primum.** The point where the lower part of the atrial septum meets the upper part of the ventricular septum and where the atrioventricular valves insert is called the cardiac "crux." The lower rim of atrial tissue in this location is called the septum primum, and this area should always be identified during scanning (Figure 25-13). Septum primum defects can occur in isolation but usually are part of a more complex CHD called an **atrioventricular septal defect (AVSD)**. This is of particular importance because AVSDs can be associated with Down syndrome, the most common chromosomal anomaly.

○ **Pulmonary veins.** Pulmonary veins should be seen entering the left atrium (see Figure 25-13). When possible, it is recommended that two of these veins be identified. Nonvisualization of the pulmonary veins that normally enter the left atrium may be associated with **total anomalous pulmonary venous**

return (TAPVR). With careful inspection, if no pulmonary veins can be seen draining into the left atrium, the patient should be referred for a complete fetal echocardiogram, because this condition is fatal in the neonate after closure of the foramen ovale and the ductus arteriosus.

○ **Atrioventricular valve alignment.** The atrioventricular valves, the right-sided tricuspid valve and left-sided mitral valve, should be seen to open separately. The leaflets should be thin and able to move freely. The tricuspid valve septal leaflet should always insert more apically into the interventricular septum than the mitral valve leaflet (Figure 25-14). This offset is normal. A key sonographic finding for an AVSD is the absence of this normal offset.

○ **Normal rate and rhythm.** Along with assessing the above elements a normal heart rate and rhythm should be confirmed. In the second trimester the normal rate ranges between 120 and 160 beats per minute (bpm). Transient episodes of bradycardia commonly occur in the second trimester. Fixed bradycardia, below 110 bpm, should be referred for further evaluation for the possibility of heart block. Mild tachycardia with rates of over 160 bpm can be seen as a normal variant during fetal movements. Persistent tachycardia of greater than 180 bpm requires further investigation. M-mode should be utilized to obtain the fetal heart rate measurement. Doppler techniques should not be used when a technique utilizing lower amounts of ultrasonic energy can be used to obtain the same information.

○ **Three types of four-chamber views.** It is necessary to utilize differing angles of insonation in order to

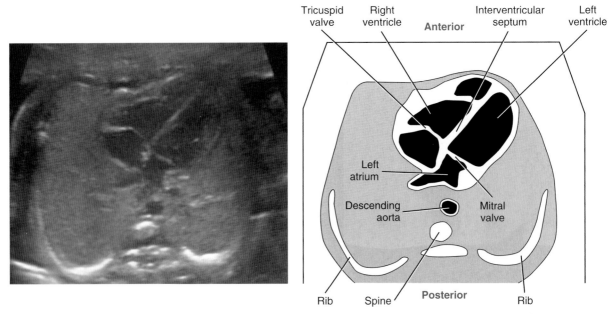

FIGURE 25-14 In this breech presentation the right-sided tricuspid valve is seen most anteriorly. The septal leaflet of the tricuspid valves clearly inserts more apically than the mitral valve leaflet insertion to the interventricular septum.

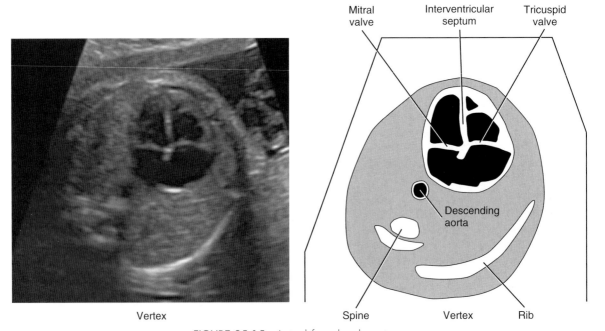

FIGURE 25-15 Apical four-chamber view.

visualize all of the above elements necessary to assess the four-chamber view. There are 3 types of four-chamber views that are commonly used to do this. Each view has the beam insonating from a different angle in order to best view the cardiac anatomy:

1. **Apical four-chamber view.** In the apical four-chamber view (Figure 25-15) the beam insonates the apex of the heart first. The beam

hits the AV valves in a perpendicular fashion, giving excellent axial resolution to evaluate the normal offset of the AV valves.

2. **Basal four-chamber view.** In the basal four-chamber view the beam insonates the base of the heart (the atria) first (Figure 25-16). The septum primum is usually easily seen. The pulmonary veins entering the left atrium are also usually nicely seen in this view.

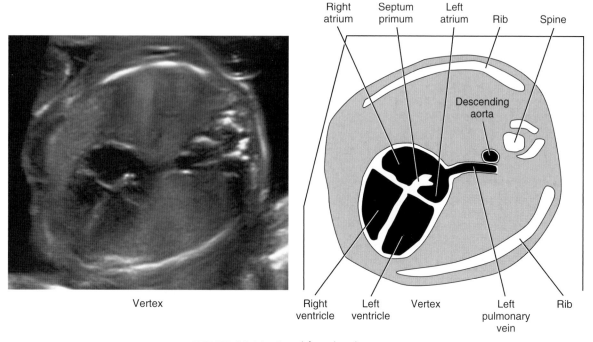

FIGURE 25-16 Basal four-chamber view.

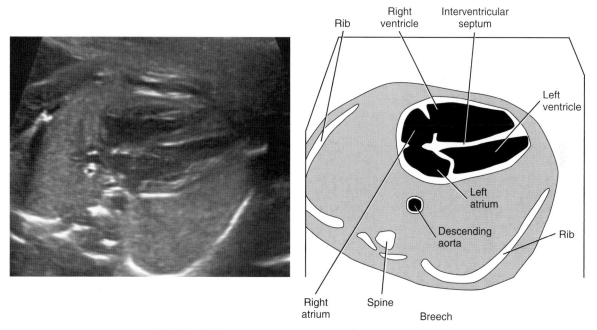

FIGURE 25-17 Subcostal or long axis four-chamber view.

3. **Subcostal or long axis four-chamber view.** In the subcostal or long axis four-chamber view the beam insonates the interventricular septum in a perpendicular fashion, providing the best resolution to interrogate it (Figure 25-17).
3. **Left Ventricular Outflow Tract (LVOT).** A technically correct four-chamber view (see Figure 25-9) is

necessary for the LVOT to be visualized. This view confirms the presence of a great vessel originating from the left ventricle. This view does not by itself confirm that it is the aorta, and not the pulmonary artery, that is arising from the left ventricle. As the beam angles superiorly in the fetal chest the atria are only partially seen and the aorta is seen to

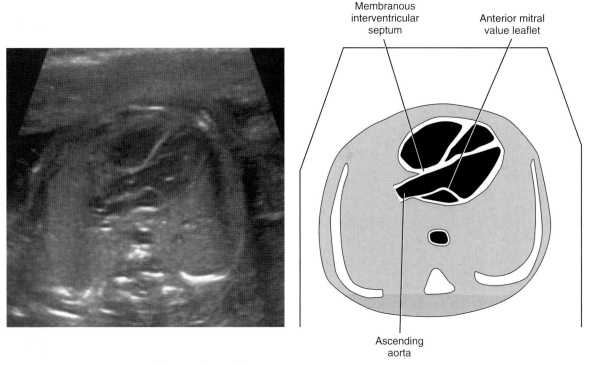

FIGURE 25-18 **Left Ventricular Outflow Tract View.** Continuity of the anterior aortic wall to the interventricular septum and, the posterior aortic wall to the anterior mitral valve leaflet, is necessary to demonstrate in this view.

communicate with the left ventricle (Figure 25-18). There are two elements that are necessary to evaluate in this view.

○ Continuity of the interventricular septum to the anterior wall of the aorta.

○ Continuity of the anterior mitral valve leaflet with the posterior wall of the aorta.

Documentation of these two elements helps to identify ventricular septal defects and conotruncal abnormalities. The direction of the anterior wall of the ascending aorta and the ventricular septum creates a wide angle (Figure 25-19). This angle is commonly absent in great vessel anomalies. The shape of the left ventricle and the outflow tract, leading into the ascending aorta, has been likened to the shape of a ballerina's foot. The aortic valve should be seen to freely open and the diameter of the ascending aorta should be the same or slightly smaller than that of the main pulmonary artery.

Superior to the LVOT view the ascending aorta is seen to course toward the fetal right shoulder before beginning a tight arch posteriorly and back toward the left (Figure 25-20). This is called the aortic arch. The brachiocephalic artery is the first branch coming off of this arch, followed by the left common carotid artery and the left subclavian artery.

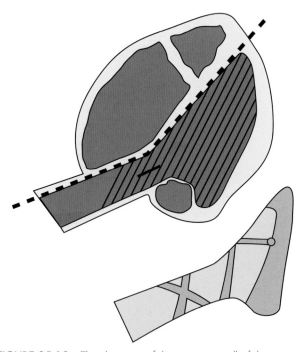

FIGURE 25-19 The direction of the anterior wall of the ascending aorta and the ventricular septum creates a wide angle that is commonly absent in great vessel anomalies. The shape of the left ventricle and the outflow tract, leading into the ascending aorta, has been likened to the shape of a ballerina's foot.

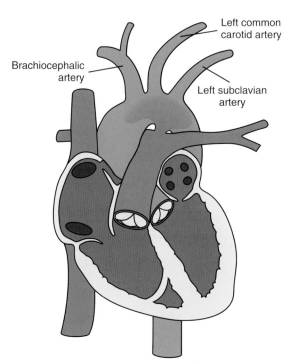

FIGURE 25-20 As one continues to angle superiorly from the LVOT view the ascending aorta is seen to course toward the fetal right shoulder before beginning a tight arch posteriorly and back toward the left. This is called the aortic arch. The brachiocephalic artery is the first branch coming off of this arch, followed by the left common carotid artery and the left subclavian artery.

4. **Right Ventricular Outflow Tract (RVOT).** In real time the main pulmonary artery can be seen to cross leftward over the ascending aorta anteriorly at a near 90-degree angle (see Figure 25-20). This view confirms the presence of a great vessel originating from the right ventricle. At this superior level the ventricles of the heart are no longer in view. Three vessels can be seen lined up from the left side to the right: the pulmonary artery, the aorta, and the superior vena cava (Figure 25-21). The pulmonary artery comes off the most anterior chamber, the right ventricle, and in the RVOT view this will be the most anterior structure. The main pulmonary artery is seen in its entirety and is a constant diameter until after the branch pulmonary arteries are given off. It proceeds a short distance posteriorly and then narrows as it continues as the ductus arteriosus to join the aortic arch. The right and left pulmonary arteries may or may not be seen in this view depending on slight movements of the transducer or the fetus. Variations of the branching of the main pulmonary artery into the two branches and the ductus arteriosus should be understood so that they are not confusing to the examiner. Ideally, one would like to visualize the right pulmonary branch as it comes off the main pulmonary artery and courses posterior to the aorta and SVC in a transverse direction to the right lung (Figure 25-22).

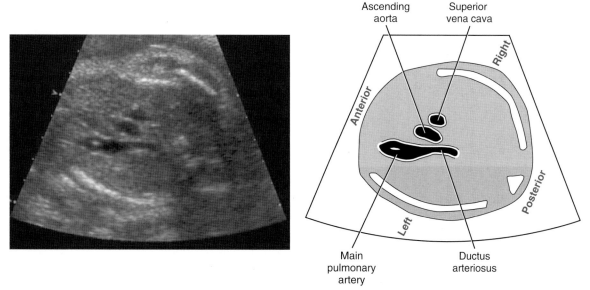

FIGURE 25-21 **RVOT View.** At this level, just superior to the chambers of the heart, the great vessels and the SVC can be seen lined up from the left to the right, being the main pulmonary artery, the ascending aorta, and the SVC.

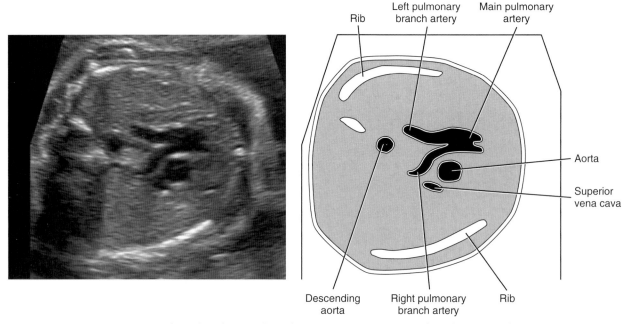

FIGURE 25-22   The right pulmonary branch artery is seen originating from the main pulmonary artery and coursing posterior to the aorta and the SVC. Seeing this branching pattern confirms that the vessel arising from the RVOT is the pulmonary artery.

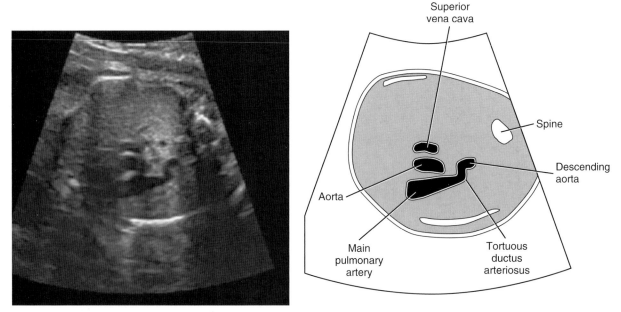

FIGURE 25-23   The main pulmonary artery narrows as it gives off the right and left branches. The ductus arteriosus in this case is somewhat tortuous as it continues posteriorly to meet the aorta.

Visualizing this branch confirms that the vessel arising from the RVOT is truly the main pulmonary artery and not the aorta, as is seen in complete transposition of the great arteries. The left pulmonary branch artery comes off the main artery just after the right branch and courses to the left lung. The ductus

arteriosus continues posteriorly to meet with the aortic arch. It can be difficult sometimes to determine where the ductus arteriosus divides from the main pulmonary and the left pulmonary branch because this position is variable and the ductus can be somewhat tortuous (Figures 25-23 and 25-24). The

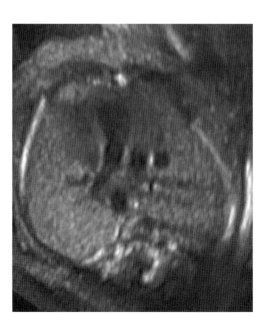
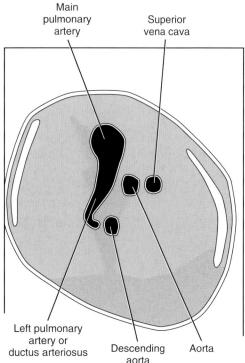

Main pulmonary artery

Superior vena cava

Left pulmonary artery or ductus arteriosus

Descending aorta

Aorta

FIGURE 25-24 The main pulmonary artery narrows in this image and moves slightly to the left. It is not clear if this area is the left pulmonary artery or the ductus arteriosus because the vessel cannot be seen to join the aorta.

diameter of the main pulmonary artery, before it gives off branches, should be equal to or slightly larger than the diameter of the ascending aorta. Because they are seen next to each other in this view, a quick comparison of sizes can be made. Anomalies that restrict the flow of blood into or out of their respective ventricles will change the volume of blood entering the great vessels and thus their size. The ascending aorta will be seen at this level as a rounded or oblong vessel as it has just left the LVOT and is coursing mostly superior at this point. Its position should be just to the left of the main pulmonary artery and its diameter similar or just smaller than the main pulmonary artery. The SVC should be seen just to the right of the aorta and normally will have a diameter just smaller than the aorta (see Figure 25-24). Abnormalities that may have a normal appearing four-chamber view, such as complete transposition of the great arteries, tetralogy of Fallot, and pulmonary atresia with a ventricular septal defect, will have an abnormal RVOT view.

With high-frequency imaging it is not uncommon to visualize the thymus gland seen anteriorly to the great vessels and SVC. It will be seen as a rounded mass that is slightly hypoechoic, as compared to lung tissue (Figure 25-25).

The RVOT view is similar to the three-vessel view, first described in the literature by Yoo et al in 1997 and published in the *Journal of Obstetrics and Gynecology*. The article was titled "Three-vessel view of the upper mediastinum: an easy means of detecting abnormalities of the ventricular outflow tracts and great arteries during obstetric screening." This view came to be known unofficially as the "line-dot-dot" view.

Elements that should be evaluated in the RVOT view include:

- **Vessel number.** Three vessels should be seen in this view. The presence of only two vessels at this level can indicate complete transposition of the great arteries, an atretic great artery, or persistent truncus arteriosus. The presence of four vessels at this level can be associated with persistent left superior vena cava.
- **Pulmonary artery bifurcation.** The vessel that is originating from the RVOT should be seen to bifurcate to the lungs. This confirms that this vessel is the main pulmonary artery.
- **Vessel size.** The pulmonary artery should be similar in size or up to 20% larger than the aorta. If this relationship does not exist it may indicate a flow-restricting anomaly.

5. **Three Vessels and Trachea (3VT).** Similar to the RVOT view, this view demonstrates the great arteries and SVC and their size and relationship to each other. Because the beam is now at a very cephalic

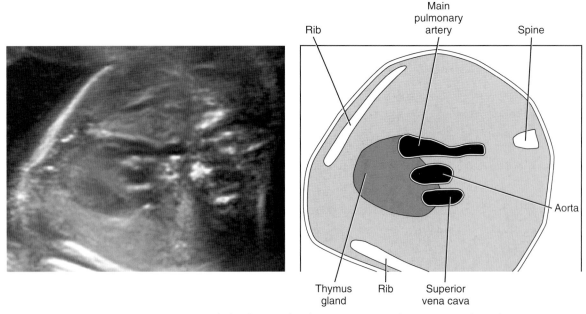

FIGURE 25-25 RVOT view with the thymus gland seen anterior to the great vessels and SVC as a slightly hypoechoic rounded mass.

position, the trachea is seen in this plane before it bifurcates and is important as a constant structure that can be used as a reference point for the location of the great artery arches (Figure 25-26). This was first described in the literature by Yagel et al in 2002 and published in the *Journal of Obstetrics and Gynecology.* The article was titled "The three vessels and trachea view (3VT) in fetal cardiac scanning."

The 3VT view shows the ductal and aortic arches in a transverse oblique plane. The pulmonary artery is seen on the left with the ductus arteriosus joining with the aorta arch. The aortic arch is seen as it courses posteriorly to meet the ductus arteriosus in a "V" pattern. The trachea is seen as a low-gray space surrounded by a bright echogenic ring (Figure 25-27). The position of the trachea is posterior to the aorta, and the aortic arch should be seen to the left of the trachea meeting with the ductus arteriosus. In some abnormal situations the aorta will course straight posteriorly and to the right of the trachea. The pulmonary artery may remain to the left of the trachea and connect posterior to the trachea with the aorta via the ductus arteriosus. This is called a "vascular ring." Both the pulmonary artery and the aorta may also be found to the right of the trachea. Any of these situations is abnormal and needs to be further evaluated for coexisting anomalies.

Elements that should be evaluated in the 3VT view include:

○ **Vessel size.** The main pulmonary artery should be similar in diameter or up to 20% larger than the aorta.

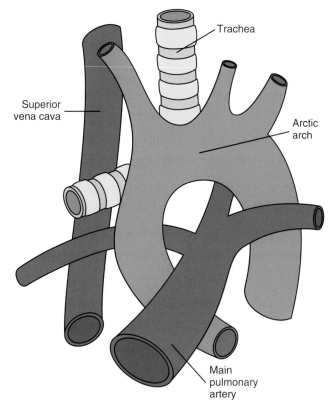

FIGURE 25-26 The trachea is seen posterior and slightly right of the aortic arch before it bifurcates.

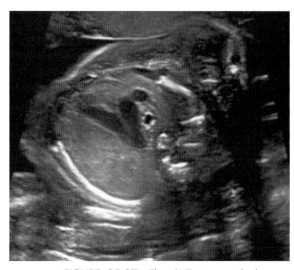
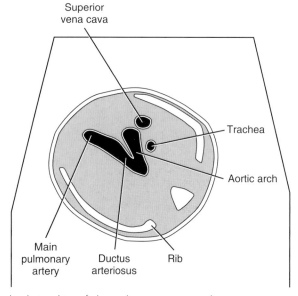

FIGURE 25-27 The 3VT view with the normal relationship of the pulmonary artery, ductus arteriosus, aortic arch, trachea, and the SVC.

○ **Vessel location.** The ductus arteriosus and the aorta should meet in a "V" formation to the left of the trachea.
○ **Vessel alignment.** The three vessels should form an oblique line with the main pulmonary artery, assuming a more anterior location, the aortic arch in the middle and the SVC more inferior and to the right (Figure 25-28).

SUMMARY

Careful attention should be taken during the cardiac screening exam to examine each of the five views. Each view has individual elements that need to be identified in order to consider the view "normal." If any element of a view is not optimally seen it is appropriate to have the patient return at a later date to reevaluate that view. It is prudent to remember that some cardiac anomalies are progressive in nature and may not be identified during the 20-week screening examination.

The screening examination of the fetal heart utilizes 2-dimensional techniques with still images and the use of cine clips. Doppler techniques, including pulsed wave Doppler, continuous wave Doppler, and color Doppler are utilized when performing a complete fetal echocardiogram to obtain information regarding blood flow velocities, flow direction, and flow timing. The use of m-mode can also be used to evaluate specific heart arrhythmias and for obtaining measurements of the cardiac chambers.

SONOGRAPHIC APPLICATIONS

The use of ultrasound for screening the fetal heart during the second-trimester anatomy evaluation is recommended to ascertain the normal appearance of the following:

- Situs solitus determination
- Size, location, and position of the fetal heart in the thorax
- The flap of the fossa ovalis in the left atrium, which documents right to left blood flow across the foramen ovale
- The moderator band situated in the right-sided ventricle
- Intact ventricular septum
- The atrial septum primum presence
- Pulmonary venous drainage into the left atrium
- The normal offset of the atrioventricular valves
- Rate and rhythm
- Continuity of the membranous IVS with the anterior aortic wall
- Continuity of the posterior aortic wall with the anterior mitral valve leaflet
- Aorta and pulmonary sizes and position in the mediastinum
- Evidence of intracardiac masses and tumors

NORMAL VARIANTS

- The axis of the fetal heart may be found at an approximate 45-degree angle to the left of a midsagittal plane. There is a normal approximate 20-degree variation in this angle.
- At the time of the screening exam of the fetal heart the right ventricle should be similar in size to the left ventricle. However, it may be normal for the right ventricle to be up to 20% wider than the left ventricle, especially as pregnancy progresses.

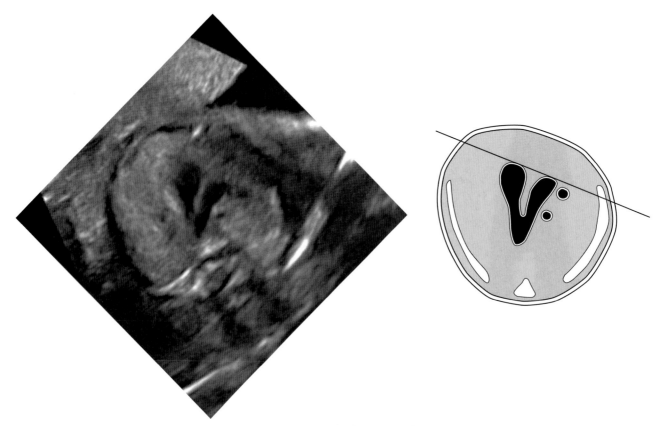

FIGURE 25-28 *Normal vessel alignment in the 3VT view.*

REFERENCE CHARTS

■ ■ ■ ASSOCIATED PHYSICIANS

- **Maternal fetal medicine physician/High-risk obstetrician:** Specializes in the preterm management of women whose pregnancies are at risk because of various medical conditions.
- **Obstetrician:** Specializes in the branch of medicine that addresses care of women during pregnancy, childbirth, and recovery.
- **Pediatric cardiologist:** A pediatrician who has received extensive training in diagnosing and treating children's cardiac problems. Evaluation and treatment may begin with the fetus because heart problems can now be detected before birth using ultrasound.
- **Sonologist/Radiologist:** Specializes in performing and/or interpreting sonograms (ultrasound examinations).

■ ■ ■ COMMON DIAGNOSTIC TESTS

- **Doppler ultrasound:** Various Doppler ultrasound techniques including color Doppler, pulsed-wave Doppler, and continuous-wave Doppler can be used to assess fetal blood flow.
- **Magnetic resonance imaging (MRI):** MRI can be used for a fetal cardiac evaluation.

■ ■ ■ LABORATORY VALUES

Nonapplicable

■ ■ ■ VASCULATURE

- Venous—umbilical vein, ductus venosus, inferior vena cava, superior vena cava, pulmonary veins
- Arteries—main pulmonary artery, right and left branch pulmonary arteries, ductus arteriosus, aorta, coronary arteries

■ ■ ■ AFFECTING CHEMICALS

- **Prostaglandin E:** A drug used in maintaining a patent ductus arteriosus in newborns. This is primarily useful when there is threat of premature closure of the ductus arteriosus in an infant with ductal-dependent congenital heart disease, including cyanotic lesions (e.g., pulmonary atresia/stenosis, tricuspid atresia/stenosis, transposition of the great arteries) and acyanotic lesions (e.g., coarctation of the aorta, hypoplastic left heart syndrome, critical aortic stenosis, interrupted aortic arch).

Introduction to Specialty Sonography

■ **CHAPTER 26**

The Neonatal Brain

ANGIE RISH, BETTY BATES TEMPKIN, AND REVA ARNEZ CURRY

OBJECTIVES

Identify the major structures in the neonatal brain.

Describe basic brain function and identify its location in the brain.

Describe the sonographic appearance of the neonatal brain in coronal and sagittal scanning planes.

Describe normal structural variants seen sonographically.

Describe the arterial supply and venous drainage of the brain.

Describe associated physicians, diagnostic tests, laboratory values, and normal measurements.

■

KEY WORDS

Anterior Fontanelle — Unossified, soft, membrane-covered space between the sutures of the skull, at the top of the head.

Aqueduct of Sylvius — Small channel for the passage of cerebrospinal fluid between the third and fourth ventricles.

Arachnoid Mater — Middle layer of three meningeal protective and supportive tissues surrounding the brain and spinal cord.

Basal Ganglia — Collection of structures coordinating movement; located in the telencephalon ("forebrain").

Brain Stem — Consists of the midbrain, pons, and medulla oblongata, which provide a pathway for ascending and descending fiber tracts. Involved with vital body functions such as breathing and heart rate.

Caudate Nucleus — Forms the inferolateral margin of the lateral ventricle's anterior horns. Represents the more superior aspect of the gray matter of the basal ganglia, a group of structures coordinating movement; located in the telencephalon ("forebrain").

Cavum Septum Pellucidum — Small cavity filled with cerebrospinal fluid that filters from the ventricles through the septal laminae. Has no connection or communication with the ventricular system. Does communicate with the cavum septum vergae. Situated between the frontal horns of the lateral ventricles. Closes before birth.

Cavum Septum Vergae — Small cavity filled with cerebrospinal fluid that filters from the ventricles through the septal laminae. Has no connection or communication with the ventricular system. Does communicate with the cavum septum pellucidum. Situated between the bodies of the lateral ventricles. Closes at the beginning of the sixth month of gestation.

Central Fissure — Separates the frontal and parietal brain lobes.

Cerebellum — Second largest portion of the brain. Occupies most of the posterior fossae. Inferior to the tentorium and posterior to the pons and medulla oblongata. Composed of symmetrical, bilateral hemispheres connected by the vermis, its medial

portion. Responsible for motor coordination and maintaining posture and equilibrium.

Cerebral Cortex — An approximately 2 mm, convoluted layer of gray matter covering each hemisphere of the cerebrum. Responsible for balancing information from different sources to maintain cognitive function.

Cerebral Hemispheres — Two identical, symmetrical right and left "halves" of the cerebrum that fill the superior cranial vault. Together they make up the cerebrum, the largest portion of the brain.

Cerebrospinal Fluid (CSF) — Clear liquid produced daily by the choroid plexi (specialized blood vessels located in the ventricles) that continually circulates through the ventricles and subarachnoid space to distribute nutrients and serve as a shock absorber against injury for the brain and spinal cord.

Cerebrum — Largest portion of the brain. Divided into two identical right and left hemispheres that communicate through a "neural bridge," the corpus callosum. Controls cognitive and motor function.

Continued

475

Choroid Plexus — Special blood vessels located in the ventricles that produce cerebrospinal fluid.

Circle of Willis — Intracranial arterial conglomeration of anastomotic or communicating collateral vessels located near the base of the brain.

Cisterna Magna — Largest expanded subarachnoid space in the brain. Filled with cerebrospinal fluid. Located at the base of the cerebellum in the posterior portion of the brain.

Corpus Callosum — A "neural bridge" or network of nerve fibers through which the cerebral hemispheres communicate.

Cranium — Protective bony vault of the skull; consists of 8 bones: 1 frontal, 1 occipital, 1 ethmoid, 1 sphenoid, 2 temporal, 2 parietal.

Diencephalon — Part of the midbrain; located just inferior to the corpus callosum. Encloses the third ventricle and includes the thalamus, hypothalamus, and epithalamus.

Dura Mater — Outer layer of three meningeal protective and supportive tissues surrounding the brain and spinal cord.

Epithalamus — Situated in the anterosuperior portion of the diencephalon. Contains the choroid plexus of the third ventricle and the pineal gland.

Falx Cerebri — Double fold of dura mater that lies in the interhemispheric fissure.

Foramen of Magendie — Middle of three holes on the floor of the fourth ventricle providing passage of cerebrospinal fluid directly into the subarachnoid space.

Foramen of Monro — Bilateral foramina that lie inferomedial to the bodies of the lateral ventricles and mark the communication between the lateral and third ventricles.

Foramina of Luschka — Lateral two of three holes on the floor of the fourth ventricle providing passage of cerebrospinal fluid directly into the subarachnoid space.

Fourth Ventricle — One of four brain cavities containing cerebrospinal fluid. Located below and connected to the third ventricle by a small channel, the aqueduct of

Sylvius, a narrow opening for the passage of cerebrospinal fluid. Directs cerebrospinal fluid into the subarachnoid space through the foramen of Magendie and foramina of Luschka, three small holes in the floor of the fourth ventricle.

Frontal Lobe — Most anterior brain lobe of the cerebral cortex. Contains sensory receptors involved with speech, movement, emotions, and problem solving.

Germinal Matrix — Composed of a fine network of blood vessels and neural tissue. Highly susceptible to hemorrhage in the premature infant.

Gyrus (pl., gyri) — Elevated or convoluted fold on the surface of the cerebral hemispheres separated by sulci or fissures.

Hypothalamus — Diencephalon structure located just inferior to the thalamus at the base of the brain. Composed of several different areas, even though it is just the size of a pea. Communicates directly with the pituitary gland.

Interhemispheric Fissure — Deep groove or indentation separating the right and left cerebral hemispheres. Contains the falx cerebri.

Lateral Ventricles — Cerebrospinal fluid–filled cavities within each cerebral hemisphere. Lie just below the corpus callosum and separated from each other by the septum pellucidum, a thin partition. Each lateral ventricle is divided segmentally into a frontal horn, body, occipital horn, and temporal horn.

Medulla Oblongata — Extends inferiorly from the pons to form the inferior portion of the brain stem that projects out of the skull through the foramen magnum (a large opening in the posterior portion of the occipital bone of the skull) and connects to the spinal cord.

Midbrain — Superior portion of the brain stem situated where the cerebellum and pons unite.

Occipital Lobe — Cerebral brain lobe located posteriorly in the brain; involved with vision.

Parietal Lobe — Cerebral brain lobe located posterior to the frontal cortex. Contains the body's sensory receptors, which interpret the impulses that allow one to recognize sensations such as pain, cold, or a light touch.

Pia Mater — Innermost layer of three meningeal protective and supportive tissues surrounding the brain and spinal cord. Adjacent to the brain and spinal cord surfaces.

Pons — Middle portion of the brain stem situated at the midline, anterior to and between the bilateral cerebellar hemispheres. It is inferior to the midbrain and superior to the medulla oblongata, to which it is directly connected.

Subarachnoid Space — Space between the arachnoid mater and pia mater containing cerebrospinal fluid it receives from the fourth ventricle.

Sulcus (pl., sulci) — Trench or groove separating the gyri on the surface of the brain.

Sylvian/Lateral Fissure — Groove or indentation separating the frontal and temporal brain lobes.

Temporal Lobe — Cerebral brain lobe located inferior to the frontal and parietal lobes; involved in recognition and perception.

Tentorium — Flap of dura mater that separates the cerebral hemispheres from the superior structures in the brain.

Thalami — A pair of large, symmetrical ovoid organs situated one (thalamus) on either side of the third ventricle, forming most of its lateral walls. Together they compose the largest portion of the diencephalon.

Third Ventricle — One of four brain cavities containing cerebrospinal fluid. Located below and connected to each lateral ventricle by the foramen of Monro, a narrow opening for the passage of cerebrospinal fluid.

Trigone — Region of the lateral ventricles where the bodies, occipital horns, and temporal horns converge.

Vermis — Medial portion of the cerebellum; connects cerebellar hemispheres.

Over the past decades, sonography has become the primary imaging method in evaluation of the neonatal brain, especially when assessing ventricular size. Currently, intracranial ultrasound imaging, including 3-dimensional (3-D) imaging of the brain is performed exclusively using compact, high-resolution, real-time transducers. Its portability, low cost, and relative noninvasive ease of performance make ultrasound particularly advantageous, especially when evaluating unstable premature infants.

Sonographic cross-sectional anatomy of the neonatal brain is best depicted with a series of both modified coronal and sagittal planes. In the past, axial scanning was also utilized, especially for obtaining accurate ventricular dimensions. However, now it is reserved primarily for Doppler imaging to investigate the circle of Willis, an intracranial arterial conglomeration of communicating collateral vessels located near the base of the brain.

The **anterior fontanelle**, commonly referred to as the "soft spot," is a membranous space on the top of the head at the midline, between the still-developing sutures of the skull. It is an area of cartilage between the bones of the skull that has not yet ossified (developed into bone). This area typically closes up by 18 months of age in a full-term baby, although it can close as early as 9 months. It is used as the primary acoustic window or approach when scanning the neonatal brain (Figures 26-1 and 26-2). From this approach, sonographic scanning plane results differ from standard cross-sections produced by computed tomography (CT) or magnetic resonance imaging (MRI).

Like the anterior fontanelle, the **posterior fontanelle** is also a "soft spot"; however, it is found on the posterior aspect of the skull (Figures 26-3 and 26-4). On a normal neonate this area ossifies much faster than the anterior fontanelle. This happens around the age of 8 weeks on a full-term baby. The posterior fontanelle can be helpful in identifying pathology near the posterior fossa when not seen well with the anterior fontanelle approach. Early closing of both the anterior and posterior fontanelles can be a sign of a problem.

LOCATION

The locations of neonatal brain structures routinely visualized with ultrasound are listed in Table 26-1.

SIZE

The bodies of the lateral ventricles can be measured from wall to wall (see Figure 26-2, *B*). This measurement is the widest line perpendicular to the longest axis of the ventricles and should measure 4 mm or less. Another measurement is the horizontal distance from

Text continued on p. 481

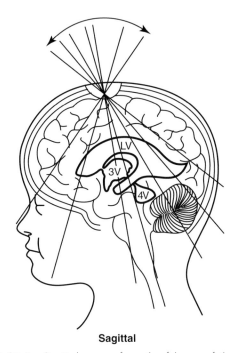

Sagittal

FIGURE 26-1   Sagittal survey from the fulcrum of the anterior fontanelle. *LV,* Lateral ventricle; *3V,* third ventricle; *4V,* fourth ventricle.

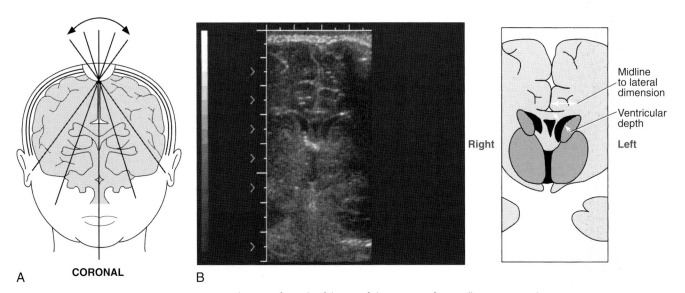

FIGURE 26-2   **A,** Coronal survey from the fulcrum of the anterior fontanelle. **B,** Coronal image at the level of the foramen of Monro. Correct level for measuring the lateral ventricles as shown.

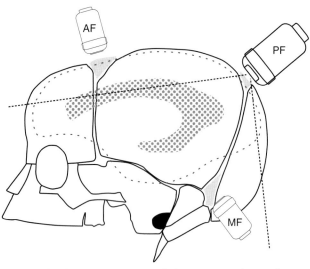

FIGURE 26-3 Demonstration of the posterior fontanelle (PF) approach. Note the locations of the anterior and mastoid fontanelles as well (AF, MF). (From Correa F, et al: Posterior fontanelle sonography: an acoustic window into the neonatal brain. *Am J Neuroradiol*, 2004;25:1274-1282.)

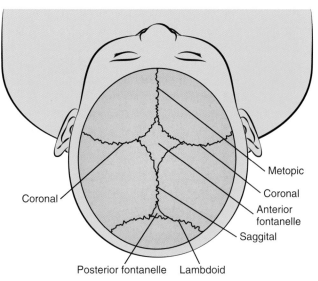

FIGURE 26-4 Demonstration of the posterior and anterior fontanelles to include the cranial sutures.

■ ■ ■ **Table 26-1** Location of Neonatal Brain Structures Routinely Visualized With Ultrasound

	Third Ventricle	Thalamus	Fourth Ventricle	Cerebellar Vermis	Aqueduct of Sylvius	Cavum Septum Pellucidum
Anterior to	Occipital lobe, fourth ventricle, cerebellar vermis, massa intermedia, aqueduct of Sylvius, corpus callosum, cavum septum vergae	Trigone, occipital lobe, choroid plexus, body lateral ventricle, occipital horn lateral ventricle	Cerebellar vermis	Occipital lobe	Cerebellar vermis, occipital lobe	Occipital lobe, corpus callosum
Posterior to	Frontal lobe, corpus callosum, massa intermedia		Medulla oblongata	Fourth ventricle, aqueduct of Sylvius, medulla oblongata, third ventricle	Medulla oblongata	Corpus callosum, frontal lobe
Superior to	Fourth ventricle, cerebellar vermis, massa intermedia, aqueduct of Sylvius, medulla oblongata	Cerebellum, choroid plexus, temporal horn lateral ventricle, occipital horn	Cisterna magna, cerebellum		Fourth ventricle	Third ventricle, massa intermedia, aqueduct of Sylvius, thalamus, basal ganglia
Inferior to	Cavum septum pellucidum, corpus callosum, caudate nucleus, foramen of Monro, cavum vergae, thalamus	Caudate nucleus, caudothalamic groove, germinal matrix, body lateral ventricle, anterior horn lateral ventricle	Aqueduct of Sylvius, third ventricle, tentorium, quadrigeminal plate	Third ventricle, corpus callosum, cavum septum pellucidum	Third ventricle, massa intermedia, cavum septum pellucidum, corpus callosum	Corpus callosum, interhemispheric fissure

Table 26-1 Location of Neonatal Brain Structures Routinely Visualized With Ultrasound—cont'd

	Third Ventricle	Thalamus	Fourth Ventricle	Cerebellar Vermis	Aqueduct of Sylvius	Cavum Septum Pellucidum
Medial to	Thalamus, caudate nucleus	Tentorium	Tentorium, temporal horn lateral ventricle			Frontal horn lateral ventricle, caudate nucleus, germinal matrix, thalamus, basal ganglia
Lt lateral to		Third ventricle				
Rt lateral to		Third ventricle				

	Corpus Callosum	Massa Intermedia	Caudate Nucleus	Choroid Plexus	Trigone	Germinal Matrix
Anterior to	Occipital lobe	Cavum septum pellucidum, corpus callosum, third ventricle	Germinal matrix, body lateral ventricle, choroid plexus	Occipital horn lateral ventricle, occipital lobe, trigone	Occipital lobe	Choroid plexus, body lateral ventricle
Posterior to	Cavum septum pellucidum, frontal lobe	Third ventricle, frontal lobe		Germinal matrix, caudate nucleus, thalamus, anterior horn lateral ventricle	Choroid plexus, thalamus	Caudate nucleus
Superior to	Cavum septum pellucidum, third ventricle, massa intermedia, aqueduct of Sylvius	Aqueduct of Sylvius, fourth ventricle, cerebellar vermis, third ventricle	Thalamus, choroid plexus, temporal horn lateral ventricle, cerebellum, trigone	Temporal horn lateral ventricle, occipital horn lateral ventricle, cerebellum	Occipital horn lateral ventricle	Thalamus, choroid plexus
Inferior to	Interhemispheric fissure	Cavum septum pellucidum, corpus callosum, third ventricle	Anterior horn lateral ventricle	Body lateral ventricle, caudate nucleus	Body lateral ventricle	Anterior horn lateral ventricle, caudate nucleus
Medial to	Caudate nucleus, thalamus, frontal horn lateral ventricle		Thalamus			Thalamus, caudate nucleus
Lt lateral to			Cavum septum pellucidum, germinal matrix, frontal horn lateral ventricle			
Rt lateral to			Cavum septum pellucidum, germinal matrix, frontal horn lateral ventricle			

Continued

Table 26-1 Location of Neonatal Brain Structures Routinely Visualized With Ultrasound—cont'd

	Medulla Oblongata	Cavum Vergae	Quadrigeminal Plate	Basal Ganglia	Cerebellum
Anterior to	Fourth ventricle, aqueduct of Sylvius, cerebellar vermis, occipital lobe				
Posterior to					Pons, medulla oblongata, temporal lobe
Superior to		Third ventricle, thalamus, cerebral peduncle	Tentorium, fourth ventricle, cisterna magna, cerebellum	Temporal lobe	
Inferior to	Third ventricle, massa intermedia, pons	Interhemispheric fissure	Thalamus, cavum vergae, body lateral ventricle	Caudate nucleus, cavum septum pellucidum, frontal horn lateral ventricle	Fourth ventricle, tentorium, quadrigeminal plate, occipital lobe, occipital horn lateral ventricle, temporal horn lateral ventricle
Medial to		Body caudate nucleus, body lateral ventricle	Choroidal fissure, temporal horn lateral ventricle		
Lt lateral to				Caudate nucleus, frontal horn lateral ventricle	
Rt lateral to				Caudate nucleus, frontal horn lateral ventricle	

	Pons	Anterior Horn Lateral Ventricle	Body Lateral Ventricle	Temporal Horn Lateral Ventricle	Temporal Horn Lateral Ventricle
Anterior to	Cerebellum	Choroid plexus, body lateral ventricle	Occipital lobe	Occipital horn lateral ventricle	
Posterior to			Caudate nucleus, germinal matrix, anterior horn lateral ventricle		
Superior to	Medulla oblongata	Thalamus, caudate nucleus, germinal matrix	Trigone, choroid plexus, thalamus, cerebellum, pons, occipital horn lateral ventricle	Cerebellum, tentorium	Caudate nucleus, germinal matrix, temporal lobe
Inferior to	Thalamus, temporal lobe, third ventricle, cerebral peduncle			Choroidal fissure, choroid plexus, thalamus	
Medial to					
Lt lateral to			Cavum vergae	Cerebral peduncle, fourth ventricle, tentorium, quadrigeminal plate	Cavum septum pellucidum
Rt lateral to			Cavum vergae	Cerebral peduncle, fourth ventricle, tentorium, quadrigeminal plate	Cavum septum pellucidum

the midline to the most lateral aspect of the lateral ventricles (see Figure 26-2, *B*). This measurement should be 12 mm or less.

Reference ranges established by a research study of preterm infants with normal ventricles at the time of imaging indicated the sizes shown in the box below.

■ ■ ■ NORMAL MEASUREMENTS

Structure	Measurement
Lateral ventricle: anterior horn width	0 to 2.9 mm
Lateral ventricle: thalamo-to-occipital distance	8.7 to 24.7 mm
Third ventricle: width	0 to 2.6 mm
Fourth ventricle: width	3.3 to 7.4 mm
Fourth ventricle: length	2.6 to 6.9 mm

However, another research study comparing ultrasound and MRI measurements of ventricular size found "small but significant" differences in ventricular measurements between the two modalities. Sonographers should therefore be careful in measuring ventricular size and related anatomy and refer to cranial measurements taken with other modalities on the same patient, when available, for comparison.

GROSS ANATOMY

Neurons are the cells that create brain activity. They form a dense, vast network. Motor neurons carry information to glands and muscles. Sensory neurons carry information from the sense organs to the central nervous system. Connector or interneurons are connections between the motor and sensory neurons. To the naked eye, neurons appear as "gray matter."

The Brain

The brain sits inside the skull. It is an approximately 3 lb spongy mass of nerve and supportive tissue. The base of the brain is connected to the spinal cord. The main parts of the brain include the *cerebrum, cerebellum,* and *brain stem.* The brain also contains 4 ventricles or cavities: 2 *lateral ventricles,* the *third ventricle,* and the *fourth ventricle.*

The brain is covered by the **cranium**, a protective bony vault of the skull; the cranium consists of 8 bones:
- One frontal
- One occipital
- One ethmoid
- One sphenoid
- Two temporal
- Two parietal

The brain is also covered by the meninges, which are 3 membranes enveloping the brain and spinal cord

Table 26-2 Major Brain Fissures

Fissure	Other Names	Separates ...
Interhemispheric	Medial longitudinal, longitudinal cerebral	Right and left cerebral hemispheres
Sylvian	Lateral fissure, lateral sulcus	Frontal and temporal lobes
Central	Fissure of Rolando	Frontal and parietal lobes
Parieto-occipital	N/A	Parietal and occipital lobes
Transverse	N/A	Cerebrum and cerebellum

that serve to support and protect. The meninges consist of the *pia mater, arachnoid mater,* and *dura mater:*
- **Pia mater**: Innermost layer; adjacent to the brain and spinal cord surfaces.
- **Arachnoid mater**: Middle layer; **subarachnoid space** filled with cerebrospinal fluid is between this layer and the pia mater.
- **Dura mater**: Outer layer; potential subdural space between this layer and the arachnoid may abnormally fill with fluid or blood (subdural hematoma). The **tentorium** is a flap of dura mater that separates the cerebral hemispheres from other major structures in the brain. The **falx cerebri** is a double fold of dura mater located in the **interhemispheric fissure** ("cerebral fissure") between the cerebral hemispheres, at the midline of the brain (Table 26-2).

The Ventricles

Cerebrospinal fluid (CSF) circulates around the brain and spinal cord to serve as a shock absorber against injury and a distributor of nutrients. It is a clear liquid produced daily by the **choroid plexus** (series of specialized blood vessels located in the ventricles) and continually circulates through the ventricles and subarachnoid space. The subarachnoid space (the space between the pia mater and the arachnoid mater) is very small in most areas, but in certain areas it is enlarged, and CSF will pool there. These pools of CSF are called cisterns. The lumbar cistern is the largest of these spaces and is found in the distal end of the spine. Other such cisterns are found in various locations within the brain. The largest of these cisterns is the **cisterna magna**, which is located at the base of the cerebellum in a posterior portion of the brain. As mentioned, there are 4 ventricles located in the brain: two *lateral ventricles,* the *third ventricle,* and the *fourth ventricle:*
- **Lateral ventricles**: Both hemispheres of the cerebrum contain a lateral ventricle. Each lies just below the

corpus callosum. The two lateral ventricles are separated from each other by the cavum septum pellucidum, a small, midline cavity filled with cerebrospinal fluid that filters from the ventricles through the septal laminae. It has no direct communication with the ventricular system. Each lateral ventricle consists of 4 segments: frontal horn, body, occipital horn, and temporal horn.

- Third ventricle: Inferior to and connected to each lateral ventricle by the foramen of Monro, a narrow opening for the passage of cerebrospinal fluid.
- Fourth ventricle: Inferior to and connected to the third ventricle by the aqueduct of Sylvius, a small channel for the passage of cerebrospinal fluid. The foramen of Magendie and foramina of Luschka are three holes on the floor of the ventricle that open into the subarachnoid space for the passage of cerebrospinal fluid.

The Cerebrum

The largest component of the human central nervous system is the cerebrum, the main portion of the brain. It is divided into two identical, right and left, symmetrical cerebral hemispheres that communicate through the corpus callosum (a "neural bridge" or network of nerve fibers), located between them at the midline of the brain. Each cerebral hemisphere is divided functionally and physically into four lobes, named after the overlying cranial bones:

- Frontal lobe
- Parietal lobe
- Temporal lobe
- Occipital lobe

If you could look down through the top of your head to the brain's cortex, you would see the two hemispheres (or right and left halves) of the cerebrum filling the superior cranial cavity. The outermost surface of the cerebral hemispheres, the cerebral cortex, or "gray matter," would appear convoluted with raised ridges called gyri that are separated from each other by sulci (grooves or indentations in the cortex). Except for the previously noted corpus callosum, the cerebral hemispheres are separated from each other at the midline by the previously mentioned, interhemispheric fissure (see Table 26-2).

Cerebral gray matter is composed of densely packed neurons (nerve bodies) with no myelin covering (in contrast to cerebral white matter discussed below) that control brain activity. Gray matter structures include the:

- Cerebral cortex: Highly convoluted external surface of the cerebrum.
- Basal ganglia: Highly specialized collection of cell clusters just superior to the thalamus. Functions in motor skills and includes the caudate nucleus, globus pallidus, and putamen.

Cerebral white matter is composed of myelinated or fat-insulated nerve cell axons that carry information between the neurons in the brain and spinal cord. White brain matter is situated between the cerebellum and brain stem, beneath the cerebral cortex. It consists of structures at the center of the brain, such as the:

- Corpus callosum: Flat, broad, nerve fibers between the right and left cerebral hemispheres that form the roof of the lateral ventricles.
- Diencephalon: Just inferior to the corpus callosum; extends to the base of the brain. Encloses the third ventricle and includes the:
  - Thalami: A pair of large, symmetrical ovoid organs situated on either side of the third ventricle, forming most of the ventricle's lateral walls. They make up the largest portion of the diencephalon.
  - Hypothalamus: Located just inferior to the thalamus at the base of the brain. Composed of several different areas, even though it is just the size of a pea. Communicates directly with the pituitary gland.
  - Epithalamus: Situated in the anterosuperior portion of the diencephalon. Contains the choroid plexus of the third ventricle and the pineal gland.

The Cerebellum

The cerebellum constitutes the second largest portion of the brain. Occupying most of the posterior fossae, the cerebellum is inferior to the tentorium and posterior to the pons and medulla oblongata. It is composed of symmetrical, bilateral hemispheres connected by the vermis, its medial portion.

The cerebellar peduncles are three pairs of nerve tracts that connect the cerebellum to the rest of the brain. The inferior cerebellar peduncle connects with the medulla, the middle cerebellar peduncle connects with the pons, and the superior cerebellar peduncle connects with the midbrain.

The Brain Stem ("Hindbrain")

If you could look through the side of your head you would see a cross-section of brain anatomy demonstrating how the brain stem connects the cerebral hemispheres to the spinal cord. The brain stem consists of the *midbrain, pons,* and *medulla oblongata:*

- Midbrain: The superior portion of the brain stem situated where the cerebellum and pons unite. Anteriorly it has a cerebral peduncle. Posteriorly it includes the tectum, which is made up of superior and inferior colliculi that form parts of the visual and auditory systems.
- Pons: The middle portion of the brain stem situated at the midline, anterior to and between the bilateral cerebellar hemispheres. It is inferior to the midbrain and superior to the medulla oblongata, to which it

is directly connected. The pons' posterior surface forms the floor of the fourth ventricle. The superior surface includes bilateral cerebral peduncles. The pons consists of many long nerve tracts that pass through the brain stem.

- **Medulla oblongata**: Extends inferiorly from the pons to form the inferior portion of the brain stem that projects out of the skull through the foramen magnum (a large opening in the posterior portion of the occipital bone of the skull) and connects to the spinal cord. The medulla's anterior surface includes two protruding longitudinal nerve tracts called the pyramids.

PHYSIOLOGY

The human brain, the body's largest and most complex mass of nervous tissue, functions with remarkable abilities.

The Cerebrum

The cerebral cortex is responsible for such functions as speech, memory, voluntary movement, logical reasoning, and emotional response. As mentioned, each cerebral hemisphere is divided functionally and physically into 4 lobes: *frontal lobe, parietal lobe, temporal lobe,* and *occipital lobe*.

The **parietal lobe** of the brain contains the body's sensory receptors, which interpret the impulses that allow one to recognize such sensations as pain, cold, or a light touch (Figure 26-5). Because the sensory pathways are crossed pathways, the impulses from the body's right side are received by the left hemisphere's sensory cortex. This somatic sensory area is located posterior to the **central fissure**.

Other cortical areas are responsible for interpreting impulses from the special sense organs. For example, the auditory area is adjacent to the sylvian fissure in the **temporal lobe**, and the olfactory area is deeper in the same lobe. The posterior part of the **occipital lobe** interprets visual impulses (see Figure 26-5).

The primary motor area is located anterior to the central fissure in the **frontal lobe** (see Figure 26-5). This area controls the movements of the conscious skeletal muscles, such as those in the face, mouth, and hands. The motor pathways are crossed pathways, as in the somatic sensory cortex.

The anterior part of the frontal lobes is believed to house the higher intellectual reasoning function. Complex memories are probably stored in both the temporal and frontal lobes. The speech function is located at the junction of the temporal, parietal, and occipital horns (see Figure 26-5).

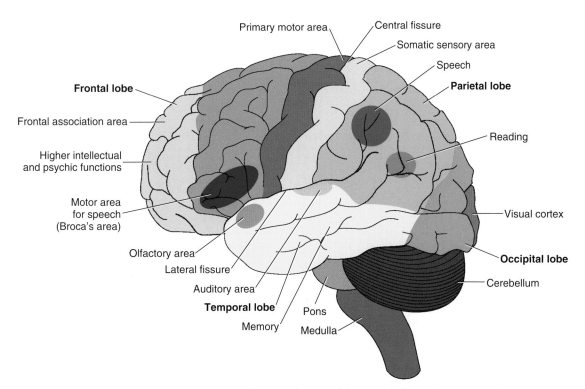

FIGURE 26-5 **Brain Function.** Various functional areas of the cerebral hemispheres. Lateral view of the brain.

The Diencephalon

The diencephalon rests superior to the brain stem and is enclosed by the cerebral hemispheres. As previously mentioned, three distinct structures make up the diencephalon: the *thalamus*, *hypothalamus*, and *epithalamus*.

The *thalamus* serves as a relay station for upward-moving sensory impulses. As a result, we can experience a crude recognition of both pleasant and unpleasant sensations. The *hypothalamus*, lying under the thalamus, plays a role in regulating body temperature, fluid balance, and metabolism. Additionally, it functions as the center for such drives as thirst, appetite, and sex. The *epithalamus* lies at the midline and is behind the third ventricle and contains the pineal gland, which synthesizes enzymes related to daylight sensitivity.

The Brain Stem

The structures of the brain stem—the *midbrain, pons,* and *medulla oblongata*—provide a pathway for ascending and descending fiber tracts. Additionally, they have small areas (i.e., nuclei) that are involved in such vital activities as swallowing and blood pressure. The pons, for example, contains nuclei involved in the control of breathing, and the medulla oblongata helps control heart rate, breathing, and vomiting, among other functions.

The Cerebellum

The cerebellum functions to provide balance and equilibrium to the body by adjusting the timing of skeletal muscle activity. As a result, body movements are coordinated and smooth.

SONOGRAPHIC APPEARANCE

When the neonatal brain is sonographically examined, the relative echogenicity of various intracranial structures, along with their locations, can be described. Sonographic appreciation of the normal anatomic brain structures becomes essential when ruling out intracranial pathology.

The bones comprising the cranial vault appear highly echogenic, whereas the parenchyma of the large cerebral hemispheres reveals a mostly homogeneous texture of relatively low echogenicity. Interspersed throughout the cerebral cortex are thin, bright lines representing various sulci and/or fissures that separate the gyri (cerebral folds).

Modified Coronal Plane Cross-Sections

When the neonatal brain is viewed in modified coronal plane cross-sections, the normal frontal horns and bodies of the lateral ventricles appear as thin, crescent-like, anechoic, fluid-filled, bilateral spaces. The corpus callosum forms their superior margin and appears low-gray at the midline of the brain. The bright, longitudinal section of the falx cerebri is also seen at this level extending from the superior edge of the brain at the midline, within the interhemispheric fissure (Figure 26-6).

Anterior to the frontal horns, in the frontal lobe of the cerebral cortex, a bright, symmetric area can be noted. Commonly referred to as the normal periventricular "blush" or "halo," this area corresponds to the frontal periventricular white matter area. The bright orbital ridge and very low-gray orbital cones (eye area) can be seen inferiorly (Figure 26-7).

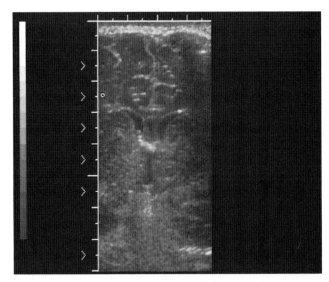
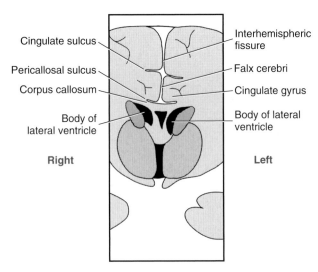

FIGURE 26-6 Coronal image of the brain at the level of the bodies of the lateral ventricles.

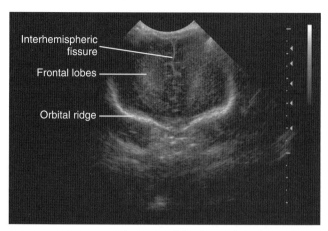

FIGURE 26-7 Coronal image of the brain through the frontal lobes. The orbital ridge forms the inferior boundary of this image.

The frontal horns of the lateral ventricles are separated by the moderately gray-appearing cavum septum pellucidum, which forms their medial margins at the midline of the brain. The cavum septum pellucidum is a normal variant sometimes noted in the neonate. It is a septum pellucidum that has a separation between its two leaflets (septal laminae) and appears anechoic due to its small cavity that is filled with CSF that filters from the ventricles through the septal laminae (Figure 26-8).

The moderately echogenic head of the **caudate nucleus** forms the inferolateral margin of the anterior horns (Figure 26-9). It represents the more superior aspect of the gray matter of the basal ganglia, a group of structures coordinating movement. The caudate

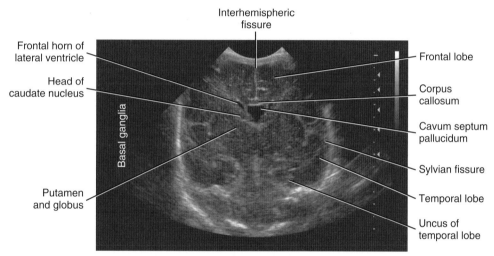

FIGURE 26-8 Coronal image of the brain at the level of the frontal horns of the lateral ventricles. The CSF in the frontal horns appears anechoic. The cavum septum pellucidum sits between the lateral ventricles and is often large in preterm infants. The corpus callosum appears above the cavum.

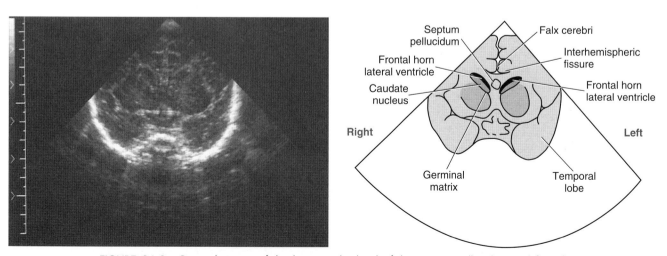

FIGURE 26-9 Coronal image of the brain at the level of the septum pellucidum and frontal horns of the lateral ventricles, showing the head of the caudate nucleus.

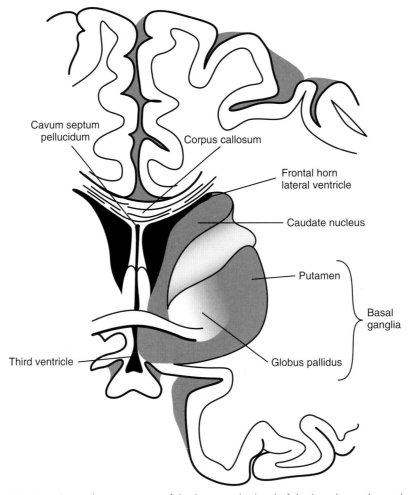

Cavum septum pellucidum

Corpus callosum

Frontal horn lateral ventricle

Caudate nucleus

Putamen

Basal ganglia

Third ventricle

Globus pallidus

FIGURE 26-10 Coronal cross section of the brain at the level of the basal ganglia and corpus callosum.

nucleus is located in the telencephalon ("forebrain"). Immediately lateral and inferior to the caudate nucleus, the putamen and globus pallidus of the basal ganglia can be noted as areas of increased echogenicity relative to the surrounding parenchyma (see Figure 26-8).

The anterior corpus callosum forms the superior margin of the frontal horns (Figure 26-10). The superior margin of the corpus callosum is marked by the echogenic pericallosal sulcus. Superior to this is the low-gray cingulate gyrus and then the bright cingulate sulcus (see Figure 26-6).

The area of the foramen of Monro can be identified just posterior to the level of the frontal horn of each lateral ventricle. The bilateral foramina lie inferomedial to the bodies of the lateral ventricles and mark the communication between the lateral and third ventricles. The third ventricle, filled with CSF, lies inferior to the foramina in the midline (Figure 26-11). It can be difficult to visualize in its axial dimension when normal in size; however, it is clearly noted as an anechoic structure

when dilated. The moderately echogenic body of the caudate nucleus marks the inferolateral margin of the bodies of the lateral ventricles. Also noted at this level are the echogenic lateral sylvian fissures, which divide the frontal and temporal lobes of the cerebral cortex (see Figure 26-11). The middle cerebral arteries lie here and are frequently seen pulsating on a real-time image.

At a level just inferior to the foramen of Monro, the bright appearance of the interpeduncular cistern makes it easy to identify. Near this cistern, the pulsations of the basilar artery are frequently seen during real-time examination.

Figure 26-12 illustrates a coronal view of the brain that shows the bilateral, homogeneous thalami, which can be seen lying inferior to the bodies of the lateral ventricles. The posterior aspect of the slit-like third ventricle lies between them. The anterior extent of the highly echogenic choroid plexus can be noted in the groove between the lateral ventricles and thalami. The choroid plexus also lies in the roof of the third and

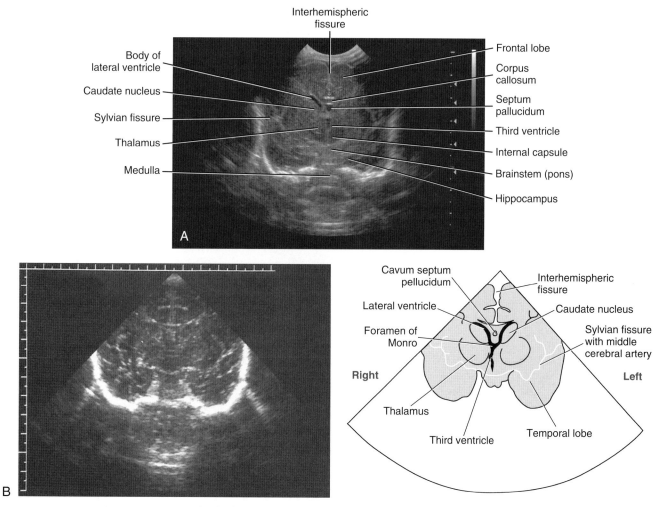

FIGURE 26-11 **A,** The third ventricle appears below both lateral ventricles and the septum pellucidum. It is often small and difficult to see but can vary considerably in size. The brainstem may be seen as a tree-like shape; **B,** The foramen of Monro may be clearly seen. The bilateral foramina lie inferomedial to the bodies of the lateral ventricles and mark the communication between the lateral and third ventricles.

fourth ventricles. A pair of low-gray structures can be identified inferior to the thalami. These represent the cerebral peduncles. This view also reveals the moderately echogenic pons and medulla oblongata of the brain stem (seen inferiorly).

A coronal view through the quadrigeminal plate cistern reveals the highly echogenic, tent-shaped tentorium cerebelli that separates the cerebellum from the more superior structures in the brain (Figure 26-13). Sometimes evident at this level is the fourth ventricle, a rectangular anechoic space in the midline. It lies just anterior to the vermis of the cerebellum in the posterior fossa (see Figure 26-13). Sonographically, the vermis, the midline portion of the cerebellum, is quite echogenic, whereas the lateral cerebellar hemispheres are noticeably hypoechoic in comparison. The anechoic cisterna magna may be seen in the space between the inferior vermis and the occipital bone.

At a more posterior level the **trigone** region of the lateral ventricles (where the bodies, occipital horns, and temporal horns converge) can be visualized. Most noticeable is the highly echogenic glomus of the choroid plexus within the trigones (Figure 26-14).

The level posterior and cephalad to the trigones reveals the symmetric, echogenic "blush" of the posterior periventricular white matter (i.e., centrum semiovale). This area is visible on either side of the reflective interhemispheric fissure (Figure 26-15).

Modified Sagittal Plane Cross Sections

Viewing the neonatal brain in sagittal sections from the fulcrum of the anterior fontanelle reveals several

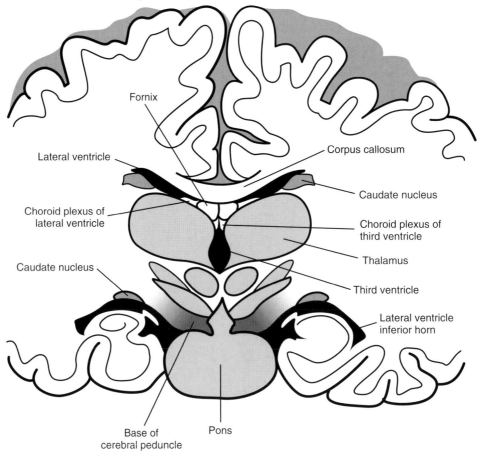

FIGURE 26-12 Coronal cross-section of the brain at the level of the thalamus.

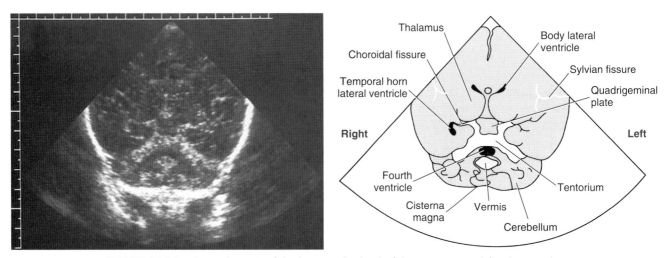

FIGURE 26-13 Coronal image of the brain at the level of the tentorium and fourth ventricle.

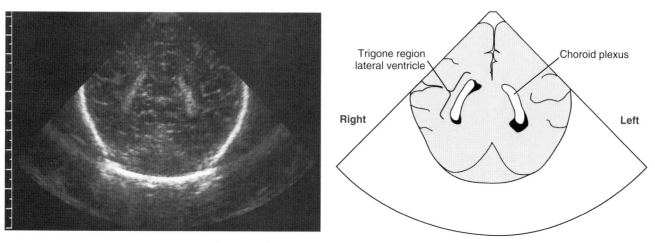

FIGURE 26-14 Coronal image of the brain at the level of the trigone region of the lateral ventricles. The choroid plexus is prominent in preterm infants; notice how it fills the lateral ventricles in this view.

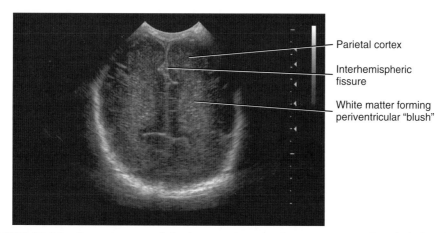

FIGURE 26-15 Coronal image of the brain at the a level just posterior and cephalad to the trigones. The white matter around the lateral ventricles may appear quite echo dense (bright) in this plane and is sometimes called a "blush" or "flare."

important anatomic landmarks. Figures 26-16 and 26-17 show some of these landmarks that include the classic crescent-shaped corpus callosum. It is clearly identified in the midline and lies just superior to the septum pellucidum. Pulsations from the anterior cerebral arteries are often seen just anterior to the corpus callosum during real-time scanning. Lying inferior to the cavum septum pellucidum and vergae (when present) is another important landmark, the third ventricle. The massa intermedia is a small gray-matter mass located in the midline of the third ventricle with no known function. Not all humans have a massa intermedia. When present, it appears homogeneous and moderately echogenic. The quadrigeminal plate cistern lies posterior to the third ventricle. The inferior end of

this cistern is marked by the highly echogenic cerebellar vermis. Indenting the anterior vermis is the anechoic fourth ventricle, which appears triangular at this level. The moderately echogenic pons and medulla oblongata of the brain stem occupy the area anterior to the fourth ventricle.

Another significant anatomic landmark, the caudothalamic groove, is clearly distinguished sonographically from a sagittal plane. This groove appears as a thin, bright arc located between the head of the caudate nucleus and the thalamus (Figure 26-18). It marks the area of **germinal matrix**, which is found more anterosuperiorly. Being composed of a fine network of blood vessels and neural tissue, the germinal matrix is highly susceptible to hemorrhage in the premature

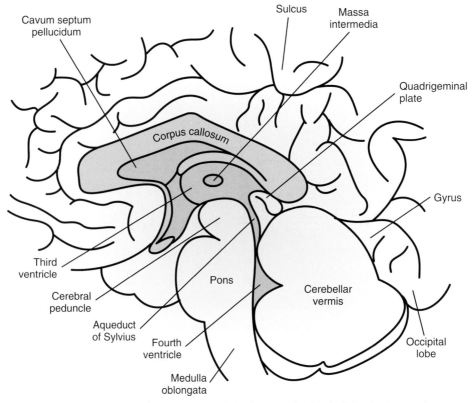

FIGURE 26-16   Sagittal cross-section of the brain at the level of the third ventricle.

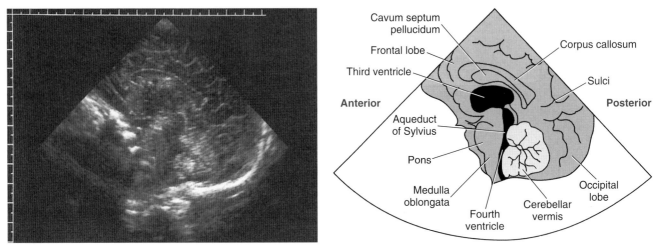

FIGURE 26-17   Sagittal image of the midline of the brain.

infant (pressure and metabolic changes can lead to rupture of these small vessels). Although the germinal matrix lies in the subependymal layer of the ventricular system in early fetal life, it regresses to the area over the head of the caudate nucleus by 6 months' gestation. It cannot be seen as a distinct structure at term by ultrasound. The caudate nucleus, lying more anteriorly, is

normally slightly more echogenic than the thalamus (see Figure 26-18).

All of the lateral ventricle horns are simultaneously seen on the sagittal image in Figure 26-19, taken at the level of the head of the caudate nucleus. On ultrasound, the CSF-filled chambers of the ventricles appear anechoic with bright reflective walls. The size of the ventricles

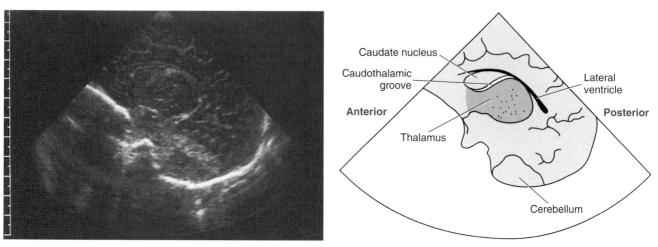

FIGURE 26-18 Sagittal image of the brain at the level of the caudothalamic groove.

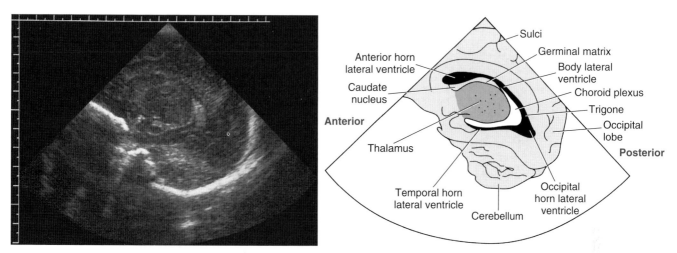

FIGURE 26-19 Sagittal image of the brain in which all the horns of the lateral ventricle can be identified.

varies, depending on how much CSF is present. This level of the brain is also characterized by the highly echogenic glomus of the choroid plexus present in the trigone region of the lateral ventricles. The normal choroid tapers as it courses anteriorly toward the foramen of Monro and should display a smooth contour. Surrounding the lateral ventricles are the frontal, parietal, temporal, and occipital lobes of the cerebrum. The echogenic periventricular "blush" should again be noted posterior to the occipital horns. This corresponds to an area of the posterior periventricular white matter.

Figure 26-20 is a sagittal image of the brain taken to the far right or left of the midline. It shows the reflective appearance of the sylvian fissure and the low to moderate echogenicity of the cerebral cortex's temporal lobe. Again, the middle cerebral arteries can commonly be

seen pulsating in the sylvian fissures. Numerous echogenic linear and curvilinear sulci can be seen in the term infant at this level. The echogenic blush from the periventricular area can be noted. A summary of some of the major brain structures and their sonographic presentations is provided in Table 26-3.

SONOGRAPHIC APPLICATIONS

Common considerations when performing sonography of the neonatal brain include:
- Doppler evaluation of cerebral blood flow abnormalities
- Detection of:
  - Ventricular size
  - Hydrocephalus (ventricular dilatation)
  - Congenital anomalies

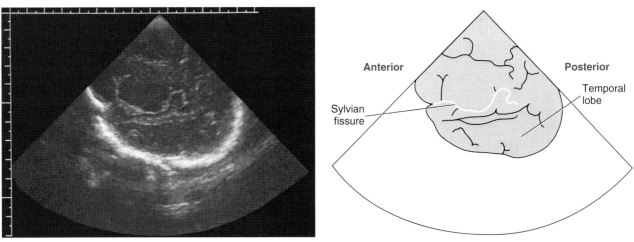

FIGURE 26-20 Sagittal image of the brain either to the far right or far left of the midline. Reveals the temporal lobe and sylvian fissure.

■ ■ ■ **Table 26-3** Sonographic Appearance of Major Brain Structures in the Neonate

Structure	Echogenicity	Location
Corpus callosum	Hypoechoic relative to adjacent structures	Unites cerebral hemispheres; forms superior margin of lateral ventricles in the midline
Falx cerebri	Bright, reflective	Lies within interhemispheric fissure
Periventricular "blush" (area of white matter)	Bright, reflective	Anterior to the frontal horns of the lateral ventricles
Caudate nucleus	Moderately hyperechoic relative to adjacent structures	Forms inferolateral margin of anterior horns of lateral ventricles
Pericallosal sulcus	Bright, reflective	Forms superior margin of the corpus callosum
Cerebral peduncles	Hypoechoic relative to adjacent structures	Lies inferior to the thalamus
Lateral ventricles	Bright, reflective walls surround anechoic cavities	Produces CSF and communicates with third ventricle through foramen of Monro
Cranial vault bones	Bright, reflective	Encloses and protects the brain
Cerebral parenchyma	Low-level echogenicity	Forms cerebrum and divided into lobes
Sulci and fissures	Bright, reflective	Separates cerebral folds
Pons and medulla oblongata	Moderately echogenic	Anterior to fourth ventricle; forms part of the brain stem
Caudothalamic groove	Bright, reflective	Lies between caudate nucleus and thalamus; marks germinal matrix, a network of blood vessels highly susceptible to bleeding in the premature infant
Cavum septum pellucidum	Anechoic	Normal variant of septum pellucidum, which separates the frontal horns of the lateral ventricles

- ○ Intracranial hemorrhage
- ○ Interventricular hemorrhage
- ○ Intracranial masses
- ○ Venous malformations
- ○ Intracranial infections
- ○ Infarction and/or edema

NORMAL VARIANTS

Normal variants of the neonatal brain are typically associated with gestational immaturity.

- **Lateral ventricles**
  - ○ Asymmetry in the size of the lateral ventricles is a common normal variant. Approximately 40% of

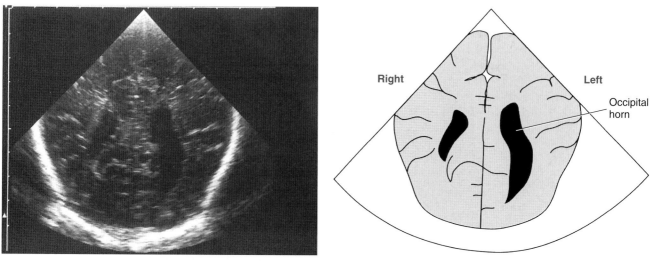

FIGURE 26-21 Coronal image showing asymmetry in the size of the occipital horns of the lateral ventricles. Considered a normal variant that corrects itself with time.

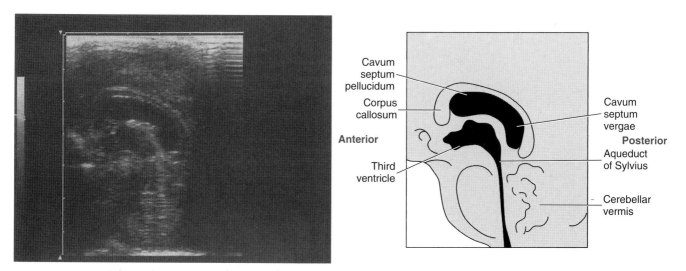

FIGURE 26-22 Sagittal image of the brain showing temporary normal variations, the cavum septum pellucidum and cavum septum vergae that close before a baby's birth.

premature infants and less than 20% of term infants reveal some asymmetry. The left lateral ventricle is generally larger than the right. The occipital horns are particularly susceptible (Figure 26-21). Ventricular size varies with the age of the infant. As the infant matures, the lateral ventricular size decreases in relation to the size of the cerebral cortex.

- **Cavum septum pellucidum and cavum septum vergae**
  - The cavum septum pellucidum is seen as an anechoic, fluid-filled space between the anterior horns

of the lateral ventricles, whereas the cavum septum vergae lies more posteriorly, between the bodies of the lateral ventricles (Figure 26-22). Although these structures communicate with each other, they do not connect with the ventricular system. The cavum septum vergae closes from posterior to anterior beginning in month 6 of gestation. Although this structure can be seen in a premature infant, it is infrequently seen in the term infant. On the other hand, the cavum septum pellucidum begins to close near term. Therefore it can be noted alone until approximately 2 months of postnatal life.

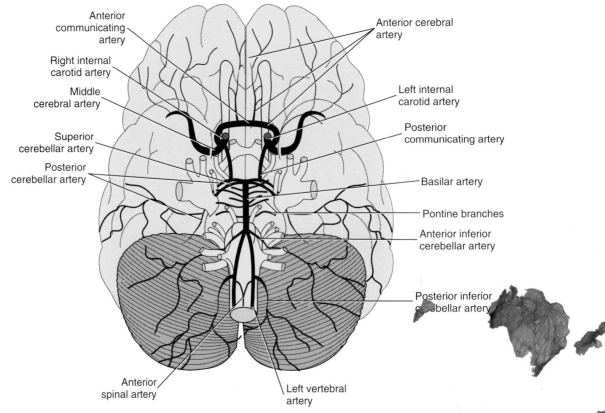

FIGURE 26-23   Blood supply to the brain as seen from the inferior surface.

REFERENCE CHARTS

■ ■ ■   ASSOCIATED PHYSICIANS

- **Radiologist:** Specializes in the diagnostic interpretation of imaging modalities that assess central nervous system pathology.
- **Neurologist:** Specializes in the diagnosis and treatment of disorders of the nervous system.
- **Neonatologist:** Specializes in the diagnosis and treatment of disorders of the newborn infant.

■ ■ ■   COMMON DIAGNOSTIC TESTS

- **Computed axial tomography (CT) scan:** Provides cross-sectional (i.e., axial) x-ray images of the brain to assess anatomy. A contrast medium is often administered to differentiate between pathology and normal anatomy. This test is performed by a radiologic technologist or radiologist. Interpretation of the test is by the radiologist.
- **Magnetic resonance imaging (MRI):** Provides valuable information about the body's biochemistry when the patient is placed in a magnetic field. Provides axial, sagittal, and coronal images of the brain directly. This diagnostic imaging technique does not require exposure to ionizing radiation. The test is performed by a radiologic technologist or radiologist and interpreted by the radiologist.

- **Electroencephalography (EEG):** Records changes in electric potential (i.e., activity) in various locations of the brain by means of electrodes placed on the scalp. This test is performed by a technologist and interpreted by a neurologist.

■ ■ ■   LABORATORY VALUES

- **Hematocrit:** This laboratory test measures the percentage of blood that is composed of red blood cells, expressed as volume percent. A decreasing hematocrit can be an indication of a possible intracranial hemorrhage.

■ ■ ■   NORMAL MEASUREMENTS

VENTRICULAR SIZE

- **Ventricular depth:** In a coronal plane at the level of the foramen of Monro, the bodies of the lateral ventricles are measured from wall to wall (see Figure 26-2). This measurement is the widest line perpendicular to the longest axis of the ventricles. Normal measurement: 4 mm or less.
- **Midline to lateral dimension:** In the same coronal plane, this measurement is the horizontal distance from the midline (i.e., falx) to the most lateral aspect of the lateral ventricles. Normal measurement: 12 mm or less.

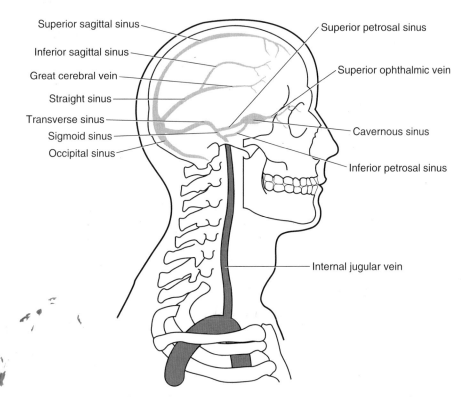

Superior sagittal sinus
Inferior sagittal sinus
Great cerebral vein
Straight sinus
Transverse sinus
Sigmoid sinus
Occipital sinus

Superior petrosal sinus
Superior ophthalmic vein
Cavernous sinus
Inferior petrosal sinus
Internal jugular vein

FIGURE 26-24 Lateral view of the head showing the major venous drainage of the brain.

■ ■ ■   VASCULATURE

The internal carotid and vertebral arteries supply blood to the brain (Figure 26-23).
- Aorta—brachiocephalic (rt.)—common carotid artery—INTERNAL CAROTID ARTERY—anterior cerebral artery—anterior communicating artery—middle cerebral artery-posterior communicating artery.
- Aorta—brachiocephalic (rt.)—rt. subclavian artery—VERTEBRAL ARTERY—anterior spinal artery—basilar artery—posterior inferior cerebellar artery—anterior inferior cerebellar artery—superior cerebellar artery—posterior cerebral artery.

Large veins, called *sinuses,* located in the brain's tough covering (i.e., the dura mater), drain the brain (Figure 26-24).
- Superior sagittal sinus—inferior sagittal sinus—great cerebral vein of Galen—straight sinus—occipital sinus—transverse sinus—sigmoid sinus—superior ophthalmic vein—cavernous sinus—superior petrosal sinus—inferior petrosal sinus—internal jugular vein.

■ ■ ■   AFFECTING CHEMICALS

Nonapplicable.

Small Parts Sonography

■ **CHAPTER 27**

The Thyroid and Parathyroid Glands

WAYNE C. LEONHARDT

OBJECTIVES

Describe the anatomy and sonographic appearance of the normal thyroid, parathyroid gland (locations), and relevant adjacent anatomic structures in the neck.

Describe the nodal zones (anatomic landmarks) when mapping abnormal cervical nodes.

Describe the physiology of the thyroid and parathyroid glands.

Describe the vascular supply of the thyroid and parathyroid glands.

Describe various shapes of normal parathyroid glands.

Describe anatomic pitfalls when scanning the thyroid and parathyroid glands.

Describe clinical laboratory tests, related diagnostic tests, normal laboratory values, and associated physicians in the workup of thyroid and parathyroid glands.

Describe the sonographic indications for thyroid and parathyroid gland studies.

■

KEY WORDS

Anterior Scalene Muscle (ASM) — Paired muscles in the lateral neck that run deep to the sternocleidomastoid muscle.

Calcitonin — Hormone secreted by the thyroid gland. Its primary function is to decrease blood calcium levels, preventing hypercalcemia.

Ectopic Parathyroid Glands — Abnormal locations of parathyroid adenomas including the thymus gland, carotid bulb, retroesophageal, intrathyroidal, and the carotid sheath.

Extrathyroidal Veins and Arteries — Vessels found at the upper and lower poles of the thyroid gland.

Hypercalcemia — Increase in serum calcium of >10.5 mg/dL.

Hypocalcemia — Low blood calcium levels.

Inferior Thyroid Artery — Largest branch of the thyrocervical trunk, which comes off the subclavian artery. Paired arteries supply the lower half of the thyroid gland. At the base of the thyroid gland it branches into 2 arteries supplying the posterior and inferior portions of the gland.

Inferior Thyroid Veins — Arise in the venous plexus of the thyroid gland, communicate with the superior and middle thyroid veins, and empty into the left and right innominate veins.

Infrahyoid Muscles — Double-layered muscle planes located anterior in the neck and superficial to the larynx, trachea, and thyroid gland. Also called "strap muscles"; include the sternohyoid (SH), sternothyroid (ST), and omohyoid (OH).

Isthmus — Unites the lower third of the right and left lobes at the level of the second, third, and fourth tracheal rings.

Longus Colli Muscle (LCM) — Wedge-shaped muscle posterior to the thyroid lobes.

Major Neurovascular Bundle (MAJNB) — Posterolateral to the thyroid gland. Consists of the common carotid artery, internal jugular vein, and the vagus nerve. Encased by the carotid sheath, which consists of areolar tissue.

Minor Neurovascular Bundle (MINB) — Posterior to the thyroid gland. Consists of the inferior thyroid artery and recurrent laryngeal nerve.

Omohyoid (OH) Muscle — One of the infrahyoid (or strap) muscles.

Parathyroid Hormone (PTH) — Also called parathormone. Secreted by parathyroid glands to maintain homeostasis of serum calcium and phosphorous levels.

Primary Hyperparathyroidism — Common endocrine disorder (1 to 2 per 1000

KEY WORDS—cont'd

population in the United States) characterized by an excess secretion of PTH by 1 or more of the parathyroid glands.

Pyramidal Lobe — Accessory thyroid lobe.

Recurrent Laryngeal Nerve — Part of the minor neurovascular bundle (MINB), which marks the posterior border of the thyroid.

Secondary Hyperparathyroidism — Endocrine disorder characterized by an excess secretion of parathyroid hormone (PTH) by all the parathyroid glands, in response to hypocalcemia and associated hypertrophy of the glands. This disorder is especially seen in patients with chronic renal failure.

Sternocleidomastoid Muscle — Large neck muscle anterolateral to the thyroid gland.

Sternohyoid Muscle (SH) — One of the infrahyoid (or strap) muscles.

Sternothyroid Muscle (ST) — One of the infrahyoid (or strap) muscles.

Strap Muscles — Infrahyoid muscles.

Superior Thyroid Artery — First branch of the external carotid artery. Paired arteries that supply the upper poles of the thyroid gland and larynx.

Superior Thyroid Veins — Arise superior to the anterolateral surface of the thyroid gland, cross the CCA, and then empty into the IJVs above the thyroid cartilage.

Thyroid-Stimulating Hormone (TSH) — Secreted by thyrotrope cells in the anterior pituitary gland to control thyroid hormone secretions; also known as thyrotropin.

Thyroxine (T₄) — Hormone produced and secreted by the thyroid gland to regulate metabolism.

Triiodothyronine (T₃) — Hormone produced and secreted by the thyroid gland to regulate metabolism.

Vagus Nerve — Part of the major neurovascular bundle (MAJNB). Located in the posterior angle formed between the internal jugular vein and the common carotid artery.

■■■ NORMAL MEASUREMENTS

Structure	Measurement
Adult thyroid gland	4 to 6 cm in length, 1.3 to 1.8 cm in anteroposterior diameter, 1.5 to 2.0 cm in width
Isthmus (adult)	4 to 6 mm in anteroposterior diameter
Thyroid gland in newborns and children	2 to 3 cm in length, 0.2 to 1.2 cm in anteroposterior diameter, 1.0 to 1.5 cm in width

(handwritten notes):
Endocrin gland.
2 lat lobes connecting isthmus.
Rt lobe > Lf lobe.
Secrete:
- Thyroxine T4
- Trii T3
- Calcitonin.
By: hypothalamus + pituitary gland.

■■■ Thyroid Gland

The thyroid gland is an endocrine gland (one of the ductless glands that release their secretions directly into the blood) consisting of 2 lateral lobes and a connecting portion called the **isthmus** (Figure 27-1). The thyroid gland secretes 3 significant hormones—thyroxine (T₄), triiodothyronine (T₃), and calcitonin—that affect body metabolism, growth, and development.

LOCATION

The thyroid (Table 27-1) is composed of right and left lobes connected across the midline by the isthmus. It is

(handwritten notes):
- Coverd by 2 layers of connective tissue.
- 2nd layer is thyroid capsule, adherent to gland surface.

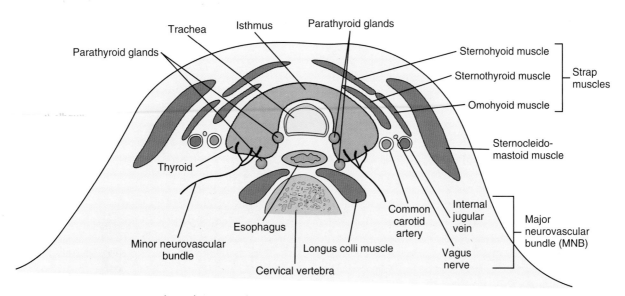

FIGURE 27-1 **Thyroid Anatomy.** Note the parathyroid glands and relevant adjacent structures.

■ ■ ■ **Table 27-1** Location of Thyroid and Parathyroid Glands Routinely Visualized With Ultrasound

	Right and Left Lobes	Isthmus	Vagus Nerve	Pyramidal Lobe	Parathyroid Glands
Anterior to	Fifth or sixth tracheal ring, esophagus (primarily on lt side), superior and inferior thyroid arteries, Rt & Lt CCA, parathyroid glands, longus colli muscle	Second & third tracheal rings		First & second tracheal rings, cricoid cartilage, thyroid cartilage, hypothyroid membrane, larynx	Longus colli muscle
Posterior to	Skin, fascia, SCM muscle, omohyoid muscle, sternohyoid muscle, sternothyroid muscle	Skin, fascia	Skin, fascia, SCM muscle, omohyoid muscle, sternohyoid muscle, sternothyroid muscle	Skin, fascia	Thyroid gland
Superior to	Innominate artery	Innominate artery		Isthmus, Rt & Lt thyroid lobes	
Inferior to	Hyoid bone, larynx, isthmus	Hyoid bone, larynx		Hyoid bone	Cricoid cartilage
Medial to	Rt & Lt CCA, Rt & Lt IJV, Rt & Lt vagus nerves	Rt & Lt thyroid lobes	Rt & Lt IJV	Rt & Lt CCA & IJV	Lateral edges of thyroid gland
Lt lateral to	Isthmus		Lt CCA		
Rt lateral to	Isthmus		Rt CCA		

CCA, Common carotid arteries; IJV, internal jugular veins; SCM, sternocleidomastoid muscle.

located in the anteroinferior part of the neck below the larynx and anterior to the trachea. The isthmus unites the lower third of the lobes at the level of the second, third, and fourth tracheal rings (see Figure 27-1). The thyroid gland is generally shaped like a U or a low-slung H (see Figure 27-7, A). In the latter the cross bar represents the isthmus and the vertical bars represent two conical lateral (right and left) lobes, rounded below and tapered above.

In short axis the thyroid gland has a saddlebag appearance, with two lobes located along either side of the trachea, connected across the midline by the isthmus (Figure 27-2). In longitudinal sections the thyroid lobes are sandwiched between musculature anteriorly and posteriorly or muscles anteriorly and the trachea posteriorly (Figure 27-3).

The thyroid is outlined posterolaterally by the common carotid artery (CCA), the internal jugular vein (IJV), the vagus nerve (VN), and the **anterior scalene muscle (ASM)**; medially by the trachea (T); and anterolaterally by the infrahyoid or **strap muscles** and **sternocleidomastoid muscles. Infrahyoid muscles** are double-layered muscle planes located anterior in the neck and superficial to the larynx, trachea, and thyroid gland. They include the **sternohyoid (SH), sternothyroid (ST)**, and **omohyoid (OH)**. The **longus colli muscle**

(LCM), esophagus (E), and **minor neurovascular bundle (MINB)**, consisting of the **inferior thyroid artery** and **recurrent laryngeal nerve**, mark the posterior border of the thyroid. The **major neurovascular bundle (MAJNB)** located posterolateral to the thyroid gland consists of the CCA, IJV, and the **vagus nerve**. It is encased by the carotid sheath, which consists of areolar tissue. The vagus nerve is located posterolateral to the thyroid lobes between the CCA and IJV (see Figures 27-1 and 27-5).

SIZE

The size and shape of the thyroid gland vary in normal patients. Tall, thin individuals generally have elongated lateral lobes that can measure up to 7 to 8 cm in the longitudinal plane. Shorter, obese patients tend to exhibit oval lateral lobes measuring less than 5 cm. As a result, normal thyroid gland measurements vary widely. The adult thyroid gland measures approximately 4 to 6 cm in length, 1.3 to 1.8 cm in anteroposterior (AP) diameter, and 1.5 to 2 cm in width (Figures 27-4 and 27-5). The isthmus measures approximately 4 to 6 mm in AP diameter (Figure 27-6). In newborns and children the gland measures approximately 2 to 3 cm in length, 0.2 to 1.2 cm in AP diameter, and 1 to 1.5 cm in width. The right lobe is often slightly larger than the left. The average weight of the thyroid is approximately 25 g.

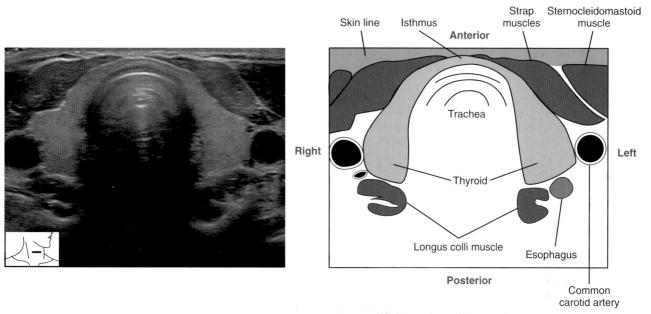

FIGURE 27-2 Transverse plane sonogram showing an axial section of normal thyroid lobe anatomy. Notice how the thyroid lobes are connected in the middle by the longitudinal section of the isthmus.

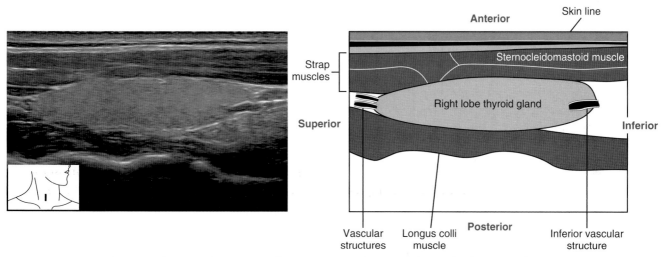

FIGURE 27-3 Sagittal scanning plane sonogram showing a longitudinal section of normal thyroid lobe anatomy and adjacent structures.

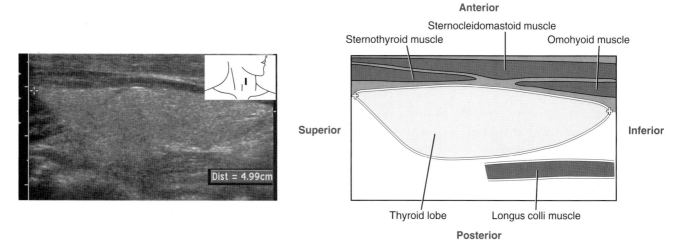

FIGURE 27-4 Sagittal scanning plane image showing a longitudinal section of the left thyroid lobe. Note caliper placement measuring the length.

Physiology:
1) Growth + development.
2) Regulates metabolism, controls memory,
weight loss/gain, heart rate, cholestrol level.
skin condition, energy level by - synthesis
- storage
- secretion of Thy hormone

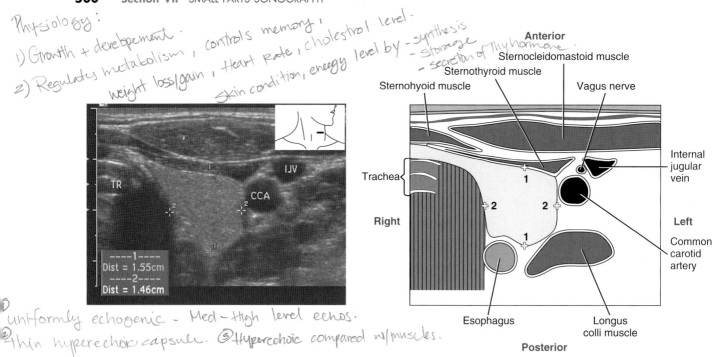

① uniformly echogenic - Med - High level echos.
② thin hyperechoic capsule. ③ Hyperechoic compared w/muscles.

FIGURE 27-5 Transverse scanning plane image showing an axial section of the left lobe of the thyroid gland. Note caliper placement (*Dist 1* and *Dist 2*) measuring the anteroposterior (AP) diameter and width.

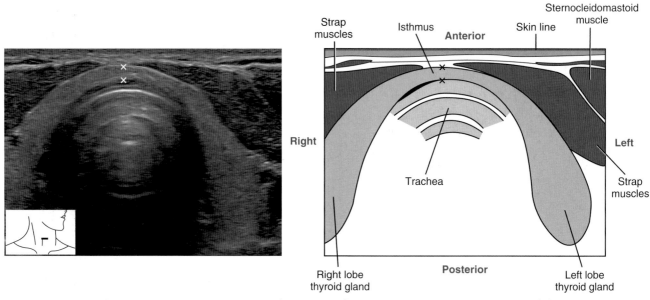

FIGURE 27-6 Transverse scanning plane image showing anteroposterior measurement of the isthmus. Note the placement of the calipers.

THYROID VOLUME

The normal mean thyroid volume is 18.6 ± 4.5 mL ($\pm$SD), which converts to an 18.6 g gland. Thyroid volumes increase with age and body weight, in patients living in regions with iodine deficiency, and in patients who have acute hepatitis or chronic renal failure. Patients who have chronic hepatitis or have been treated with thyroxine or radioactive iodine have a decreased thyroid volume.

Thyroid volume is calculated using linear parameters or, more precisely, with mathematical formulas. Among the linear parameters the anteroposterior diameter is the most accurate because it is relatively independent of dimensional asymmetry between the two lobes. When the anteroposterior diameter exceeds 2 cm the thyroid gland may be considered enlarged.

The mathematical method to calculate thyroid volume is based on the ellipsoid formula with a correction factor (length × width × thickness × 0.529 for each lobe). The mean volume per thyroid lobe is approximately 8.91 mL (range, 1.33 to 21.96 mL; SD, 5.1 mL).

GROSS ANATOMY

As mentioned, the thyroid gland is composed of right and left lobes connected by an isthmus. It is covered by two thin layers of connective tissue. The first layer is the pretracheal fascia, or false thyroid capsule, which surrounds the gland. The second layer is the true thyroid capsule, adherent to the gland surface. Thyroid parenchyma is composed of follicles (glandular epithelium and colloid), connective tissue, stroma, blood vessels, nerves, and lymphatics.

PHYSIOLOGY

The thyroid plays a major role in growth and development. It regulates basal metabolism and controls various functions of the body, including memory, weight loss or gain, heart rate, cholesterol levels, skin conditions and energy levels by the synthesis, storage, and secretion of thyroid hormones. It produces and secretes 3 hormones: triiodothyronine (T_3), thyroxine (T_4), and calcitonin. The secretion of these hormones is regulated by the hypothalamus and the pituitary gland. Thyroid secretion is primarily controlled by thyroid-stimulating hormone (TSH), which is secreted by the anterior pituitary gland. Thyroxine (T_4) is the primary hormone (90%) secreted by the thyroid. Triiodothyronine (T_3) represents a small portion (approximately 10%).

Calcitonin is secreted by the parafollicular cells (C cells) of the normal thyroid. Its primary function is to decrease blood calcium levels, preventing hypercalcemia. This hormone serves the opposite purpose of parathormone, discussed later in this chapter. Plasma calcitonin concentration level is elevated in a number of conditions; more important, it is elevated in the majority of patients with medullary thyroid carcinoma. The thyroid is composed of follicles filled with colloid, which is secreted by cuboidal epithelioid cells lining the periphery of the follicle. Colloid consists mainly of the glycoprotein thyroglobulin, which contains thyroid hormones within its molecule. When thyroid hormone is needed, TSH, or *thyrotropin*, secreted by the anterior pituitary gland, triggers the release of hormones into the bloodstream. The secretion of TSH is regulated by the thyrotropin-releasing factor, produced by the hypothalamus. The level of thyrotropin-releasing factor is controlled by the basal metabolic rate (BMR). A decrease in BMR results from a low concentration of thyroid hormones, causing an increase in thyrotropin-releasing factor. This causes an increase in TSH secretion and an increase in the release of these hormones. Once the blood level of hormones is returned to normal, the BMR stabilizes and TSH secretion ceases.

BLOOD SUPPLY

The thyroid is a highly vascular gland. Its blood supply consists of paired superior and inferior thyroid arteries and veins and, often, middle thyroid veins. Thyroid vessels are best seen at the upper and lower poles of the gland. The superior thyroid artery is the first branch of the external carotid artery. It runs superficially over the anterior border of the upper pole, sending a branch deep into the gland. It divides into an anterior branch curving toward the isthmus to anastomose with the contralateral artery and a posterior branch running down the back of the lobe to anastomose with an ascending branch of the inferior thyroid artery. The inferior thyroid artery supplies the lower half of the thyroid and is the largest branch of the thyrocervical trunk, which comes off the subclavian artery. It ascends to the inferior pole of the gland and divides into several branches, supplying the inferior portion of the thyroid and anastomosing posteriorly with the superior thyroid branches. Superior thyroid veins accompany the superior thyroid arteries (Figure 27-7, *A*). The mean diameter of major thyroid arteries is between 1 and 2 mm. Normal peak systolic velocities range between 20 and 40 cm/sec. Intraparenchymal arteries exhibit peak systolic velocities between 15 and 30 cm/sec (Figure 27-7, *B–D*). Superior thyroid veins arise above the anterolateral surface of the gland, cross the CCA, and empty into the IJVs above the thyroid cartilage. Inferior thyroid veins arise in the venous plexus of the thyroid gland, communicate with the superior and middle thyroid veins, and empty into the left and right innominate veins. The middle thyroid veins arise from the venous plexus on the lateral surface of the gland and empty into the lower end of the jugular vein. Similar to thyroid arteries, thyroid veins measure approximately 1 to 2 mm in diameter. Lower or inferior veins can measure up to 7 to 8 mm in diameter (Figure 27-7, *E*). Current high-sensitivity color Doppler imaging demonstrates the rich vascularity within the thyroid gland (Figure 27-7, *F*).

SONOGRAPHIC APPEARANCE

The normal thyroid gland is uniformly echogenic, with medium- to high-level echoes similar to those of the liver and testes. A thin, bright line (specular reflector) that bounds the thyroid lobes and isthmus is the thyroid capsule. Normal thyroid parenchyma is more echogenic than the surrounding contiguous muscular structures and vasculature (see Figure 27-10). Branches of the inferior and superior thyroid arteries and veins appear as anechoic structures with bright, thin walls (Figure 27-8).

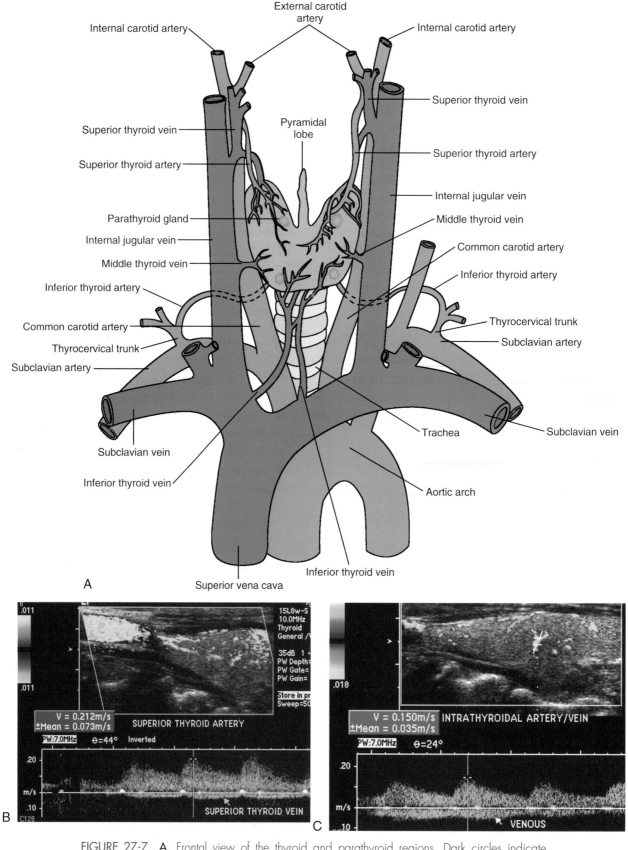

FIGURE 27-7 **A,** Frontal view of the thyroid and parathyroid regions. Dark circles indicate normal parathyroid location. **B,** Color duplex, longitudinal section of the thyroid gland and superior thyroid artery, demonstrating arterial flow with a peak systolic velocity of 0.212 m/s. Note superior thyroid vein flow below the baseline. **C,** Color duplex, longitudinal section of an intrathyroidal artery and vein. The peak systolic velocity of the intrathyroidal artery is 0.150 m/s.

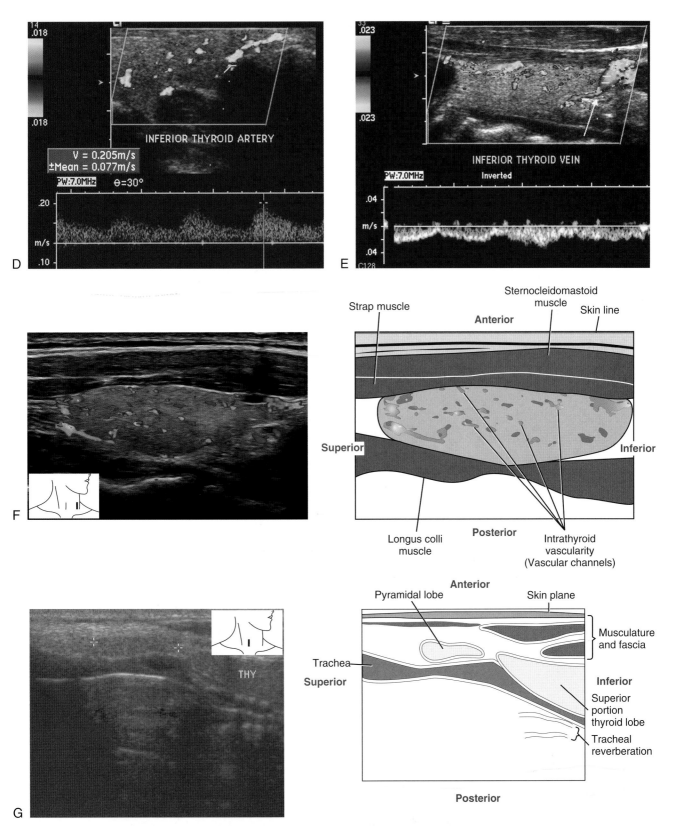

FIGURE 27-7, cont'd **D,** Color duplex, longitudinal section of the inferior thyroid artery, demonstrating arterial flow with a peak systolic velocity of 0.205 m/s. **E,** Color duplex, longitudinal section of the inferior thyroid vein, demonstrating normal phasic flow. **F,** Power Doppler, longitudinal section of the thyroid gland, demonstrating normal intrathyroid vascularity. **G,** Longitudinal section of the upper pole of the thyroid and pyramidal lobe (between calipers).

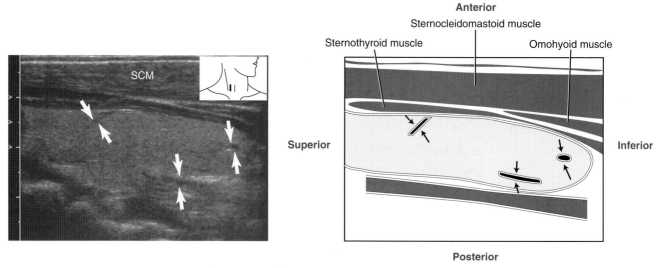

FIGURE 27-8 Longitudinal section of the right lobe of the thyroid gland; 1-mm to 2-mm tubular structures *(arrows)* represent intrathyroidal vessels.

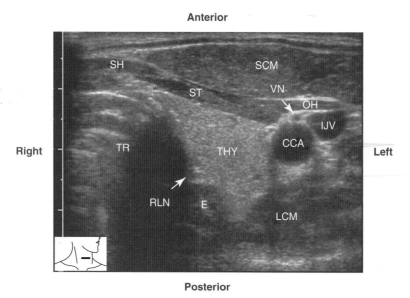

FIGURE 27-9 Transverse scanning plane image of the left lobe of the thyroid gland and adjacent anatomic structures: common carotid artery (CCA), esophagus (E), internal jugular vein (IJV), longus colli muscle (LCM), omohyoid muscle (OH), recurrent laryngeal nerve (RLN), sternocleidomastoid muscle (SCM), sternohyoid muscle (ST), sternothyroid muscle (SCM), thyroid (THY), trachea (TR), and vagus nerve (VN).

Color and power Doppler sonography are helpful in identifying intrathyroidal and extrathyroidal arteries and veins (see Figure 27-7, *B* to *D*).

On transverse plane images, axial sections of the CCA and IJV are seen as circular anechoic areas with bright walls, adjacent to the lateral border of the thyroid gland. The neck muscles (infrahyoid, sternocleidomastoid, and longus colli) are hypoechoic relative to the thyroid gland. The LCM appears triangular in shape. The esophagus, primarily a midline structure, is usually visualized to the left of midline. It is clearly identified by the target appearance of bowel in the transverse plane and by its peristaltic movements when the patient swallows. The vagus nerve lies in the posterior angle formed between the internal jugular vein and common carotid artery. On transverse images it is seen in axial sections as a small, very dark gray circular structure. The recurrent laryngeal nerve is a circular low-gray structure with an echogenic rim located between the esophagus, trachea, and posterior thyroid lobe (Figures 27-9 and 27-10).

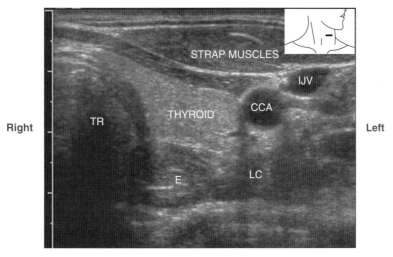

FIGURE 27-10 Transverse scanning plane image showing an axial section of the left lobe of the thyroid gland. Observe how thyroid parenchyma appears hyperechoic compared to surrounding structures. Note the anatomic relationship and shapes of the thyroid lobe, strap muscles, trachea (TR), esophagus (E), longus colli muscle (LCM), thyroid (T), common carotid artery (CCA), and internal jugular vein (IJV).

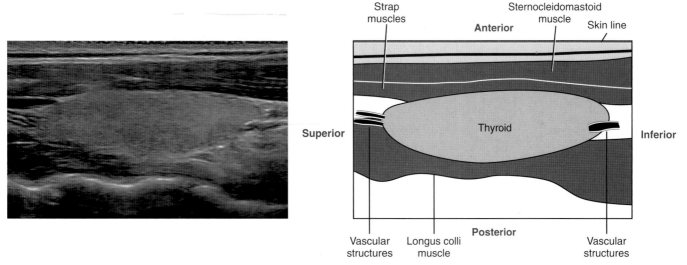

FIGURE 27-11 Longitudinal section of the strap muscles and longus colli muscle (LCM). Note their relationship to the thyroid gland.

The infrahyoid muscles (strap muscles) and sternocleidomastoid muscles are seen anterior to the thyroid, and the LCM is posterolateral (Figure 27-11).

SONOGRAPHIC APPLICATIONS

- Evaluation of the thyroid gland for suspicious nodules before surgery (Figure 27-12)
- Determining the nature of a neck mass(es) (origin, number, composition, size)
- Determining thyroid agenesis or dysgenesis in neonates
- Detecting recurrent carcinoma after thyroidectomy or regional nodal metastases in patients with proven or suspected thyroid carcinoma
- Evaluating abnormalities detected by other imaging modalities or laboratory studies (e.g., a thyroid nodule detected on computed tomography, positron emission tomography, nuclear scintigraphy, magnetic resonance imaging, or seen on another ultrasound exam of the neck [e.g., carotid ultrasound])
- Evaluation of patients at high risk for occult thyroid malignancy

TECHNIQUE: Standard longitudinal and transverse 2D grayscale and color duplex images were obtained of the neck with compartment mapping, as defined below.

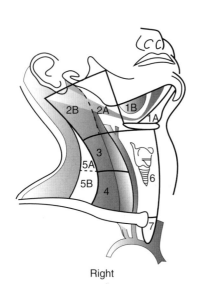
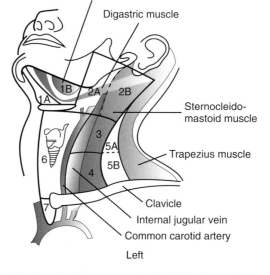

Right   Left

	NODAL GROUP	LANDMARKS
1A	SUBMENTAL	Midline, anterior to digastric muscle and superior to hyoid bone
1B	SUBMANDIBULAR	Lateral to zone 1A but medial or anterior to submandibular gland
2A	UPPER IJV CHAIN	Anterior or medial to IJV vein but lateral/posterior to submandibular gland; superior to hyoid bone
2B	UPPER IJV CHAIN	Posterior to the IJV and SCM and above the carotid bifurcation
3	MIDDLE IJV CHAIN	From level of carotid bifurcation to the inferior cricoid arch; lateral to the CCA
4	LOWER IJV CHAIN	From the level of the cricoid arch inferiorly to the clavicle: lateral to the CCA
5A	SUPRACLAV FOSSA/POST TRIANGLE	Posterior to SCM, from the base of the skull to the cricoid arch
5B	SUPRACLAV FOSSA/POST TRIANGLE	Posterior to the SCM from the cricoid arch to the clavicle
6	ANT CERVICAL PARATRACHEAL	Anterior-medial to the CCA from the level of the hyoid to the manubrium
7	ANT CERV UPPER MEDIASTINAL	Anterior-medial to the CCA; deep to the sternum
	SUPRACLAVICULAR	Lateral to the CCA; located above the clavicle

Schematic drawing of zone anatomic landmarks adapted from Scanning the post-thyroidectomy neck: Appearance and technique, JDMS 26:(5), 215-223, 2010.

FIGURE 27-12 Sample worksheet used by Summit Medical Center for identification of nodule location. Reprinted with permission, courtesy Alta Bates Summit Medical Center, Berkeley, California.

[Handwritten annotations:] Parathyroid anatomy:
1) Posterior to thyroid, anterior to LCM
2) appear in area of an anatomic "triangle" formed by thyroid gland, LCM, CCA, IJV.

- Monitoring the size of nodules under treatment (thyroid-suppression therapy)
- Evaluation for regional nodal metastasis in patients with proven or suspected thyroid carcinoma before thyroidectomy
- Evaluation of the location and characteristics of palpable neck masses, including an enlarged thyroid gland
- Ultrasound-guided thyroid cyst aspiration(s), fine needle aspiration/biopsy (FNAB), core-needle biopsy, and guidance for percutaneous treatment (ethanol injection) (PEI) of nonfunctional and hyperfunctioning benign thyroid nodules and of lymph node metastases from papillary carcinoma
- Follow-up of previously detected thyroid nodules, when indicated

NORMAL VARIANTS

Normal anatomic variations may mimic both intrathyroidal and extrathyroidal pathology.

- Small branches of superior and inferior thyroid arteries and veins may appear very low gray on gray-scale imaging and be potentially mistaken for small nodules. The use of color Doppler confirms vascular flow in these structures. Large inferior parathyroid adenomas may be mistaken for a thyroid nodule; clinical history and detection of polar or feeding artery helps distinguish the two (see Figures 27-16, 27-19).
- The cervical esophagus is normally situated posterior to the left lobe of the thyroid, and may simulate a thyroid nodule on transverse scanning plane views (Figure 27-13); observing peristalsis in both longitudinal and axial sections enables distinction of the esophagus from a true nodule.
- Another anatomic pitfall is an esophageal diverticulum, which is rare and can mimic a thyroid mass. An esophageal diverticulum is a pouch that protrudes outward in a weak portion of the esophageal lining. Esophageal diverticula are classified by their location within the esophagus. Two specific types are *Killian-Jamieson* and *Zenker's*:
  - **Killian-Jamieson diverticulum** is a rare esophageal diverticulum that protrudes in the anterolateral wall of the cervical esophagus inferior to cricopharyngeus and lateral to the longitudinal tendon of the esophagus.
  - **Zenker's diverticulum** is located posterior and midline, in the back of the throat just above the esophagus. Symptoms include dysphasia (difficulty swallowing, characterized by a feeling of food caught in the throat).

Like thyroid nodules, esophageal diverticula are oval to round. Trapped food, debris, and air may manifest as echogenic foci mimicking microcalcifications of papillary carcinoma (see Figure 27-13, *A*). To avoid this pitfall, the extrathyroidal location of the diverticulum should be confirmed with visualization of a connection to the esophagus (see Figure 27-13, *B*). Real-time imaging will demonstrate peristalsis, or movement of air and debris when the patient swallows. To accentuate the peristalsis connection between the esophagus and the diverticulum, have the patient hold a small amount of water in his or her mouth and then ask him or her to swallow using cine-clips to capture the peristalsis.

- An accessory lobe called the **pyramidal lobe** is present in approximately 10% to 40% of the population. It extends cephalad from the isthmus and ascends as far as the hyoid bone. A pyramidal lobe may extend from the right or left side of the isthmus; however, it arises more frequently on the left (see Figure 27-7, *A* and *G*).
- Other normal variations include:
  - Absence of the isthmus
  - Asymmetry (right lobe may be twice the size of the left lobe)
  - Absence of lateral lobes

Parathyroid Glands

Parathormone

Parathyroid glands are small, encapsulated, oval structures attached to the posterior surfaces of the lateral lobes of the thyroid gland (see Table 27-1). Most people have four symmetric parathyroid glands (see Figures 27-1 and 27-7, *A*). Parathyroid glands secrete **parathyroid hormone (PTH)** to maintain homeostasis of serum calcium and phosphorous levels.

LOCATION

Parathyroid glands are typically located posterior to the thyroid gland and anterior to the LCM. Superior parathyroid glands develop from the fourth branchial pouch and can be found posterior to the thyroid at the cricothyroid junction (in 77%) or behind the upper pole of the thyroid (in 22%). Inferior parathyroid glands derive from the third branchial pouch and descend further with the primordial thyroid during development. Because of their greater caudal migration, inferior parathyroid glands are more variable in location. The majority of inferior parathyroid glands (>60%) are found at or just inferior to the posterior aspect of the lower pole of the thyroid. Inferior parathyroid glands may also be imbedded within the thyroid tissue.

The majority of parathyroid masses appear in the area of an anatomic "triangle" formed by the thyroid gland, LCM, CCA, and IJV (see Figures 27-1 and 27-9). The minor neurovascular bundle (MINVB) is the only anatomic structure that lies in this region; it measures 5 mm in diameter.

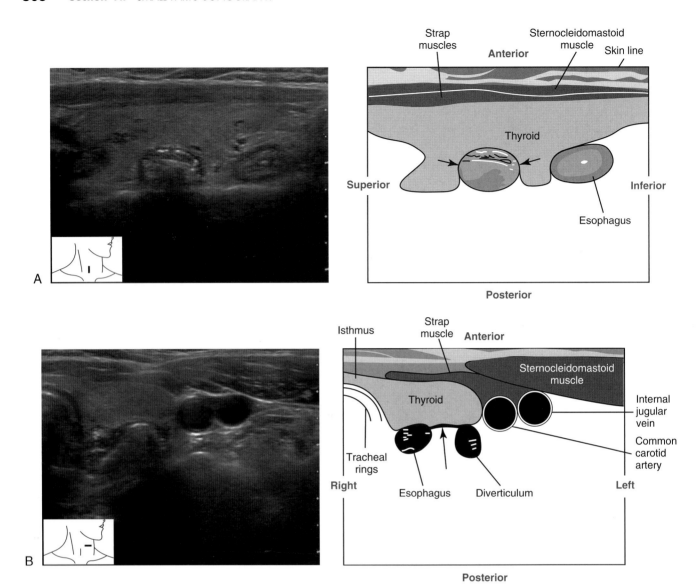

FIGURE 27-13 **A,** Sagittal scanning plane, longitudinal image section of left thyroid lobe showing a "mass" pitfall (between arrows) of "Killian-Jamieson" diverticulum. **B,** Transverse scanning plane, axial image section of left thyroid lobe demonstrating connection (arrow) between esophageal Killian-Jamieson" diverticulum when the patient swallows water.

SIZE

Normal parathyroid glands measure approximately 5 to 7 mm in length, 3 to 4 mm in width, and 1 to 2 mm in thickness ($5 \times 3 \times 1$ mm). They weigh between 10 and 78 mg, with a mean average of 35 to 40 mg.

GROSS ANATOMY

Parathyroid glands are composed of masses of chief cells, with some wasserhelle (water-clear) and oxyphil cells arranged in a columnar fashion. The color of parathyroid glands varies from light yellow in older patients to a reddish or light brown in young patients, depending on the amount of fat within the gland.

The shape of parathyroid glands varies. They are most often oval, bean shaped, or spherical (83%); however, they are sometimes elongated (11%), bilobulated (5%), or multilobulated (1%) (Figure 27-14).

The nerve supply is abundant; it arises from the thyroid branches of the cervical sympathetic ganglia.

PHYSIOLOGY

absorption of Ca+ to blood.

Parathyroid glands secrete parathyroid hormone (PTH), also called parathormone. As mentioned, their primary function is to help maintain homeostasis of blood calcium concentration by promoting calcium absorption into the blood, preventing hypocalcemia. When

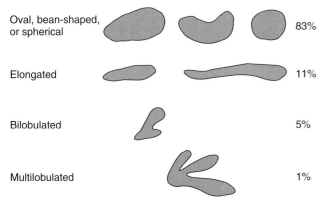

Oval, bean-shaped, or spherical — 83%

Elongated — 11%

Bilobulated — 5%

Multilobulated — 1%

FIGURE 27-14 Parathyroid gland variations.

serum calcium levels are low, the parathyroid hormone raises serum calcium by releasing calcium from the bone, increasing calcium absorption in the gut, and decreasing renal calcium by decreasing renal phosphate excretion.

BLOOD SUPPLY

The superior and inferior parathyroid glands are supplied by separate small branches of the superior and inferior thyroid arteries and by branches from the longitudinal anastomoses between these vessels (see Figure 27-7, *A*). Venous drainage is into the thyroid plexus of the veins. The lymphatic channels drain with those of the thyroid gland.

SONOGRAPHIC APPEARANCE

Normal parathyroid glands are small and similar in echogenicity to the thyroid and surrounding tissues,

making them difficult to visualize. They are not generally identified with ultrasound unless they are abnormal. The typical sonographic appearance of a parathyroid adenoma is uniformly hypoechoic relative to the normal thyroid gland. The characteristic hypoechoic appearance is caused by the uniform hypercellularity of the gland with little fat content. The rare functioning parathyroid lipoadenomas are more echogenic than the adjacent thyroid gland because of their high fat content. Parathyroid adenomas are oval or bean-shaped homogeneous structures, without through transmission, that measure between 0.8 to 1.5 cm long and weigh 500 to 1000 mg (Figure 27-15). Giant adenomas can measure greater than 5 cm in length and weigh more than 10 g. With parathyroid enlargement, changes appreciated sonographically include lobulation, acoustic inhomogeneity (heterogeneous echo texture), cystic degeneration, and occasional calcifications (Figures 27-16 to 27-18).

Parathyroid adenomas are highly vascular lesions supplied by enlarged feeding arteries that arise from the branches of the inferior and superior thyroid arteries. Enlarged parathyroid glands demonstrate intraparenchyma hypervascularization with prominent diastolic flow (Figures 27-19 and 27-20).

Color and power Doppler have a reported sensitivity of 88% in locating parathyroid adenomas. The presence of an enlarged extrathyroidal feeding artery leading to an abnormal parathyroid gland aids in the detection of an otherwise inconspicuous parathyroid adenoma (Figure 27-21).

It is of paramount importance to have a thorough understanding of the normal sonographic appearance of relevant adjacent anatomic structures in the

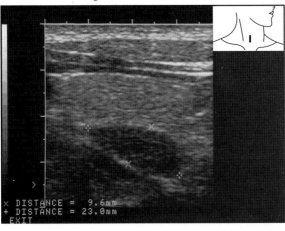

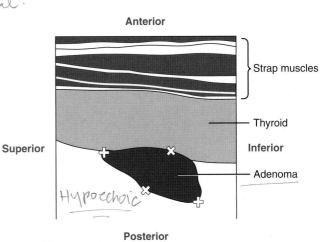

FIGURE 27-15 Longitudinal section of the right thyroid lobe, demonstrating a typical oval-shaped parathyroid adenoma. Notice how the adenoma is hypoechoic relative to the thyroid, oval, and located posterior to the lobe. Calipers measuring the length and anteroposterior (AP) diameter. Note the placement of the calipers (+, x).

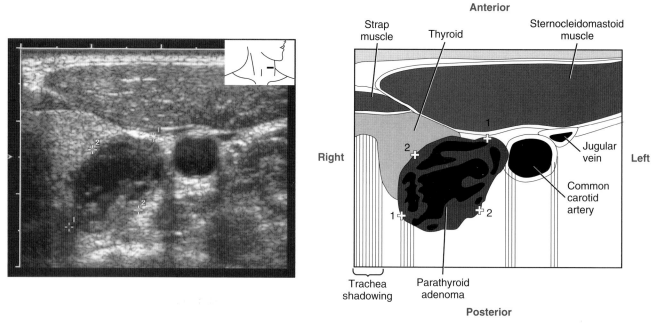

FIGURE 27-16   Transverse scanning plane image through the mid-left lobe of the thyroid, demonstrating a heterogeneous parathyroid adenoma. Calipers measuring the width and anteroposterior diameter. Note the placement of the calipers (Dist 1 and Dist 2).

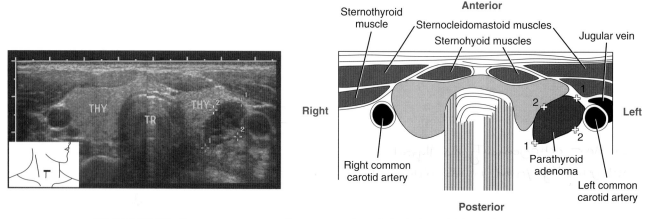

FIGURE 27-17   Transverse scanning plane image through both thyroid lobes, showing a left parathyroid adenoma. Calipers measuring the width and anteroposterior diameter. Note the placement of the calipers (Dist 1 and Dist 2). Note the heterogeneity of the thyroid gland.

neck, to avoid pitfalls when imaging the parathyroid glands. Normal cervical structures and coexisting thyroid nodules can mimic parathyroid adenomas, producing false-positive results.

In the sagittal imaging plane the LCM runs the length of the thyroid gland and is hypoechoic compared with the normal thyroid (see Figure 27-12). In the transverse imaging plane the LCM appears triangular in shape and can be mistaken for a parathyroid adenoma, particularly when the gland is elongated (see Figure 27-10). An anechoic parathyroid adenoma located medial to a collapsed jugular vein could be mistaken for the normal IJV. The esophagus has also been mistaken for a large parathyroid adenoma (see Figure 27-10).

Other cervical structures that may simulate parathyroid adenomas include small extrathyroidal veins and arteries (that lie adjacent to the posterior and lateral aspects of the thyroid), enlarged cervical lymph nodes, and any coexisting thyroid nodules. Color Doppler imaging can be helpful to differentiate vascular from nonvascular structures in the neck (Figure 27-22, A and B on p. 513). Enlarged cervical lymph nodes appear

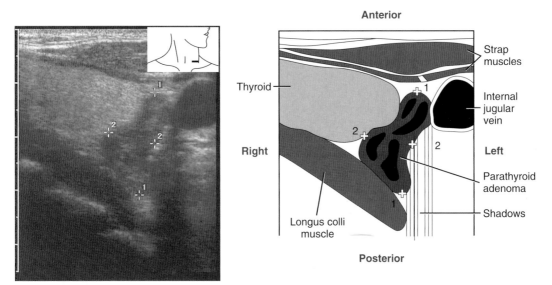

FIGURE 27-18 Transverse scanning plane showing an axial section of the left lower lobe of the thyroid gland and a lobulated parathyroid adenoma. Note how the adenoma lies postero-lateral to the thyroid and anterior to the longus colli muscle. Note the placement of the calipers (*Dist 1* and *Dist 2*). Note that the longest axis of the adenoma is seen anteroposteriorly.

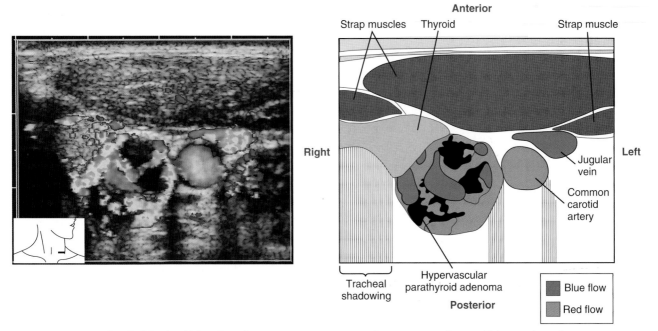

FIGURE 27-19 Color Doppler, transverse scanning plane image of a mid-left parathyroid adenoma. Note the hypervascularization of the adenoma. Color void areas represent cystic areas. Note the relationship of the adenoma to the thyroid gland, common carotid artery, and jugular vein.

oval and exhibit low-intensity echoes. They often have an echogenic band or hilum composed of fat, vessels, and fibrous tissue. These nodes usually lie laterally in the neck adjacent to the jugular vein, away from the thyroid gland (Figures 27-23 and 27-24). Occasionally, parathyroid adenomas can be found laterally in the carotid sheath, and percutaneous biopsy may be necessary to distinguish a parathyroid adenoma from an abnormal lymph node.

When a thyroid nodule protrudes from the posterior aspect of the thyroid, it can mimic a parathyroid adenoma. An imaging sign that is helpful in this situation is a thin echogenic line that separates the parathyroid adenoma from the gland itself. Thyroid nodules, which arise from within the gland, do not demonstrate this tissue plane of separation. Also, the sonographic appearance of many thyroid nodules is heterogeneous or mixed, compared with parathyroid adenomas, which tend to be homogeneous and hypoechoic relative to the normal thyroid gland.

SONOGRAPHIC APPLICATIONS

- Localization of parathyroid adenomas in patients with suspected primary or secondary hyperparathyroidism (abnormality due to increased calcium levels found in the blood)
- Localization of autologous parathyroid gland implants
- Assessment of the number and size of enlarged parathyroid glands in patients who have undergone previous parathyroid surgery or ablative therapy with recurrent symptoms of hyperparathyroidism
- Localization of thyroid/parathyroid abnormalities or adjacent cervical lymph nodes for (FNA) biopsy, and ablation

NORMAL VARIANTS

- Most people (approximately 80%) have 4 parathyroid glands located in a symmetric position

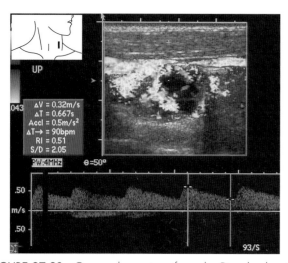

FIGURE 27-20 Gray-scale version of a color Doppler, longitudinal section of a left parathyroid adenoma, demonstrating hypervascular arterial flow.

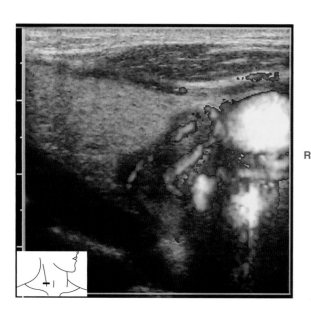

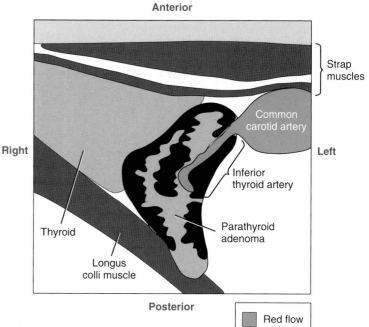

FIGURE 27-21 Power Doppler image of a parathyroid adenoma. Note the feeder inferior thyroid artery supplying the adenoma.

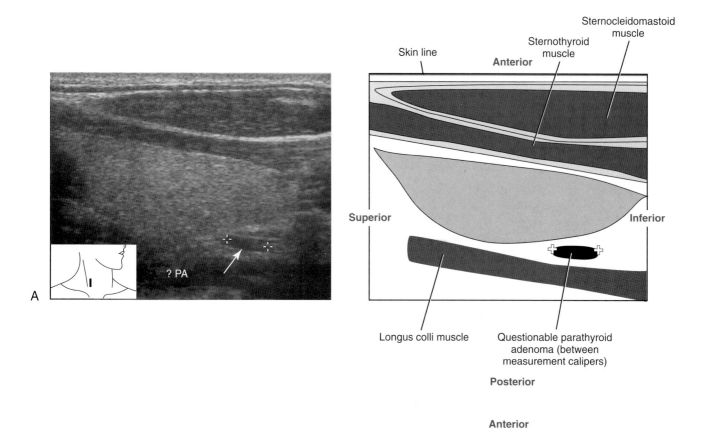

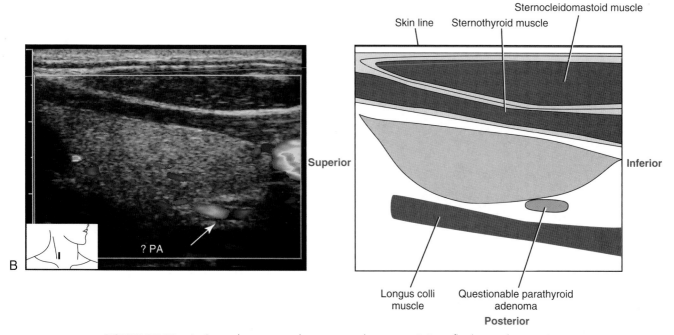

FIGURE 27-22   **A,** Sagittal scanning plane image showing a 0.6-cm flat hypoechoic structure simulating a small parathyroid adenoma, posterior to the lower pole of the right thyroid lobe. Note the placement of the calipers. **B,** Color Doppler image of **A.** Notice how the very low-gray structure fills with color, indicating a vascular structure and not a parathyroid adenoma.

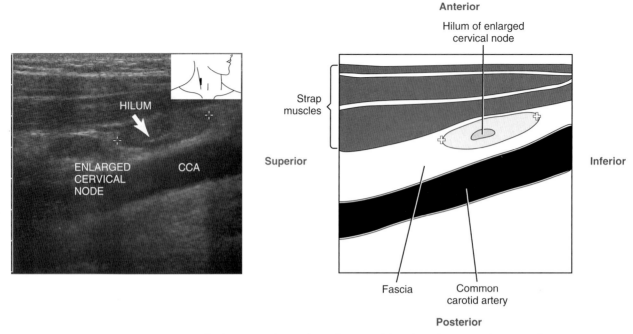

FIGURE 27-23 Longitudinal section of an enlarged, cervical lymph node seen adjacent to the common carotid artery. Notice how the node appears very low gray with an echogenic hilum (*arrow*). Note the placement of the calipers.

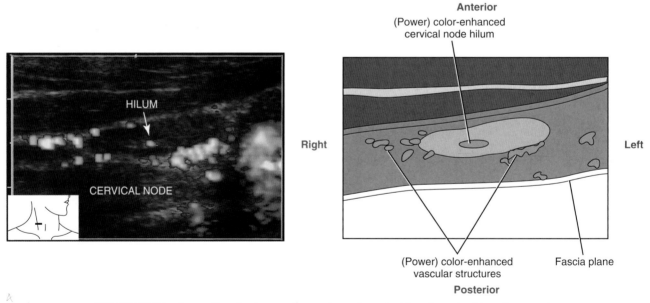

FIGURE 27-24 Power Doppler image of an enlarged cervical lymph node. Note the vascular flow within the hilum.

contiguous with the thyroid gland (see Figures 27-1, 27-2, and 27-7, *A*).

- As many as 13% to 15% of individuals have more than five parathyroid glands, and 5% will have only three glands.

- **Ectopic parathyroid glands** are frequently found within the thymus or perithymic tissues (10%). Other aberrant locations include intrathyroidal (1%), the carotid bifurcation and sheath (1%), and in the retroesophageal space (1% to 3%) (Figure 27-25).

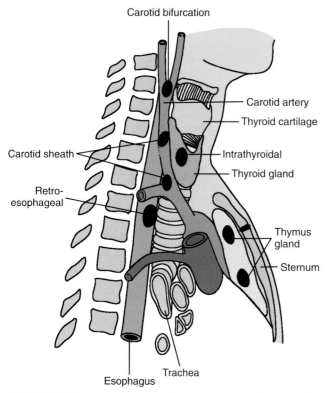

Carotid bifurcation

Carotid artery

Thyroid cartilage

Carotid sheath

Intrathyroidal

Thyroid gland

Retro-esophageal

Thymus gland

Sternum

Esophagus

Trachea

FIGURE 27-25 Lateral section of mediastinum and neck, illustrating aberrant locations of parathyroid glands. Black circles indicate aberrant locations: thymus gland, carotid bifurcation, retroesophageal, intrathyroidal, carotid sheath.

REFERENCE CHARTS

■ ■ ■ ASSOCIATED PHYSICIANS

- **Surgeon:** Specializes in surgery, a branch of medicine that treats diseases, deformities, and injuries by operative methods.
- **Endocrinologist:** Specializes in medical diseases of the endocrine system. Principal endocrine glands include the thyroid, parathyroid, adrenal, pituitary, testes, and ovaries.
- **Radiologist:** Specializes in the diagnostic interpretation of imaging modalities that assess thyroid and parathyroid abnormalities.
- **Interventional radiologist:** Specializes in invasive radiographic and sonography procedures for diagnosis and treatment.
- **Pathologist:** Specializes in the interpretation of tissue biopsies and blood tests.

■ ■ ■ COMMON DIAGNOSTIC TESTS AND PROCEDURES

Evaluation of the thyroid and parathyroid glands requires both physiologic and morphologic information to diagnose thyroid and parathyroid disease. Various diagnostic tests

available to achieve diagnostic efficacy include scintigraphy (radionuclide scanning), single photon emission computed tomography (SPECT), positron emission tomography (PET), high-resolution sonography, computed tomography (CT), magnetic resonance imaging (MRI), and fine-needle aspiration biopsy (FNAB). Two newer imaging advances for evaluating the thyroid gland are contrast-enhanced ultrasound and elastography.

- **Scintigraphy:** Scintigraphy is the diagnostic modality of choice for patients with palpable thyroid masses. It is the most common screening technique used in conjunction with ultrasound for the evaluation of thyroid function and morphology. A radioactive tracer or agent (^{123}I, ^{131}I, or ^{99m}Tc pertechnetate) is administered that targets the thyroid gland. It is monitored and photographed to assess thyroid function and differentiate between normal and abnormal thyroid tissue. This test is performed by a nuclear medicine technologist. Interpretation of the test is by the radiologist. The spatial resolution of this technique makes it difficult to delineate and characterize small nodules. Multiple nodules may be present within the gland when scintigraphy indicates only a solitary nodule. A major role of scintigraphy is to determine whether a lesion is "hot" (hyperfunctioning or more uptake than the normal thyroid gland) or "cold" (nonfunctioning or less uptake than the normal thyroid gland). On ^{123}I scintigraphy, hot nodules have a 1% to 4% risk for malignancies, whereas cold nodules have a 10% to 25% risk for malignancies. On ^{99m}Tc scintigraphy, 29% of hot nodules have malignancies. ^{131}I scintigraphy is often used to detect metastasis in patients with a thyroid cancer.
- **Single photon emission computed tomography (SPECT):** Single photon emission computed tomography is a nuclear medicine tomographic imaging technique using gamma rays. It is similar to conventional nuclear medicine planar imaging using a gamma camera. However, it is able to provide true 3-dimensional (3-D) information. This information is typically presented as cross-sectional slices through the patient, but can be reformatted as required. Because SPECT is very similar to planar gamma imaging, the same radiopharmaceuticals may be used. To acquire SPECT images, the gamma camera is rotated around the patient. Projections are acquired at defined points during the rotation, typically every 3 to 6 degrees. A full 360-degree rotation is used to obtain an optimal reconstruction. The time taken to obtain each projection is also variable; 15 to 20 seconds is typical. This gives a total scan time of 15 to 20 minutes. SPECT imaging with technetium ^{99m}Tc sestamibi (MIBI SPECT) has a reported sensitivity of 95% and specificity of 100% in the evaluation of parathyroid glands and correctly identified malignant thyroid nodules in 4 of 5 patients with concomitant multinodular goiter. This test is performed by a nuclear medicine technologist. Interpretation of the test is by the radiologist.
- **Positron emission tomography (PET):** PET is a nuclear medicine functional imaging technique that produces a 3-D image or map of functional processes in the

body. The system detects pairs of gamma rays emitted indirectly by a positron-emitting radionuclide (tracer), which is introduced into the body on a metabolically active molecule. 3-D images of tracer concentration within the body are then reconstructed by computer analysis. In modern PET-CT scanners, 3-D imaging is often accomplished with the aid of a CT x-ray scan performed on the patient during the same session, in the same machine. To conduct the scan, a short-lived radioactive tracer isotope, which decays by emitting a positron that also has been chemically incorporated into a metabolically active molecule, is injected into the patient. There is a waiting period while the metabolically active molecule becomes concentrated in the tissues of interest; then the patient is placed in the imaging scanner. The molecule most commonly used for this purpose is fluorodeoxyglucose (FDG), a sugar, for which the waiting period is typically an hour. The concentrations of tracer imaged will indicate tissue metabolic activity by virtue of the glucose uptake. PET imaging produces images that detail biochemistry changes in the body and, consequently, is useful in thyroid cancer diagnosing and staging. This test is performed by a nuclear medicine technologist. Interpretation of the test is by the radiologist.

- **Sonography:** Sonography uses high-frequency (8 to 16 MHz) sound waves to image and characterize thyroid parenchyma, abnormal parathyroid glands, and adjacent anatomic structures. Resolution is between 0.7 to 1.0 mm. Linear transducers with either rectangular or trapezoidal scan format are preferred to sector transducers because of the wider field of view and the capability to combine high-frequency gray-scale and color Doppler images. In patients with large necks and/ or an enlarged thyroid gland, a 5- to 8-MHz convex transducer provides a quick and accurate assessment of thyroid size and volume. Thyroid lobes, isthmus, and adjacent muscles and vasculature are assessed for normal and abnormal echogenicity and structure. The examination includes the central neck from the lower border of the mandible to the sternal notch and bilateral cervical nodal chains, including nodal levels I to VII, to detect adenopathy, tumor invasion, and thrombosis (refer to nodal zone worksheet, Figure 27-12). Ultrasound is the most definitive imaging technique used for determining whether a lesion is cystic or solid and whether it is intrathyroidal or extrathyroidal. It is excellent for localizing thyroid nodules and parathyroid adenomas for aspiration, ethanol ablation, and/or percutaneous biopsy. The accuracy of ultrasound in detecting parathyroid disease is approximately 74% to 94%. Acoustic penetration is limited when evaluating the retrotrachea and substernal regions because acoustic walls or air-containing structures such as the trachea and lung preclude through sound transmission. In the above setting, the combined use of scintigraphy, MRI, and CT increases the diagnostic efficacy. This test is performed by a sonographer. Interpretation of the test is by the radiologist.

- **Computed axial tomography (CT) scan:** CT imaging consists of contiguous axial 2- to 3-mm sections throughout the thyroid gland and adjacent anatomy. Images are acquired from the hyoid bone down to the carina. A contrast material is usually administered to differentiate between pathology and normal anatomy. CT is less specific than sonography for establishing the cystic nature of nodules. However, it overcomes sound penetration limitations and provides anatomic definition in the substernal and retrotracheal regions. CT, like magnetic resonance imaging (MRI), is useful in assessing the overall extent of a mass. Less desirable features of CT imaging include streak artifacts from the shoulder girdle, use of intravenous iodinated contrast material, and exposure to ionizing radiation. This test is performed by a CT technologist. The test is interpreted by the radiologist.

- **Magnetic resonance imaging:** MRI involves magnetism, radio waves, and a computer to produce images of body structures. A surface coil is centered over the thyroid gland, providing high-quality, 3-mm thick images. Axial and sagittal views are acquired from the hyoid bone to the lung apices. MRI provides multiplane imaging and a contrast scale between normal and pathologic thyroid anatomy and adjacent anatomic structures. For some procedures, contrast agents such as gadolinium are used to increase the accuracy of the images. This technique permits excellent delineation of anatomic structures in the neck and thorax. For example, blood vessels are easily identified from adjacent lymph nodes. MRI is an excellent imaging modality for monitoring disease processes pretherapy and posttherapy. This test is performed by an MRI technologist. Interpretation of the test is by the radiologist. CT and MRI are particularly useful when thyroid tissue extends into the mediastinum and cervical region.

- **Fine-needle aspiration/biopsy (FNAB):** Fine-needle aspiration biopsy may provide the definitive diagnosis of thyroid nodules, cervical lymph nodes, and parathyroid adenomas. With sonographic guidance, lesions a few millimeters in size can be biopsied. For FNAB most physicians use a 25-gauge needle, 1½ inches long, with a disposable 10 mL plastic syringe and pistol-grip syringe holder. Once the needle tip is in the nodule, gentle suction is applied while the needle is moved back and forth within the nodule vertically. This maneuver allows the dislodging of cellular material and easy suction into the needle. As the name indicates, the biopsy technique uses aspiration to obtain cells or fluid from a thyroid mass. Such biopsies are easy to perform and well tolerated by the patient. With an experienced pathologist and physician who have mastered the biopsy technique, a diagnostic sensitivity of 99% can be achieved. Complications are unusual, a small hematoma being the most common. This procedure is performed by an interventional radiologist, an endocrinologist, or a surgeon. Interpretation of the test is by a pathologist.

- **Ultrasound-guided percutaneous ethanol injection:** Percutaneous ethanol injection (PEI) is a nonsurgical procedure involving the injection of absolute ethanol into thyroid cysts, benign thyroid and autonomously functioning nodules, enlarged parathyroid glands for chemical ablation, and cervical nodal metastases from papillary carcinoma. Results from PEI include cellular dehydration and protein denaturation, followed by coagulative necrosis, reactive fibrosis, vascular thrombosis, and hemorrhagic infarction. For treatment of thyroid nodules and cysts, ethanol is injected through a 21- or 22-gauge spinal needle with a closed conical tip and three terminal side holes allowing for large amounts of ethanol, thereby reducing the total number of sessions. Several treatment sessions are needed (usually four to eight), generally performed at 2-day to 2-week intervals. The total amount of ethanol delivered is usually 1.5 times the nodular volume. PEI is generally well tolerated. A common side effect is a burning sensation for a short period of time at the injection site, radiating to the mandibular or retroauricular regions. The efficacy of response is inversely proportional to the thyroid volume—the smaller the nodule, the more complete the response. Complete cure is reported to be achieved in 68% to 100% of pretoxic nodules and in 50% to 89% of toxic nodules. Delivery of ethanol to cervical nodal metastases is via a 25-gauge needle with a tuberculin syringe containing up to 1 mL of 95% ethanol. Color Doppler imaging is paramount to assess decreased or absent blood flow after ethanol injection. For parathyroid adenoma ablation, ethanol is injected into multiple sites of the mass, with a volume of about half that of the mass, typically 0.1 to 1.0 mL. The tissue becomes echogenic at the moment of injection; the echogenicity slowly disappears over 1 minute. There is also a marked decrease in vascularity of the parathyroid adenoma, secondary to thrombosis and occlusion of the parathyroid vessels. The injections are repeated every day or every other day until the serum calcium reaches the normal range. Ethanol ablation is most often used in postoperative patients with recurrent or persistent hyperparathyroidism who have sonographically visible, biopsy-proven hyperfunctioning parathyroid tissue and who are poor surgical candidates. Ethanol ablation has been shown to be very useful in patients with MEN I who have had previous subtotal parathyroidectomy with recurrent disease in their remaining residual half-gland in the neck. This procedure is performed by an interventional radiologist, an endocrinologist, or a surgeon. The color Doppler portion of the test is performed by a sonographer. Interpretation of the test is by the interventional radiologist.

- **Contrast-enhanced ultrasound:** Contrast enhanced ultrasound (CEUS) imaging is a major breakthrough for ultrasound. By using a microbubble contrast agent and contrast-specific imaging software it is able to visualize the micro- and macrocirculation of the targeted organ. Ultrasound contrast agents are gas-filled microbubbles that are administered intravenously into the systemic circulation. Microbubbles have a high degree of echogenicity, which is the ability of an object to reflect the ultrasound waves. The echogenicity difference between the gas in the microbubbles and the soft tissue surroundings of the body is immense.

   Sonographic imaging using microbubble contrast agents enhances the ultrasound backscatter, or reflection of the ultrasound waves, to produce a unique image with increased contrast due to the high echogenicity difference. Recent articles have shown that CEUS is a highly sensitive and cost-effective method for localization of pathologic parathyroid glands in patients with primary hyperparathyroidism. Other articles mentioned that CEUS was helpful for detecting malignant thyroid nodules. The test is performed by the sonographer. Interpretation of the test is by the radiologist.

- **Elastography:** Ultrasound elastography is a dynamic technique used to estimate and display elastic properties (tissue stiffness) by measuring the degree of tissue distortion under external pressure by the ultrasound probe. Thyroid gland elastography is used to study hardness/elasticity of a thyroid nodule to differentiate malignant from benign. Benign nodules are softer and deform more easily, whereas malignant nodules are harder and deform less when compressed by ultrasound. The elastography technique determines the amount of tissue displacement at various depths, by assessing the ultrasound signals reflected from the tissues before and after compression. Dedicated software provides an accurate measurement of tissue distortion and displays it visually as an elastographic image. The elastogram displayed over the B-mode is color coded. Blue represents the softest tissue, and red represents the hardest tissue. Real-time shear elastography is the latest technique that characterizes and quantifies tissue stiffness better than conventional elastography. Cystic lesions and calcified nodules are excluded from ultrasound elastographic evaluation. Ultrasound elastography helps in characterizing a cystologically indeterminate nodule as malignant or benign with a high accuracy that is almost comparable to FNAB. The major limitation of ultrasound elastography is that it cannot assess lesions which are not surrounded by adequate normal tissue. The test is preformed by a sonographer. Interpretation of the test is by the radiologist.

■ ■ ■ LABORATORY TESTS

THYROID

Thyroid hormone production is modulated by a feedback-control mechanism effected through the hypothalamus and the pituitary gland. Thyrotropin (TSH), secreted by the anterior pituitary, controls thyroid hormone production. Several laboratory tests are performed to evaluate thyroid function. No one clinical test can be used alone to diagnose hypothyroidism or hyperthyroidism. Common tests include T_4, T_3, TSH (thyroid-stimulating hormone), T_3 resin uptake, and RAI (radioactive iodine uptake). The following laboratory tests are performed by a licensed laboratory technologist. Tests are interpreted by the pathologist.

- **Thyroxine:** T_4, with four iodine atoms, is the most abundant thyroid hormone produced. T_4 is commonly used for screening and follow-up of patients whose diagnosis is either hypothyroidism or hyperthyroidism. The test measures both free thyroxine and the portion carried by the thyroid-binding plasma protein. T_3 (triiodothyronine) contains three iodine atoms and represents a small portion of thyroid hormone, but it is more potent than T_4. Both T_3 and T_4 can also be measured indirectly by radioimmunoassay. This is a very sensitive method of determining the concentration of hormones in blood plasma. A venous blood sample is drawn and "tagged" with specific radioactive substances that specifically bind with either T_3 or T_4. The amount of radioactivity measured indirectly indicates the concentration of thyroid hormone indirectly. Increased levels of T_3 and T_4 are associated with hyperthyroidism, whereas decreased levels indicate hypothyroidism.
- **T_3 resin uptake:** Indirectly measures the amount of T_4 by measuring the amount of T_3 that can be attached to the proteins that bind the thyroid hormones. The resin uptake test measures the amount of T_3 remaining and free to bind to the resin added to the blood sample. A measured amount of radioactive-tagged T_3 and resin is added to a sample of the patient's blood. The resin is placed in a test tube to absorb any of the radioactive-tagged T_3 that cannot be taken up by the thyroid-binding globulin in the blood sample. Increased T_3 into the resin indicates hyperthyroidism; decreased T_3 into the resin indicates hypothyroidism.
- **Thyroid-stimulating hormone:** TSH, or thyrotropin, which is produced by the pituitary gland, controls the serum levels of the thyroid hormones. Measurement of TSH is useful in determining whether hypothyroidism is due to primary hypofunction of the thyroid gland (intrinsic thyroid disease) or to secondary hypofunction of the anterior pituitary gland, caused by insufficient stimulation by the pituitary. TSH also measures a patient's response to thyroid medication, particularly a patient with primary hypothyroidism or pituitary hypothyroidism.
- **Radioactive iodine test:** RAI uptake test evaluates thyroid function by measuring the amount of orally ingested ^{123}I or ^{131}I that accumulates in the thyroid gland after 6 and 24 hours. The largest portion of iodine is transported via the circulatory system to the thyroid gland. An external counting probe (gamma detector) measures the radioactivity in the thyroid as a percentage of the original dose, indicating the ability of the gland to trap and retain iodine. The normal range is about 10% to 15% at 6 hours and 15% to 30% at 24 hours. This test is performed by a nuclear medicine technologist. Interpretation of the test is done by the radiologist.

PARATHYROID

- The most common clinical situation for parathyroid imaging is **hypercalcemia** (serum calcium levels greater than 10.5 mg/dL).

- **Primary hyperparathyroidism** is caused by a solitary parathyroid adenoma in 80% to 90% of cases, by multiple glands in 10% to 20%, and by parathyroid cancer in less than 1%. **Secondary hyperparathyroidism** refers to the excessive secretion of parathyroid hormone (PTH) by the parathyroid glands in response to **hypocalcemia** (low blood calcium levels) with associated hypertrophy of the parathyroid glands. This disorder is especially seen in patients with chronic renal failure. Secondary hyperparathyroidism can also result from malabsorption (chronic pancreatitis, small bowel disease, malabsorption–dependent bariatric surgery) in that the fat-soluble vitamin D cannot get reabsorbed. This leads to hypocalcemia and a subsequent increase in PTH in an attempt to increase serum calcium levels. In secondary hyperparathyroidism all four glands are usually abnormal.

■■■ **LABORATORY VALUES**

- Resin T_3 uptake (RT_3U) (specimen S): 25% to 35%
- Thyroid-stimulating hormone (specimen S): 5 to 10 units/mL
- Thyroxine (T_4) (specimen S): 4.5 to 13 mcg/dL
- Triiodothyronine: 75 to 195 mcg/dL (pregnancy and oral contraceptives tend to increase values)
- Calcium: 8.5 to 10.5 mg/dL, the normal range may vary slightly between laboratories
- Parathyroid hormone (PTH): 10 to 55 pg/mL, the normal range may vary slightly between laboratories

■■■ **VASCULATURE**

- **Superior supply:** External carotid artery → superior thyroid artery → superior thyroid veins → internal jugular veins.
- **Inferior supply:** Thyrocervical artery → inferior thyroid artery → inferior thyroid veins → middle thyroid veins → right and left innominate veins.

■■■ **AFFECTING CHEMICALS**

- **Thyroid-stimulating hormone (TSH):** Stimulates the thyroid to make and release thyroid hormones.
- **Serum parathyroid hormone (PTH):** Homeostatic metabolic function supporting serum calcium and phosphorous levels, includes activating osteoclasts, which influences the release of calcium by the bones, augmenting the absorption of calcium in the gut, increasing renal tubular reabsorption of calcium that conserves free calcium, increasing conversion of vitamin D to its active dihydroxy form in the kidneys, and increasing urinary phosphate excretion that lowers the serum phosphate level.

CHAPTER 28

Breast Sonography

LISA STROHL

OBJECTIVES

Describe the function of the breast.
Define the location of anatomy related to the breast.
Describe the size relationships of normal breast anatomy.
Describe the sonographic appearance of normal breast anatomy.

Discuss advanced breast imaging technique(s).
Describe the associated physicians, diagnostic tests, and laboratory values related to breast sonography.

KEY WORDS

3-D/4-D — Sonography that provides multiplanar imaging.

Acini — Small, grape-shaped secretory portions of a gland (singular, *acinus*).

Alveoli — Glandular tissue elements within mammary lobules.

Anterior Pituitary Gland — Located in the brain and influenced by the hypothalamus. Secretes prolactin, which stimulates development of the secretory system of the breast after childbirth to prepare for lactation.

Breast — Mammary gland that produces milk after pregnancy for suckling.

Breast Parenchyma — Mammary layer that contains glandular tissues and ducts.

Connective Tissues — Supportive structures located in the mammary layer.

Cooper's Ligaments — Suspensory ligaments that run between each 2 lobules from the deep muscle fascia to the skin surface.

Elastography — Also known as *strain imaging* or *elasticity*, elastography helps determine the stiffness of a mass relative to its surrounding tissue. Another type of elastography referred to as *shear wave elastography* uses a focused ultrasound beam to create an acoustic radiation force impulse. This type of elastography allows for a quantitative measurement of tissue stiffness.

Estrogen — Hormone that stimulates breast tissue development during puberty, childbearing years, and pregnancy.

Exocrine — Glands with ducts; mammary glands secrete milk through lactiferous ducts after pregnancy.

Fatty Breast — Normal variant characterized by increased fatty components throughout the breast. Deposition of fat increases with age and parity.

Fibrocystic Breast — Normal variant common in women of childbearing age.

Hypothalamus — Region in the brain that controls hormones and the anterior pituitary gland. Produces prolactin-inhibiting factor, which prevents release of prolactin until milk production becomes necessary following childbirth.

Lactation — Secretion of milk from mammary glands (breasts).

Lactiferous Ducts — Ducts in the parenchyma of the breast that secrete milk after pregnancy.

Mammary Layer — Second of the 3 breast layers; contains glandular tissues, ducts, and connective tissues.

Mammography — Radiographic examination of the breast.

Montgomery's Glands — Ampulla or expanded region for each lactiferous duct near the nipple, where milk can be stored until released by suckling.

Oxytocin — Hormone produced by the posterior pituitary gland, which stimulates contraction of the lactiferous ducts for milk secretion. Secretion is stimulated by infant suckling during breastfeeding.

Parenchymal Elements — Lobes, lobules, ducts, and acini components of the breast.

Pectoralis Major Muscle — Large chest muscle located in the retromammary layer.

Progesterone — Elevated levels of this hormone during pregnancy stimulate development of breast lobules and alveoli to prepare the breast for lactation.

Prolactin — Hormone released from anterior pituitary gland that stimulates development of the secretory system of the breast after childbirth to prepare for lactation.

Prolactin-Inhibiting Factor — Inhibiting factor released by hypothalamus that prevents release of prolactin until after milk production becomes necessary following childbirth.

Retromammary Layer — Most posterior of the 3 breast layers; contains retromammary fat, muscle, and deep connective tissues.

Stromal Elements — Connective tissue and fat components of the breast.

Subcutaneous Layer — Most anterior of the 3 breast layers; contains skin and subcutaneous fat.

■■■ NORMAL MEASUREMENTS

Structure	Measurement
Lactiferous ducts	Nonpregnant women: 2 mm
	Nursing women: 8 mm

The mammary glands are modified sweat glands. They are **exocrine** organs whose main function is the secretion of milk via the **lactiferous ducts** after childbirth. This function is called **lactation** (Figure 28-1).

LOCATION

The **breast** is anterior to the pectoralis major, serratus, and external oblique muscles and the sixth rib (Figure 28-2 and Table 28-1). It is bounded medially by the sternum and bordered laterally by the margin of the axilla. The superior border consists of the second and third ribs. The inferior border is the seventh costal cartilage. The breast is bordered laterally by the axilla. The purpose of the breast is to provide nourishment to the suckling infant.

SIZE *Estrogen : Breast Grow*

The size of the normal breast varies depending on the age, functional state, and amount and arrangement of stromal and parenchymal elements of the individual.

There is an increase in development of breast tissue owing to stimulation by **estrogen** during puberty and, later, during childbearing years and pregnancy. With the decrease in hormonal stimulation after menopause, the normal breast will atrophy to some degree.

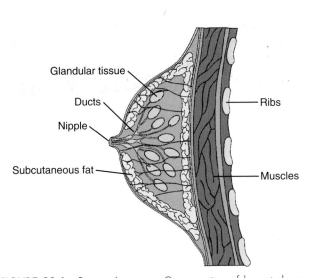

FIGURE 28-1 **Breast Anatomy.** Cross-section of breast demonstrating basic anatomy.

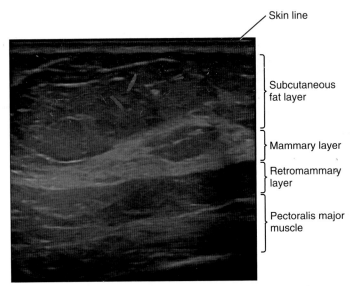

FIGURE 28-2 **Breast Anatomy.** Image of breast anatomy also showing the pectoralis muscle (posteriorly).

■■■ Table 28-1 Location of Breast Structures Routinely Visualized With Ultrasound

	Breast	Subcutaneous Layer	Mammary Layer	Retromammary Layer	Pectoralis Major Muscle
Anterior to	Pectoralis major muscle, serratus muscle, external oblique muscle, sixth rib	Mammary layer, retromammary layer, pectoralis major muscle	Retromammary layer, pectoralis major muscle	Pectoralis major muscle	
Posterior to	Skin	Skin	Subcutaneous layer, skin	Mammary layer, subcutaneous layer, skin	Retromammary layer, mammary layer, subcutaneous layer, skin
Superior to	Seventh rib				
Inferior to	First or second rib				Clavicle
Medial to	Axilla				
Lt lateral to	Sternum				Sternum
Rt lateral to	Sternum				Sternum

Prolactin Ant Pit → produce milk.
oxytocin Post Pit → eject milk by contraction of
after child birth myoepithelial of mamary glands.
Hypothalamus → Prolactin-inhibiting.

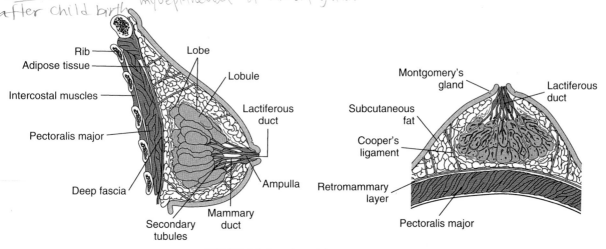

FIGURE 28-3 Normal breast anatomy.

GROSS ANATOMY

connective tissue

Functional part

Supportive/Structural

Anatomically, the breast is composed of parenchymal and stromal elements. The **parenchymal elements** include the lobes, lobules, ducts, and **acini**, which are small, grape-like secretory structures. The normal breast is composed of 15 to 20 mammary lobes separated by adipose tissue. Each lobe has an external drainage pathway into the nipple. The lobes are further divided into lobules, each of which contains glandular tissue elements (**alveoli**). Each lobule consists of up to 100 acini clustered around a collecting duct. Many lobules make up a mammary lobe, from which secondary tubules form mammary ducts, which lead to lactiferous ducts that exit at the nipple (Figure 28-3).

The **stromal elements** include fat and all of the **connective tissue**, which helps provide support and structure. Support of breast tissue is provided by the suspensory ligaments of Cooper (**Cooper's ligaments**), which run between each two lobules from the deep muscle fascia to the skin surface (see Figure 28-3).

The breast has 3 layers. The **subcutaneous layer** contains the skin and all of the subcutaneous fat; the **mammary layer** contains the glandular tissues, ducts, and connective tissues; and the **retromammary layer** contains the retromammary fat, muscle, and deep connective tissues.

PHYSIOLOGY

Breast development is stimulated by estrogen, as stated earlier. This stimulation causes the development of stromal and parenchymal elements throughout the breast. The glandular tissues of the breast become active as a result of hormonal stimulation during pregnancy. Increased levels of **progesterone** stimulate the development of the breast lobules and alveoli.

Both the production of milk and its absence are controlled by hormones produced within the **hypothalamus**

and **anterior pituitary gland**, located deep within the brain. The hypothalamus produces many hormones and influences the anterior pituitary gland. The hypothalamus produces **prolactin-inhibiting factor**, which prevents the release of prolactin until milk production becomes necessary after childbirth. At that time the anterior pituitary gland will secrete **prolactin**, which stimulates development of the secretory system of the breast.

Prevents lactating during Pregnancy

After the placenta has been expelled and estrogen levels have decreased, the prolactin levels will begin to increase to a level that allows the production of milk. The infant's suckling stimulates the secretion of **oxytocin** from the posterior pituitary gland. This causes contraction of the lactiferous ducts, and lactation begins.

The function of the alveoli is to secrete milk into the secondary tubules. All secondary tubules from each lobule converge to form a lactiferous duct. Each lactiferous duct has an ampulla or expanded region called **Montgomery's glands** near the nipple, where milk can be stored until released during suckling. Secretions from the areolar glands keep the nipple area pliant.

SONOGRAPHIC APPEARANCE

SOFT/lubricated.

The sonographic appearance of the breast depends on several factors, primarily the age of the woman and the functional state of the breast.

The 3 breast layers are very distinct and easy to differentiate. The most anterior layer, the *subcutaneous layer*, contains the skin, the most anterior connective tissue components, and fat lobules. The skin line and connective tissue appear bright and reflective. As a general rule, fat usually appears bright and reflective; however, fat lobules in the breast are the exception because they appear hypoechoic relative to the skin and connective tissue components. The middle layer is the *mammary layer*, which contains glandular tissue or **breast**

ligaments : Echogenic.
Skin : Echogenic.
in Breast ONLY ← Fat : Hypoechoic.

parenchyma. Fat can be seen between the parenchymal elements, which vary in appearance according to maternal age and breast function. The most posterior layer is the *retromammary layer*, which can be similar in size and appearance to the subcutaneous layer. It contains fat lobules and the deeper connective tissue components. The retromammary layer is bordered posteriorly by the **pectoralis major muscle**, which appears distinctly hypoechoic in comparison with adjacent structures (Figure 28-4).

Although all three layers of breast tissue are affected by natural processes, the mammary layer demonstrates the greatest changes sonographically. The younger breast has a higher percentage of parenchyma compared with the percentage of fat within the breast. This higher percentage causes the younger breast to be denser. Dense parenchyma is difficult to visualize with mammography, a radiological examination of the breast; therefore younger patients presenting with possible masses are often first evaluated by sonography.

With age, the breast parenchyma becomes replaced by fatty tissues. This causes the anterior subcutaneous layer to become more prominent as the mammary layer atrophies and occupies a smaller percentage of overall breast size.

The fat components appear hypoechoic to surrounding parenchymal breast tissue (Figure 28-5, *A*). Breast ducts and ductules appear as anechoic tubular structures (Figure 28-5, *B*). The fibrous components, such as Cooper's ligaments, demonstrate increased echogenicity and are seen as bright, linear echoes (Figure 28-5, *C*). The glandular or parenchymal tissues tend to appear homogeneous in texture, with medium-level to low-level echogenicity (Figure 28-5, *D*). When scanning directly anterior to the nipple, posterior shadowing is visualized (Figure 28-5, *E*).

The overall sonographic appearance should be consistent throughout each breast and between the two breasts. When the sonographic appearance is heterogeneous throughout the breast, it allows for differentiation of pathology.

FIGURE 28-4 Anatomic Layers of the Breast.

Handwritten annotations on Figure 28-4:
Appearance:
Fat: hypoechoic
ligaments: hyperechoic
Ducts: Anechoic.
Glandular: Homogeneous mid to low-level.
Parenchyma:
Skin: Hyper
connective tissue: Hyper.

Figure labels: Skin line, Subcutaneous layer, Mammary layer, Retromammary layer, Pectoralis major muscle

Margin annotation: more hypoechoic

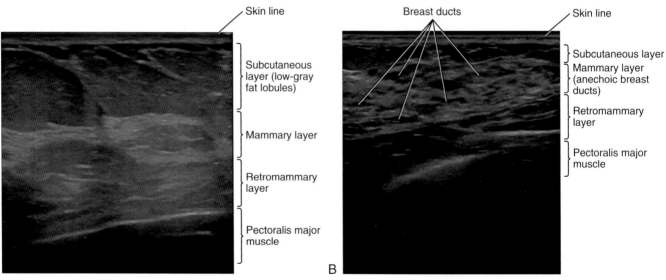

FIGURE 28-5 **Sonographic Appearance of the Breast. A,** Fatty component of the breast. **B,** Ducts of the breast.

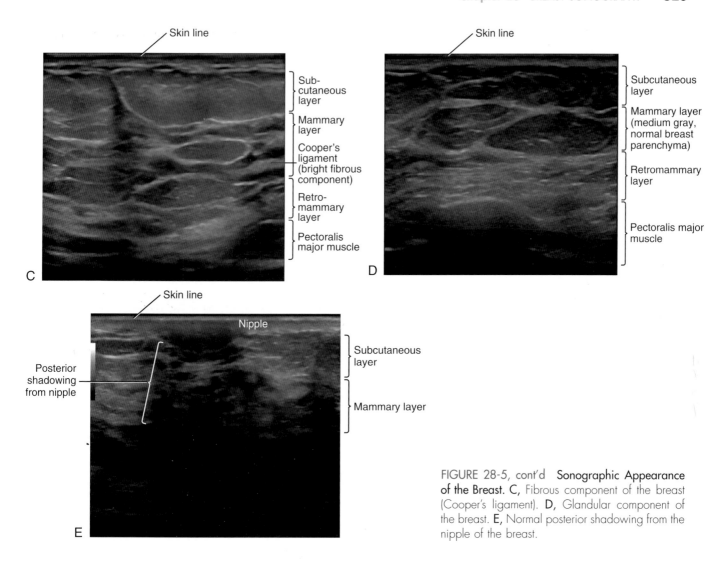

FIGURE 28-5, cont'd **Sonographic Appearance of the Breast. C,** Fibrous component of the breast (Cooper's ligament). **D,** Glandular component of the breast. **E,** Normal posterior shadowing from the nipple of the breast.

SONOGRAPHIC APPLICATIONS

- Determining breast mass composition (Figure 28-6, A to F): Note that the presence of large collections of calcifications in the breast may be detected sonographically. However, each collection or individual calcification must be at least a few millimeters in diameter. It is important to remember that ultrasound is not capable of detecting the very small (approximately 1 mm) calcifications that are visible with mammography and often represent the first signs of breast cancer.
- Ruling out the presence of lymph node masses that often accompany breast cancer.
- Ruling out palpable masses.
- Ruling out cysts.
- Correlating mammography findings.
- Evaluating breast implants (Figure 28-7).

- In many cases, ultrasound-guided procedures such as breast cyst aspirations and breast biopsies are used as alternatives to surgery (Figure 28-8).

NORMAL VARIANTS

- **Fibrocystic breast:** A variant common in women of childbearing age. Various fibrotic components and cystic areas may be distributed throughout the entire breast.
- **Fatty breast:** Characterized by increased fatty components throughout the breast, with decreased echogenicity. Deposition of fat increases with age and parity. Breasts often appear more fatty after menopause because the fat components become more prominent as the mammary ducts begin to atrophy. Fatty breasts may demonstrate areas of bright echogenicity due to the connective tissues surrounding the mammary ducts.

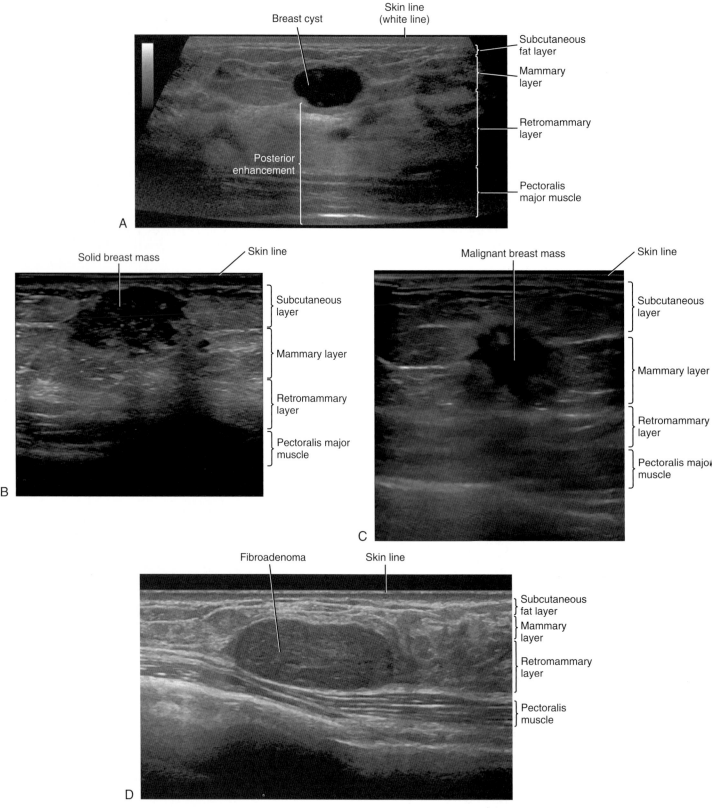

FIGURE 28-6 **Breast Masses and Dilated Subareolar Ducts. A,** Breast cyst. **B,** Solid breast mass. **C,** Malignant mass. **D,** Fibroadenoma (fibrous and glandular benign tumor). (**A** and **D** courtesy GE Imaging, Waukesha, Wisconsin.)

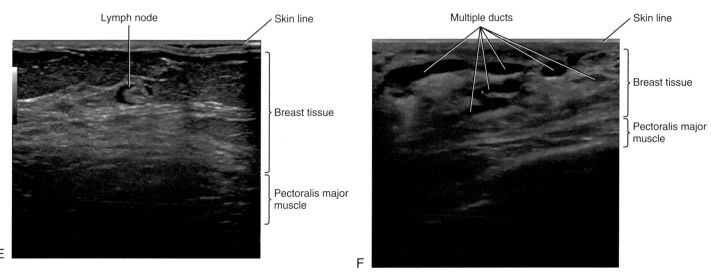

FIGURE 28-6, cont'd **Breast Masses and Dilated Subareolar Ducts. E,** Lymph node. **F,** Dilated subaerolar ducts.

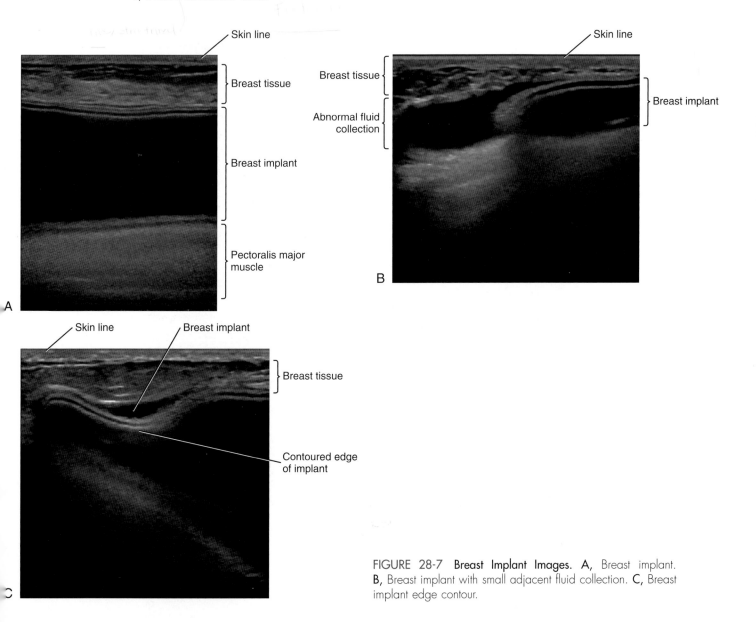

FIGURE 28-7 **Breast Implant Images. A,** Breast implant. **B,** Breast implant with small adjacent fluid collection. **C,** Breast implant edge contour.

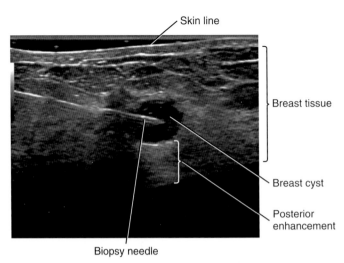

FIGURE 28-8 Ultrasound-Guided Fine-Needle Cyst Aspiration.

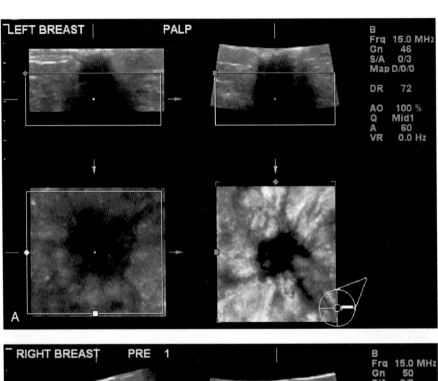

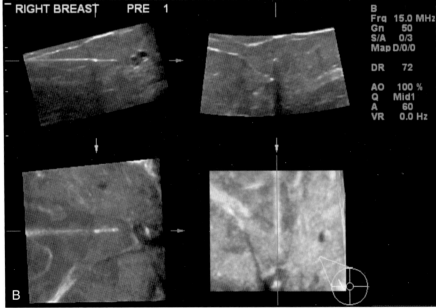

FIGURE 28-9 3-D/4-D Breast Images. **A,** 3-D/4-D breast lesion. **B,** 3-D/4-D breast biopsy.

ADVANCED TECHNIQUES IN BREAST IMAGING

- **Elastography**: The fibrous breast has increased amounts of connective tissue and therefore increased echogenicity. Compression sonography is most helpful in assessing the fibrous breast because it eliminates some of the posterior shadowing resulting from the increase in dense connective tissues. Using palpation and compression, this technique has evolved into elasticity imaging, also known as strain imaging or elastography, and helps determine the relative stiffness of a mass relative to the surrounding tissue. Another type of elastography referred to as *shear elastography* uses a focused ultrasound beam to create an acoustic radiation force impulse. This type of elastography allows for a quantitative measurement of tissue stiffness in kilopascals or meters per second based on the propagation speed of the shear wave through the breast tissue.

- **3-D/4-D**: Sonography provides multiplanar imaging. 3-D provides images in three planes, the third plane being the C-plane (coronal), and 4-D provides real-time 3-D imaging. The C-plane provides additional diagnostic information not traditionally imaged in traditional 2-D imaging (Figure 28-9, *A* and *B*).

BREAST SELF-EXAMINATION

The American Medical Association strongly urges women to perform breast self-examinations every month. This is the first step to breast care, followed by yearly clinical examinations performed by a gynecologist, and yearly mammogram screenings for women over age 40 (Figure 28-10).

HOW TO EXAMINE YOUR BREASTS

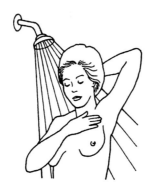

1 In the shower:

Examine your breasts during bath or shower; hands glide easier over wet skin. Fingers flat, move gently over every part of each breast. Use right hand to examine left breast, left hand for right breast. Check for any lump, hard knot or thickening.

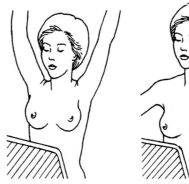
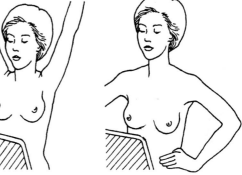

2 Before a mirror:

Inspect your breasts with arms at your sides. Next, raise your arms high overhead. Look for any changes in contour of each breast, a swelling, dimpling of skin or changes in the nipple.

Then, rest palms on hips and press down firmly to flex your chest muscles. Left and right breast will not exactly match – few women's breasts do.

Regular inspection shows what is normal for you and will give you confidence in your examination.

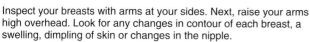
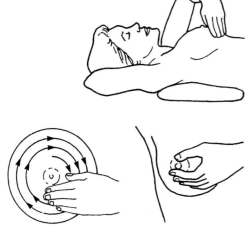

3 Lying down:

To examine your right breast, put a pillow or folded towel under your right shoulder. Place right hand behind your head – this distributes breast tissue more evenly on the chest. With left hand, fingers flat, press gently in small circular motions around an imaginary clock face. Begin at outermost top of your right breast for 12 o'clock, then move to 1 o'clock, and so on around the circle back to 12. A ridge of firm tissue in the lower curve of each breast is normal. Then move in an inch, toward the nipple, keep circling to examine every part of your breast, including nipple. This requires at least three more circles. Now slowly repeat procedure on your left breast with a pillow under your left shoulder and left hand behind head. Notice how your breast structure feels.

Finally, squeeze the nipple of each breast gently between thumb and index finger. Any discharge, clear or bloody, should be reported to your doctor immediately.

FIGURE 28-10 **Breast Self-Examination.** The correct procedure for self-examination of the breast. (Courtesy the American Cancer Society.)

REFERENCE CHARTS

■ ■ ■ ASSOCIATED PHYSICIANS

- **Gynecologist/Obstetrician:** Specializes in the examination and treatment of women, including during pregnancies. The physician often performs yearly breast examinations as part of a physical examination. Diagnostic tests based on the breast examination may be ordered. Often a referral to a surgeon will be made if follow-up is necessary.
- **Internist:** Specializes in general health care. The physician may be involved in diagnostic testing or in referrals for further follow-up. The physician may be involved in surgical follow-up, if necessary.
- **Surgeon:** Specializes in decision making and in surgical procedures, as well as follow-up made necessary by pathologic findings. This physician is generally responsible for performing surgical procedures such as biopsies, mastectomies, and lumpectomies.
- **Radiologist:** Specializes in interpreting the diagnostic tests used to image the breast. The radiologist may perform procedures such as fine-needle biopsies if questionable areas are seen on mammography.
- **Pathologist:** Determines the presence of pathology through typing tissue obtained at biopsy or other surgical procedures, by means of microscopic cellular analysis.

■ ■ ■ COMMON DIAGNOSTIC TESTS

- **Self-examination:** Should be performed regularly by all women more than 30 years of age or by any woman whose family physician has determined that she is at risk for developing breast cancer. Changes of any sort should be reported and assessed by a physician as soon as possible (see Figure 28-10).
- **Mammography:** A compression x-ray test used to visualize breast tissue. It easily demonstrates the small clusters of calcification that often indicate early breast cancer. It is recommended that women receive a baseline study at between 35 and 40 years of age, and then according to their physician's guidelines. The test is performed by a radiologic technologist and interpreted by a radiologist.
- **Sonography:** A nonionizing imaging modality that uses sound waves to obtain diagnostic information; often done in conjunction with mammography. It is performed by a sonographer and interpreted by a radiologist.
- **Thermography:** Assesses breast tissue by indicating skin temperature; rarely used in the United States. Based on the theory that the presence of cancerous tumors will cause the overlying skin to have a different temperature than normal areas. This test would be performed by a technologist and interpreted by a physician, most likely a radiologist.

■ ■ ■ LABORATORY VALUES

- **Carcinoembryonic antigen (CEA):** This antigen level is used after a diagnosis of breast cancer. It is secreted by the liver and may be elevated in cancer removal to rule out tumor recurrence. A decrease in the antigen level represents tumor removal. Antigen levels are then monitored to detect an increase in baseline levels, which would indicate tumor recurrence.
- **Alkaline phosphatase:** This enzyme may help rule out tumor metastasis in patients with identified breast cancer. It is secreted by the liver and may be elevated in liver diseases, as well as in bone, lung, and pancreatic carcinomas. Alkaline phosphatase is normally elevated during pregnancy and during the first year of life.

■ ■ ■ VASCULATURE

- **Arterial blood:** Supplied through the internal thoracic or the internal mammary artery. The internal mammary artery originates off the subclavian artery and enters the breast through the second, third, and fourth intercostal spaces medially and through the lateral thoracic artery. That artery becomes the superficial mammary artery and supplies the more superficial breast structures.
- **Venous drainage:** Occurs through a combination of superficial and deep venous systems. The veins course parallel to the arteries.
- **Lymph drainage:** The breast's lymphatic system originates in lymph capillaries within breast connective tissues. Lymph drainage from the breast originates in the connective tissues of the breast and follows 3 main pathways: 75% of lymph drainage occurs through the axillary lymph nodes, which are in close proximity to the axillary tail of the breast, which extends superolaterally to border the axilla; 20% of lymph drainage occurs medially through the thoracic nodes; and 5% occurs subcutaneously through the intercostal nodes.

■ ■ ■ AFFECTING CHEMICALS

- **Prolactin:** A hormone secreted by the anterior pituitary gland that stimulates development of the breast's secretory system. Prolactin secretion is controlled by prolactin-inhibiting hormone, which is produced by the hypothalamus. After the decrease in estrogen that follows childbirth, prolactin levels increase and lactation becomes possible.
- **Estrogen:** A hormone produced in the ovaries that stimulates the development of breast tissues and duct systems during puberty.
- **Oxytocin:** A hormone produced in the hypothalamus and stored in the posterior pituitary gland; causes duct contraction and allows for the flow of milk during nursing.
- **Progesterone:** A hormone produced by the placenta that stimulates development of the breast lobules and alveoli during pregnancy.

- **Insulin:** A hormone produced by the pancreas that is necessary for breast development during pregnancy.
- **Cortisol:** A hormone produced by the adrenal cortex that is necessary for breast development during pregnancy.
- **Thyroxine:** A hormone produced by the thyroid gland that is necessary for breast development during pregnancy.
- **Caffeine:** Reduced caffeine intake may lessen breast lumps, swelling, and soreness, especially in women with fibrocystic breast changes. Such a reduction will not affect risk factors for breast cancer.
- **Vitamin E:** Affects the levels of fat and hormones in the blood and may help relieve pain and swelling of breast tissues.
- **Danazol:** A male hormone that may help to decrease pain and swelling of the breast. It suppresses activity of the anterior pituitary gland and is used to treat women with endometriosis. This hormone may be associated with side effects.

CHAPTER 29

Scrotal and Penile Sonography

TIMOTHY L. OWENS, MICHAEL J. KAMMERMEIER, AND ZULFIKARALI H. LALANI

OBJECTIVES

Describe the location of the scrotum, testicles, epididymis, ductus (vas) deferens, and penis.

Identify the gross anatomy of the scrotum, testicles, ducts, and penis.

Describe the normal size of the testicles.

Describe the sonographic appearance of the testicles, epididymis, and penis.

Identify the associated physicians, related diagnostic tests, and laboratory values.

KEY WORDS

Buck's Fascia — Thick, fibrous loosely applied covering of skin that envelops the penis.

Convoluted Seminiferous Tubules — Tubules that produce and transport sperm.

Corpora Cavernosa — Two of three cylindrical masses of erectile tissue that constitute the penis.

Corpus Spongiosum — One of three cylindrical masses of erectile tissue that comprise the penis. Surrounds the male urethra.

Cremaster Muscle — Surrounds each testicle and extends into the abdomen over the spermatic cord. Contraction of the cremaster muscle performs the important function of regulating the temperature of the testicles.

Ductus (Vas) Deferens — Thicker, less convoluted continuation of the ductus epididymis. Each joins with its corresponding seminal vesicle to form an ejaculatory duct.

Ductus Epididymis — See Epididymis.

Ejaculatory Ducts — Two ducts that course through the prostate gland and empty into the prostatic urethra.

Epididymis — Single, tightly wrapped tube that is also called the *ductus epididymis*. Empties into the ductus deferens.

Median Raphe — Median ridge that externally divides the scrotum into lateral portions.

Mediastinum Testis — Partial division or septum of each testis formed by a continuation of the tunica albuginea.

Pampiniform Plexus — Network of veins that drain the testes and become the spermatic veins.

Penis — Male organ of copulation and urination.

Rete Testis — Network of seminiferous tubules formed in the mediastinum testis.

Scrotum — Pouch of skin that is continuous with the abdomen. It is suspended from the base of the male pelvis, between the perineum and the penis. Contains the testicles, epididymis, and proximal portion of the ductus (vas) deferens.

Semen — Fluid composed of sperm and secretions of glands associated with the male urogenital tract.

Spermatic Cord — Two cords that contain the ductus deferens, testicular arteries, venous pampiniform plexus, lymphatics, autonomic nerves, and fibers of the cremaster muscle.

Spermatogenesis — Process of sperm production.

Testicles/Testes — Paired organs (male gonads) of reproduction. They are classified as both endocrine and exocrine glands that produce testosterone and sperm.

Testosterone — Hormone produced by the testes at the onset of puberty; causes growth in the male sex organs and development of secondary male sex characteristics such as body hair and voice deepening (endocrine function).

Tunica Albuginea — Dense, white fibrous tissue that covers each testis and forms the mediastinum testis and interlobar septa.

Tunica Dartos — Internal septum that divides the scrotum into two sacs.

Tunicae Vaginalis — Covering layers of the testicles. Consists of two layers derived from the perineum: an outer parietal layer that is closely attached to the internal spermatic fascia and an inner visceral layer that is closely attached to the testicle.

Urethra — Membranous canal that transports urine from the bladder to the exterior of the body. In the male, it also serves to discharge semen.

■ ■ ■ NORMAL MEASUREMENTS	
Structure	**Measurement**
Normal adult testicle	3 to 5 cm in length; 2 to 3 cm in width; 2 to 3 cm anteroposterior
Epididymis	3.8 cm in length; uncoiled, 6 m
Ductus (vas) deferens	45 cm in length

This chapter includes the scrotum, testicles, penis, and related structures (Figure 29-1). Other structures within the male pelvis, the prostate gland and seminal vesicles, are described in Chapter 20. The ureters, urinary bladder, and related muscles and vasculature are described in Chapter 17.

LOCATION

The scrotum is suspended from the base of the male pelvis between the perineum and the penis. The scrotum contains the testicles, epididymis, and proximal portion of the ductus (vas) deferens (Table 29-1).

The epididymis is connected to the superior portion of the testis and runs along the posterior aspect to the base of the testis. The epididymis drains into the ductus (vas) deferens at the base of the testis. The ductus deferens courses superiorly and exits the scrotum through the inguinal canal. Once inside the abdominal cavity, each ductus deferens courses along the lateral aspect of the urinary bladder and turns medially and posteriorly to connect with the seminal vesicles.

SIZE
Testis

The normal adult testicle measures approximately 3 to 5 cm (1.5 to 2 inches) in length, 2 to 3 cm (1 inch) in anteroposterior dimension, and 2 to 3 cm (1 inch) in width. When a male is between the ages of 12 and 17 years, the testicle undergoes rapid growth. Before age 12, the average testicular volume is less than 5 mL. After the male reaches maturity, the average testicular volume is approximately 25 mL, with the testicle weighing between 10 g and 15 g. The testicle gradually decreases in size with advancing age.

Epididymis

The epididymis is actually a single, tightly wrapped tube called the ductus epididymis. When unwrapped, the ductus epididymis measures approximately 6 m (20 feet) in length and about 1 mm in diameter. The epididymis (head, body, and tail combined), as seen

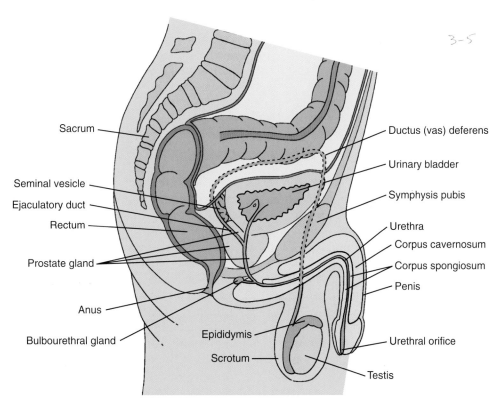

FIGURE 29-1   **Male Pelvis.** Sagittal cross section of the male pelvis, illustrating the relationships of genital organs to surrounding structures.

■ ■ ■ **Table 29-1** Location of Male Pelvis Structures Routinely Visualized With Ultrasound

	Prostate Gland	Seminal Vesicles	Testicles	Epididymis	Corpus Spongiosum	Corpora Cavernosa	Cavernosal Arteries
Anterior to	Rectum					Cavernosal arteries	
Posterior to	Peritoneum, symphysis pubis	Urinary bladder	Tunica albuginea, tunica vaginalis, scrotum, skin	Testicle	Skin	Corpus spongiosum, cavernosal arteries, skin	
Superior to	Urinary bladder (at proximal urethra), ejaculatory duct, seminal vesicles	Prostate gland		Testicle			
Inferior to	Obturator internus muscle, levator ani muscle						
Medial to		Rt and lt ureters			Corpora cavernosa		Corpora cavernosa
Lt lateral to						Cavernosal arteries	
Rt lateral to						Cavernosal arteries	

grossly, measures only 3.8 cm (1.5 inches) in length. The epididymis empties into the ductus deferens, which measures approximately 45 cm (18 inches) in length.

GROSS ANATOMY

Scrotum

The scrotum is a sac of cutaneous tissue that supports the testicles, or testes, the paired organs of reproduction. The skin and superficial fascia of the scrotum are continuous with those of the abdomen (Figure 29-2). Externally, the scrotum is divided into lateral portions by a median ridge called the median raphe. Internally, the scrotum is divided into sacs by a septum called the dartos or tunica dartos. The dartos contains superficial fascia and contractile tissue, which is also continuous with the subcutaneous tissue of the abdominal wall and is abundantly supplied by small blood vessels. Just posterior to the dartos lies the external spermatic fascia, which is a continuation of the external oblique fascia of the abdominal wall. The cremaster muscle surrounds each testicle and extends into the abdomen over the spermatic cord. The cremaster muscle is covered by the cremasteric fascia; this is continuous with the internal oblique fascia of the abdomen. Contraction of the cremaster muscle performs the important function of regulating the temperature of the testicles. Deep to the cremaster muscle is the innermost fascial layer of the scrotum, the internal spermatic fascia or infundibuliform fascia. This inner fascia surrounds the covering layers of the testicles, the tunica vaginalis. The tunica vaginalis consists of two layers derived from the perineum: an outer parietal layer that is closely attached to the internal spermatic fascia, and an inner visceral layer that is closely attached to the testicle.

Testis

Figure 29-3 illustrates the testis, epididymis, and ductus (vas) deferens. Each testis is covered by a dense, white fibrous tissue called tunica albuginea. The tunica albuginea extends into the posterior wall of the testicle and forms the mediastinum testis and interlobar septa. The septa of the mediastinum radiate into the testicle and separate into 200 to 300 lobules. Each lobule contains one to three convoluted seminiferous tubules. The seminiferous tubules are connected to straight tubules, which lead to a network of ducts called the rete testis. The rete testis is located within the mediastinum testis and exits the mediastinum as a series of coiled efferent ducts.

The blood supply to the testicles is via the internal spermatic arteries, which arise from the midabdomen as branches of the aorta just inferior to the renal vessels. The right testicular vein drains into the inferior vena cava at the level near the renal veins. The left testicular vein drains into the left renal vein.

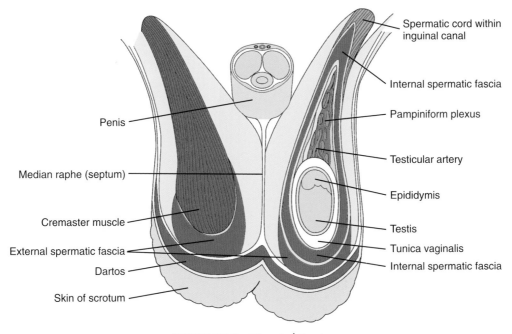

Spermatic cord within inguinal canal

Internal spermatic fascia

Pampiniform plexus

Testicular artery

Epididymis

Testis

Tunica vaginalis

Internal spermatic fascia

Penis

Median raphe (septum)

Cremaster muscle

External spermatic fascia

Dartos

Skin of scrotum

FIGURE 29-2 Dissected Scrotum.

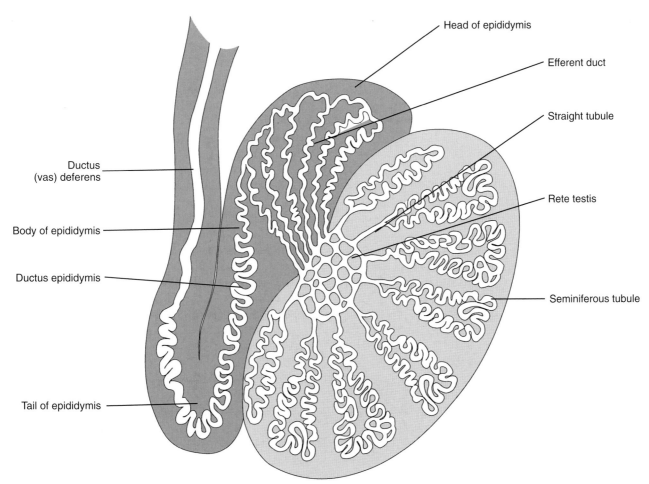

Head of epididymis

Efferent duct

Straight tubule

Rete testis

Seminiferous tubule

Ductus (vas) deferens

Body of epididymis

Ductus epididymis

Tail of epididymis

FIGURE 29-3 Enlarged longitudinal cross-section of testis, epididymis, and ductus (vas) deferens, illustrating the complex network of ducts needed to transport sperm.

Epididymis

The epididymis is composed mostly of a single convoluted tube, the ductus epididymis, encapsulated by a serosal layer. The ductus epididymis is lined by pseudostratified columnar epithelium, and its walls contain a thin layer of smooth muscle. The ductus epididymis is subdivided into a head (globus major), body, and tail (globus minor). The head of the epididymis is the larger, superior portion consisting mostly of the efferent ducts that empty into the ductus epididymis. The body runs along the posterior aspect of the testis and contains the ductus epididymis. The tail is the smaller, inferior portion, where the ductus epididymis empties into the ductus deferens.

Ductus (Vas) Deferens

The ductus deferens is a thicker, less convoluted continuation of the ductus epididymis. Three smooth muscle layers contribute to this duct's increased thickness. At its terminal portion near the seminal vesicles, the ductus deferens dilates; this area is referred to as the ampulla of the deferens.

Spermatic Cord

The two spermatic cords extend from the inguinal canals and internal inguinal rings into the pelvis. Each **spermatic cord** contains the ductus deferens, testicular arteries, venous **pampiniform plexus** (network of veins that drain the testes and become the spermatic veins superiorly), lymphatics, autonomic nerves, and fibers of the cremaster muscle.

Penis

The **penis** is composed of three cylindrical masses of tissue. There are two **corpora cavernosa** situated dorsolaterally and a single **corpus spongiosum** in the midventral region, which contains the spongy **urethra** (Figure 29-4). The three corpora are bound and separated by the fibrous tissue called the tunica albuginea. Superficial to the tunica albuginea is **Buck's fascia**, a thick, fibrous, loosely applied covering of skin that envelops the penis. The three corpora are composed of smooth muscle and erectile tissue that enclose vascular cavities. The penis becomes enlarged and erect when engorged with venous blood.

The blood supply to the penis and urethra is via the paired internal pudendal arteries, which are branches of the internal iliac arteries. These arteries divide into a deep artery of the penis and the bulbourethral artery. The deep artery of the penis supplies the corpora cavernosa. Branches of the dorsal artery and bulbourethral artery supply the corpus spongiosum, glans penis, and urethra.

The main veins of the penis are the superficial dorsal vein and the deep dorsal vein. The superficial dorsal vein is located outside Buck's fascia, and the deep dorsal vein is beneath Buck's fascia. The superficial and deep dorsal veins connect with the pudendal venous plexus, which drains the penis via the internal pudendal vein.

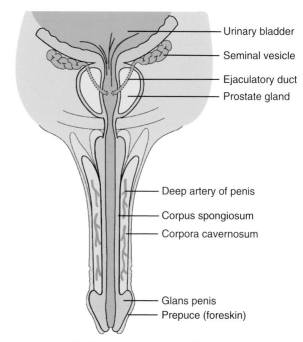

FIGURE 29-4 Anatomy of the Penis.

PHYSIOLOGY

The testicles (testes) are the male gonads and are classified as both endocrine and exocrine glands. At the onset of puberty the testes produce **testosterone**, which causes growth in the male sex organs and development of secondary male sex characteristics, such as body hair and voice deepening (endocrine function). The testes also produce sperm, which are transported through a network of ducts (exocrine function) that store and transport the sperm. The process by which genetic information is passed from one generation of a species to the next is called *reproduction*. In human reproduction, 23 chromosomes are passed from the male gamete, or sperm cell, to the female gamete, or ovum, which also contains 23 chromosomes. Through the union of these gametes, a zygote is formed, containing a total of 46 chromosomes. Multiple divisions of the zygote develop into a new organism. The male gametes, or spermatozoa, are produced in the testes by the process of meiosis. The seminiferous tubules within the testicle are lined with spermatogonia. These spermatogonia develop into mature spermatozoa through the process of **spermatogenesis**. The entire process takes approximately 2 to 3 weeks. Approximately 300 million spermatozoa mature every day. The spermatozoa are transported out of the testes through the efferent ducts into the ductus epididymis, where the final maturation of the sperm occurs. The spermatozoa can remain viable in storage for up to 4 weeks, after which time they are reabsorbed. The function of the ductal system is to store and help propel the sperm during ejaculation.

The production of sperm might be considered the most important function of the male reproductive system, but without the secretions of the accessory organs the sperm could not survive to complete the process of reproduction. The seminal vesicles secrete an alkaline, viscous fluid rich in fructose, which contributes to sperm viability. This fluid constitutes approximately 60% of the volume of semen.

The prostate (see Chapter 20) also produces and secretes an alkaline fluid. Its secretions constitute between 13% and 33% of the volume of semen. This alkaline fluid is believed to neutralize the acid environment of the vagina, uterus, and fallopian tubes, where fertilization of the ovum takes place.

The reproductive function of the penis is to eject semen into the vagina. Sexual stimulation increases the blood supply to the penis. The penile arteries dilate as the penis is engorged with blood. Expansion of these arteries and blood sinuses within the corpora cavernosa causes compression of the veins that drain the penis; thus most of the blood is retained, resulting in an erection. During ejaculation, increased pressure within the urethra causes the urinary bladder sphincter to close. This mechanism prevents urine from being expelled during ejaculation and semen from entering the bladder.

SONOGRAPHIC APPEARANCE
Scrotal Contents

Sonographically, normal testicular parenchyma is homogeneous, containing medium-level echoes similar in appearance to those of the thyroid gland (Figures 29-5, A and B, and 29-6).

The normal testis is also very vascular. Color Doppler is often used to rule out testicular torsion. Figure 29-7 demonstrates the normal testicular vascular pattern.

The highly echogenic line running along the long axis of the testis demonstrates the mediastinum testis. This is a normal finding and should not be mistaken for pathology (Figures 29-8 and 29-9).

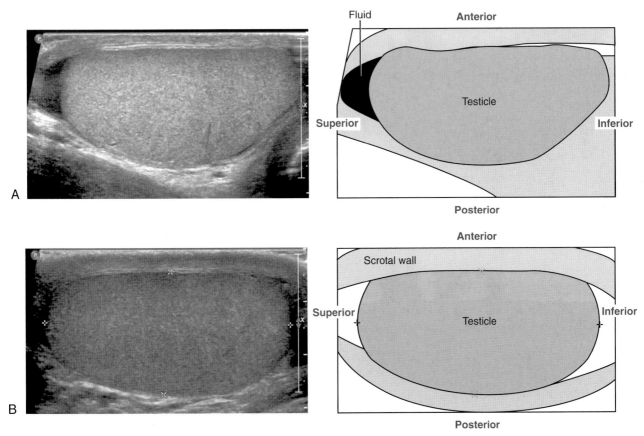

FIGURE 29-5 **A,** Longitudinal section of the testis in the sagittal scanning plane. **B,** Longitudinal section of the testis with anteroposterior and superior to inferior (length) measurements in the sagittal scanning plane.

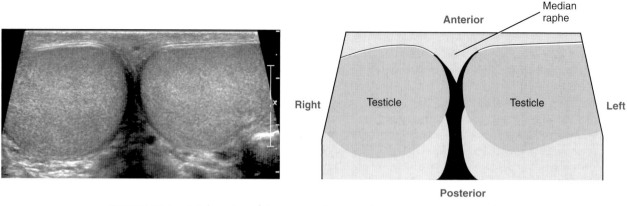

FIGURE 29-6   Axial section of the scrotum/testes in the transverse scanning plane.

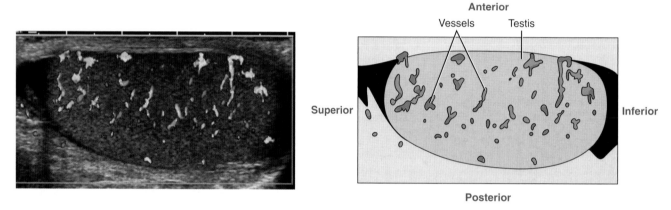

FIGURE 29-7   Color Doppler in a longitudinal section of testis.

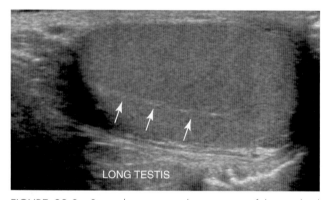

FIGURE 29-8   Sagittal scanning plane image of longitudinal section of testis, demonstrating the mediastinum testis (arrows).

A few millimeters of anechoic fluid are also normally seen between the two layers of the tunica vaginalis (see Figures 29-6 and 29-7). Excess fluid may indicate pathology (hydrocele) (Figure 29-10).

The head of the epididymis is seen superior and posterior to the testicle. The body of the epididymis courses posterior, and the tail lies at the inferior aspect of the testis. The echogenicity of the epididymis is equal to or slightly less than that of the normal testicle. However, the texture of the epididymis is generally coarser in appearance (Figures 29-11 to 29-13).

The various layers of the scrotum are not normally differentiated on ultrasound. The combination of the scrotal wall layers typically appears as a single, highly echogenic stripe.

The spermatic cord may be visualized as it courses through the inguinal canal (Figures 29-14 and 29-15).

Color-flow Doppler is useful in identifying the blood vessels within the cord (Figure 29-16).

Penis

The most extensive role of penile ultrasonography is in the evaluation of vasculogenic impotence. The advent of duplex ultrasound has made this diagnosis possible. Another use of penile ultrasound is detection of pathologic abnormalities such as fibrosis, tumors, and periurethral diseases.

In the transverse scanning plane the corpus spongiosum will be seen in the midline, compressed

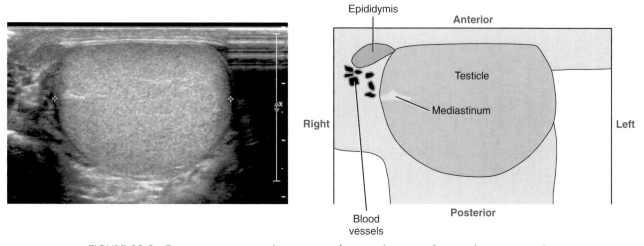

FIGURE 29-9   Transverse scanning plane image of an axial section of testis, demonstrating the mediastinum testis.

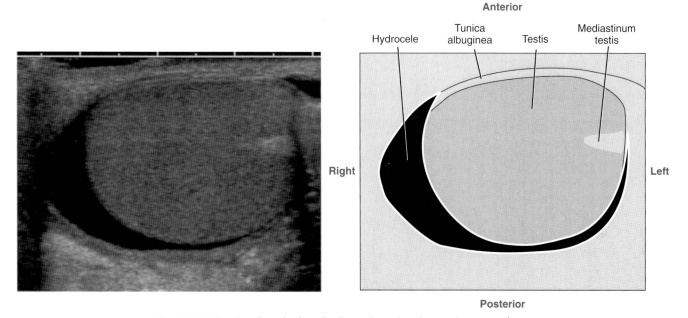

FIGURE 29-10   Anechoic hydrocele shown lateral to the axial section of testis.

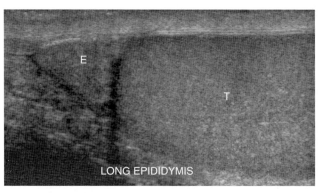

FIGURE 29-11   Head of epididymis, denoted by *E,* is shown in this longitudinal section of the testis (T).

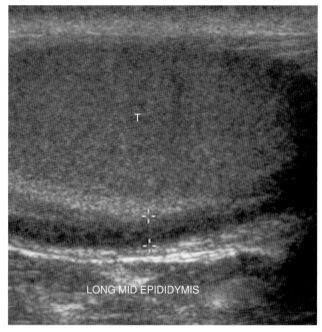

FIGURE 29-12 Longitudinal section of testis shows midportion of the epididymis. Note calipers identifying the walls of the epididymis.

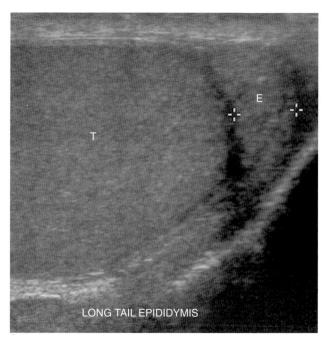

FIGURE 29-13 Tail of the epididymis, denoted by *E*, is shown in this longitudinal section of the testis *(T)*.

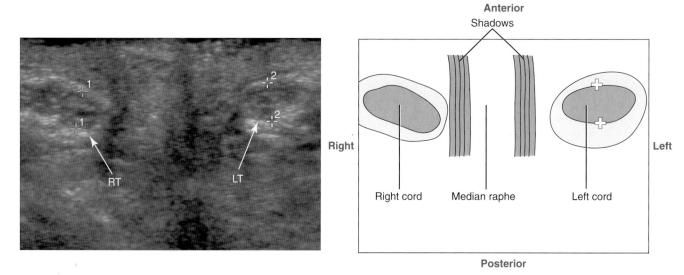

FIGURE 29-14 Transverse scanning plane image demonstrating both right and left spermatic cords as they pass through the inguinal canal.

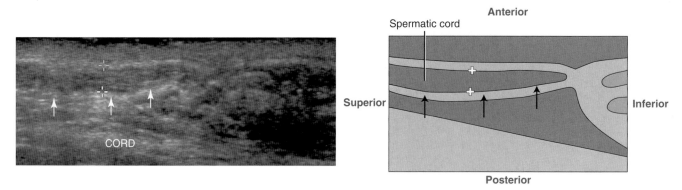

FIGURE 29-15 Longitudinal section of the spermatic cord.

by the transducer, and will appear elliptical in shape (Figure 29-17).

Sonographically, the normal corpus spongiosum should be of homogeneous texture composed of medium-level echoes. The paired corpora cavernosa are posterior to the corpus spongiosum and appear symmetrically round or oval, also with a medium-level homogeneous echo texture. The corpora cavernosa are covered by the highly echogenic tunica albuginea. The echogenic plane dividing the two corpora cavernosa is an extension of the tunica albuginea called the septum penis (Figure 29-18).

Centrally located within the corpora cavernosa are cavernosal arteries, which can be identified by their echogenic walls and pulsations as seen in real time (Figure 29-19).

In a sagittal scanning plane each corpus cavernosum appears homogeneous with highly echogenic tunica albuginea visualized anteriorly and posteriorly.

In a sagittal scanning plane the cavernosal arteries will be imaged in their long axis and appear as parallel echogenic lines, representing the walls of the artery, coursing through the middle of the corpora cavernosa. Figure 29-20 illustrates a longitudinal section of the penis and cavernosal artery. Figures 29-21 and 29-22 demonstrate the cavernosal arteries using color Doppler and power Doppler, respectively.

SONOGRAPHIC APPLICATIONS
Scrotum
- Testicular size
- Inflammatory processes (epididymitis, orchitis)
- Presence and composition of masses

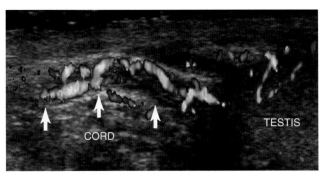

FIGURE 29-16 Color Doppler image demonstrating blood flow within the spermatic cord.

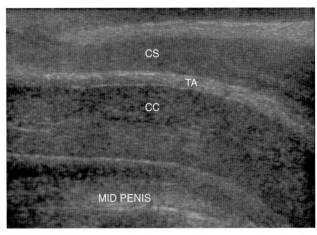

FIGURE 29-18 Longitudinal section of the penis, showing the corpus spongiosum (CS) and corpus cavernosum (CC) separated by the echogenic tunica albuginea (TA).

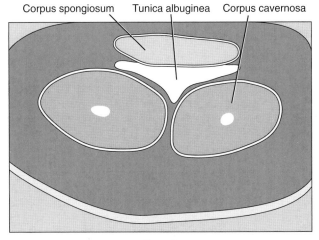

FIGURE 29-17 Transverse scanning plane image of an axial section of the penis, showing the corpus spongiosum compressed by the transducer and the corpora cavernosa dorsal to the corpus spongiosum.

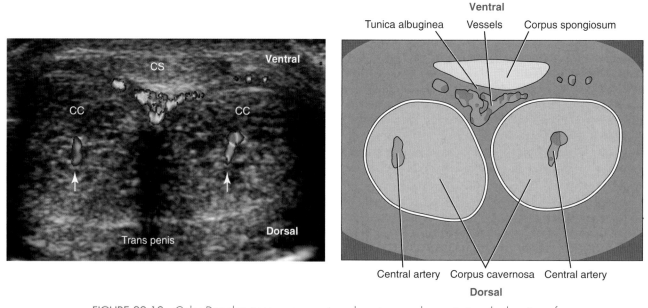

FIGURE 29-19 Color Doppler, transverse scanning plane image, demonstrating the location of the cavernosal arteries *(arrows)*.

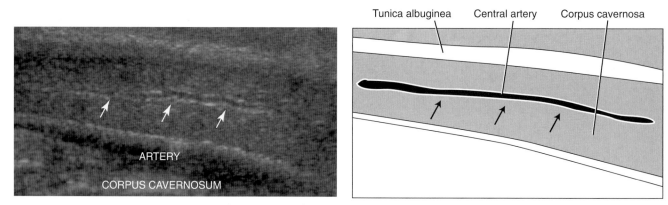

FIGURE 29-20 Longitudinal section of the corpus cavernosum, demonstrating the centrally located cavernosal artery *(arrows)*.

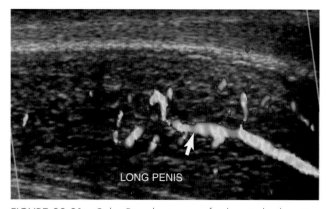

FIGURE 29-21 Color Doppler image of a longitudinal section of the cavernosal artery.

- Detection of peritesticular fluid collections (hydrocele)
- Evaluation of scrotal trauma
- Doppler evaluation to rule out testicular torsion
- Evaluation of scrotal pain
- Location of undescended testicles

Penis
- Detection of fibrosis (Peyronie's disease)
- Detection of scar tissue and plaques
- Evaluation of tumors
- Penile hematoma
- Evaluation of periurethral disease
- Doppler evaluation of vasculogenic impotence

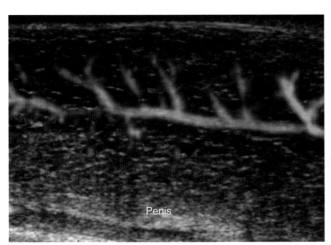

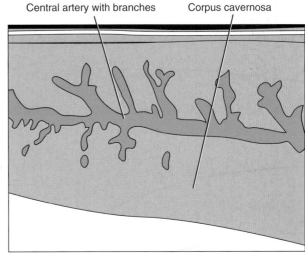

Central artery with branches   Corpus cavernosa

Penis

FIGURE 29-22 Doppler image of a longitudinal section of the cavernosal artery.

NORMAL VARIANTS

- **Cryptorchidism:** Failure of the testicles to descend into the scrotum. Common locations of undescended testes include the abdomen, inguinal canal, and at the external inguinal ring.

REFERENCE CHARTS

■ ■ ■ ASSOCIATED PHYSICIAN

- **Urologist:** Specializes in surgical diseases of the male genitourinary tract and female urinary system.

■ ■ ■ COMMON DIAGNOSTIC TESTS

- **Magnetic resonance imaging (MRI):** A noninvasive imaging modality that is very useful in identifying soft tissue structures. It is performed by a radiologic technologist and interpreted by a radiologist.
- **Ultrasonography:** Second to direct physical palpation by a urologist, this is the method of choice for evaluating the male genitourinary system. It is typically performed by a sonographer and interpreted by a radiologist.

■ ■ ■ LABORATORY VALUES

- Nonapplicable.

■ ■ ■ VASCULATURE

- Nonapplicable.

■ ■ ■ AFFECTING CHEMICALS

- Nonapplicable.

CHAPTER 30

Pediatric Echocardiography

VIVIE MILLER AND VIVIAN G. DICKS

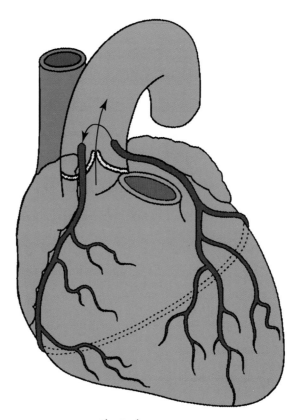

The Pediatric Heart.

OBJECTIVES

Describe the function of the heart.

Describe the size and position of the heart in the normal child.

Name the chambers, great veins, and great arteries of the heart.

Describe the flow of blood through the heart of a fully developed fetus, including the fetal shunts and their purpose.

Describe the flow of blood through the heart of a normal neonate after closure of the fetal shunts.

Describe the sonographic appearance of the pediatric heart.

Describe the associated physicians.

Describe the associated diagnostic tests.

KEY WORDS

Aorta — Great artery originating from the left ventricle of the heart. It is described as the ascending (proximal) aorta, transverse (arch) aorta, and descending (thoracic and abdominal) aorta.

Aortic Valve — Semilunar valve with 3 leaflets or cusps; so named because of the half-moon or crescent shape of the cusps.

Apex — Bluntly pointed inferior or caudal end of the heart that is directed to the left and anteriorly. It is partially obscured by the left lung.

Ascending Aorta — Proximal portion of the aorta that arises from the left ventricle of the heart. Its branches include the right and left coronary arteries. Continues as the transverse (arched) aorta.

Atria — The two upper, filling chambers of the heart. They are separated by the interatrial septum.

Atrioventricular (AV) Node — Part of the heart's conduction system. When the AV node fires, it sends impulses along the bundle of His. Then the impulses travel through the Purkinje fibers into the myocardium. The ventricles contract at once from above downward.

Atrioventricular (AV) Valves — Valves (the tricuspid valve on the right; the mitral valve on the left) that control the openings through which the atria and ventricles on each side of the heart communicate.

Base — Broad end of the heart directed to the right posterosuperiorly.

Bundle of His — Part of the heart's conduction system. A band of cardiac muscle fibers that connect the atria and ventricles and serve to rapidly transmit impulses in the heart to assist with heart contractions.

Cardiac Conduction System — Mechanism by which the heart is made to effectively pump blood through the vessels. The muscle fibers of the heart have the inherent ability to contract without a nerve stimulus.

Cardiac Veins — Veins that drain the heart. Most drain into the coronary sinus, a large vein that acts as a reservoir.

Chordae Tendineae — Tendinous cords connecting each atrioventricular valve (tricuspid and mitral valves) to papillary muscles of the heart.

Common Carotid Arteries — Arteries that distribute oxygenated blood to the head and neck. The right common carotid artery is a branch of the brachiocephalic trunk (or innominate artery). The left common carotid artery is a branch of the transverse (arched) aorta. These arteries branch into right and left internal and external carotid arteries.

Coronary Arteries — Arteries that perfuse the heart muscle and inner structures. So named because they form a corona, or crown, around the heart. There are two main coronary arteries: the right coronary artery arising from the right sinus of Valsalva and the left coronary artery arising from the left sinus.

Coronary Sinus — Large cardiac vein draining the heart muscle.

Descending (Thoracic and Abdominal) Aorta — Multiple-branched aorta. The thoracic aorta is the proximal portion of the descending aorta. It is a continuation of the aorta from the arch of the transverse aorta to the aortic hiatus of the diaphragm. The abdominal aorta is the lower portion of the descending aorta from the aortic hiatus of the diaphragm to the bifurcation into right and left common iliac arteries. Branches are multiple throughout the chest and abdomen.

Diastole — Period of dilation of the ventricles of the heart.

Ductus Arteriosus — Connection between the dorsal aorta and the left pulmonary artery.

Ductus Venosus — One of three fetal shunts; enables oxygenated blood from the mother to pass almost directly into the fetal heart, bypassing the liver. After birth it will fibrose and become the ligamentum venosum.

Endocardium — Inner lining of the cavities of the heart.

Epicardium — Outer covering of the myocardium, or muscle of the heart. Composed of two linings or membranes: the inner visceral pericardium and the outer parietal pericardium. The space between them is the pericardial cavity.

Foramen Ovale — Opening between the heart's atria in the fetus.

Inferior Vena Cava (IVC) — One of the two great veins normally connected to the right atrium. The other is the superior vena cava.

Innominate Artery — Also called the brachiocephalic trunk; a branch of the transverse aortic arch. Its branches include the right common carotid and right subclavian arteries.

Interatrial Septum — Partition separating the right and left atria.

Interventricular Septum — Partition separating the right and left ventricles.

Mitral Valve — The left atrioventricular (AV) valve with two fan-shaped or triangular leaflets inserted more superiorly on the septum toward the base of the heart. Normally has two sets of chordae tendineae that are, in turn, connected to two papillary muscles.

Myocardium — Muscle of the heart.

Papillary Muscles — Muscular projections from ventricle walls attached to the cusps of the atrioventricular (AV) valves by chordae tendineae.

Parietal Pericardium — Outer of the two linings composing the epicardium (outer covering of the heart).

Pulmonary Artery (Main, Right, Left) — Main pulmonary artery that receives blood from the right ventricle and then branches into a right pulmonary artery to the right lung and a left pulmonary artery to the left lung.

Pulmonary Valve — Semilunar valve with three leaflets or cusps; so named because of the half-moon or crescent shape of the cusps.

Pulmonary Veins — Four veins that return oxygenated blood to the left atrium from the lungs.

Purkinje Fibers — Part of the heart's conduction system. Cardiac muscle fibers that rapidly transmit impulses in the heart to coordinate heart contractions.

Semilunar Valves — Aortic valve and pulmonary valve; so named because of the half-moon or crescent shape of their three leaflets or cusps.

Sinoatrial (SA) Node — Sets the pace of the heart and is therefore called the pacemaker of the conduction system. As the SA node fires, electrical impulses travel through internodal tracts to both atria.

Sinuses of Valsalva — Recessed pockets, or outpouchings, of the aorta that house the openings of the coronary arteries. There are three sinuses, each of which is associated with one cusp of the aortic valve. The sinuses protect the openings from the rush of blood through the aortic valve and prevent the valve leaflets from occluding the openings.

Subclavian Arteries — Arteries that distribute oxygenated blood to the head, neck, chest wall, and spinal cord. The right subclavian artery is a branch of the brachiocephalic trunk (or innominate artery). The left subclavian artery is a branch of the transverse (arched) aorta.

Superior Vena Cava (SVC) — One of the two great veins normally connected to the right atrium. The other is the inferior vena cava.

Systole — Period of contraction of the ventricles of the heart.

Transverse (Arched) Aorta — Continuation of the ascending (proximal) aorta. Its branches include the innominate artery (or brachiocephalic trunk), left subclavian artery, and left common carotid artery. Continues as the descending (thoracic and abdominal) aorta.

Tricuspid Valve — Right atrioventricular (AV) valve with three fan-shaped leaflets connected to three sets of chordae tendineae that are, in turn, connected to three papillary muscles.

Ventricles — The two lower, pumping chambers of the heart. The right and left ventricles are separated by the interventricular septum.

Visceral Pericardium — Inner of the two linings composing the epicardium (outer covering of the heart).

■ ■ ■ NORMAL VALUES FOR CHILDREN ARRANGED BY WEIGHT

Weight (lb)	Mean (cm)	Range (cm)	Number of Subjects	Weight (lb)	Mean (cm)	Range (cm)	Number of Subjects
RVD				**LA Dimension**			
0 to 25	0.9	0.3 to 1.5	26	0 to 25	1.7	0.7 to 2.3	26
26 to 50	1.0	0.4 to 1.5	26	26 to 50	2.2	1.7 to 2.7	26
51 to 75	1.1	0.7 to 1.8	20	51 to 75	2.3	1.9 to 2.8	20
76 to 100	1.2	0.7 to 1.6	15	76 to 100	2.4	2.0 to 3.0	15
101 to 125	1.3	0.8 to 1.7	11	101 to 125	2.7	2.1 to 3.0	11
126 to 200	1.3	1.2 to 1.7		126 to 200	2.8	2.1 to 3.7	5
5LVID				**Aortic Root**			
0 to 25	2.4	1.3 to 3.2	26	0 to 25	1.3	0.7 to 1.7	26
26 to 50	3.4	2.4 to 3.8	26	26 to 50	1.7	1.3 to 2.2	26
51 to 75	3.8	3.3 to 4.5	20	51 to 75	2.0	1.7 to 2.3	20
76 to 100	4.1	3.5 to 4.7	15	76 to 100	2.2	1.9 to 2.7	15
101 to 125	4.3	3.7 to 4.9	11	101 to 125	2.3	1.7 to 2.7	11
126 to 200	4.9	4.4 to 5.2	5	126 to 200	2.4	2.2 to 2.8	5
LV and IV Septal Wall Thickness				**Aortic Valve Opening**			
0 to 25	0.5	0.4 to 0.6	26	0 to 25	0.9	0.5 to 1.2	26
26 to 50	0.6	0.5 to 0.7	26	26 to 50	1.2	0.9 to 1.6	26
51 to 75	0.7	0.6 to 0.7	20	51 to 75	1.4	1.2 to 1.7	20
76 to 100	0.7	0.7 to 0.8	15	76 to 100	1.6	1.3 to 1.9	15
101 to 125	0.7	0.7 to 0.8	11	101 to 125	1.7	1.4 to 2.0	11
126 to 200	0.8	0.7 to 0.8	5	126 to 200	1.8	1.6 to 2.0	5

The structures of the heart include four chambers, four main valves, two great veins, four smaller veins, two great arteries, septa, and muscle.

The heart is the muscular pump of the body's cardiovascular system, providing the force that propels blood through all the vessels. The heart and vessels are a distribution and collection system in general, providing transportation for the distribution of nutrients, gases, minerals, vitamins, hormones, and blood cells to the tissues and collection of waste products for excretion from the body.

1. The tissues of the body receive oxygen and nutrients.
2. The tissues of the body have a disposal service for the collection and excretion of waste products such as carbon dioxide and other toxic materials.
3. The tissues of the body can release secretory materials or hormones that can quickly exert an influence on body parts distant from the source.
4. Medications injected into the body are distributed quickly throughout all areas of the body.
5. The body's defense system, which includes antibodies and white blood cells, moves to areas of infection and inflammation.

PRENATAL DEVELOPMENT

An understanding of prenatal development of the heart is critical in assessing the normal fetal heart (see Chapters 22 and 23 on first, second, and third trimester obstetrics).

In the 3-week-old embryo, the heart arises as two cords, called *cardiogenic cords*. These cords will canalize to form two heart tubes. The heart tubes will gradually move toward each other and fuse to form a single heart tube (Figure 30-1). The tube elongates and develops alternative dilatations and constrictions, which indicate the development to come. The bulbus cordis and ventricle grow faster than other regions, causing the heart tube to bend upon itself and form a bulboventricular loop. Normal looping is toward the right. The result is that the atrium and the sinus venosus (which will later form right and left horns) come to lie posterior and superior to the bulbus cordis, truncus arteriosus, and ventricle.

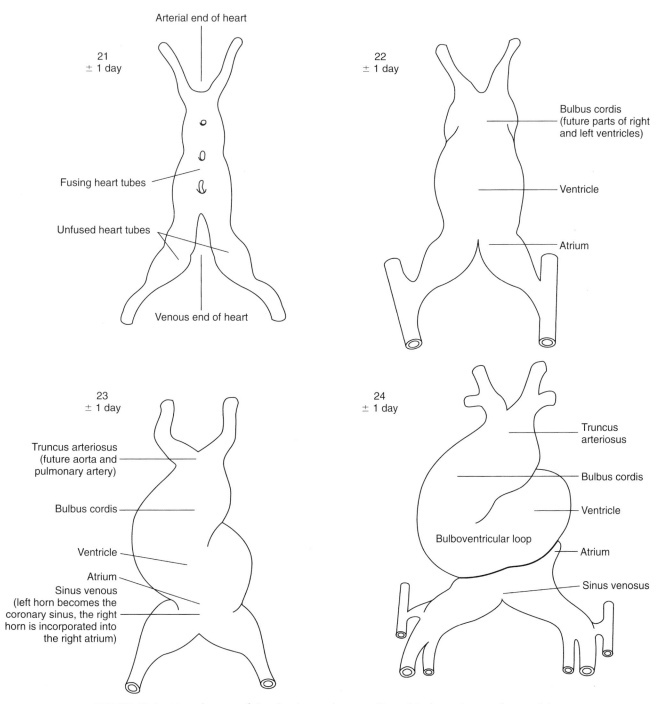

FIGURE 30-1 Ventral views of the developing heart at 20 to 25 days, showing fusion of the endocardial heart tube to form a single tube. Note bending to form the bulboventricular loop.

Beginning in week 4 of embryologic development, and by the end of week 7, the heart is completely partitioned into two atria, two ventricles, two great arteries, and veins.

Partitioning of the atrioventricular canal begins during week 4 of embryologic development (Figure 30-2). Swellings called endocardial cushions form on the dorsal and ventral walls of the atrioventricular canal. These cushions develop and grow toward each other, fusing during week 5. The heart is now divided into a right and left atrioventricular canal.

The partitioning of the common atrium is accomplished by the development of two septa, the septum primum and the septum secundum (Figure 30-3). The

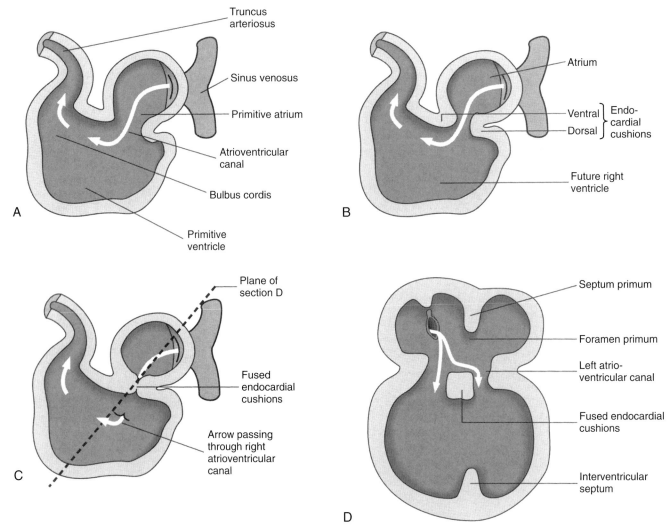

FIGURE 30-2 **A** to **C,** Sagittal sections of the heart during weeks 4 and 5, illustrating division of the atrioventricular canal. **D,** Coronal section of the heart at the plane shown in **C.** Note that the interatrial and interventricular septa have also begun to develop.

septum primum is a thin, crescent-shaped membrane (the first septum) that grows toward the fused endocardial cushions, beginning at the dorsocranial wall of the primitive atrium. As this curtain-like septum grows toward the endocardial cushions, a large opening develops called the *foramen primum.* This opening eventually closes as the septum primum continues to grow toward and fuse with the endocardial cushions. However, before the foramen primum is closed, perforations, or fenestrations, appear in the dorsal part of the septum primum to create a second opening, called the *foramen secundum.* At about this time, the septum primum joins or fuses with the left side of the endocardial cushions to completely close the foramen primum. By the end of week 5, another crescentic membrane grows from the ventrocranial wall of the atrium, immediately to the

right of the septum primum. This is the septum secundum, or second septum. As it grows, it covers or overlaps the foramen secundum that formed in the septum primum to shape an oval opening, named the **foramen ovale.** The cranial part of the septum primum gradually disappears. The remaining part of the septum attaches to the endocardial cushions to establish the flap of the foramen ovale. This is one of three fetal shunts.

Partitioning of the primitive ventricle begins with a muscular ridge in the floor of the single ventricle near the apex (Figure 30-4; also see Figure 30-7). This foramen is subsequently closed, with ridges extending from the right and left sides of the bulbus cordis, called *bulbar ridges,* and the endocardial cushions (Figure 30-5). The thin, small, membranous interventricular septum is derived from an extension of tissue from the right side

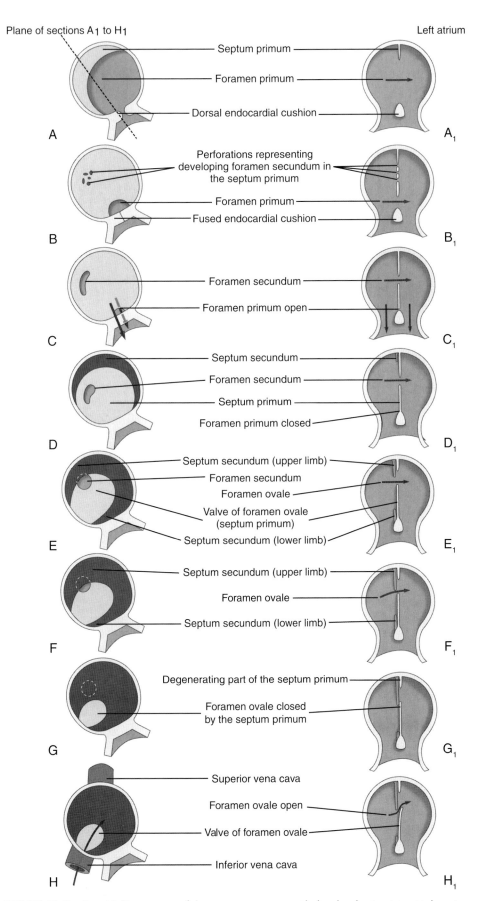

Plane of sections A₁ to H₁

Left atrium

A — Septum primum / Foramen primum / Dorsal endocardial cushion — **A₁**

B — Perforations representing developing foramen secundum in the septum primum / Foramen primum / Fused endocardial cushion — **B₁**

C — Foramen secundum / Foramen primum open — **C₁**

D — Septum secundum / Foramen secundum / Septum primum / Foramen primum closed — **D₁**

E — Septum secundum (upper limb) / Foramen secundum / Foramen ovale / Valve of foramen ovale (septum primum) / Septum secundum (lower limb) — **E₁**

F — Septum secundum (upper limb) / Foramen ovale / Septum secundum (lower limb) — **F₁**

G — Degenerating part of the septum primum / Foramen ovale closed by the septum primum — **G₁**

H — Superior vena cava / Foramen ovale open / Valve of foramen ovale / Inferior vena cava — **H₁**

FIGURE 30-3 **A** to **H,** Partitioning of the primitive atrium, with the developing interatrial septum viewed from the right side. **A₁** to **H₁,** Coronal sections of the developing interatrial septum at the plane shown in **A.** Note that as the septum secundum develops, it overlaps the opening in the septum primum (foramen secundum). The valve-like nature of the foramen ovale is illustrated in **G** and **H.** When pressure in the right atrium exceeds that in the left atrium (as in the fetus), blood passes from the right to the left side of the heart. When the pressures are equal or higher in the left atrium (as is normal after birth), the septum primum closes the foramen ovale.

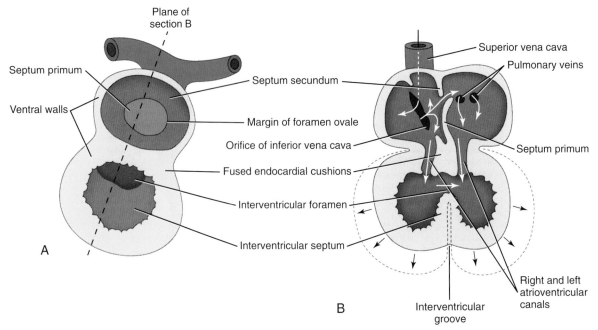

FIGURE 30-4 **Partitioning of the Primitive Heart. A,** Sagittal section in week 5, showing the cardiac septa and foramina. **B,** Coronal section at a slightly later stage, illustrating the direction of blood flow through the heart and expansion of the ventricles. Note the formation of the interventricular septum and the interventricular foramen in both diagrams.

of the fused endocardial cushions. This tissue merges with the aorticopulmonary septum (fused bulbar ridges) and the thick muscular interventricular septum. After closure of the interventricular septum, the aorta communicates with the left ventricle, and the pulmonary trunk communicates with the right ventricle. There is now no direct communication between the newly formed right and left ventricles.

The bulbus cordis and truncus arteriosus begin partitioning into the aorta and pulmonary artery during week 5. The growth of cells in the wall of the bulbus cordis results in bulbar ridges. Truncal ridges form in the truncus arteriosus and are continuous with the bulbar ridges (Figure 30-6). The spiral formation of these ridges results in a spiral aorticopulmonary septum. In Figure 30-6, *B* and *F,* this septum is shown oriented right/left at level 3. At level 2, it is oriented dorsoventrally or anterior/posterior. It twists again, and at level 1 it is again oriented right/left. In Figure 30-6, *E* and *H,* the septum has divided the bulbus cordis and truncus arteriosus into the aorta and pulmonary trunk. Because of the spiraling of the aorticopulmonary septum, the pulmonary trunk twists around the aorta.

The bulbus cordis is absorbed into the ventricles (Figure 30-7). It becomes the conus arteriosus, or infundibulum, of the right ventricle. In the left ventricle it is called the *aortic vestibule,* which is the part just proximal to the aortic valve.

Another fetal shunt, the ductus arteriosus, is a connection between the dorsal aorta and the left pulmonary artery. Both the ductus arteriosus and the left pulmonary artery are derivatives of the left sixth aortic arch (see Figures 30-6, *A,* and Figure 30-9).

The inferior vena cava is derived from four segments of the primitive veins of the embryonic trunk. It enters the inferior posterior part of the right atrium. The superior vena cava is derived from two primitive veins of the embryo, the right anterior cardinal vein and the right common cardinal vein. It enters the posterior superior part of the right atrium.

The four pulmonary veins are derived from the primitive pulmonary vein and its four main branches (Figure 30-8). As the primitive vein is incorporated into the left atrium, the four main branches remain, each one entering the left atrium separately.

Fetal Circulation

Circulation through the fully developed normal fetal heart is shown in Figure 30-9 on p. 552. Oxygenated blood from the mother, via the placenta, enters the umbilical vein and passes through the ductus venosus to the inferior vena cava and into the right atrium of the fetal heart. The ductus venosus, one of the three fetal shunts, enables oxygenated blood from the mother to pass almost directly into the fetal heart, bypassing the liver. After birth it will fibrose and become the ligamentum venosum.

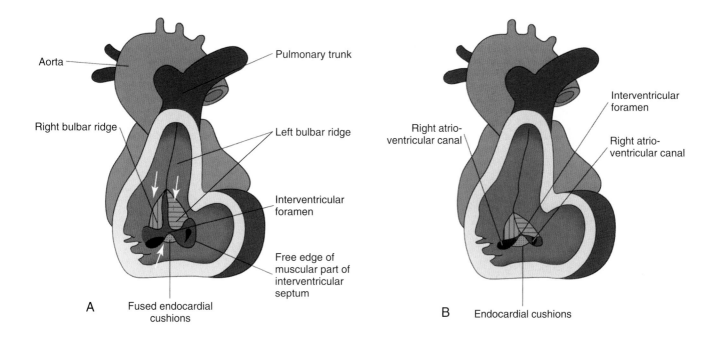

A — labels: Aorta, Pulmonary trunk, Right bulbar ridge, Left bulbar ridge, Interventricular foramen, Free edge of muscular part of interventricular septum, Fused endocardial cushions

B — labels: Right atrio-ventricular canal, Interventricular foramen, Right atrio-ventricular canal, Endocardial cushions

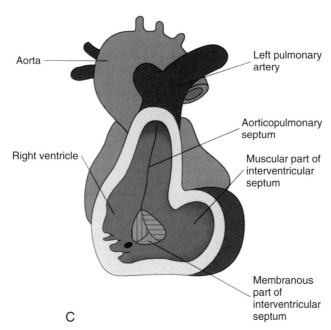

C — labels: Aorta, Left pulmonary artery, Aorticopulmonary septum, Right ventricle, Muscular part of interventricular septum, Membranous part of interventricular septum

FIGURE 30-5 **Closure of the Interventricular Foramen and Formation of the Membranous Part of the Interventricular Septum.** The walls of the truncus arteriosus, bulbus cordis, and right ventricle have been removed. **A,** At 5 weeks, showing the bulbar ridges and the fused endocardial cushions. **B,** At 6 weeks, showing that proliferation of subendocardial tissue diminishes the interventricular foramen. **C,** At 7 weeks, showing the fused bulbar ridges and the membranous part of the interventricular septum formed by extensions of tissue from the right side of the endocardial cushions.

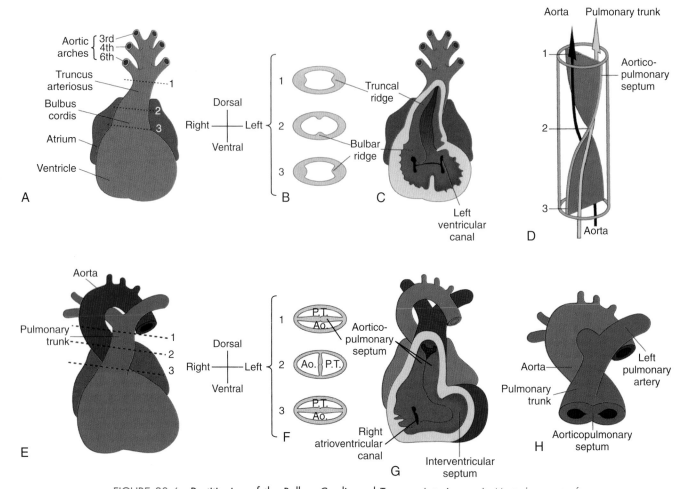

FIGURE 30-6 *Partitioning of the Bulbus Cordis and Truncus Arteriosus.* **A,** Ventral aspect of the heart at 5 weeks. **B,** Transverse sections through the truncus arteriosus and bulbus cordis, illustrating the truncal and bulbar ridges. Note that the orientation is of looking down into the truncus arteriosus from above, keeping in mind the dorsal and ventral aspects of the truncal tube as the aorticopulmonary septum spirals within it. **C,** The ventral wall of the heart and truncus arteriosus have been removed to demonstrate these ridges. **D,** Spiral form of the aorticopulmonary septum. **E,** Ventral aspect of the heart after partitioning of the truncus arteriosus. **F,** Sections through the newly formed aorta (Ao.) and pulmonary trunk (P.T.), showing the aorticopulmonary septum. **G,** At 6 weeks, the ventral wall of the heart and pulmonary trunk have been removed to show the aorticopulmonary septum. **H,** The great arteries twisting around one another as they exist in the normal neonatal heart.

Much of the blood from the inferior vena cava is directed across the foramen ovale, the second shunt, into the left atrium. From here the blood enters the left ventricle and then exits through the aorta.

Some blood from the inferior vena cava remains in the right atrium and mixes with blood from the superior vena cava and **coronary sinus** (the large cardiac vein draining the heart muscle) and passes into the right ventricle. This blood then exits the pulmonary trunk, some going to the lungs for development, but most going through the ductus arteriosus, the third shunt, to the aorta.

Fetal to Adult Circulation

The ductus venosus, ductus arteriosus, and the placenta are the three anatomic structures that differentiate fetal circulation from adult circulation. During childbirth and elimination of the placenta, blood flow increases in the lungs. It is thought that because of the low temperature from the removal of the placenta and cooling of the umbilical cord that a vasoactive polypeptide named *bradykinin* is responsible for the vasodilatation of the pulmonary arterioles. The combination of oxygen and bradykinin causes the alveoli in the lungs to expand and fill with air.

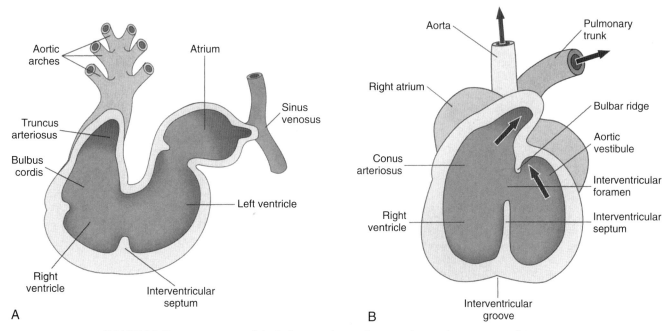

A

B

FIGURE 30-7 Incorporation of the bulbus cordis into the ventricles, and partitioning of the bulbus cordis and truncus arteriosus into the aorta and pulmonary trunk. **A,** Sagittal section at 5 weeks, showing the bulbus cordis as one of the five primitive chambers of the heart. **B,** Coronal section at 6 weeks, after the bulbus cordis has been incorporated into the ventricles to become the conus arteriosus (infundibulum) of the right ventricle and the aortic vestibule of the left ventricle.

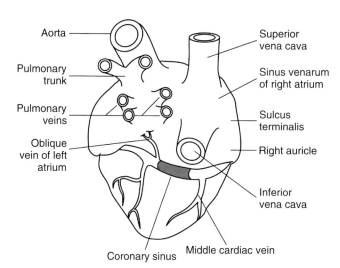

FIGURE 30-8 Dorsal view at 8 weeks, showing the positions of the superior and inferior venae cavae with respect to the right atrium. The pulmonary veins, each with separate openings into the left atrium, are also shown.

LOCATION

As its name implies, the heart is roughly heart-shaped. It is positioned in the lower anterior chest, posterior to the sternum and anterior to the thoracic vertebrae and esophagus. It rests on the diaphragm in the middle mediastinum, bounded laterally by the right and left lungs. Two thirds of the heart lies to the left of midline and one third lies to the right. The **apex** of the heart is the bluntly pointed inferior or caudal end that is directed to the left and anteriorly. It is partially obscured by the left lung. The **base** is the broad end directed to the right posteriorly and cranially (Figure 30-10).

SIZE

The heart is approximately the size of an individual's clenched fist. The pediatric internal dimensions of the structures vary with age and weight. Normal values for these structures are presented in the Normal Measurements box at the beginning of this chapter.

GROSS ANATOMY

Structurally the heart is divided into upper and lower chambers and divided into right-sided and left-sided chambers (Figure 30-11).

The two upper chambers, the **atria**, are the filling chambers of the heart. There is a right atrium and a left atrium, roughly equal in size, thin walled, and separated by a partition called the **interatrial septum**. After birth, there is normally no direct communication between these two chambers.

The two lower chambers, the **ventricles**, are the pumping chambers of the heart. The right ventricle and left ventricle are separated by the **interventricular septum**.

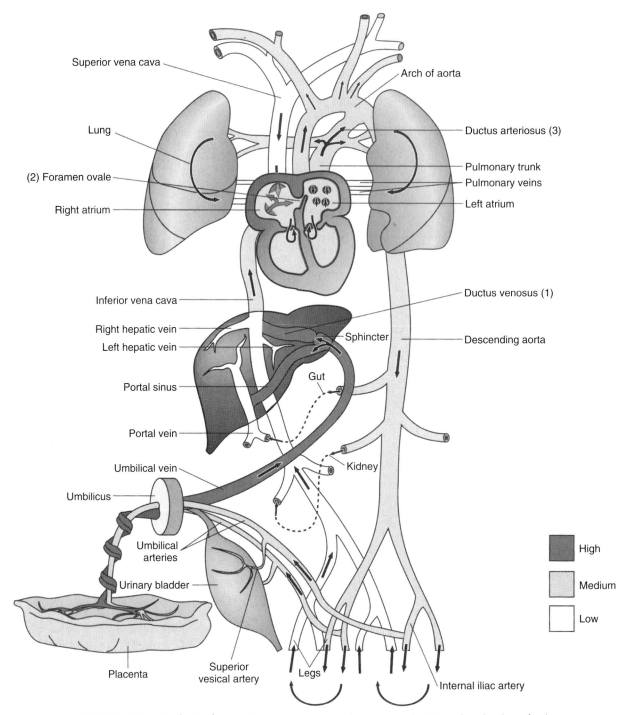

FIGURE 30-9 **Fetal Circulation.** The organs are not drawn to scale. Note that the three fetal shunts permit most of the blood to bypass the liver and the lungs: *(1)* the ductus venosus, *(2)* the foramen ovale, and *(3)* the ductus arteriosus.

The atrium and the ventricles on each side are separate; however, they communicate through openings controlled by an **atrioventricular (AV) valve.** The ventricles, in turn, are connected to outflow tracts with semilunar (half-moon–shaped) valves controlling the exit of blood from the heart.

The inner lining of the cavities of the heart is called the **endocardium.** The outer covering of the **myocardium,** or muscle of the heart, is called the **epicardium.** It is composed of two linings or membranes. The inner membrane, the **visceral pericardium,** adheres to the myocardium. The outer membrane is the **parietal**

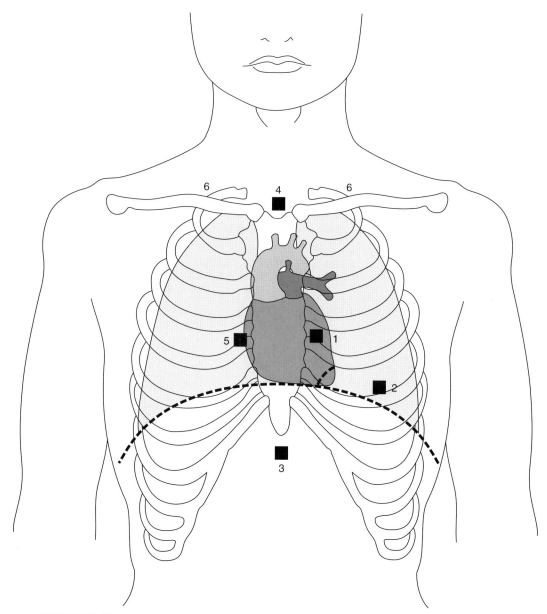

FIGURE 30-10   Relative position of the heart with respect to other organs within the chest cavity. Note blocks denoting transducer positions that provide "windows" for imaging the heart. (1) Parasternal long axis and parasternal short axis positions. (2) Apical four chamber, apical five chamber, and apical long axis. (3) Subcostal or subxiphoid position. (4) Suprasternal notch position. (5) Right parasternal position. (6) Although not indicated by blocks, the supraclavicular fossa (right and/or left) is also sometimes used in obtaining echocardiographic images.

pericardium. The space between them is the pericardial cavity containing a thin, watery fluid that allows the heart to move easily as it beats.

The beating heart makes distinctive sounds. There are two major heart sounds. The first sound, S_1, is caused by closure of the AV valves; the second, S_2, is caused by the semilunar valves closing. There is a normal splitting of the second sound, the first being that of the aortic valve before the closure of the pulmonary valve component.

Structural differences of the chambers are very helpful in evaluating the pediatric heart. These differences help to determine situs (position), atrioventricular concordance, and ventriculoarterial concordance. The right atrium is normally connected to the two great veins, the **superior vena cava (SVC)** and the **inferior vena cava (IVC)**. The left atrium normally receives four pulmonary veins. The right ventricle is normally connected to the pulmonary artery and the left ventricle to the aorta.

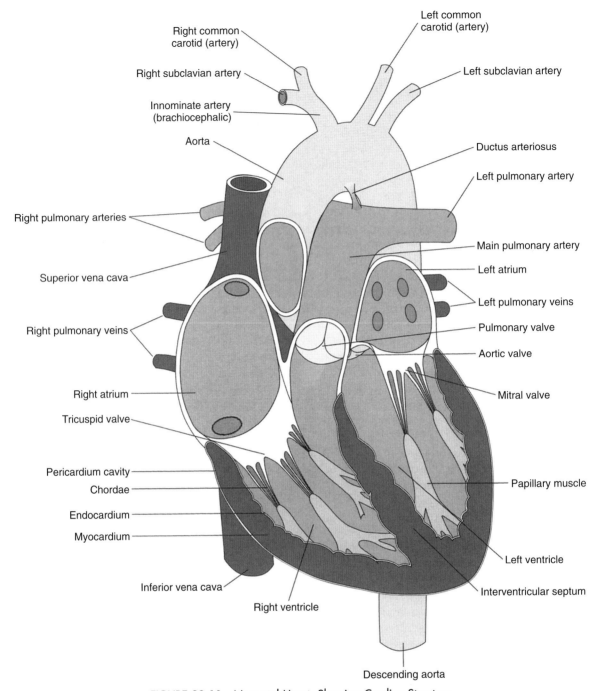

FIGURE 30-11 Neonatal Heart, Showing Cardiac Structure.

The right AV valve, called the **tricuspid valve**, has three fan-shaped leaflets connected to three sets of **chordae tendineae** that are, in turn, connected to three **papillary muscles**. The tricuspid valve has a more inferior or apical insertion point than its counterpart on the left side. The right ventricle is triangular. It has a more heavily trabeculated endocardial surface, a moderator band in the lower third of the chamber, and an infundibular muscle band, or conus, in the right ventricular outflow tract.

On the other side, the left AV valve, called the **mitral valve**, has two fan-shaped or triangular leaflets inserted more superiorly on the septum toward the base of the heart. Normally, the mitral valve has two sets of chordae and two papillary muscles. The left ventricular myocardium is relatively thicker than its counterpart on the right because it is pumping against higher pressures. The left ventricle has an ellipsoid shape and smooth endocardial surface. All of these characteristics help differentiate the right heart from the left heart.

The semilunar valves, which are the aortic valve and pulmonary valve, have three leaflets or cusps, so named because they are shaped like crescents or half-moons. The aorta has a right coronary cusp, a left cusp, and a noncoronary cusp. Immediately distal to these cusps are recessed pockets, or outpouchings, of the aorta, called sinuses of Valsalva. These sinuses house the openings, or ostia, of the coronary arteries. The sinuses help protect the ostia from the rush of blood through the aortic valve and prevent the valve leaflets from occluding the openings. There are three sinuses, each of which is associated with one cusp of the aortic valve. The right sinus is related to the coronary cusp, where the ostium of the right coronary artery is located. The left sinus is behind the left cusp and houses the ostium of the left coronary artery. The noncoronary cusp is so named because no coronary artery is associated with its sinus.

The greatest volume of blood entering the right and left atria from their respective veins flows passively through the open AV valves into the ventricles. The pressure in the ventricles begins to rise. As the pressure rises, the AV valves begin to close. The atria contract, forcing the AV valves to reopen and the remainder of blood in the atria to be propelled into the ventricles. This is diastole.

The pressure in the ventricles is now greater than that in the atria. The AV valves close, the semilunar valves open, and blood is ejected from the ventricles. This is systole. The ventricular pressure is now less than the atrial pressure because blood is continuously filling the atria. The semilunar valves close, the AV valves open, and the cycle continues.

The right heart is concerned with the pulmonary circulation, moving blood to the lungs for oxygenation. The left heart is concerned with the systemic circulation, delivering oxygenated blood to the tissues (Figure 30-12; see Figure 30-11).

Blood from the head and neck are drained by the right and left innominate veins into the SVC. The flow of blood from the SVC, the IVC (draining the body), and coronary sinus (draining the heart) empty into the right atrium. It then flows through the tricuspid valve into the right ventricle. From here the blood flows through the pulmonary valve into the main pulmonary artery. The main pulmonary artery branches into a right pulmonary artery to the right lung and a left pulmonary artery to the left lung. This is the pulmonary circulation.

Oxygenated blood returns to the left atrium via four pulmonary veins. From the left atrium it passes through the mitral valve into the left ventricle and through the aortic valve into the ascending aorta. Blood fills the head and neck vessels, the innominate, the left common carotid, and left subclavian arteries and continues down the descending aorta. This is systemic flow.

Cardiac Perfusion and Drainage

The coronary arteries perfuse the heart muscle and inner structures and are so named because they form a corona, or crown, around the heart. There are two main coronary arteries: the right coronary artery arising from the right sinus of Valsalva and the left coronary artery arising from the left sinus (Figure 30-13, A).

The right coronary artery courses in the atrioventricular groove separating the atria from the ventricles. It gives off a muscular branch and a marginal branch and continues around the heart posteriorly until it anastomoses with, or joins, the left circumflex coronary artery. At this anastomosis the right coronary artery gives off a branch called the *posterior descending coronary artery*, which travels along the posterior interventricular septum.

The left main coronary artery divides almost immediately into the left circumflex and the left anterior descending coronary arteries. The left circumflex extends around the heart posteriorly until it joins the right coronary artery, as mentioned. The left anterior descending coronary artery travels downward anteriorly along the interventricular septum, giving off muscular branches, or septal perforators. It curves posteriorly to meet the posterior descending coronary artery.

The veins that drain the heart do not form a corona, though they usually course with the arteries. They are simply called cardiac veins (Figure 30-13, B). Most of the veins drain into the coronary sinus, a large vein that serves as a reservoir. From here it empties into the right atrium through the thesbian valve. The veins that do not drain into the sinus drain directly into the right atrium.

Normal variations in coronary artery anatomy and perfusion must be taken into account when an evaluation of them is needed for diagnostic purposes.

Cardiac Conduction System

The cardiac conduction system is the mechanism by which the heart is made to effectively pump blood through the vessels. The muscle fibers of the heart have the inherent ability to contract without a nerve stimulus. However, if each fiber contracted independently, the heart would not be very effective in getting blood to the tissues.

The cardiac conduction system is a specialized group of cardiac muscle, nodes, tracts, and fibers that can generate and conduct electrical impulses through heart muscle, causing a synchronous, coordinated contraction or heartbeat (Figure 30-14).

The sinoatrial node, or SA node, sets the pace of the heart. It is therefore called the pacemaker of the conduction system. The electrocardiogram (ECG, or sometimes called EKG) measures the electrical activity of the conduction system and indirectly myocardial activity. As the SA node fires, electrical impulses travel through

Text continued on p. 559

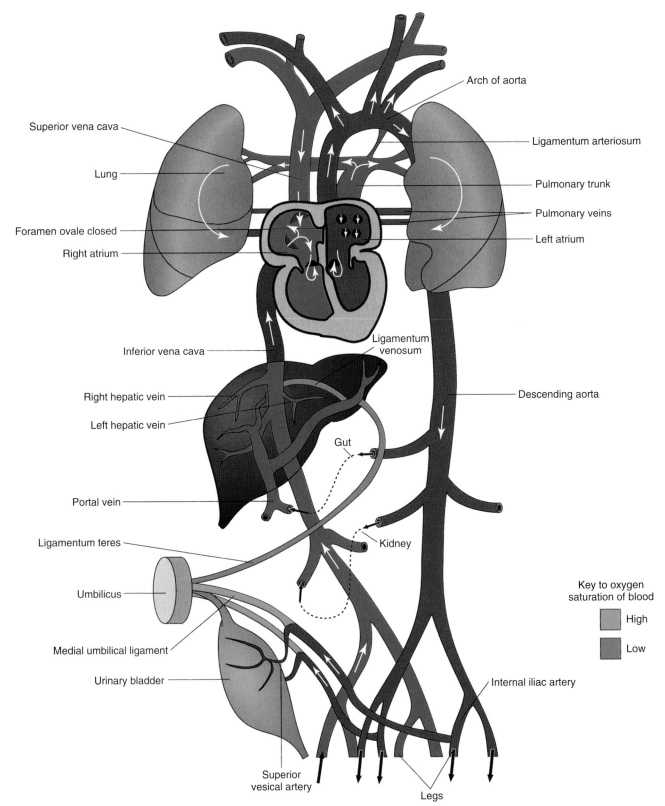

FIGURE 30-12 **Neonatal Circulation.** Adult derivatives of the fetal vessels and structures that become nonfunctional at birth are also shown. Arrows indicate the course of the neonatal circulation. The organs are not drawn to scale. After birth, the three shunts that short circuited the blood during fetal life cease to function, and the pulmonary and systemic circulations become separated.

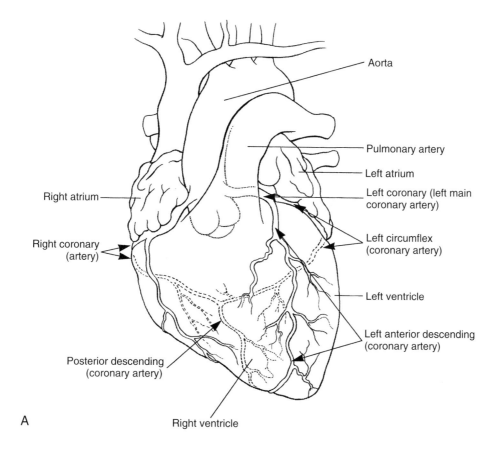

Aorta

Pulmonary artery

Left atrium

Right atrium

Left coronary (left main coronary artery)

Left circumflex (coronary artery)

Right coronary (artery)

Left ventricle

Left anterior descending (coronary artery)

Posterior descending (coronary artery)

A

Right ventricle

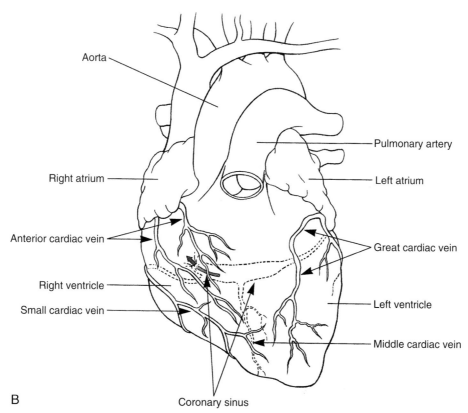

Aorta

Pulmonary artery

Right atrium

Left atrium

Anterior cardiac vein

Great cardiac vein

Right ventricle

Small cardiac vein

Left ventricle

Middle cardiac vein

B

Coronary sinus

FIGURE 30-13 **A,** Coronary arteries and their positions on the heart. **B,** Cardiac veins. These are anterior, or ventral, views. The dashed lines indicate the position of the vessels as viewed from the posterior, or dorsal, surface of the heart.

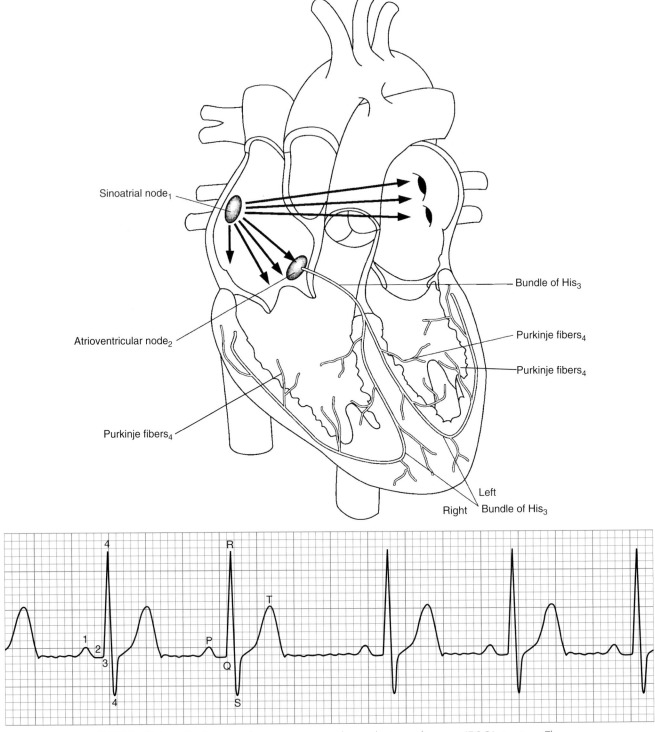

FIGURE 30-14   Cardiac conduction system and an electrocardiogram (ECG) tracing. The numbers on the ECG corresponding with the numbers indicated on the heart diagram relate the electrical activity of the heart to the waveform of the ECG.

internodal tracts to both atria, SA_1. On the ECG this is reflected by the P-wave signaling that atrial contraction is about to take place. Contraction occurs at once.

At the same time that impulses are passing through the atria, they also travel to the **atrioventricular node**, or **AV node**, located in the medial wall of the right atrium. There is a very brief delay in the activation and transmission of the AV node. This is reflected on the ECG as the end of the P-wave, labeled *2* on the tracing and AV_2 on the heart diagram. After this delay the AV node fires, sending impulses along the **bundle of His** located superficially on the interventricular septum. From here the impulses travel through the **Purkinje fibers** into the myocardium. The ventricles contract at once from above downward. The QRS deflection on the ECG reflects this transmission and is numbered *3* and *4* on the tracing. BH_3 and Pf_4 on the heart diagram reflect this electrical activity.

The T-wave indicates a recovery of electrical charge in the ventricles or return of the myocardium to a resting state. The next cycle begins with another P-wave.

Normal pacemaker (SA node) rates (beats/min) at various ages are as follows:

SA Node Rate	Age
100 to 180	0 to 1 month
110 to 180	1 year
60 to 120	5 years
55 to 110	10 years
50 to 100	Adult

Cardiac muscle, as mentioned earlier, has the inherent ability to contract without a nerve stimulus. However, stimulation by the autonomic nervous system (ANS) affects the rate of SA node firing and also the coronary arteries.

The sympathetic fibers of the ANS cause an increase in the heart rate. The parasympathetic division, specifically the vagus nerve, or tenth cranial nerve, causes the heart rate to slow down.

PHYSIOLOGY

The heart is the primary organ of the circulatory system, providing the force that propels blood through all the vessels of the body.

The basic functions of the heart are to distribute oxygenated blood to all parts of the body and to receive deoxygenated blood from the head and body for transportation to the lungs.

SONOGRAPHIC APPEARANCE

In sonography of the heart, we use 2-D (2-dimensional), 3-D (3-dimensional), M-mode, Doppler (color, tissue imaging, and contrast), pulsed-wave (PW) Doppler, and continuous-wave (CW) Doppler ultrasonic techniques to get the most complete, accurate diagnostic information.

In color-flow imaging the color sector is usually narrowed or "coned" as much as possible to see only the area of interest. This yields better resolution or detail. Structures outside of the coned area may be poorly visualized or not seen at all, depending on the equipment used and how the color wedge is presented.

Doppler tissue imaging uses the same principles of color Doppler, except the target is the heart muscle rather than blood flow within the heart. Contrast echocardiography used along with a perfluorocarbon-based agent to opacify the blood in the heart was developed to improve resolution of the heart wall.

These various techniques have their advantages and disadvantages. However, in doing an echocardiogram, all are needed to perform a thorough examination that will give the clinician the information needed to properly diagnose the patient.

When performing 2-D sonography, it is important that the equipment is set to as wide a gray scale (shade of gray) as possible. This will greatly aid in recognizing and differentiating normal tissue from disease tissue (intramural masses).

On the 2-dimensional image, the heart muscle (myocardium) has a soft, homogeneous, even-textured echogenicity. The appearance ranges from medium- to low-gray intensity. The valves and chordae appear more echogenic than the myocardium. The valves will appear as thin, flexible lines that are freely mobile. The pericardium is the most echogenic structure, having a smooth, fluid-like, linear appearance.

Figure 30-15 shows the plane of sound through the heart in the parasternal long axis view. Figure 30-16 shows echocardiographic images in the parasternal long axis view and their schematic representations, respectively. Note the structures and their positions relative to one another. Also note that the left ventricular apex is not seen in this view.

Basic M-mode (for time-motion mode) scanning includes measurements taken at the aortic valve level, the mitral valve level, and the chordal level in the left ventricle (Figure 30-17).

Figure 30-18 shows an M-mode tracing of the left ventricle. Note the chordae on the inner surface of the left ventricular posterior wall. Figure 30-19 is a tracing at the mitral valve level. The echogenic areas seen in the right ventricle after each QRS complex are artifacts caused by inspiration of air into the lungs. The tracing of the aortic valve is shown in Figure 30-20, taken from the short axis view.

The planes of the short axis views through the heart are shown in Figure 30-15.

Figure 30-21 shows the echocardiographic image in the parasternal short axis view at the aortic valve level. Note that the commissure, or closure line, between the noncoronary and left coronary cusp of the aortic valve

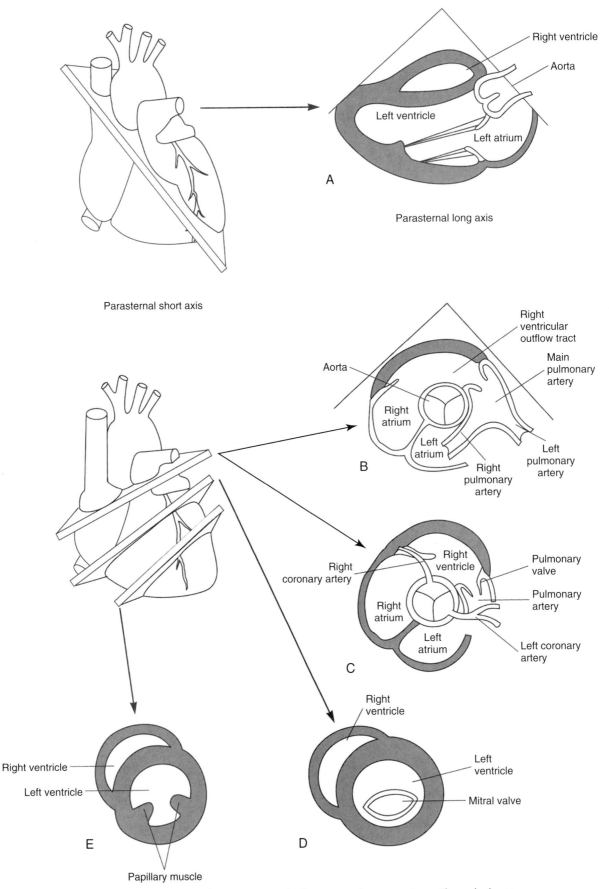

FIGURE 30-15 Parasternal Long Axis and Short Axis Planes, or Cuts, Through the Heart. A, Echocardiographic sketch of the parasternal long axis view. B, Parasternal short axis view at the level of the aortic valve. C, Short axis view showing the coronary arteries. D, Short axis view at the level of the mitral valve. E, Short axis view at the level of the papillary muscles.

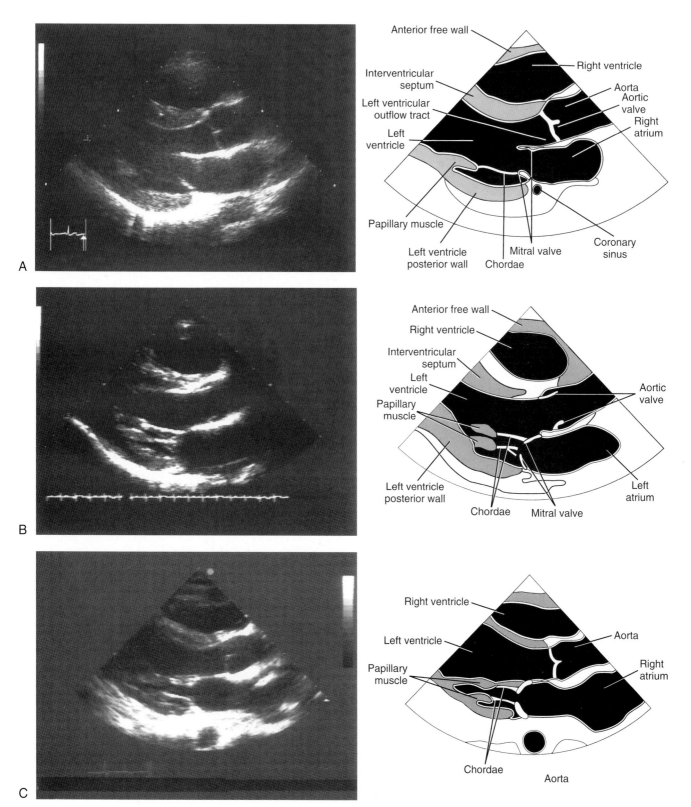

FIGURE 30-16 Echocardiographic Images in the Parasternal Long Axis View. **A,** Diastolic frame. **B,** Systolic frame. **C,** Late diastolic frame.

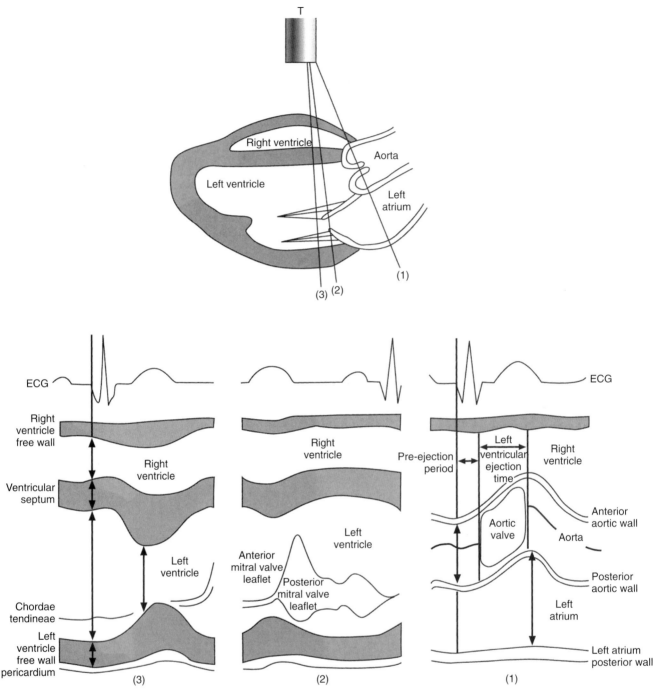

FIGURE 30-17 Parasternal long axis view, indicating cuts at the various levels where M-mode tracings will be recorded. The lower diagram is a schematic of an M-mode tracing at the various levels shown in the upper diagram. Currently, M-mode tracings are also being done in parasternal short axis views. (Redrawn from Park MK: *Pediatric cardiology for practitioners*, ed 5, St. Louis, 2008, Mosby.)

is not well visualized. This occurs because of the orientation of the plane of sound, which strikes the structure parallel rather than perpendicularly. However, all three commissures are usually very well seen in this view. Figure 30-21, *C* and *D*, show color flow in this short axis view. Flow is seen in the right atrium passing through the tricuspid valve into the right ventricular outflow tract. It then moves through the pulmonary valve into

the main pulmonary artery. From here, the blood flows into the right and left pulmonary artery branches toward their respective lung. Figure 30-21, *E*, is a pulsed-wave (PW) Doppler tracing of the pulmonary valve. The velocity is within normal limits.

The mitral valve level is seen in Figure 30-22. The left ventricle should appear as a concentric circle; the anterior and posterior mitral valve leaflets should appear

Text continued on p. 566

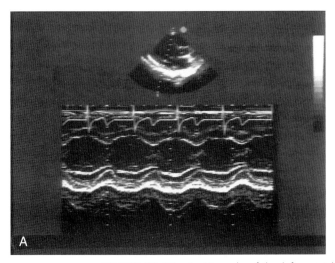

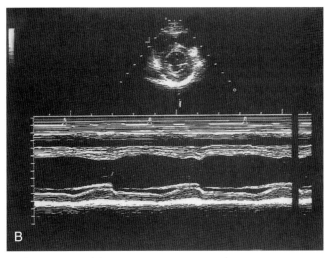

FIGURE 30-18 **A**, M mode of the left ventricle in the parasternal long axis view. **B**, M mode of the left ventricle in the parasternal short axis view.

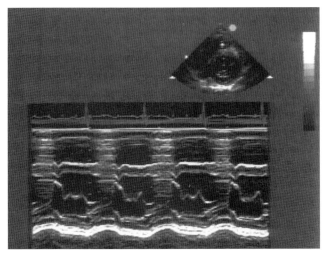

FIGURE 30-19 M-mode tracing of the mitral valve in the parasternal short axis view.

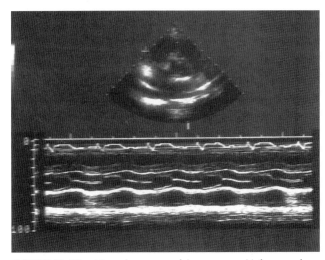

FIGURE 30-20 M-mode tracing of the aorta and left atrium from the parasternal short axis view.

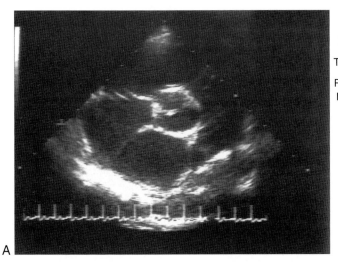

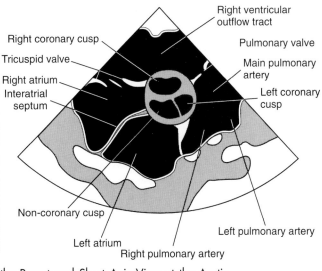

FIGURE 30-21 Echocardiographic Images in the Parasternal Short Axis View at the Aortic Valve Level. **A**, With the valve closed.

Continued

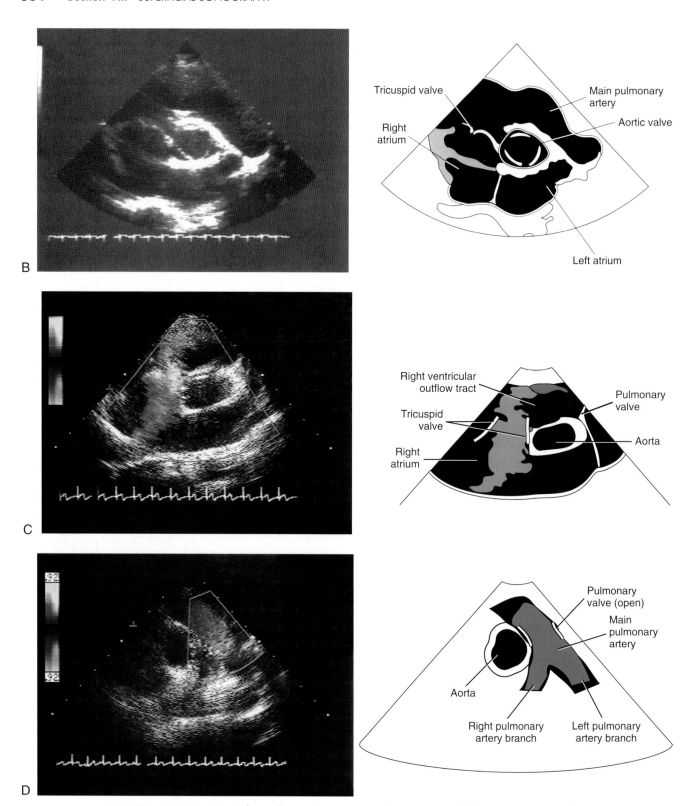

FIGURE 30-21, cont'd Echocardiographic Images in the Parasternal Short Axis View at the Aortic Valve Level. **B,** With the valve open. **C,** Parasternal short axis view showing color flow through the tricuspid valve. Note the blue color as the flow turns to move away from the transducer. **D,** As flow continues from **C,** it is going away from the transducer through the pulmonary valve and into the right and left pulmonary branches.

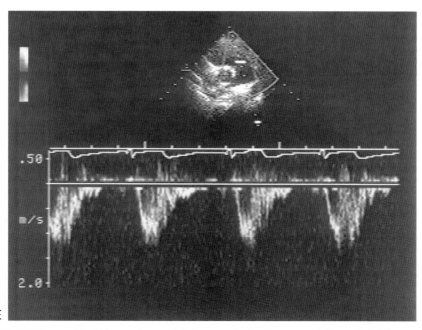

FIGURE 30-21, cont'd Echocardiographic Images in the Parasternal Short Axis View at the Aortic Valve Level. E, Pulsed-wave Doppler at the pulmonary valve with normal velocity.

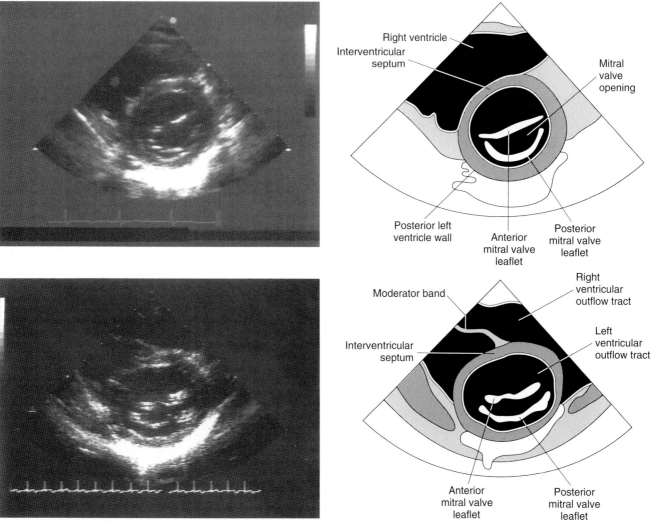

FIGURE 30-22 Echocardiographic Images in the Short Axis Plane at the Level of the Mitral Valve.

within the circle toward the posterior aspect of the cavity. In real time the leaflets should open symmetrically and appear unrestricted in their movement. The left ventricular outflow tract is seen anterior to the mitral valve. The left ventricular walls should contract and relax concentrically and smoothly. The right ventricle is often seen in this view. It should look like a half-moon, adjacent to the interventricular septum. The moderator band may also be visualized.

The echocardiographic image and schematic of the papillary muscle level are shown in Figure 30-23. Again, the left ventricle should appear as a concentric circle. The anterolateral papillary muscle is seen at its usual position, 3 or 4 o'clock. The posteromedial papillary muscle is most often positioned at 8 o'clock. Note the areas of the interventricular septum, the anterior and anterolateral walls, the posterior lateral wall, and the inferoposterior wall of the left ventricle.

The apical views include the apical four-chamber and the apical long axis (Figure 30-24). There is also an apical two-chamber view, not shown, visualizing the left atrium and ventricle only. The apical four-chamber view is great for Doppler interrogation of the mitral valve. The apical long axis puts the aortic valve in an excellent position for a Doppler study.

Echocardiographic images of the four-chamber view are shown in Figure 30-25. All four cardiac chambers are visualized, as well as the tricuspid and mitral valves. There may be an artifactual dropout of echoes in the midportion of the interatrial septum. The interventricular septum is usually seen in its entirety. It is usually possible to visualize the four pulmonary veins entering the left atrium. However, confirmation can be realized only by Doppler examination. Figure 30-25, *A*, shows a color-flow image in this view. The flow is across the mitral valve. Figure 30-25, *B*, is an image of

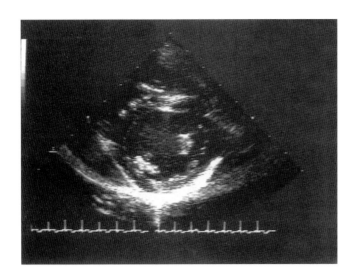
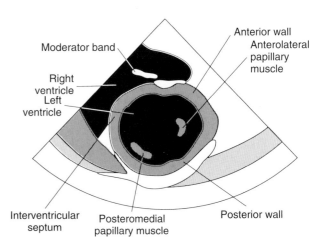
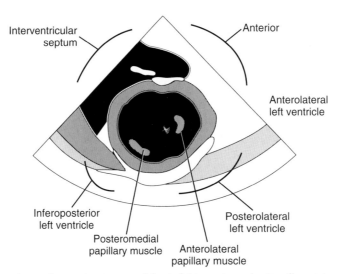

FIGURE 30-23 Echocardiographic Image of the Left Ventricle at the Papillary Muscle Level.

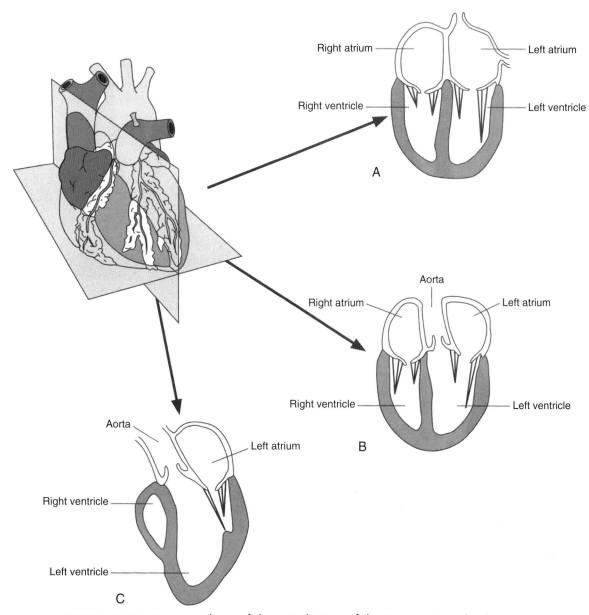

FIGURE 30-24 Scanning Planes of the Apical Views of the Heart. **A,** Four-chamber view. **B,** Five-chamber view. **C,** Apical long axis view. (Redrawn from Park MK: *Pediatric cardiology for practitioners,* ed 5, St. Louis, 2008, Mosby.)

the PW Doppler tracing of the mitral valve in a different patient. In the apical long axis view note the left atrium, mitral valve, left ventricle, left ventricular outflow tract, aortic valve, and ascending aorta (Figure 30-26).

Subcostal views provide a wealth of information (Figure 30-27). The subcostal four-chamber view is used mainly to interrogate the interatrial septum. In this view the septum is perpendicular to the plane of sound, giving the best possible image of the structure (Figure 30-28). The entire heart and surrounding area can be seen very well in this view, making it excellent for determining situs and optimum for detecting pericardial effusions (Figure 30-29).

Figure 30-30 visualizes the suprasternal planes; see Figure 30-30, *A,* for the long axis view of the aorta. Figure 30-31 shows echocardiographic images and simplified diagrams, respectively, of the long axis of the aorta. The ascending aorta, transverse arch, and descending aorta are shown. The innominate artery, left common carotid artery, and left subclavian artery are visualized leaving the arch. The right pulmonary artery is cut in cross section and is seen as a circular structure in the inner curvature of the arch.

Figure 30-32 offers an excellent image of the long axis of the right ventricular inflow tract. In some patients all

Text continued on p. 574

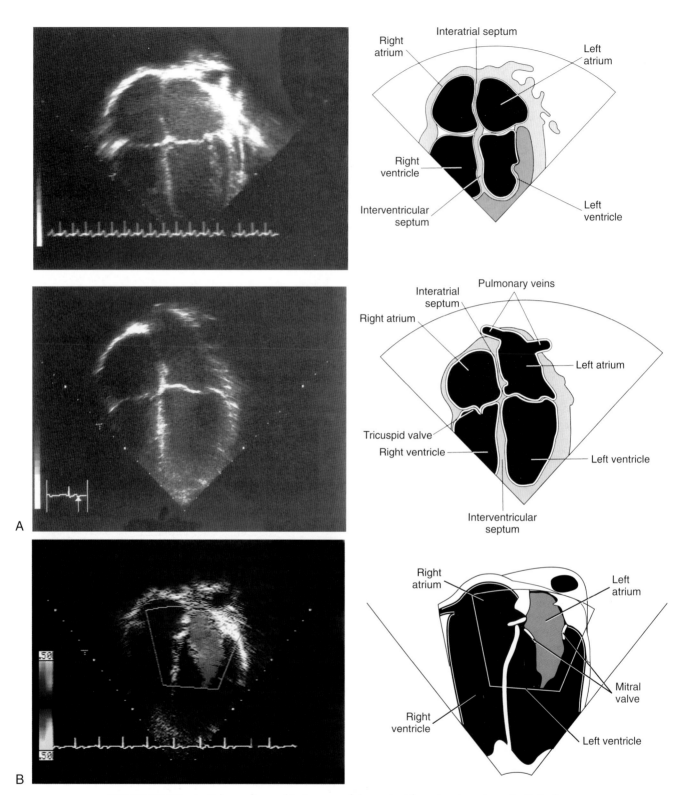

FIGURE 30-25   **A,** Echocardiographic images of the apical four-chamber view. **B,** Color-flow Doppler of the mitral valve. Echocardiographic image of inflow from the left atrium through the mitral valve into the left ventricle. The flow is red because it is moving toward the transducer positioned at the apex. Note the laminar flow (no turbulence).

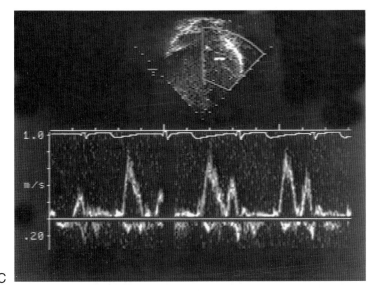

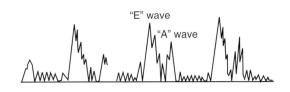

FIGURE 30-25, cont'd C, Pulsed-wave Doppler of the mitral valve. Pulsed-wave Doppler of mitral inflow. Again, note the laminar flow indicated by lack of echoes between the waves.

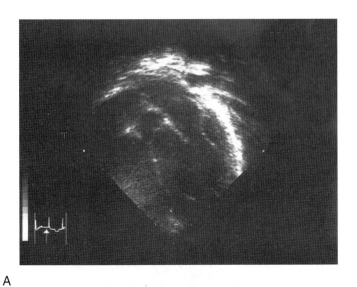

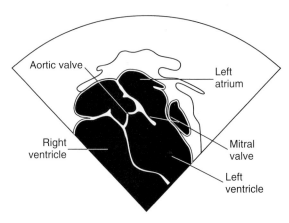

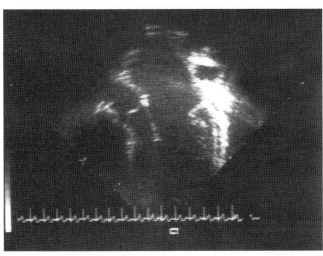

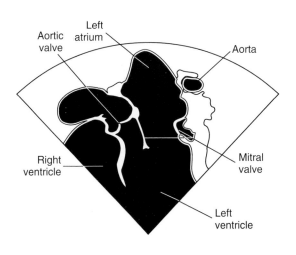

FIGURE 30-26 A, Echocardiographic images in the apical long axis view of two patients. Both are shown in the anatomically correct position.   *Continued*

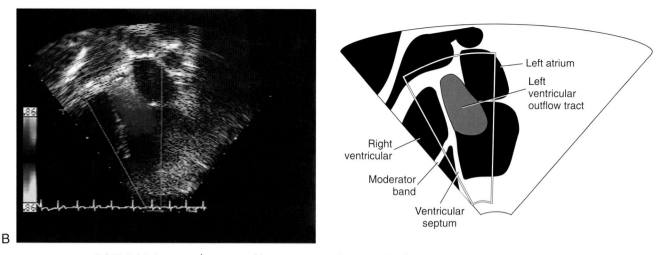

B

FIGURE 30-26, cont'd   B, Apical long axis view showing color flow in the left ventricular outflow tract, through the aortic valve and a limited section of the ascending aorta. The transducer is at the apex of the heart, with the flow moving away from it. Therefore the blood flow is shown in blue.

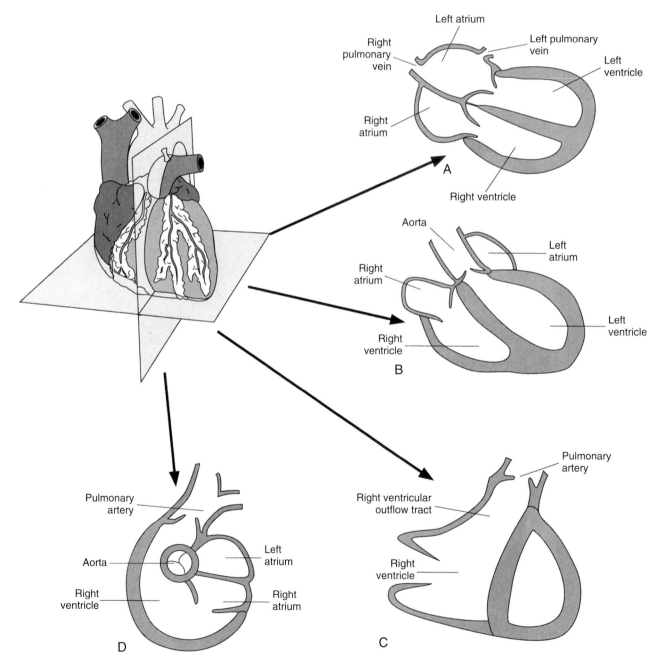

FIGURE 30-27   Four Planes in the Subcostal Position. A, Four-chamber. B, Five-chamber. C, Long axis of right ventricular outflow tract. D, Short axis at aortic valve level. (Redrawn from Park MK: *Pediatric cardiology for practitioners,* ed 5, St. Louis, 2008, Mosby.)

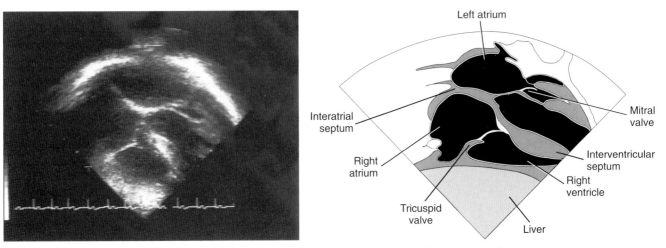

FIGURE 30-28 Echocardiographic Image in the Subcostal Four-Chamber View for Interrogation of the Interatrial Septum.

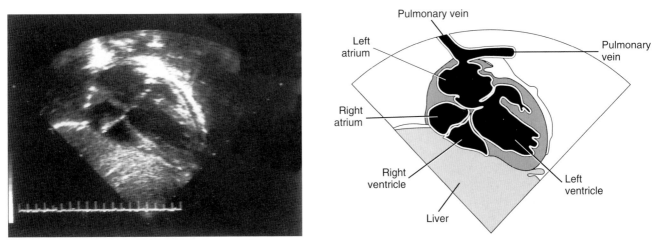

FIGURE 30-29 Subcostal Four-Chamber View Showing the Heart and Surrounding Area.

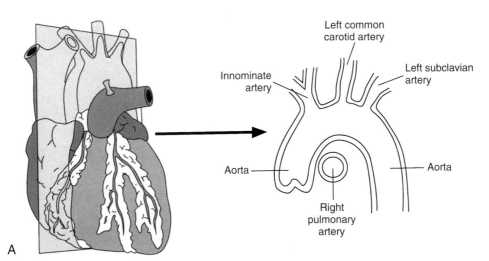

FIGURE 30-30 Schematic of the Planes of Sound Through the Heart in the Suprasternal Position. A, Long axis view.

Continued

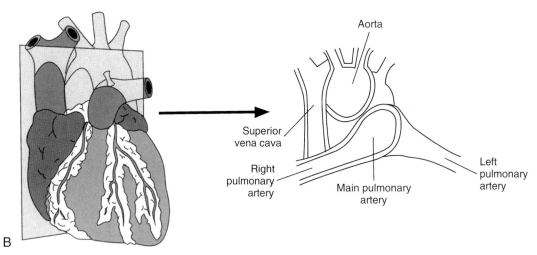

FIGURE 30-30, cont'd   Schematic of the Planes of Sound Through the Heart in the Suprasternal Position. **B,** Short axis view. (Redrawn from Park MK: *Pediatric cardiology for practitioners,* ed 5, St. Louis, 2008, Mosby.)

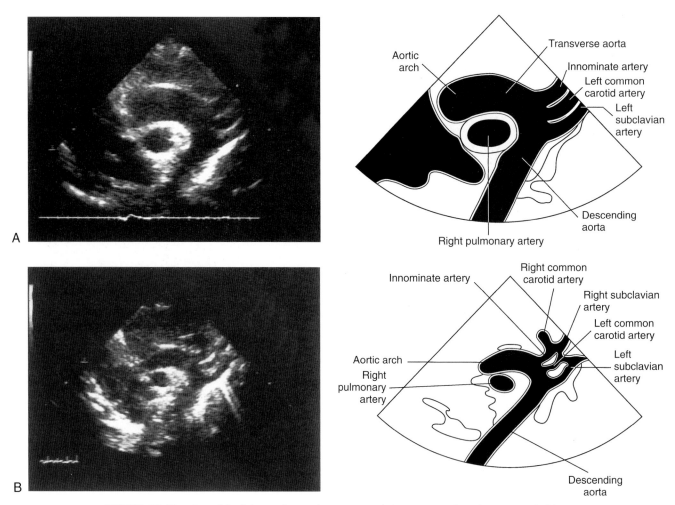

FIGURE 30-31   **A** and **B,** Echocardiographic images of the aortic arch in long axis. **B,** Note the bifurcation of the innominate artery into the right subclavian and right common carotid arteries.

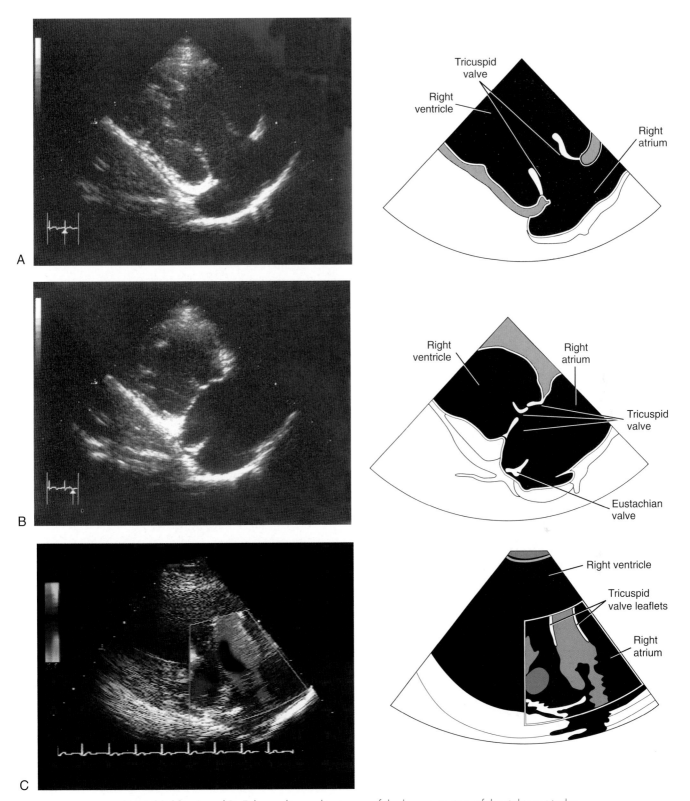

FIGURE 30-32 **A** and **B**, Echocardiographic image of the long axis view of the right ventricular inflow tract. **A**, Diastolic image. **B**, Systolic frame. **C**, Color-flow Doppler of the right ventricular inflow tract. The flow is toward the transducer from the right atrium through the tricuspid valve into the right ventricle.

three papillary muscles and chordae may be seen. Note the eustachian valve in the right atrium marking the entrance of the inferior vena cava.

See Figure 30-32, *C*, for a color-flow image across the tricuspid valve. The long axis view of the right ventricular outflow tract is shown in Figure 30-33. It includes the right ventricular outflow tract, pulmonary valve, main pulmonary artery, and the right and left pulmonary artery branches.

Views of the coronary arteries from the parasternal, short axis view, aortic valve level are shown in Figure 30-34. This view, with minor angulations, should yield excellent images of the right and left coronary artery ostia and their positions in the sinuses. The long axis of the coronary sinus as it empties into the right atrium is seen in Figure 30-35.

Figure 30-36 shows sagittal plane sections of the heart. Figure 30-36, *A*, is at the level of the long axis view of the left ventricular outflow tract, aortic valve, and ascending aorta. Figure 30-36, *B*, is of the right ventricular outflow tract and the pulmonary valve. Figure 30-36, *C*, is a short axis view of the heart at the aortic valve level. The long axis of the superior and inferior venae cavae entering the right atrium is shown in Figure 30-37.

All first-time studies should include subxiphoid views for general orientation, a view of the positions of the coronary artery ostia in the parasternal short axis view, and the suprasternal notch view for the arterial and venous head/neck vessel connections and positions, if possible.

SONOGRAPHIC APPLICATIONS

Echocardiography is an aid in diagnosing congenital structural and flow abnormalities of the heart, including:

- Atria septal defects/patent foramen ovales
- Ventricular septal defects
- Patent ductus arteriosus
- Coarctation of the aorta
- Tetralogy of Fallot
- Transposition of the great arteries
  Echocardiography also helps:
- Rule out intracardiac masses and tumors
- Assess and monitor heart size and function in patients on continual medical therapy that may affect the heart, such as chemotherapeutic drugs
- Monitor patients with conditions that directly or indirectly affect the heart, such as sickle cell anemia and Kawasaki disease

Text continued on p. 578

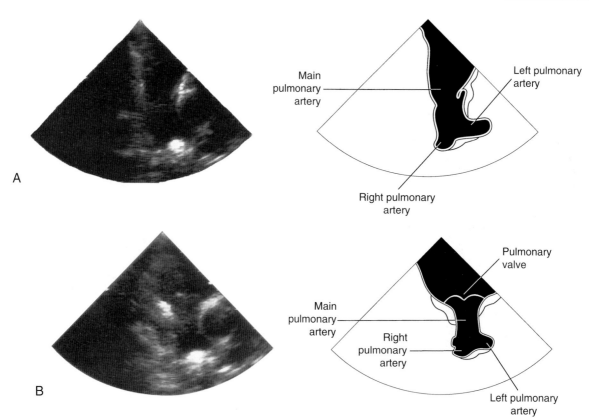

FIGURE 30-33 Echocardiographic Image of the Parasternal Long Axis of the Right Ventricular Outflow Tract. **A,** Systolic frame with the pulmonary valve open. **B,** Diastolic frame with the pulmonary valve closed.

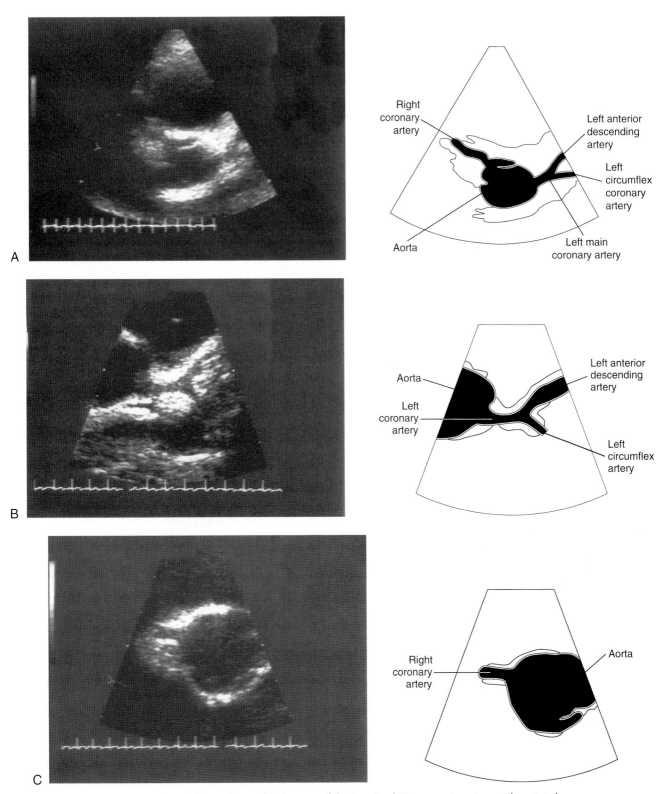

FIGURE 30-34 **Echocardiographic Images of the Proximal Coronary Arteries as They Exit the Aorta. A,** View of the RCA, LCA and bifurcation, LAD, and LCX. Part of the aortic valve leaflets is seen within the aorta. **B,** Image of the LCA and branches. **C,** RCA. *LAD,* Left anterior descending coronary artery; *LCA,* left coronary artery; *LCX,* left circumflex coronary artery; *RCA,* right coronary artery.

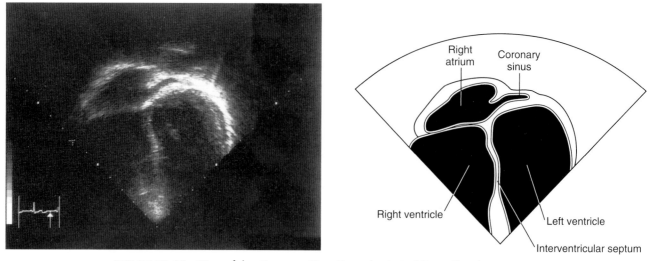

FIGURE 30-35   View of the Coronary Sinus From the Apical Four-Chamber Position.

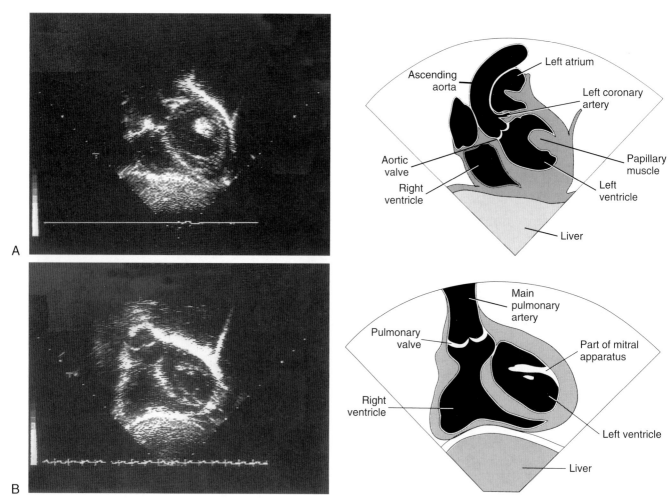

FIGURE 30-36   **A,** Subcostal short axis, or sagittal, view of the heart showing the left ventricular outflow tract, aortic valve, and ascending aorta. Note the left main coronary artery. **B,** Subcostal or subxiphoid short axis view demonstrating the right ventricular outflow tract, pulmonary valve, and main pulmonary artery.

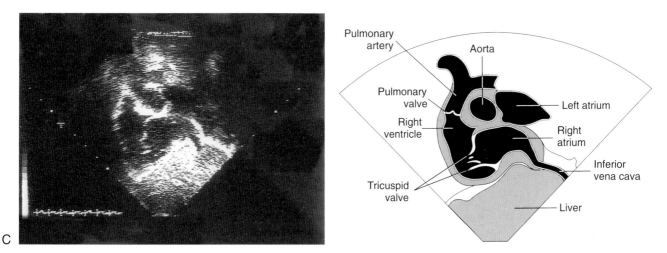

FIGURE 30-36, cont'd   C, Subxiphoid short axis, aortic valve level, showing left and right atrium, tricuspid valve, right ventricular outflow tract, and main pulmonary artery.

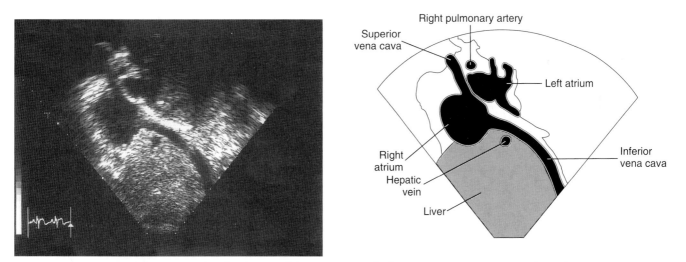

FIGURE 30-37   Subxiphoid View of the Superior and Inferior Venae Cavae Entering the Right Atrium.

- Evaluate the results of medical treatment and surgical repair of diseases of the heart
  Using pulsed- and continuous-wave Doppler:
- Congenital valvular stenosis can be diagnosed. The valvular velocities in the pediatric heart range from approximately 0.8 m/s to not over 1.5 m/s. Color-flow imaging will show the stenosis as turbulence (mosaic pattern). Valvular regurgitation (backflow) can also occur and can be seen with color-flow Doppler.

NORMAL VARIANTS

- **Dextrocardia:** A condition in which the heart is located in the mediastinum as a mirror image of its normal position, the ventricular apex being rightward.
- **Mesocardia:** A condition in which the apex is directed to the left as normal but with the heart itself being more medially positioned within the chest.

REFERENCE CHARTS

■ ■ ■   ASSOCIATED PHYSICIANS

- **Radiologist:** Specializes in the diagnostic interpretation of imaging modalities that aid in the diagnosis of heart disease.
- **Cardiologist:** Specializes in the diagnosis and treatment of the diseases of the heart and related vessels.
- **Thoracic surgeon:** Specializes in the structural modification of the heart in the treatment of heart disease.

■ ■ ■   COMMON DIAGNOSTIC TESTS

- **Chest x-ray:** This test, recorded on photographic film, provides a picture of the ribs, lungs, and heart. If the possibility of congestive heart failure is considered, this study aids in determining whether the heart is abnormally enlarged and whether there is fluid in the lungs. The test is performed by a radiologic technologist and interpreted by a radiologist.
- **Electrocardiogram (ECG; sometimes called EKG):** This test monitors or measures the electrical activity of the heart and indirectly the heart muscle. Electrodes are placed on various positions on the chest and on each wrist and ankle. The electrodes are connected to a machine that amplifies the electrical impulses of the heart and records them on graph paper. A stress ECG may be done to measure the electrical activity of the heart during exertion, such as exercise on a treadmill. This test is usually performed by an ECG technician or a cardiologist and interpreted by a cardiologist.

- **Cardiac scan:** This scan involves the injection of a radioactive substance while a special camera traces its movement through the heart. By identifying increased activity, "hot spot" imaging shows areas of heart muscle damage resulting from an infarct. A thallium scan will indicate areas where heart muscle is not receiving oxygen. A blood pool scan will reveal how efficiently blood is moving through the heart. This test is performed by a nuclear medicine technologist and interpreted by a radiologist or cardiologist.
- **Electrophysiologic study (EPS):** A catheter with electrodes attached to the end is placed through the femoral vein and guided to the heart. One electrode is placed near the sources of electrical activity, the SA node, and the bundle of His. Another electrode may be guided through the subclavian vein into the right ventricle. This study maps the electrical activity of the heart and is used to help diagnose patients with various arrhythmias. It is more accurate than an ECG because the electrodes are closer to the source of the electrical activity. This test is performed by an EPS technician and cardiologist. It is a sterile procedure.
- **Cardiac catheterization:** Catheterization is a sterile procedure in which 1 or more catheters are introduced into a vein or artery and guided to the heart. The catheter can be used to assess intracardiac pressures, retrieve samples of blood for testing (oxygen content), and inject a contrast agent to render the heart visible on film. This test is used to evaluate chambers, valves, and coronary arteries. Cardiac catheterization is performed by cardiologists assisted by radiologic/cardiac technicians. The examination is interpreted by the cardiologist.
- **Transesophageal echocardiography (TEE):** In this procedure a very small probe (transducer/endoscope combination) is placed in the mouth and advanced into the esophagus down to the stomach. Images of the heart in multiple planes are taken from the stomach and the esophagus. From these positions within the body, the view of the heart is unobstructed by bone, small rib spaces, increased body mass, and air in the lungs. Heart structures are well visualized, especially posterior structures that are not well seen from a transthoracic approach. The study is performed by a cardiologist with the help of a sonographer who operates the ultrasound equipment. The cardiologist interprets the study.
- **Stress echocardiography:** This is a procedure in which the echocardiogram is performed while the patient is stressed (the heart rate is caused to be increased by some method). There are 3 basic types or methods of increasing the heart rate: treadmill, bicycle, and pharmacologic. There are many indications for doing a stress echocardiogram. A major indication is visualization of wall-motion abnormalities in coronary artery disease. The study is performed by a cardiologist or designate, a treadmill technologist, and a sonographer. A cardiologist interprets the study.

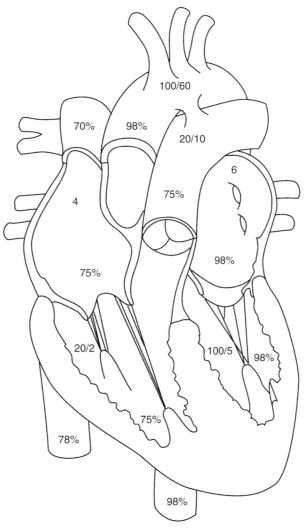

■ ■ ■ LABORATORY VALUES

The laboratory values for the heart are shown below in Figure 30-38. Note that the oxygen content in the pulmonary circuit is lower than in the systemic circuit. Normal oxygen content on the right side is usually between 65% and 80%. Oxygen content on the left side ranges between 95% and 100%. The pressures on the left side are normally higher than those on the right side, with right-sided systolic pressures being about one fourth to one fifth of those on the left.

FIGURE 30-38 Laboratory Values for the Heart. The percentages show the relative oxygen saturations of the blood in the various vessels and cavities of the heart. The numbers with the slash between them show the normal systolic and diastolic pressures, respectively. The pressure values in the atria are diastolic since they have no systolic pressure.

■ ■ ■ VASCULATURE

Aorta—right and left coronary arteries—right and left coronary artery branches—heart muscle and structures—capillaries—cardiac veins—right atrium or coronary sinus—to right atrium.

■ ■ ■ AFFECTING CHEMICALS

- **Epinephrine:** A hormone secreted by the adrenal medulla that causes increased heart rate and blood pressure.
- **Thyroid hormone:** A hormone secreted by the thyroid gland that regulates overall body metabolism and causes an increase in the heart rate.

CHAPTER 31

Adult Echocardiography

J. CHARLES POPE III

OBJECTIVES

Describe the location of the heart in the chest.

Describe the sonographic appearance of the heart.

Describe the imaging planes of the heart.

Identify cardiac anatomy in the various imaging planes.

Describe cardiac hemodynamics and physiology.

Describe the phases of the cardiac cycle and relate them to intracardiac events.

Learn the normal values for heart chamber sizes, wall thickness, and Doppler flow velocities.

Identify normal Doppler flow patterns.

Discuss the indications for transesophageal echocardiography (TEE).

Identify the most common reasons for obtaining a TEE.

Discuss the intraoperative use of TEE.

Describe the standard TEE echocardiographic images.

■

KEY WORDS

Aortic Valve — Semilunar valve between the left ventricle and aorta.

Apical View — Can visualize all 4 heart chambers in this view; also known as *subcostal* or *subxiphoid* view.

Atrioventricular (AV) Node — Second section of the conduction system; located near the inferior portion on the right side of the interatrial septum.

Atrioventricular Valves — Valves located between atria and ventricles.

Atria — The two upper cavities of the heart.

Bundle of His — Part of the final segment of the conduction system; divides into the right and left bundle branches, which run down the interventricular septum and help distribute the electrical impulse to the ventricular muscle fibers, thereby causing mechanical contraction.

Chordae Tendineae — Fibrous bands that attach the tips of the atrioventricular valve (tricuspid and mitral) leaflets to papillary muscles located in the ventricles.

Continuous Wave (CW) — Form of spectral Doppler used to provide hemodynamic information. Transducer sends out continuous sound waves to record information.

Coronary Arteries — Arise from the right and left sinuses of Valsalva and provide oxygen to the heart.

Coronary Sinus — Drains deoxygenated blood from the heart and empties into the right atrium.

Doppler — Used to derive hemodynamic information about the heart. Spectral Doppler is divided into three forms: pulsed wave (PW) and continuous wave (CW) and Tissue Doppler Index (TDI).

Endocardium — Thin layer of endothelial tissue lining the internal surface of the heart.

Epicardium — Smooth, thin outer layer of the heart.

Eustachian Valve — Can be seen in the right atrium near the entrance of the inferior vena cava.

Inferior Vena Cava — Major blood vessel that drains lower extremities and abdominal pelvic cavity; empties into the right atrium.

Mitral (Bicuspid) Valve — Valve between left atrium and left ventricle.

M Mode — Tool for evaluating subtle changes or rapid movements of the heart that the eye may not see during the real-time examination.

Myocardium — Thick layer of contractile muscle between the endocardium and pericardium.

Parasternal — Long axis echocardiography view that transects the heart from the base to the apex.

Pericardium — Sac that contains the heart. This sac contains a small amount (10 to 20 mL) of serous fluid that lubricates the heart as it beats.

Pulmonic Valve — Valve between right ventricle and pulmonary artery.

Pulsed Wave (PW) — Form of spectral Doppler used to provide hemodynamic information about the heart. Transducer sends out pulsed sound to record information.

Purkinje Fibers — Fibers that innervate the ventricular myocardium and help distribute the electrical impulse to the ventricular muscle fibers, thereby causing mechanical contraction.

Semilunar Valves — Aortic and pulmonary valves.

Sinoatrial (SA) Node — Electrical impulses from the SA node spread over both atria by way of internodal pathways, causing them to contract at the same time (atrial systole).

Superior Vena Cava — Major blood vessel draining upper extremities and head; empties into the right atrium.

Suprasternal — Transducer placement that allows visualization of the ascending and descending aorta and the aortic arch, as well as the vessels that arise from it.

Tissue Doppler — Form of spectral Doppler that measures the motion of the myocardium.

Transesophageal Echocardiography (TEE) — Transducer inserted into esophagus to obtain echocardiographic images.

Transthoracic Echocardiography (TTE) — "Traditional" form of echocardiography in which transducer is placed on the thorax to obtain images of the heart.

Tricuspid Valve — Atrioventricular valve between right atrium and ventricle.

Ventricles — Two inferior chambers of the heart.

■

■ ■ ■ NORMAL M-MODE MEASUREMENTS

Structure	Measurement
Aortic root dimension	1.9 to 4.0 cm
Aortic cusp separation	1.5 to 2.6 cm
Left atrial dimension	1.9 to 4.0 cm
Mitral valve excursion	1.6 to 3.0 cm
Mitral valve E-F slope	70 to 150 mm/sec
Left ventricular end diastolic dimension	3.5 to 5.7 cm
Left ventricular ejection fraction	0.55%
Left ventricular fractional shortening	0.25%
Interventricular septal thickness	0.6 to 1.2 cm
Posterior left ventricular wall thickness	0.6 to 1.2 cm
Right ventricular dimension	0.7 to 2.7 cm

The heart is the center of the cardiovascular system. It is a muscular organ, nearly the size of your fist, that beats over 100,000 times every day. The heart's main function is to pump unoxygenated blood to the lungs and oxygenated blood to the vessels and tissues of the body.

The echocardiogram is a noninvasive diagnostic test used to evaluate the structural and hemodynamic relationships within the heart. It is an important tool used to assess overall cardiac function.

PRENATAL DEVELOPMENT

See Chapter 25, Fetal Echocardiography, and Chapter 30, Pediatric Echocardiography.

LOCATION

The heart lies within the thoracic cavity, obscured by bone and lung. Located posterior to the sternum, the heart is situated between the right and the left lung within a space called the *middle mediastinum* (Figure 31-1). The heart lies at a 45-degree angle, between the third and fifth intercostal spaces.

The heart sits within a sac called the **pericardium**. This sac contains a small amount (10 to 20 mL) of serous fluid that lubricates the heart as it beats.

The lower border of the heart forms a blunt point called the *apex*, which is formed by the tip of the left ventricle. It is directed to the left of the midline and sits more inferiorly and anteriorly than the base of the heart, where the great vessels arise.

The superior border of the heart is formed by the **atria**. The inferior portion is almost entirely right ventricle and only a small portion of the left ventricle.

The anterior surface of the heart is composed almost entirely of the right ventricle, though a small portion of the right atrium and left ventricle can be seen. The left heart covers the posterior surface.

The right atrium makes up the right border of the heart, and the left ventricle, along with a small portion of the left atrium, covers the left border.

SIZE

The size of the heart depends on a person's age, weight, and sex. The American Society of Echocardiography has set standards by which the heart should be measured. These measurements will be discussed further in the section on M-mode echocardiography.

GROSS ANATOMY

The heart is a muscular four-chambered pump located in the center of the chest. Internally, it is divided into two collecting chambers (atria) and two pumping chambers (ventricles). A system of connecting arteries and veins allows the heart to move blood from systemic to pulmonary circulation and back (Figure 31-2).

The walls of the heart consist of three layers: (1) the **epicardium**, the smooth, thin outer layer; (2) the **myocardium**, the thick layer of contractile muscle; and (3) the **endocardium**, the thin layer of endothelial tissue lining the internal surface.

The two upper cavities of the heart are the right and left atria. From the superior portion of each atrium is a small triangular extension called an *appendage*. The appendages are also called *auricles* (because they resemble ears). Within the appendages and extending out to the anterior surfaces of the atria are the pectinate

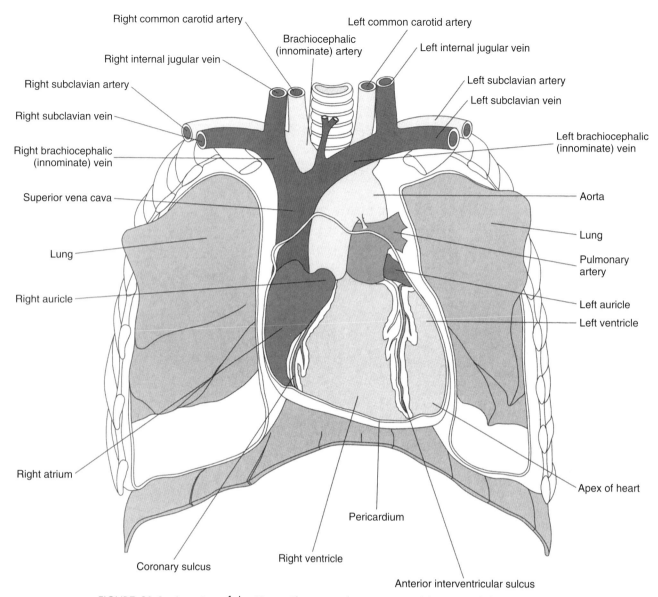

FIGURE 31-1 **Location of the Heart.** The external structures and location of the heart in the thoracic cavity.

muscles. The remaining endocardial surfaces of the atrial walls are smooth.

The atria are separated medially by the interatrial septum. Along this septum is a thinner oval region known as the *fossa ovalis*. This corresponds to the foramen ovale in the fetal heart.

The right atrium receives deoxygenated blood from all parts of the body, including itself. The blood returning from the peripheral tissues enters the heart via the inferior and superior venae cavae. The coronary sinus also enters the right atrium and drains the vessels that had supplied the heart. The left atrium, on the other hand, receives blood from the lungs via four pulmonary veins.

The two inferior chambers are the right and left **ventricles**. The ventricles have thicker walls than do the atria, and the left ventricle is almost three times thicker than the right. This is because the pressure is greater in the left heart than in the right. The right ventricle is also more trabeculated than the left and contains four prominent muscular bands: (1) parietal band, (2) crista supraventricularis, (3) septal band, and (4) moderator band (often seen with ultrasound). Medially, the ventricles are separated by the interventricular septum (IVS).

On the external surface of the heart, the ventricles are separated by the anterior and posterior interventricular sulci. The ventricles are then separated from the atria by

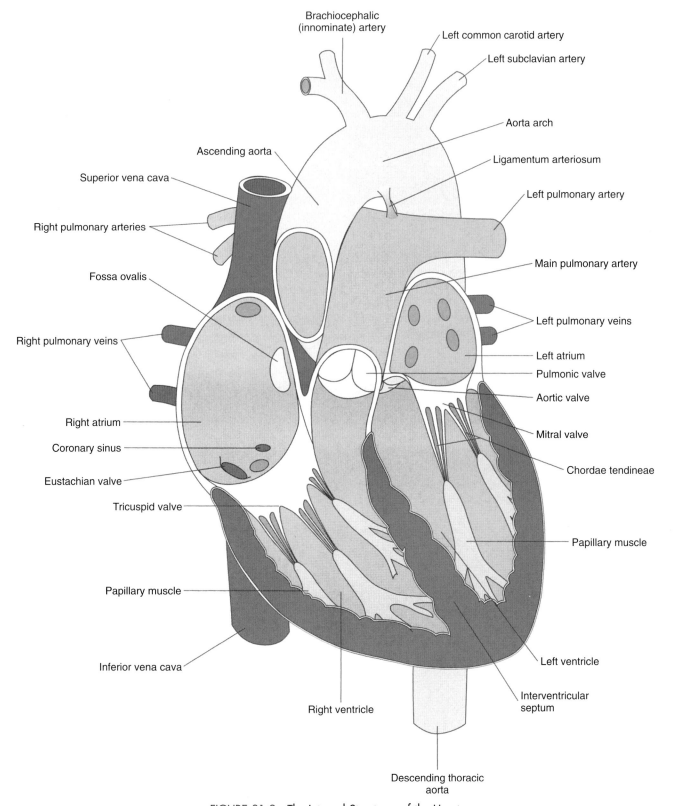

FIGURE 31-2 The Internal Structures of the Heart.

the coronary sulcus. The sulci are grooves that contain the coronary vessels, all of which are embedded in fat. The fat serves to protect the vessels.

Located within the heart are four one-way valves. Their function is to maintain a uniform direction of blood flow. These valves are divided into two groups; atrioventricular and semilunar. The atrioventricular valves are located between the atria and the ventricles and are anchored at one end to the annulosus fibrosus. Chordae tendineae attach the tips of the leaflets to papillary muscles located in the ventricles. Normally, this arrangement keeps blood flowing in one direction only.

The semilunar valves are located at the junction where the ventricles meet the great vessels. They are called *semilunar* because each of the three leaflets is shaped like a half-moon. The pocket shape of the leaflets, as well as the pressure exerted during diastole, closes the semilunar valves and prevents blood from moving backward.

The right-sided atrioventricular valve is called the tricuspid valve because it has three leaflets: anterior, posterior, and septal. The left-sided atrioventricular valve is called the mitral (or bicuspid) valve because of its similar appearance to a bishop's miter. It has two leaflets: anterior and posterior. These are composed of three scallops located both anteriorly and posteriorly.

The two semilunar valves are the aortic valve and the pulmonic valve. The aortic valve is located at the junction of the left ventricle and the aorta. Its three cusps are the right coronary cusp, the left coronary cusp, and the noncoronary cusp. The pulmonic valve is located at the junction of the right ventricle and the pulmonary artery. It has three cusps: anterior, right, and left. Just distal to the aortic valve in the proximal aortic root are outpouchings known as the *sinuses of Valsalva*.

Just as there are three cusps to the valve, there are three sinuses. This is where the coronary arteries originate. The right and left coronary arteries arise from the right and left sinuses of Valsalva. The noncoronary sinus has no artery associated with it.

PHYSIOLOGY

Circulatory System

As blood circulates throughout the body, it carries valuable nutrients and the oxygen required for survival of the tissues. Circulation of the blood is controlled by the heart.

Right heart circulation begins in the right atrium, which collects deoxygenated blood from the entire body (Figure 31-3). Blood returning from the upper portion of the body enters the right atrium via the superior vena cava. Deoxygenated blood from the lower body enters the right atrium by way of the inferior vena cava. The heart also drains deoxygenated blood from itself

through the coronary sinus. This blood also enters the right atrium.

Once the right atrium is full, the oxygen-depleted blood flows through the tricuspid valve and into the right ventricle. The right ventricle then pumps the blood past the pulmonic valve and into the main pulmonary artery. The main pulmonary artery shortly thereafter bifurcates into the right and left pulmonary arteries. These in turn enter each of the lungs, where the blood is reoxygenated in the pulmonary circuit.

Once the blood has passed through the pulmonary capillary circuit and has been reoxygenated, it needs to be collected and distributed to the heart and the rest of the body. This is the function of the left heart. Freshly oxygenated blood is returned from the lungs to the left atrium through the four pulmonary veins. The blood then passes from the left atrium, through the mitral valve, and into the left ventricle. The left ventricle then pumps the blood past the aortic valve and into the aorta. From here, the oxygenated blood is distributed to the heart and the rest of the body through the arterial system. This is the start of systemic circulation.

Cardiac muscle tissue needs a constant supply of fresh blood to remain viable. It accomplishes this through the coronary arterial system. There are two major coronary arteries: the right and the left main coronary arteries. The origin of the coronaries is the aortic root just posterior to the valve in the region of the right and left sinuses of Valsalva.

The left coronary artery differs from the right in that shortly after its origin, the left main artery bifurcates, forming the left anterior descending artery, which usually supplies the anterior left ventricular wall, apex, and a portion of the interventricular septum with oxygenated blood. The other branch is the left circumflex coronary artery, which mainly supplies the left atrium and the lateral and posterior walls of the left ventricle.

The right coronary artery also branches into the posterior descending artery, which supplies portions of the right and left ventricles with oxygenated blood, and the marginal artery, which supplies the right atrium and some of the right ventricle.

The heart also has a venous system that courses over its surface and drains into the coronary sinus. The specific pattern of the arteries and veins may vary among individuals.

Conduction System

The heart has an intricate electrical system composed of highly specialized cardiac muscle tissue. The conduction system is designed to provide continuous electrical stimulation to the heart, ensuring that the various segments of the cardiac cycle progress in the normal, sequential manner.

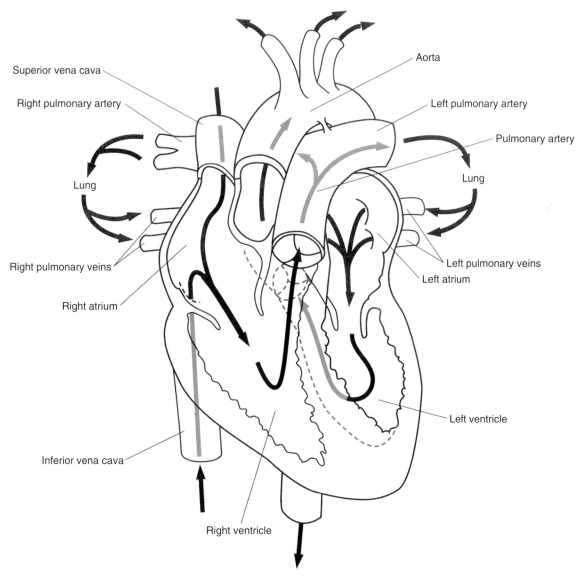

FIGURE 31-3 Cardiac circulation.

The conduction system is composed of four major sections: the **sinoatrial (SA) node**, the **atrioventricular (AV) node**, the **bundle of His** (pronounced *hiss*), and the **Purkinje fibers** (Figure 31-4). Each section has a specific task to perform in regulating the cardiac cycle. In addition to its specific tasks, each portion of the conduction system has its own intrinsic rate of discharge. This allows the different sections of the conduction system to regulate the cardiac cycle in the event of a primary pacemaker failure. The dominant pacemaker of the heart is going to be the one discharging at the highest rate.

Normally the SA node is the pacemaker. It therefore sets the basic pace for the heart rate with a discharge rate of between 60 and 100 beats per minute. Located in the upper portion of the right atrium, near the entrance of the superior vena cava, the SA node receives input from both the sympathetic and parasympathetic nervous systems. Electrical impulses from the SA node spread over both atria by way of internodal pathways, causing them to contract at the same time (atrial systole). This impulse is responsible for the P-wave of the electrocardiogram and, in turn, causes the AV node to depolarize.

The AV node is the second section of the conduction system. It is located near the inferior portion on the right side of the interatrial septum. Its primary task is to delay transmission of the SA nodal impulse long enough to give the ventricles time to repolarize and fill completely. The AV node is responsible for the P-R interval of the electrocardiogram, with an intrinsic

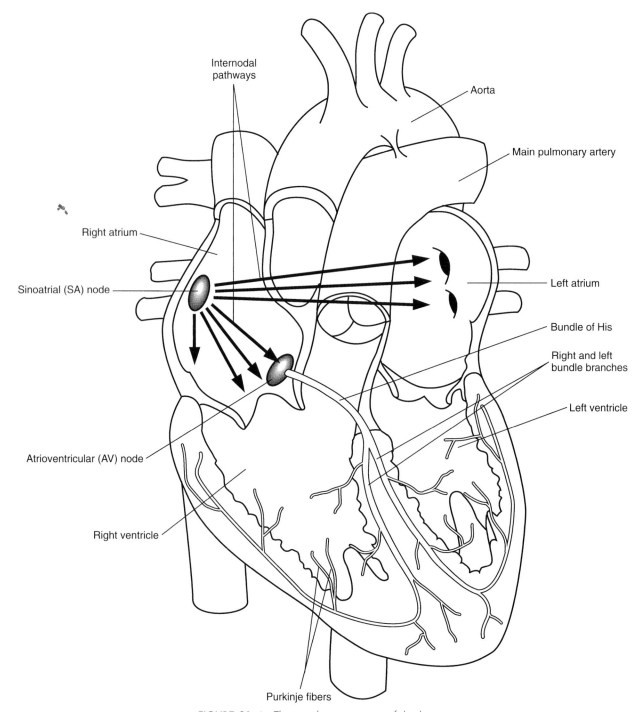

FIGURE 31-4 The conduction system of the heart.

discharge rate of 55 beats per minute. In the event of SA node failure, the AV node is the backup pacemaker for the heart.

The impulse is then delivered to the final segments of the conduction system, the bundle of His and the Purkinje fibers. The bundle of His divides into the right and left bundle branches, which run down the interventricular septum. The Purkinje fibers innervate the ventricular myocardium. Together, they are responsible for distributing the electrical impulse to the ventricular muscle fibers, thereby causing mechanical contraction. This transmission is responsible for the QRS complex noted on the electrocardiogram. The bundle of His and the Purkinje fibers (with discharge rates of 40 to 30, respectively) are next in line in the event of pacemaker failure, with the ventricular myocardium (discharge rate of 20 beats per minute) acting as a final backup in the event of total pacemaker failure.

The Electrocardiogram

The electrocardiogram (ECG, or sometimes called EKG) is composed of a number of different waveforms that represent the electrical impulses of the cardiac cycle. These impulses can be detected on the surface of the body; when electrodes are placed on the skin, the change in the electrical field can be measured. Three distinct waves are recognized and labeled with letters P, Q, R, S, and T (Figure 31-5).

The P-wave and the P-R interval represent the final portion of the cardiac cycle, known as *diastole.* The P-wave appears as a small upward bump. This reflects atrial depolarization caused by the SA node, as the electrical impulse travels through atrial muscle tissue. The atria contract, resulting in atrial systole. The P-R interval reflects the delay in transmission caused by the AV node.

The next downward deflection represents the beginning of the QRS complex, which continues in an upward direction and ends in a downward motion. This reflects the electrical stimulation of the ventricular myocardium, caused by the distribution of the electrical impulse through the bundle of His and the Purkinje fibers. The QRS complex represents the beginning of the portion of the cardiac cycle known as *systole.*

The T-wave of the ECG represents the ventricular repolarization (relaxation) phase of the cardiac cycle and marks the start of the diastolic portion of the cardiac cycle. The S-T segment is a refractory period and begins at the end of ventricular systole to the time of repolarization.

By study of the variations in the sizes of the deflections and the time intervals of the ECG, abnormal cardiac rhythms and conduction patterns can be diagnosed.

Systole/Diastole

The cardiac cycle is categorized into two separate and distinct segments: systole and diastole. Both segments

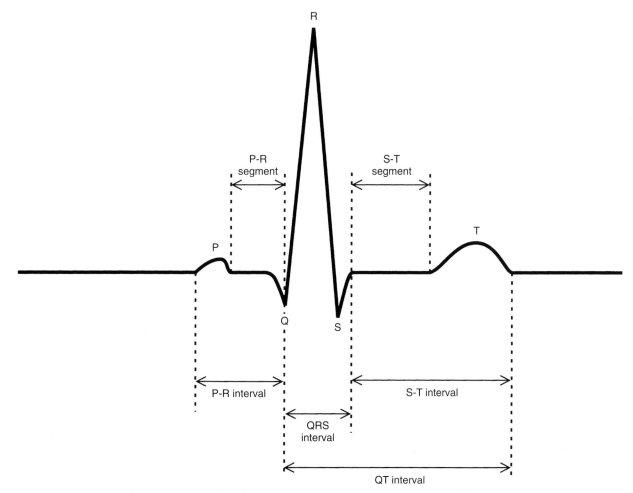

FIGURE 31-5 QRS Complex. Single beat on a normal electrocardiogram (ECG) demonstrating the QRS complex.

contribute significantly to maintaining the cardiac output. A thorough understanding of the systolic and diastolic phases of the cardiac cycle, as well as the hemodynamics (the movement of blood) associated with them, will allow the sonographer to better understand and envision the echocardiographic examination.

Diastole is the left ventricular relaxation and filling phase of the cardiac cycle. Diastole occurs from the end of the T-wave until the beginning of the next QRS complex. During this portion of the cardiac cycle the atria are filling with blood. The AV valves are closed and the ventricular pressures are at or near 0 mm Hg. As pressure in the atria rises to a point above the ventricular pressures, the AV valves open to eject the volume of blood into the ventricles. This is known as the *rapid filling phase* of the cardiac cycle. At that point, ventricular myocardium is relaxed. As pressures rise in the ventricle and fall in the atria, the AV valves begin to drift shut. Just before ventricular systole, the atria contract (corresponding to the P-wave on the ECG) to eject their final volumes of blood into the ventricles. This increases the amount of stretch on ventricular muscle fibers, thereby increasing the force of muscle contraction. During this period of time, the semilunar valves are closed and pressure in the ventricles increases just as the volume of blood increases, before systole.

Systole is the ventricular ejection phase of the cardiac cycle and occurs from the onset of the QRS complex to the end of the T-wave. The ventricular muscle fibers contract. The increase in pressure causes the AV valves to close, preventing backflow of blood and causing the semilunar valves to open. The blood is ejected from the ventricles and enters the aorta and pulmonary artery. As the blood is ejected, the pressure in the ventricles starts to decrease, and in turn, pressure in the atria starts to increase. This sets the stage for the next cardiac cycle.

SONOGRAPHIC APPEARANCE
Two-Dimensional Echocardiography
Sonographically, the pericardium is the most echogenic structure of the heart and is often seen as bright or white in color. Blood or any other fluids appear anechoic or black. The myocardium and papillary muscles are homogeneous and appear sonographically to be composed of medium-gray shades. The thin, mobile leaflets, or valve cusps, have a slightly increased echogenicity when compared with heart muscle, depending on the angle of the ultrasound beam. The views presented here reflect the standards set by the American Society of Echocardiography for two-dimensional echocardiograms.

A **parasternal** long axis view transects the heart from the base to the apex (Figure 31-6). Most anteriorly, the right ventricle will be visualized. This is separated from the left ventricle by the interventricular septum (IVS).

The IVS is continuous with the anterior portion of the aortic root. Only two of the aortic valve leaflets are visualized from this view. The more anterior leaflet is the right coronary cusp, and the more posterior leaflet is the noncoronary cusp. Posterior to the aortic root is the left atrium. The posterior portion of the aortic root is continuous with the anterior mitral valve leaflet. The posterior mitral valve leaflet attaches to the valve annulus, near the atrioventricular groove. Attached to the posterior wall of the left ventricle, the posteromedial papillary muscle may be visualized. The chordae tendineae can be seen to extend from this muscle to the tips of the mitral valve leaflets. The area from the tips of the mitral valve leaflets to the aortic valve is considered the left ventricular outflow tract (LVOT). At the level of the atrioventricular groove a small, echo-free area may be noticed. This represents the coronary sinus. Posterior to the heart another anechoic area is seen. This represents a cross-section of the descending thoracic aorta.

During diastole, the mitral valve is in the open position, allowing the left ventricle to fill with blood, and the aortic valve is closed (Figure 31-7, *A*). As the ventricle fills with blood, the distance between the septal and posterior walls increases. During systole the left ventricle contracts and the walls squeeze closer together. The mitral valve is now closed and the aortic valve is open, allowing blood to leave the left ventricle and enter the aortic root (Figure 31-7, *B*). The patient is connected to an ECG monitor that runs simultaneously along the image. This helps to assist in timing the cardiac cycle.

In a parasternal short axis view at the level of the aortic valve, the great arteries of the heart are visible (Figure 31-8). Centrally located in this view is the aortic valve. This should appear as a circle with a Y in the middle—representing the aortic valve cusps in the diastolic phase of the cardiac cycle—when the leaflets are normally closed. At this point in the cardiac cycle, the right, the left, and the noncoronary cusps are easily visualized. During systole the valve leaflets open to form a triangle (Figure 31-9). The origin of the coronary arteries may be seen at this level near the right and left coronary cusps. Posterior to the aorta, the left atrium can be seen. In some instances the left atrial appendage may be seen jutting off to the right of the screen. The right atrium can be seen on the left side of the screen separated from the left atrium by the interatrial septum (IAS). Moving anteriorly along the left side of the screen, the next structure noted is the tricuspid valve, which separates the right atrium from the right ventricle. The right ventricle is most anterior and can be seen wrapping around the aorta. The right ventricle is separated from the pulmonary artery, which is seen on the right side of the screen, by the pulmonic valve.

The mitral valve can be visualized from a parasternal short axis view. The heart appears as a circle, with the

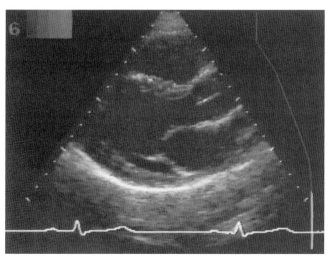

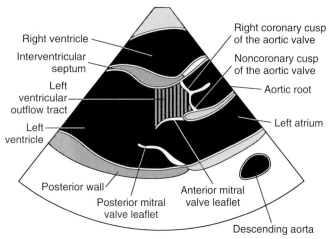

Right ventricle

Interventricular septum

Left Ventricular outflow tract

Left ventricle

Posterior wall

Posterior mitral valve leaflet

Right coronary cusp of the aortic valve

Noncoronary cusp of the aortic valve

Aortic root

Left atrium

Anterior mitral valve leaflet

Descending aorta

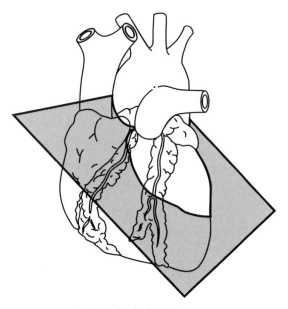

PLANE OF SECTION

FIGURE 31-6 Parasternal long axis view.

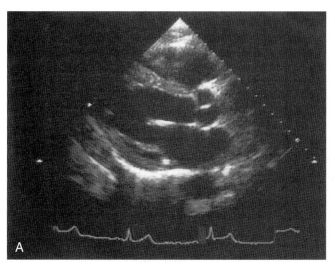

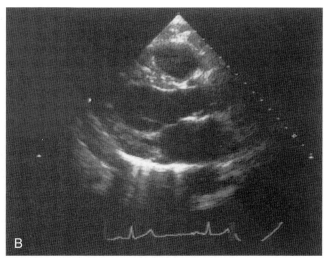

FIGURE 31-7 Parasternal long axis view in diastole (**A**) and systole (**B**).

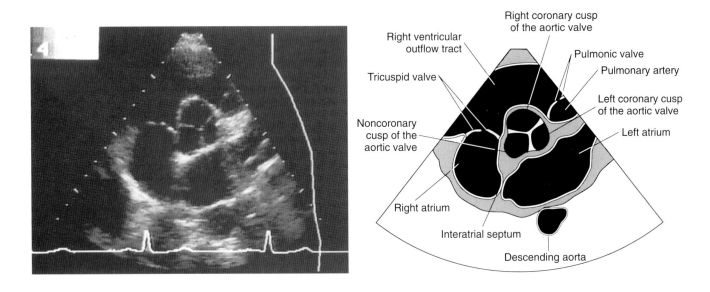

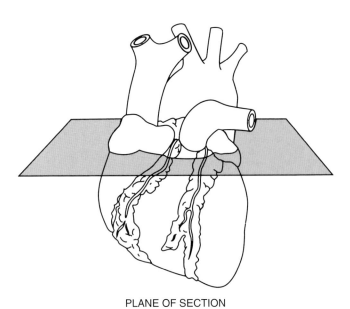

PLANE OF SECTION

FIGURE 31-8 Parasternal short axis view at the level of the aortic valve during diastole.

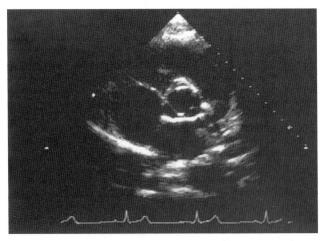

FIGURE 31-9 Parasternal short axis view at the level of the aortic valve during systole.

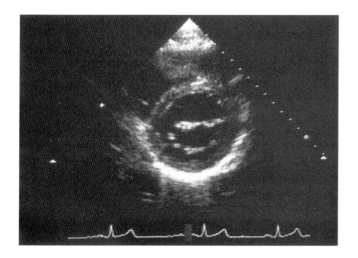

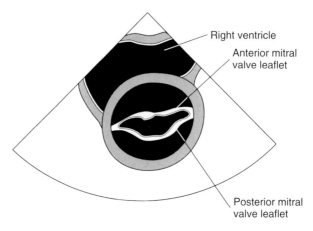

Right ventricle

Anterior mitral
valve leaflet

Posterior mitral
valve leaflet

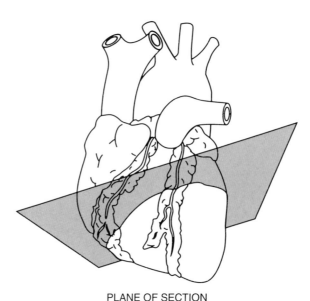

PLANE OF SECTION

FIGURE 31-10 Parasternal short axis view at the level of the mitral valve.

anterior and posterior valve leaflets seen in the center of the image (Figure 31-10). As the leaflets open and close during the cardiac cycle, they look somewhat like the mouth of a fish. Anterior to the left heart is the right ventricle. These structures are separated by the IVS.

At the level of the papillary muscles, the left ventricle again appears as a circular structure, and the papillary muscles protrude from the inner surface of the ventricular wall. Two papillary muscles are visible (Figure 31-11). The posteromedial muscle is seen on the left of the screen, and the anterolateral is seen on the right of the screen. The anechoic area within the left ventricle then takes on the shape of a mushroom. The right ventricle is again anterior to the left ventricle and is separated by the IVS.

Figure 31-12 is an **apical** four-chamber view displaying all four chambers of the heart. The ventricles are displayed at the top of the screen, and the atria are displayed at the bottom of the 2-dimensional sector image. The left ventricle and left atria are displayed on the right side of the screen. The right ventricle and right atria are displayed on the left side of the screen. Wall motion can be evaluated from the apical view by further subdividing the left ventricle into basal (proximal), mid, and apical (distal) walls (Figure 31-13). The apical window also allows views of the inferior and anterior walls in the two-chamber view.

The interventricular septum separates the left from the right ventricle. Deep in the right ventricle, near the apex, the moderator band can be seen to cross from the

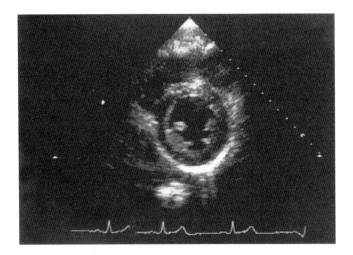

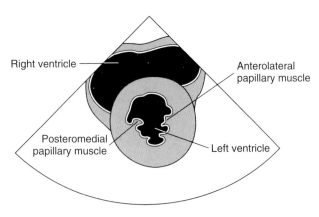

Right ventricle

Anterolateral papillary muscle

Posteromedial papillary muscle

Left ventricle

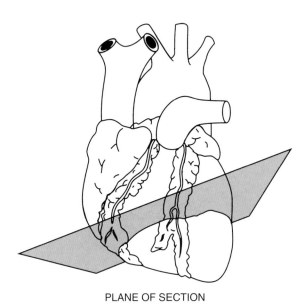

PLANE OF SECTION

FIGURE 31-11 Parasternal short axis view at the level of the papillary muscles.

right ventricular free wall to the interventricular septum. The interatrial septum separates the left from the right atria. The pulmonary veins can be seen entering the inferior portion of the left atrium. Both the anterior and posterior mitral valves can be seen in the left heart, whereas only two of the tricuspid leaflets can be seen in the right heart. The septal leaflet of the tricuspid valve is situated slightly closer to the apex of the heart (normally no more than 1 cm) than the anterior leaflet of the mitral valve.

The aortic root can be imaged along with the other four chambers. This is referred to as an apical five-chamber view (Figure 31-14).

An image of the ascending and descending aorta and the aortic arch, as well as the vessels that arise from it, can be visualized from a **suprasternal** orientation (Figure 31-15). The vessels in descending order are (1) brachiocephalic (or innominate) artery, (2) left common carotid artery, and (3) left subclavian artery. The subcostal view allows a view across the right ventricle from the area of the liver and subxiphoid area. It allows inspection of the right atrium and right ventricle, in addition to tricuspid valve morphology and interatrial septum.

Posterior to the arch, a cross-sectional view of the right pulmonary artery can be seen. In some instances the left atrium can be seen posterior to this.

M-Mode Echocardiography
Two-dimensional imaging is a very powerful diagnostic tool and has superseded the qualitative role of M mode in the echocardiographic examination. Yet M mode is

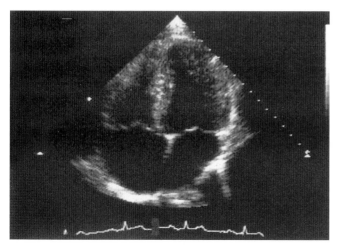

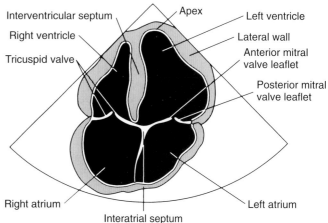

Interventricular septum — Apex — Left ventricle
Right ventricle — Lateral wall
Tricuspid valve — Anterior mitral valve leaflet
Posterior mitral valve leaflet
Right atrium — Left atrium
Interatrial septum

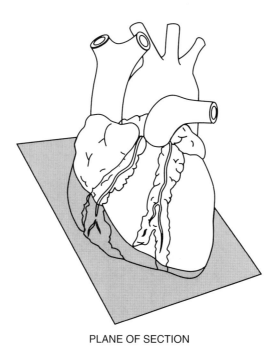

PLANE OF SECTION

FIGURE 31-12 Apical four-chamber view.

still an important supplement to the cardiac examination. It provides a quantitative system through which measurements of cardiac structures can be obtained. Where a structure should be measured and what is considered normal are based on the recommendations of the American Society of Echocardiography. This makes the practice of assessing an M-mode examination consistent.

M mode is also a tool for evaluating subtle changes or rapid movements of the heart that the eye may not see during the real-time examination. Simply put, the *M* in M mode stands for *motion.* Imagine drawing a line through the heart. Everything along that line is por-

trayed on a graph, creating a 1-dimensional reproduction of the cardiac structures.

An M mode is a measure of distance over time. Distance is presented on the X axis and is calibrated by a series of dots that are 1 cm apart. Time is displayed across the Y axis. Here, a series of dots 0.5 second apart are used for calibration (Figure 31-16).

The M mode is most commonly scrolled on paper from a strip chart and appears as a black tracing on a white background.

The anatomy seen at the level of the aortic valve includes the right ventricle anteriorly, the anterior wall of the aortic root, the posterior wall of the aortic root,

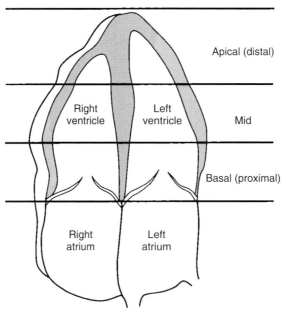

FIGURE 31-13   The subdivisions of the left ventricular walls from an apical four-chamber view.

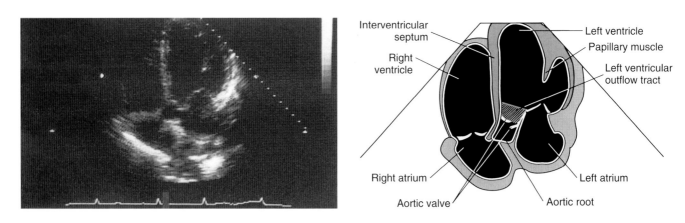

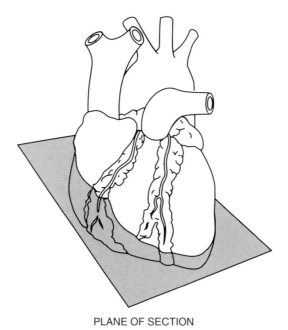

PLANE OF SECTION

FIGURE 31-14   Apical five-chamber view.

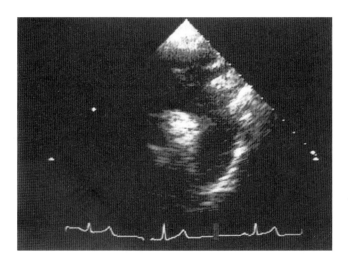

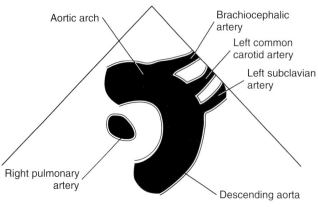

Aortic arch

Brachiocephalic
artery

Left common
carotid artery

Left subclavian
artery

Right pulmonary
artery

Descending aorta

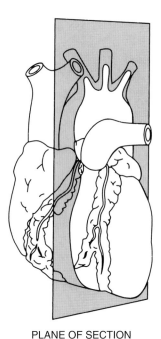

PLANE OF SECTION

FIGURE 31-15 Aortic arch from the suprasternal notch view.

and the left atrium. The aortic valve is seen with the aortic root. Only two cusps are seen from this view: the right coronary cusp anteriorly and the noncoronary cusp posteriorly (Figure 31-17). These cusps can be seen to form a sort of box during systole as blood is ejected from the left ventricle. The closed valve appears as a straight line during diastole.

The mitral valve is a biphasic valve caused by the rapid filling phase of the LV and the atrial "kick" in the latter part of the cardiac cycle (Figure 31-18). The valve is open during diastole and closed during systole. Its biphasic quality causes the motion of the anterior leaflet to appear in the shape of an M. The posterior leaflet mirrors the anterior and appears as a W.

The anterior leaflet of the mitral valve is labeled alphabetically to correspond with the various phases of diastole (Figure 31-19). To begin with, the D point represents the opening of the valve during diastole and the E point represents the maximum excursion of the leaflet. This occurs during the passive filling phase. The anterior leaflet then begins to close. The point where it stops moving posteriorly is the F point. The next peak anterior motion of the mitral valve is the A-wave. This corresponds to atrial contraction and the P-wave on the ECG.

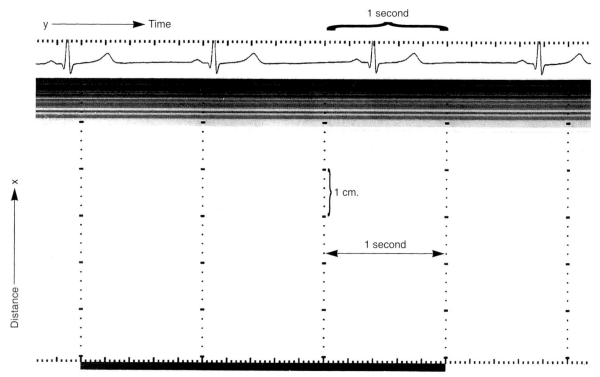

FIGURE 31-16 Proper calibration for an M mode.

Valve closure is appropriately represented by the C point. In some situations, such as diastolic dysfunction of the left ventricle, an additional bump may occur between the A and C points. This abnormal closure of the valve creates what is known as a B notch.

M-mode sampling from the left ventricle is seen in Figure 31-20 on p. 599. Starting anteriorly, the anatomy seen is the right ventricle, the IVS, the left ventricle, and the posterior wall of the left ventricle.

Other areas of the heart can be evaluated by M mode. Generally, the only other structures seen are the valve leaflets from the tricuspid and pulmonary valves. Normally, only one tricuspid valve leaflet is seen with M mode (Figure 31-21 on p. 600). The pulmonic valve is the most difficult to visualize, but it can be especially helpful in patients with pulmonary stenosis or hypertension (Figure 31-22 on p. 601). The pulmonic valve is also labeled using letters A through F.

Doppler Echocardiography

Spectral Doppler and color-flow mapping are two forms of Doppler used to derive hemodynamic information about the heart. Spectral Doppler is divided into 3 forms: pulsed wave (PW), continuous wave (CW), and tissue Doppler. Each form has its advantages and disadvantages but should be used in conjunction to realize their full potential. Tissue Doppler is a newer technique that measures the motion of the myocardium. It is sensitive in picking up diastolic abnormalities of the heart. An extension of this is strain imaging, which can allow systolic evaluation of the heart as well as ejection fraction.

Normal Doppler Waveforms

Normal flow within the heart has a characteristic appearance. When interrogating each valve, it is important to recognize these normal patterns so that any type of disturbance can be fully evaluated. Abnormal flow within the heart indicates increased velocities, regurgitation, turbulence, and abnormal diastolic function.

It is also important to note the direction of flow. Blood moving toward the transducer will be represented above the baseline on the Doppler strip, and flow moving away from the transducer will fall below the baseline. When evaluating a profile, it is important to look at the pattern, velocity, direction of flow, and timing, in accordance with the cardiac cycle.

Doppler is best evaluated when flow is parallel to the transducer. This is not necessarily where the best 2-dimensional image is obtained.

Mitral Valve. Normal mitral flow is biphasic, taking the shape of an M. Like the M-mode tracing, the E-wave is higher than the A-wave. In the apical four-chamber view, flow moves toward the transducer from the left atrium to the left ventricle. Mitral flow therefore is above the baseline and occurs during diastole (Figure 31-23 on p. 601).

Text continued on p. 602

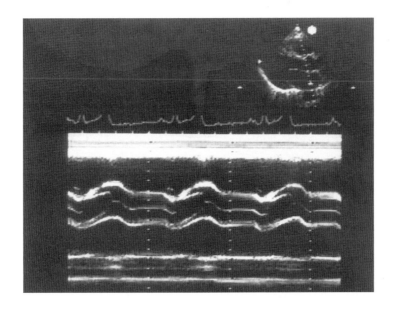

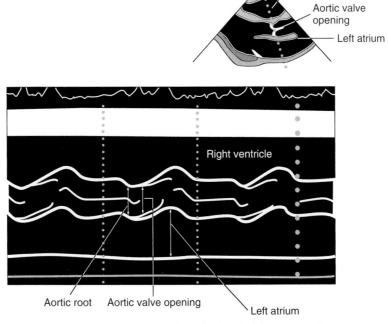

FIGURE 31-17   M mode at the level of the aortic valve.

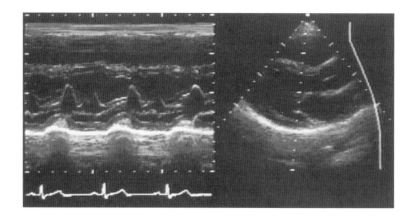

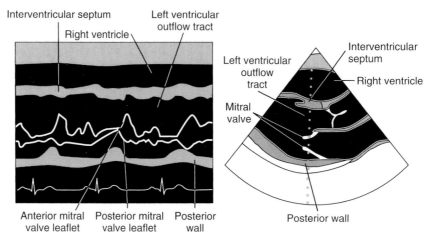

Interventricular septum
Left ventricular outflow tract
Right ventricle
Anterior mitral valve leaflet
Posterior mitral valve leaflet
Posterior wall

Left ventricular outflow tract
Interventricular septum
Right ventricle
Mitral valve
Posterior wall

FIGURE 31-18   M mode at the level of the mitral valve.

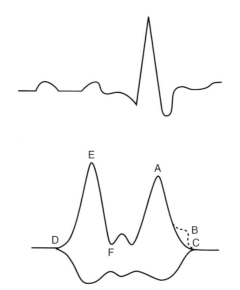

FIGURE 31-19   Proper labeling of the mitral valve.

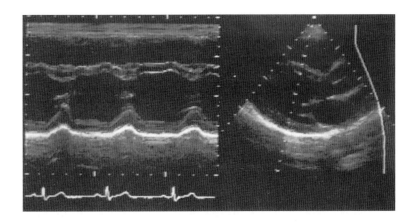

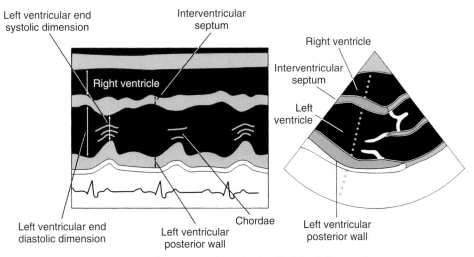

FIGURE 31-20   M mode at the level of the left ventricle.

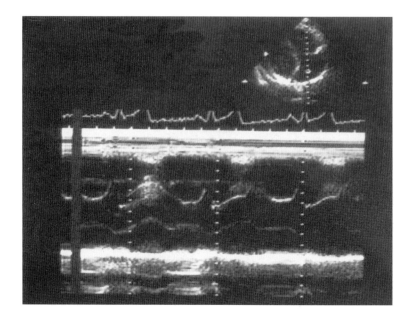

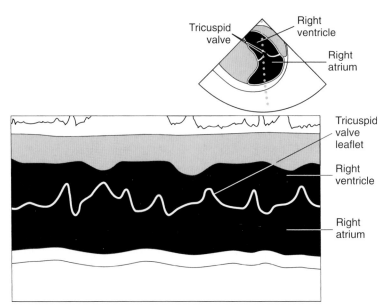

FIGURE 31-21   M mode through the tricuspid valve.

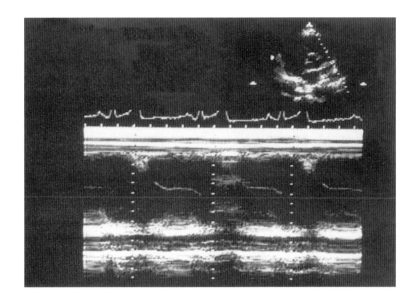

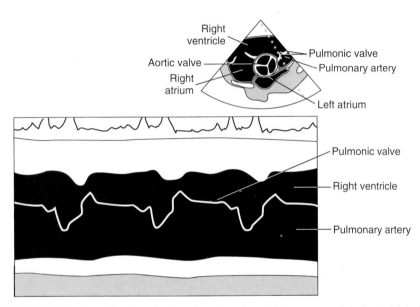

FIGURE 31-22 M mode through the pulmonic valve with its proper alphabetical labels.

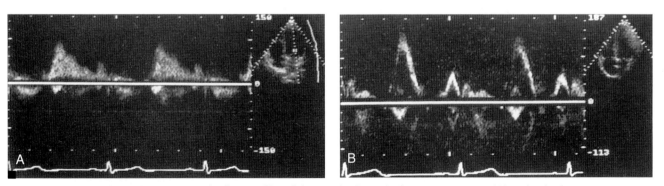

FIGURE 31-23 Doppler flow profiles of the mitral valve in both continuous wave (A) and pulsed wave (B).

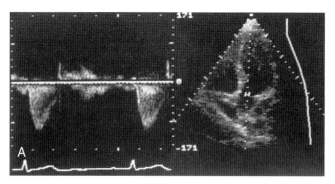
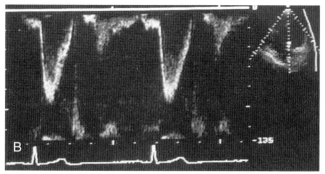

FIGURE 31-24   Doppler flow profiles of the aortic valve in both continuous wave **(A)** and pulsed wave **(B)**.

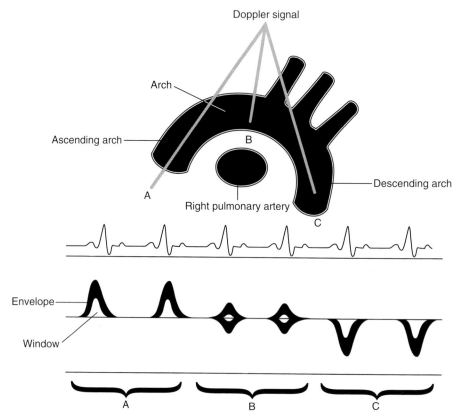

FIGURE 31-25   **Doppler Flow in the Aortic Arch.** As flow moves toward the transducer in the ascending aorta, it appears above the baseline; as flow moves away in the descending aorta, it falls below the baseline.

Aortic Valve. Normal aortic flow is systolic and is shaped like a bullet. When sampled from the apical five-chamber view, blood moves away from the transducer, from the left ventricle to the aortic root. Here, the profile would appear below the baseline (Figure 31-24).

Aortic Arch. Either the ascending or the descending aorta may be evaluated from the suprasternal notch. Depending on how the transducer is angled, flow will appear above the baseline within the ascending aorta

and below the baseline within the descending aorta. Flow will be systolic and bullet shaped (Figure 31-25).

Tricuspid Valve. Normal tricuspid flow is also shaped like an M. It occurs during diastole and appears above the baseline. The velocity range is lower than that for the mitral valve. This is caused by lower pressures found in the right heart (Figure 31-26).

Pulmonic Valve. The systolic flow of the pulmonic valve appears below the baseline and has a bullet shape (Figure 31-27).

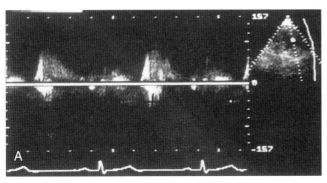

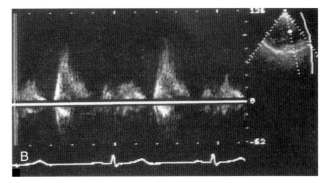

FIGURE 31-26 Doppler flow profiles of the tricuspid valve in both continuous wave **(A)** and pulsed wave **(B)**.

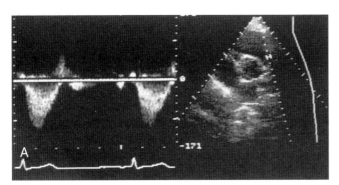

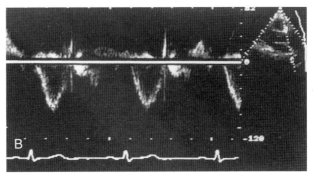

FIGURE 31-27 Doppler flow profiles of the pulmonic valve in both continuous wave **(A)** and pulsed wave **(B)**.

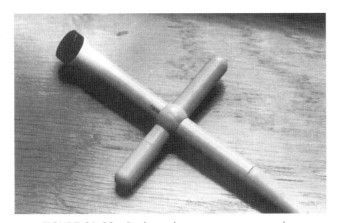

FIGURE 31-28 Dedicated continuous wave probe.

In addition to a duplex Doppler evaluation, which provides an image of the heart along with the Doppler waveform, a dedicated CW Doppler probe may be used (Figure 31-28). This specialized probe provides only the spectral waveform, without the 2-dimensional image.

Transesophageal Echocardiography

Although **transthoracic echocardiography (TTE)** remains the cornerstone of echocardiographic imaging and diagnosis, **transesophageal echocardiography (TEE)** is increasing in use because it provides information not obtainable by the transthoracic approach.

In most labs the most common indication for TEE is evaluation for a cardiac source of embolus. Other common indications include evaluation of prosthetic valves and native valvular disease, infective endocarditis, aortic pathology including aortic dissection, intracardiac masses, and congenital heart disease. Other indications include patients with lung disease, critically ill patients (especially those on a ventilator), and patients with sternal infections or thoracic deformities.

Technically inadequate surface examinations may be the result of a poor acoustic window from the patient's body habitus or other skeletal abnormalities, or chronic obstructive pulmonary disease with hyperinflated lungs. Patients on ventilators or status post open heart surgery with sternal bandages or open sternum are also candidates for TEE. Critically ill patients and patients on ventilators who often have very limited acoustical windows are good candidates for TEE.

Applying the probe requires the patient to be lying in the left lateral decubitus position or in an upright position. The probe is advanced to the oropharynx, and the patient is asked to swallow several times. The neck is flexed. The probe is advanced 30 to 35 cm from the incisors into position.

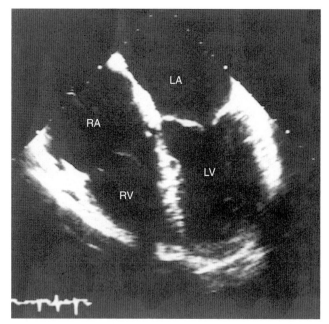

FIGURE 31-29 TEE midesophageal view with four chambers of the heart demonstrated. The left and right atria and ventricles are seen. Note the mitral valve is more visible than the tricuspid valve.

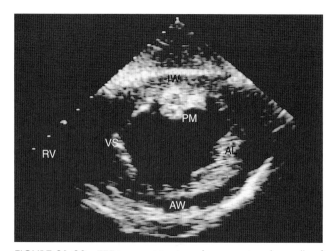

FIGURE 31-30 TEE trangastric view demonstrating the walls of the left ventricle and chamber size. Note the ventricular septum separating the left and right ventricles.

Midesophageal views are short or horizontal views from a longitudinal scan obtained at approximately 30 to 35 cm. At roughly 35 to 40 cm, the four chambers of the heart can be identified (Figure 31-29). Transgastric long axis and short axis views at the 40- to 45-cm range are where the descending thoracic aorta is evaluated with about a 180-degree counterclockwise rotation. The left ventricle and chamber size can be assessed as well (Figure 31-30). On basilar views at approximately the same range, the aorta, right and left atria, and interatrial

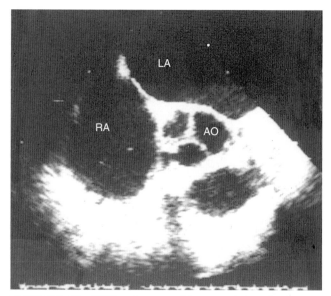

FIGURE 31-31 TEE basilar view of the aorta, left and right atria, and the interatrial septum.

septum can be demonstrated (Figure 31-31). Contrast enhancements may be performed using agitated saline with rapid intravenous injection to rule out any shunting abnormalities.

TEE is often used in the intraoperative setting. It can be used to evaluate valve replacement or repair. TEE can detect air or fat emboli (complications that may occur from operative procedures). Although not recommended as a routine procedure, TEE can also be used to monitor high-risk coronary artery disease to identify wall motion abnormalities that may indicate abnormal left ventricular function.

Three-Dimensional Echocardiography

Three-dimensional (3-D) echocardiography is a new imaging technique that provides an additional window of information regarding cardiac anatomy. The addition of an elevation plane adds X, Y, and Z planes of imaging. The ability to acquire large volumes of data provides a tool for complete 3-D presentation. Application of this new exciting technique includes the following: providing a closer inspection of the mitral valve and aortic valve for surgical planning; evaluation of masses and LV shape; evaluation of complex congenital heart disease; imaging of atrial anatomy; improved inspection of prosthetic valves; and visualization and guidance in various interventional procedures such as EP studies and cardiac catheterizations. An example of a 3-D parasternal image is provided in Figure 31-32. The depth of the LV chamber and mitral valve leaflets can be appreciated in this presentation. Three-dimensional imaging also includes a multiplane format that allows more sophisticated measurements and calculations to be performed.

SONOGRAPHIC APPLICATIONS

Echocardiography is commonly used in the evaluation of the following:

- Cardiac anatomy
- Cardiac size
- Acquired heart disease (stenosis, valve replacement)
- Congenital heart disease
- Coronary heart disease
- Pericardial diseases
- Cardiac tumors/thrombi
- Diseases of the aorta
- Cardiomyopathies
- Hemodynamic information
- Vegetations

NORMAL VARIANTS

- **Eustachian valve:** Can be seen in the right atrium near the entrance of the inferior vena cava. In the fetus, it was a functional valve covering the entrance to the IVC. Only a remnant of the valve is now seen. It is best visualized in the right ventricular inflow view (Figure 31-33).
- **Moderator band:** A normal tissue structure that extends from the anterior free wall of the right ventricle to the IVS. It provides a quick path for the conduction system to reach the ventricular wall. The moderator band is best visualized in the apical four-chamber view (Figure 31-34).
- **Chiari network:** Appears as a fine mobile fiber within the right atrium that originates near the entrance of the inferior vena cava and often extends to the crista terminalis. This can be seen in any of the views in which the right atrium is pictured (Figure 31-35).
- **Ectopic chordae:** Thin, fibrous strands that extend from one ventricular wall to another. They can be found in either ventricle and are best visualized in the apical views (Figure 31-36).
- **Interatrial septal aneurysm:** Appears as a bulge in the atrial septum that moves to and fro with respiration. This is best seen in either the apical four-chamber view or the subcostal four-chamber view (Figure 31-37).

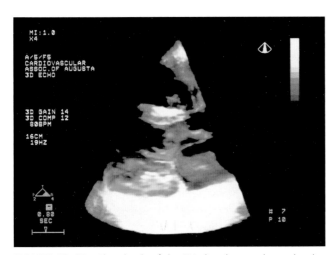

FIGURE 31-32 The depth of the LV chamber and mitral valve leaflets can be appreciated in this presentation.

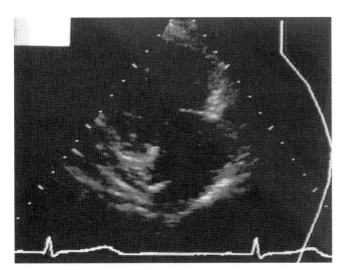
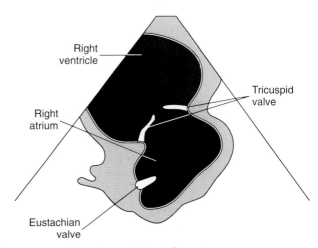

FIGURE 31-33 **Eustachian Valve.** Eustachian valve as seen in the right ventricular inflow view. Found in the right atrium, it is a normal variant.

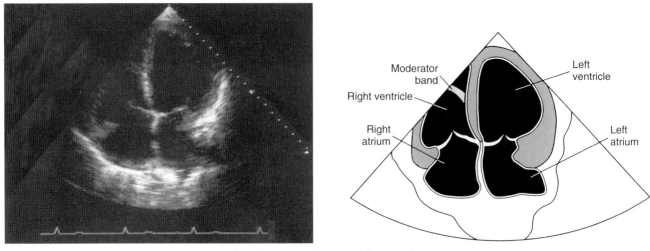

FIGURE 31-34 Moderator band as seen in the apical four-chamber view. It is a normal structure found in the right ventricle.

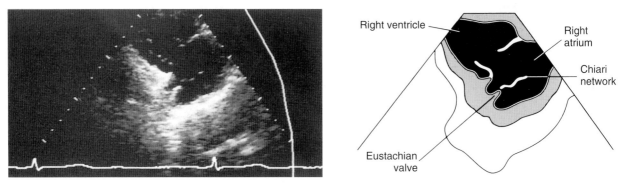

FIGURE 31-35 Chiari network as seen in the right ventricular inflow view. It is a normal variant found in the right atrium.

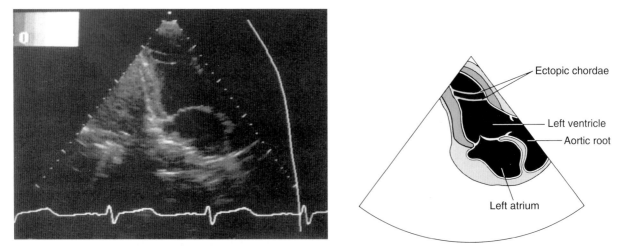

FIGURE 31-36 Ectopic chordae as seen in the left ventricle of the apical long axis view. These are normal variants and can be found in either ventricle.

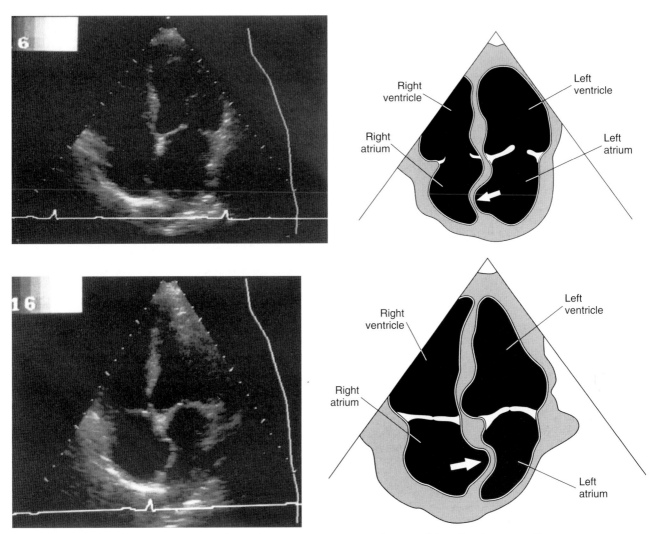

FIGURE 31-37 Interatrial septal aneurysm as seen in the apical four-chamber view. This is considered a normal variant and moves to and fro with respiration.

REFERENCE CHARTS

▪ ▪ ▪ ASSOCIATED PHYSICIANS

- **Cardiologist:** Specializes in the medical treatment of patients with heart disease.
- **Radiologist:** Specializes in the diagnostic interpretation of imaging modalities; therefore some radiologists may also read echocardiograms.

▪ ▪ ▪ COMMON DIAGNOSTIC TESTS

- **Transesophageal echocardiography (TEE):** Provides information regarding the heart and associated vessels not obtainable through the transthoracic approach. The personnel involved in TEE usually include a cardiologist, cardiac sonographer, nurse, and possibly cardiovascular physician's assistant. The laboratory should be equipped with suction equipment, oxygen, crash cart, and blood pressure monitor. Imaging equipment includes the ultrasound unit and a transesophageal probe, usually with multiplane capabilities. The probe is basically a gastroscope with an imaging PISA electric crystal at the tip. The frequency is typically between 5 and 6.5 MHz. The TEE scope consists of a control head with deflection controls. The device usually has a large inner wheel and a smaller outer wheel for antegrade and retrograde flexion and for lateral and medial angulations. The flexible shaft is similar to that seen in gastroscopy. Patient preparation includes a thorough history and cardiac examination. The patient should be asked about any gastrointestinal symptoms. Preoperative orders include approximately 4 hours of fasting before the procedure. Just before the examination, intravenous access is established, and a topical anesthesia is applied to the oropharynx to diminish the gag reflex. Sedation is also administered. Outpatients should have a responsible person drive them to and from the hospital. Risks associated with TEE are extremely low, although a few deaths have been reported when rare cardiac arrhythmias have occurred. Additional possible complications are uncommon, but these may include hypotension, laryngospasm and arterial hypoxia (rare), drug reactions, and endocarditis.

- **History and physical examination:** The cardiologist questions the patient to gather a good history and performs a full physical examination. This can help determine the diagnosis.
- **Auscultation:** Listening to the sounds of the heart with the aid of a stethoscope.
- **Chest x-ray study:** This provides information on the size and structure of the heart. At times the cardiac silhouette is diagnostic for specific abnormalities. The test is performed by a technician but is interpreted by either the radiologist or the cardiologist.
- **Electrocardiogram (ECG):** Provides information on the electrical behavior of the heart during the cardiac cycle. A technician performs the test, which is then interpreted by a cardiologist.
- **Exercise stress test:** The patient may be exercised on a bicycle or treadmill when coronary artery disease is suspected. During the stress test an ECG is done. This provides information on functional changes in the heart and determines the degree of stimulus that will provoke an adverse reaction. Thallium can also be used. It is a radionuclide that traces the path of the blood as it flows through arteries and perfuses the myocardial cells. A stress test is not performed when valvular disease is suspected. The technician performs the test in the presence of a cardiologist, who then interprets the results.
- **Computed axial tomography (CT) and magnetic resonance imaging (MRI):** These two other imaging studies can be used in the evaluation of heart disease. They are most useful in evaluating cardiac masses, tumors, or effusions. They are often performed by a technician but may be done in the presence of a physician. These tests are interpreted by a radiologist.
- **Cardiac catheterization:** An invasive technique in which the tip of a long catheter is introduced into either an artery or a vein through an arm or leg. The catheter is then threaded into the heart. This is an important clinical test used to evaluate coronary artery disease, ventricular and valvular function, pressures within the chambers and across the valves, and the oxygen content of the blood (important in cases of septal defects). The test is performed and interpreted by a cardiologist.

■ ■ ■ LABORATORY VALUES

- **Creatine phosphokinase (CPK):** An enzyme found in all muscle tissue. The MB fraction of CPK helps in assessing the presence of myocardial infarction. Elevation of CK-MB indicates that an infarct is present. The CK-MB should peak within 24 hours.
- **Lactic dehydrogenase (LDH):** LDH is also found throughout the body, and a certain percentage is used to assess myocardial infarction. LDH usually peaks within 24 to 48 hours and when elevated indicates the presence of an infarct.

■ ■ ■ VASCULATURE

Nonapplicable.

■ ■ ■ AFFECTING CHEMICALS

- **Epinephrine:** Produced by the adrenal medulla, it increases the excitability of the SA node, thereby increasing the heart rate and the strength of the contractions.
- **Potassium:** Can interfere with nerve impulse generation; therefore it decreases heart rate and the strength of the contractions.
- **Sodium:** Also may decrease heart rate and contraction strength because it tends to interfere with calcium participation in muscular contraction.
- **Calcium:** As with sodium, a high amount of calcium can increase the heart rate and the strength of its contractions.

■ ■ ■ NORMAL DOPPLER VELOCITIES IN ADULTS

- Mitral valve: 0.6 to 1.3 m/sec
- Aortic valve: 1.0 to 1.7 m/sec
- Tricuspid valve: 0.3 to 0.7 m/sec
- Pulmonic valve: 0.6 to 0.9 m/sec
- Left ventricular: 0.7 to 1.1 m/sec

CHAPTER 32

Vascular Technology

MARSHA M. NEUMYER

OBJECTIVES

Define the role of indirect and direct noninvasive techniques used for the evaluation of vascular disease.

Describe the anatomy of the extracranial and intracranial arteries, as well as the peripheral arterial and venous systems.

Describe the sonographic appearance of the extracranial and intracranial arteries, as well as the lower extremity peripheral arterial and venous vasculature.

Define the hemodynamic patterns and Doppler spectral waveforms found in the normal vasculature.

■

KEY WORDS

Accuracy — Indicates percentage (i.e., overall agreement) of all the noninvasive studies that were correctly identified when compared with the gold standard.

Area Reduction — Calculates percentage of stenosis.

Bicuspid Venous Valves — Valves that serve to promote unidirectional flow and regulate venous pressure in the distal lower extremity venous system.

Biphasic Doppler Spectral Waveform — Lacks the forward diastolic flow component associated with the high-resistance, multiphasic Doppler spectral waveform normally found in resting peripheral arteries. The biphasic waveform demonstrates systolic upstroke, systolic deceleration, and a reverse flow component.

Boundary Layer Separation — Characterizes the normal blood flow patterns in the carotid bulb.

Circle of Willis — Intracranial arterial configuration of anastomotic and communicating collateral vessels located at the base of the brain.

Color Doppler Imaging — Encodes the Doppler-shifted frequencies within a chosen region of interest; superimposed on a gray-scale anatomic image.

Diameter Reduction — Calculates size of reduced arterial lumen diameter resulting from disease or extrinsic compression.

Direct/Indirect Noninvasive Vascular Diagnostic Tests — Indirect physiologic test procedures indicate the presence of flow-limiting vascular disease by demonstrating blood pressure or volume changes distal to the site of disease. In contrast the direct procedures demonstrate tissue characteristics and flow patterns in vessels at the site of disease.

Doppler Color-Flow Imaging — Visually highlights regions of blood flow and superimposes it on the gray-scale image of surrounding tissues. This is accomplished by encoding the Doppler-shifted frequencies of the returned signals related to movement within a designated area.

Doppler Spectral Waveform — Provides information about blood flow velocity, flow direction, presence of flow disturbance or turbulence, and vascular impedance.

False Negative (FN) — Laboratory studies in which the noninvasive test is negative for the chosen category of disease, but the gold standard is positive for that degree of disease severity.

False Positive (FP) — Laboratory studies in which the noninvasive test is positive for the chosen category, but the gold standard is not in agreement.

Gosling Pulsatility Index — Calculated demonstration of variable proportions of diastolic to systolic flow.

High-Resistance Vascular Bed/End Organ/Tissues — Organs or tissues with low metabolic demands.

Linear Reflectivity — Associated with the echogenic properties of collagen fibers in the tunica intima and tunica media layers of arterial walls.

Low-Resistance Vascular Bed/End Organ/Tissues — Organs or tissues with high metabolic demands.

Negative Predictive Value (NPV) — Calculation indicating the predictive ability of a negative test to identify patients without disease.

Positive Predictive Value (PPV) — Calculation indicating the predictive capability of a positive test to identify patients with disease.

Power Doppler Imaging — Visually highlights regions of blood flow and superimposes them on the gray-scale image of surrounding tissues. This is accomplished by encoding the intensity of the returned signals within the chosen region of interest.

Prevalence — Calculation indicating when disease is truly present in the population.

Sensitivity — Calculation indicating how "sensitive" a noninvasive test is in detecting the presence of disease.

Specificity — Calculation indicating how "specific" a noninvasive test is in determining when a patient is normal, or negative, for disease.

Spectral Broadening/Spectral Bandwidth — An increase in echoes proportional to an increase in turbulence or flow disturbance.

Systolic Window — Relatively signal-free area between the arterial Doppler shift signal and the baseline during the systolic portion of a Doppler spectral display. Present in the absence of disease or vessel tortuosity.

Continued

609

Transmural Pressure — Venous wall pressure. Veins have the remarkable characteristic of undergoing tremendous volume changes with little change in transmural pressure.

Triphasic Doppler Spectral Waveform — Normally found in arteries from the level of the distal abdominal aorta to the tibial arteries at the ankle.

True Negative (TN) — Laboratory studies in which the noninvasive test is negative for the chosen category of disease, and the gold standard is also negative.

True Positive (TP) — Laboratory studies in which the noninvasive test is positive for the disease category in question, and the gold standard is also positive for the same severity of disease.

■ ■ ■ NORMAL MEASUREMENTS

Extracranial Cerebrovascular Vessels	Diameter	Lower Extremity Arteries	Diameter
Common carotid artery	5 to 6 mm	Common iliac artery	1.20 cm
Internal carotid artery/external portion	4 to 5 mm	External iliac artery	0.79 cm
External carotid artery	3 to 4 mm	Common femoral artery	0.82 cm
Vertebral arteries	2 to 3 mm, then smaller as arteries run superiorly	Superficial femoral artery/proximal portion	0.60 cm
		Superficial femoral artery/distal portion	0.54 cm
		Popliteal artery	0.52 cm
Intracranial Cerebrovascular Arteries	**Diameter**	Tibial arteries	0.45 cm
Internal carotid artery/terminal portion	3 to 4 mm	**Deep Veins**	**Diameter**
Middle cerebral artery	2 to 3 mm	Tibial veins	~ 5 mm
Anterior cerebral artery	2.0 to 2.5 mm	Popliteal vein	0.9 to 1.5 cm
Anterior communicating artery	0.5 to 1.0 mm	Femoral vein (superficial femoral vein)	0.9 to 1.0 cm
Posterior communicating arteries	1.5 to 2.0 mm	Common femoral vein	1.2 to 1.9 cm
Posterior cerebral artery	2.5 to 3.0 mm	**Superficial Veins**	**Diameter**
Basilar artery	3.5 to 4.2 mm and·at least 2 cm long	Great saphenous vein (thigh)	2 to 3 mm (calf), 4 to 6 mm
Vertebral arteries	2 mm	Small saphenous vein	4 to 7 mm

The field of noninvasive vascular diagnosis has expanded almost exponentially over the past 5 decades. Historically, indirect physiologic techniques utilizing segmental limb systolic pressure measurements and plethysmographic techniques were used to detect the presence, location, and severity of circulatory compromise. These modalities were soon followed by the introduction of gray-scale imaging and Doppler velocity spectral analysis. Vascular laboratories quickly adopted and validated sonography for the identification of pathology and evaluation of blood flow patterns in the cerebrovascular, peripheral arterial, and peripheral venous circulations. The next generations of ultrasound instruments provided enhanced gray-scale imaging and even more sophisticated Doppler technology, which made it possible to explore the vasculature of the abdomen and brain. In recent years, these modalities have been complemented with color and **power Doppler imaging**, making it possible to acquire multi-dimensional, volume information about vessels and organs. This advanced technology has greatly improved understanding of the impact of vascular disorders on blood flow within the arterial and venous circulations.

Indirect physiologic studies continue to play an important role in the modern vascular laboratory, primarily for the detection and localization of peripheral arterial disease. Duplex sonography, a morphologic study, has become the primary diagnostic tool for demonstration of tissue characteristics and blood flow patterns at the site of disease in the cerebrovascular, peripheral arterial, venous, and abdominal vascular systems. Although indirect physiologic testing and direct sonographic imaging are complementary, the choice of test, or tests, is dictated by the patient's clinical presentation. The primary focus of this chapter is on the recognition of normal structure and function and the detection of cerebrovascular, peripheral arterial, and venous disorders with direct sonographic imaging. Abdominal vascular evaluations are discussed in Chapter 13.

EXTRACRANIAL CEREBROVASCULAR SYSTEM

Common Carotid, Internal Carotid, External Carotid, and Vertebral Arteries

The extracranial cerebrovascular system consists of the common carotid arteries (CCAs), the internal carotid arteries (ICAs), the external carotid arteries (ECAs), and the vertebral arteries (VAs). The system is symmetric on each side of the neck (Figure 32-1).

The extracranial cerebrovascular system provides blood flow to the cerebral hemispheres, the eyes, and the muscles of the face, forehead, and scalp. The carotid arteries supply the eyes, via the ophthalmic arteries, and the anterior two-thirds of the brain. The VAs become confluent with the basilar artery at the level of the foramen magnum and supply blood to the brain stem, cerebellum, and undersurface of the cerebral hemispheres. Intracranially, the carotid arterial system anastomoses with the vertebral-basilar system to form the **circle of Willis**, an arterial ring at the base of the brain (Figure 32-2).

Each extracranial carotid system has a common carotid artery that bifurcates, most often at the level of the superior thyroid cartilage, into an ICA and an ECA. On the right side of the body the CCA arises from the innominate, or brachiocephalic, artery, which also branches into the subclavian artery. The subclavian artery then passes posterior to the scalenus anterior muscle. The left common carotid and subclavian arteries arise separately from the aortic arch. Variations may include absence of the innominate artery with the right subclavian and common carotid originating from the arch, a common origin of the innominate and left common carotid arteries, and the presence of a left innominate artery, or the aorta may arch to the right with the normal arterial arrangements reversed.

The CCAs pass cephalad into the anterolateral aspect of the neck slightly behind the thyroid gland and lateral to the trachea, esophagus, larynx, and pharynx. The level of the carotid bifurcation and the arrangement of the ICA and ECA may vary. In most patients the ICA is posterior and lateral to the ECA. The ICA normally has no branches in the neck, but intracranially it gives rise to the ophthalmic artery, which supplies blood flow to the eye, and to the middle and anterior cerebral arteries. The ICA is divided into four major segments: cervical, petrous, cavernous, and cerebral. The ECA has branches that supply blood flow to the neck, face, and scalp. These branches sonographically help to distinguish the ECA from the ICA and include the superior thyroid, ascending pharyngeal, lingual, facial, occipital, posterior auricular, superficial temporal, and maxillary arteries.

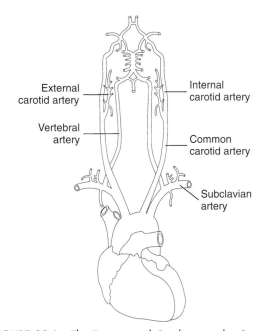

FIGURE 32-1 The Extracranial Cerebrovascular System.

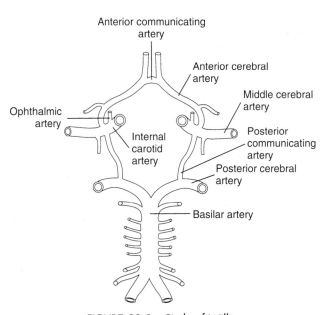

FIGURE 32-2 Circle of Willis.

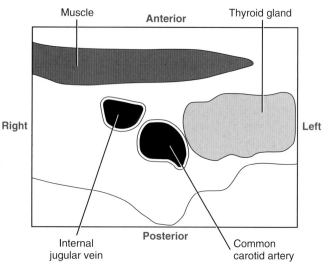

FIGURE 32-3 *Transverse scanning plane image of the common carotid artery, jugular vein, and thyroid gland.*

Anatomic variations may include the absence of the CCA, with the ICA and ECA arising directly from the aortic arch, the absence of a carotid bifurcation, or agenesis of either the ICA or ECA.

The vertebral arteries arise as the first branch of the subclavian arteries and pass cranially through the foramina of the transverse processes of the upper six cervical vertebrae. The vertebrals pass superiorly to the atlas, winding around the lateral mass of the atlas, and enter the vertebral canal anterior to the spinal cord. The two vertebral arteries enter the skull through the foramen magnum and join to form the basilar artery, which supplies structures in the posterior fossa.

Size of the Extracranial Cerebrovascular Vessels

The normal common carotid artery is approximately 5 to 6 mm in diameter. This vessel may decrease in transverse diameter as a result of atherosclerotic occlusive disease, which may compromise antegrade blood flow.

The extracranial portion of the ICA measures approximately 4 to 5 mm in diameter. The vessel decreases in diameter as it enters the brain. The ECA is usually of smaller diameter than the ICA, measuring approximately 3 to 4 mm. The vertebral arteries are approximately 2 to 3 mm in diameter at their origin, decreasing in width as they course cephalad. These vessels are often asymmetric in size.

Sonographic Appearance of the Extracranial Carotid and Vertebral Arteries

Using an anterior oblique or posterior oblique longitudinal scan plane, the skin, platysma, and fascia will lie between the probe and the carotid artery.

The lateral lobe of the thyroid gland is identified lateral to the common carotid artery. The artery is enclosed within the carotid sheath, along with the vagus nerve and the jugular vein. The jugular vein is located lateral to the CCA and displays characteristic movement that varies with respiration and cardiac activity (Figure 32-3). Transverse pulsatility of the carotid artery will be noted to be in phase with the cardiac cycle.

At the level of the carotid bifurcation, the dilation (carotid sinus) of the carotid bulb can be identified and the division into the ICA and ECA noted (Figure 32-4).* A defined dilation of the artery may not be apparent in some patients, and the bulb frequently is part of the common carotid, internal carotid, or external carotid arteries. The relationship between the internal and external carotid arteries is variable and dependent on whether an antero-oblique or a postero-oblique scan plane has been used. The vessels can be further identified by their signature Doppler waveform.

Sonographically, the normal arterial wall demonstrates **linear reflectivity** associated with the echogenic properties of collagen fibers in the tunica intima and tunica media layers of the arterial wall (Figure 32-5). This acoustic feature is not found in the walls of the jugular vein.

The vertebral arteries may be visualized using an anteroposterior approach in the midcervical segment of the neck as they course through the fossae of the transverse vertebral processes (Figure 32-6). The origin of the vertebral vessels can be documented using a transverse approach to the subclavian artery at the level of the common carotid origin (Figure 32-7).

---

*Images in this chapter courtesy Penn State Hershey Vascular Noninvasive Diagnostic Laboratory, Hershey, Pennsylvania.

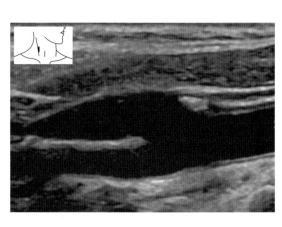

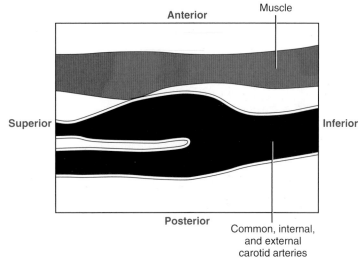

FIGURE 32-4 Image of long axis section of carotid bifurcation demonstrating the common, external, and internal carotid arteries.

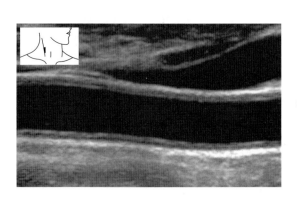

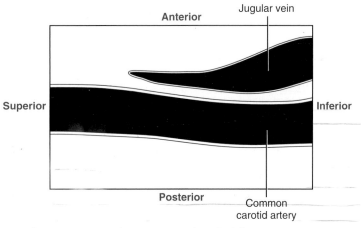

FIGURE 32-5 Image of long axis section of common carotid artery. Arterial wall definition reveals linear reflectivity resulting from the echogenicity of collagen found in the intima and media.

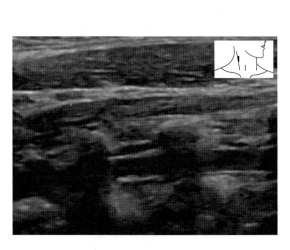

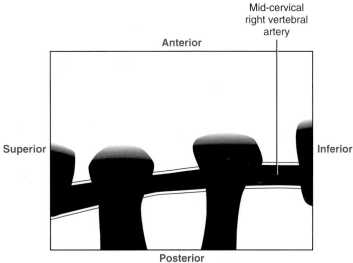

FIGURE 32-6 Image of the vertebral artery coursing through the transverse vertebral processes.

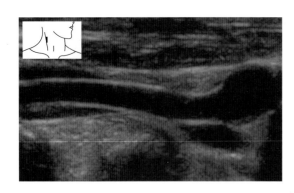

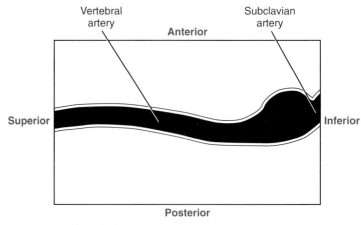

FIGURE 32-7 **Image of the Vertebral Artery Origin.** The subclavian artery is seen in the transverse plane just distal to the origin of the right common carotid artery.

Hemodynamic Patterns of the Extracranial Carotid and Vertebral Arteries

Approximately 80% of the blood flow from the CCA enters the ICA to supply the circulation of the brain and eye. The residual 20% of flow enters the ECA to supply the muscles of the face, forehead, and scalp.

The brain and eye have high metabolic demands and therefore are **low-resistance end organs**. For this reason, flow in the ICA will be cephalad throughout the cardiac cycle. In contrast, the muscles of the face, forehead, and scalp normally have low metabolic demands and are considered **high-resistance tissues**. Therefore the flow pattern for the ECA is characterized by forward flow in systole, and a low or reverse diastolic flow component.

The normal increased diameter of the carotid bulb compared to the CCA results in a pressure-flow gradient on the posterolateral wall of the bulb (wall opposite the flow divide). Because blood will normally flow from high- to low-pressure regions, the flow stream within the bulb separates into forward flow entering the ICA and flow reversal near the posterolateral wall (Figure 32-8). This is known as **boundary layer separation** and characterizes the normal blood flow patterns in the carotid bulb.

The vertebral arteries supply blood flow, by way of the basilar artery, to the posterior cerebral hemispheres. Therefore their flow patterns will be similar to those seen in the ICA with constant forward diastolic flow.

Blood moves through the arteries in layers or laminae. The laminae slide over each other, impeded by friction from within the fluid or from movement against the arterial wall. Velocity profiles generally will be influenced by tapering or curvature of the vessel, entrance and exit effects on inertia of blood as the vessel widens and dilates, and the presence of turbulence caused by anatomic abnormality or disease.

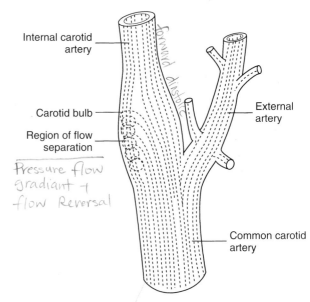

FIGURE 32-8 Carotid bifurcation demonstrating boundary layer separation in the carotid bulb.

To accurately evaluate hemodynamic patterns, the velocity spectral information must be collected at an angle of insonation of 60 degrees or less with respect to the blood flow vectors and the vessel walls. Remember the **Doppler equation**:

$$\Delta F = \frac{2VF_0 \cos \Theta}{c}$$

where ΔF = Doppler-shifted frequency, V = blood flow velocity, F_0 = carrier Doppler frequency, $\cos \Theta$ = angle of insonation with respect to the blood flow vectors, and c = constant for speed of sound in soft tissue (1540 m/sec).

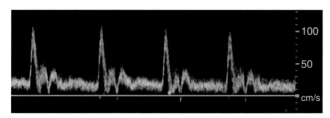

FIGURE 32-9 Doppler spectral waveform from a normal common carotid artery. Note forward diastolic flow.

Doppler Velocity Spectral Waveforms

Common Carotid Artery

The CCA has a Doppler velocity spectral waveform that mimics both the internal carotid and external carotid artery waveforms. The blood flow pattern is characterized by a sharp systolic upstroke, rapid systolic deceleration, and because most of its flow is to the low-resistance vascular beds of the brain and eye, constant forward diastolic flow. In the presence of ICA occlusion, the flow pattern in the CCA may mimic the high-resistance pattern of the ECA as the majority of its flow volume will enter the ECA circulation.

In a normal CCA the flow pattern is laminar. This flow pattern is characterized by a uniform systolic velocity; a "window," an area absent of Doppler shifts, under the systolic component; and a very narrow Doppler velocity spectrum (Figure 32-9). During the deceleration phase of systole, velocity decreases, and the viscous drag on the cells nearest the wall results in movement of these cells over a slightly broader range of velocities. This is manifested by thickening of the velocity spectral envelope. This **spectral broadening** becomes more evident during diastole as the blood cells return to their laminae.

In the absence of disease the velocity in the CCA approximates 60 cm/sec, but a wide range of normal velocities from 30 to 110 cm/sec has been documented.

Internal Carotid Artery

The ICA is characteristically a high-flow, low-resistance vessel. The **Doppler spectral waveform** from this artery demonstrates rapid systolic upstroke, a blunt systolic peak, and constant forward diastolic flow (Figure 32-10). A **systolic window** is present in the absence of disease or vessel tortuosity. Peak systolic velocity normally is less than 125 cm/sec or less than twice the velocity in the CCA (Table 32-1).

External Carotid Artery

In contrast, the ECA is a low-flow, high-resistance vessel. The Doppler velocity waveform exhibits multiphasicity with sharp systolic upstroke, rapid deceleration, and low

Table 32-1 Diagnostic Doppler Velocity Criteria for Determining Degree of Internal Carotid Artery Diameter Reduction

Diameter Stenosis (%) Category	ICA Peak Systolic Velocity (cm/sec)	ICA/CCA Peak Systolic Velocity Ratio	ICA End-Diastolic Velocity (cm/sec)
Normal	<125	<2.0	<40
<50 (with plaque)	<125	<2.0	<40
50 to 69	125 to 230	2.0 to 4.0	40 to 100
>70	>230	>4.0	>100
>80	>230	>4.0	>140
Occluded	No flow	N/A	N/A

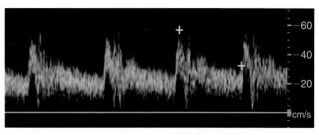

FIGURE 32-10 Doppler spectral waveform from a normal internal carotid artery demonstrating constant forward diastolic flow.

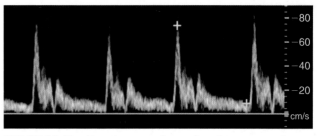

FIGURE 32-11 Doppler spectral waveform from a normal external carotid artery. Note the low diastolic flow component.

diastolic flow (Figure 32-11). A reverse flow component may be present in early diastole. In the presence of ICA occlusion, the ECA may mimic the internal carotid artery waveform because of collateral compensatory flow to the brain via ECA branches.

Carotid Bulb

The Doppler spectral waveform from the carotid bulb varies with position of the Doppler sample volume (Figure 32-12). If the sample volume is placed in the region of the flow divide, along the wall separating the ICA and ECA, the waveform will demonstrate forward diastolic flow. As the sample volume is stepped across the lumen of the bulb to the posterior wall, the waveform will exhibit reverse flow in the region where there is separation of the boundary layers.

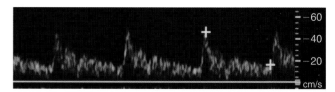

<figure><figcaption>FIGURE 32-13 Doppler spectral waveform from a normal vertebral artery.</figcaption></figure>

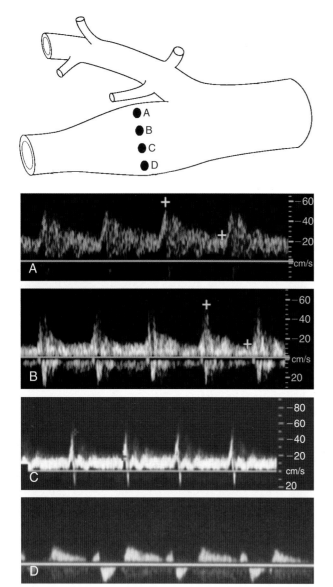

FIGURE 32-12 Montage of Carotid Bulb and Doppler Spectral Waveforms. **A,** Recorded from the region of the flow divide with primarily forward flow. **B,** Recorded from the boundary layer showing separation of the flow stream into forward and reverse flows. **C,** The beginning of the reverse flow phase. **D,** Reverse flow occurring along the posterolateral wall of the bulb.

Vertebral Arteries

The spectral display from a normal vertebral artery should resemble the waveform from the ICA with constant forward flow throughout diastole (Figure 32-13). The vertebrals are high-flow, low-resistance vessels exhibiting a velocity range of 30 to 60 cm/sec. Occasionally, high-resistance spectral waveforms are present. This finding is most often associated with extrinsic compression of the artery by bony projections (spondylosis, arthritis) as it courses through the transverse processes of the vertebral column.

THE INTRACRANIAL CEREBROVASCULAR SYSTEM

Ophthalmic, Terminal Internal Carotid, Middle Cerebral, Anterior Cerebral, Anterior Communicating, Posterior Communicating, Posterior Cerebral, Vertebral and Basilar Arteries

The intracranial cerebrovascular system comprises the arteries of the circle of Willis, which anastomoses the anterior and posterior cerebral circulations (see Figure 32-2). Arteries within the circle of Willis include the anterior communicating, anterior cerebral, supraclinoid segment of the ICA (terminal ICA), posterior communicating, and posterior cerebral arteries. It should be noted that although the middle cerebral artery (MCA) is always included in a noninvasive transcranial evaluation, anatomically it does not lie within the circle of Willis.

The carotid arteries form the anterior cerebral circulation, which supplies blood to the cerebral hemispheres, the eyes, accessory organs, forehead, and part of the nose. The ICA is divided into 4 major segments. The cervical segment of the ICA ascends in the neck anterior to the transverse processes of the cervical vertebrae, then enters the skull via the carotid canal, where it traverses the petrous portion of the temporal bone. The petrous segment of the ICA has vertical and horizontal portions. The vertical portion initially ascends in the carotid canal, passing inside the petrous bone for approximately 1 cm before curving anteromedially. The horizontal portion passes superomedially within the petrous bone to enter the cranial cavity. The cavernous segment is referred to as the *carotid siphon* because of its S-shaped configuration. This segment of the ICA initially courses anteriorly and then passes superomedially through the cavernous siphon toward the anterior clinoid process. It gives rise to cavernous, meningeal, and hypophyseal branches. The cerebral segment of the ICA traverses the dura mater medial to the anterior clinoid process and then passes superolaterally to bifurcate into the anterior cerebral artery (ACA) and middle cerebral artery. The ophthalmic artery is a principal branch of the cerebral ICA segment. The right and left anterior cerebral arteries are joined by the anterior communicating artery (ACoA).

The vertebral and basilar arteries form the posterior cerebral circulation, which perfuses the brain stem, cerebellum, and back and undersurface of the cerebral hemispheres. The vertebral arteries (VAs) are divided into the prevertebral, cervical, horizontal, and intracranial segments. The prevertebral segment arises from the subclavian artery and ascends the neck to enter the transverse foramen of the cervical vertebrae at the level of C-6, where it becomes the cervical segment. It is surrounded by the nerve plexus of the cervical sympathetic system and lies posterior to the vertebral and jugular veins and the inferior thyroid artery. Occasionally, the inferior thyroid artery and costocervical trunk may originate from the proximal segment of the vertebral artery. The cervical segment gives rise to multiple small branches providing flow to the spinal cord, cervical vertebrae, and adjacent muscles. In the presence of vertebral or carotid artery occlusive disease, these branches anastomose with ECA branches to provide collateral compensatory flow. The cervical segment courses cranially through the transverse processes to the level of C-1 or C-2, where it terminates. Along its course, it is in close contact medially with the uncinate processes of the vertebral bodies and posteriorly with the ventral rami of the cervical nerves. On each side, the VAs then course posteriorly within the vertebral sulcus and ascend anteromedially through the dura mater, looping between the atlas and axis (horizontal segment) before entering the skull. The intracranial segments ascend from the dura mater through the foramen magnum, where they join to form the basilar artery along the inferior surface of the pons.

The distal segment of the basilar artery courses posteriorly before its bifurcation into the left and right posterior cerebral arteries (PCAs). Along its course it gives rise to small anterior inferior cerebellar, internal auditory, pontine, and superior cerebellar arteries. The posterior circulation is connected to the anterior circulation on each side of the brain by the posterior communicating arteries (PCoAs).

The most common anatomic anomalies include absent or hypoplastic segments of the circle of Willis and affect the anterior cerebral artery in approximately 25% of cases.

Size of the Intracranial Cerebrovascular Arteries

The terminal internal carotid artery has a diameter of 3 to 4 mm. The diameter of the middle cerebral artery is 2 to 3 mm, whereas the diameter of the anterior cerebral artery is 2.0 to 2.5 mm. The anterior communicating artery has a small diameter, averaging 0.5 to 1.0 mm. The posterior communicating arteries have a slightly larger diameter, ranging from 1.5 to 2.0 mm. The diameter of the posterior cerebral artery averages 2.5 to 3.0 mm. The basilar artery exhibits an average diameter of 3.5 to 4.2 mm and is at least 2 cm in length in most adults. The vertebral arteries frequently differ in diameter from side to side, with one side most often being dominant. The diameter of the vertebral arteries approximates 2 mm in the normal adult.

Sonographic Appearance of the Intracranial Arteries

Given the small diameter of the intracranial arteries, it is quite difficult to detect their presence and follow their course on a sonographic B-mode examination of the brain. For this reason, **color Doppler imaging** is used to facilitate identification of vessels and for recognition of regions of disturbed flow (Figure 32-14).

The terminal internal carotid artery, carotid siphon, MCA, ACA, and occasionally the ACoA, may be insonated using a transtemporal window, directing the image plane just above the zygomatic arch and immediately anterior and slightly superior to the tragus of the ear (Figure 32-15). **Doppler color-flow imaging** will demonstrate flow toward the probe in the normal middle cerebral artery at a depth of 30 to 60 mm and away from the probe in the anterior cerebral artery at a

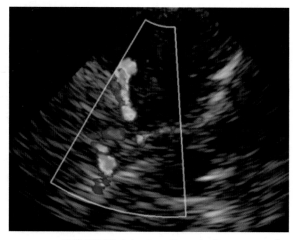
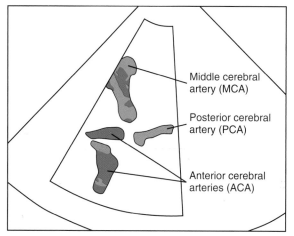

FIGURE 32-14 Doppler color-flow image of intracranial circulation from a transtemporal window. *ACA,* Anterior cerebral artery; *MCA,* middle cerebral artery; *PCA,* posterior cerebral artery.

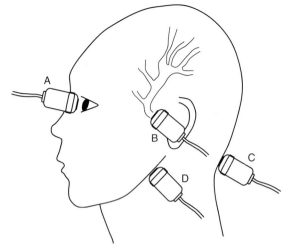

FIGURE 32-15 Acoustic windows commonly used for transcranial imaging. **A**, Transorbital window. **B**, Transtemporal window. **C**, Transoccipital window. **D**, Submandibular window.

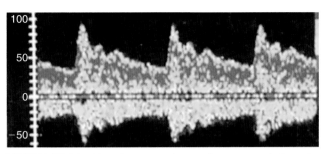

FIGURE 32-16 Doppler spectral waveforms recorded at the bifurcation of the internal carotid artery into the middle cerebral (MCA) and anterior cerebral (ACA) arteries. Note flow toward the probe in the MCA and away from the probe in the ACA.

depth of 60 to 75 mm. Bidirectional flow may be found in the carotid siphon, terminal ICA, and anterior communicating artery (ACoA).

The PCA and the PCoA can be insonated from the superior aspect of the transtemporal window using a slightly more posterior angulation of the probe. Flow in the P1 segment (initial segment) of the PCA will normally be toward the probe at a depth of 60 to 75 mm, whereas flow away from the probe is normally found in the P2 segment (segment beyond the origin of the PCoA).

The ophthalmic artery (OA) can be insonated using a transorbital scan plane, taking care to decrease the power output of the ultrasound system to a level less than 17 mW/cm^2 and a mechanical index (MI) of 0.28 (see Figure 32-15). Flow in the ipsilateral OA is normally toward the probe at a depth of 35 to 55 mm.

From a transoccipital approach, using the foramen magnum as an acoustic window, the vertebral and basilar arteries can be insonated (see Figure 32-15). The vertebral arteries should demonstrate flow away from the probe at a depth range of 60 to 90 mm. The basilar artery can be insonated at a depth range of 70 to 120 mm and normally exhibits flow direction toward the brain.

Hemodynamic Patterns of the Intracranial Arteries

Because the intracranial arteries supply blood flow to the low-resistance tissues of the brain, the Doppler spectral waveforms from the anterior and posterior circulation will normally exhibit constant forward diastolic flow. However, the proportion of diastolic to systolic flow may vary. This relationship can be demonstrated by calculation of the Gosling pulsatility index, as shown in the following equation, where PI = pulsatility index,

PSV = peak systolic velocity, EDV = end diastolic velocity, and MV = maximum of the mean velocity, which may be expressed as the time-averaged peak, or mean, velocity (TAP-V) on some instruments.

$$PI = \frac{PSV - EDV}{MV}$$

The normal range of pulsatility indices for the MCA, ACA, and PCA is between 0.5 and 1.1. Pulsatility of the Doppler spectral waveform decreases in the presence of proximal flow limiting stenosis, distal vasodilatation, apnea, arteriovenous shunts, or increased P_{CO_2} or in association with any condition that results in decreased vascular resistance. In contrast, pulsatility increases with bradycardia, aortic insufficiency, hyperventilation, or decreased P_{CO_2} or with any condition that results in increased vascular resistance and decreased diastolic flow.

Pulsatility of the Doppler spectral waveform from the ophthalmic artery is slightly increased compared with the spectral waveforms from arteries within the circle of Willis.

Doppler Velocity Spectral Data and Flow Direction
Middle Cerebral and Anterior Cerebral Arteries
Using a transtemporal window, flow in the MCA will normally be toward the probe with a mean systolic velocity of 55 ± 12 cm/sec. Flow direction at the MCA/ACA bifurcation will be bidirectional. The ACA can be insonated at a range of 60 to 75 mm depth and should demonstrate flow away from the probe at a mean velocity of 50 ± 11 cm/sec (Figure 32-16).

Posterior Cerebral Artery
Slight posterior angulation of the probe will allow interrogation of the posterior cerebral artery at a depth of 60 to 75 mm with mean velocity of 40 ± 10 cm/sec (Figure 32-17). Flow in the P1 segment will normally be toward the probe, whereas flow direction in the P2 segment will be away from the probe.

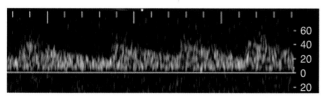

FIGURE 32-17 Doppler spectral waveforms from the posterior cerebral artery.

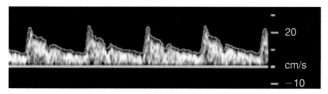

FIGURE 32-18 Doppler spectral waveforms from the ophthalmic artery. Note the slight increase in pulsatility compared to the arteries within the circle of Willis.

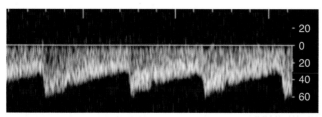

FIGURE 32-19 Doppler spectral waveforms from the proximal basilar artery. Note that flow is away from the probe.

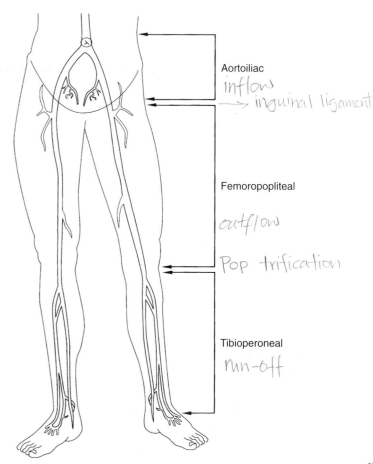

FIGURE 32-20 Lower extremity arterial tree demonstrating the aortoiliac, femoropopliteal, and tibioperoneal systems.

Ophthalmic Artery

The transorbital approach is commonly chosen for interrogation of the ophthalmic arteries. Using this window, flow direction in the ophthalmic artery is normally toward the probe at a depth of 35 to 55 mm with a mean velocity range of 21 ± 5 cm/sec (Figure 32-18).

Carotid Siphon

Within the carotid siphon, flow in the supraclinoid segment should be away from the beam at a depth of 60 to 80 mm and a mean velocity of 41 ± 10 cm/sec, whereas flow direction in the genu is bidirectional and within the parasellar segment toward the beam at a mean velocity of 47 ± 14 cm/sec.

Vertebral and Basilar Arteries

The vertebral and basilar arteries can be insonated from the transforaminal window. Flow direction in the vertebral and basilar arteries is normally away from the probe. Mean velocity range in the vertebral arteries is 38 ± 10 cm/sec, whereas the basilar artery mean velocity range is 41 ± 10 cm/sec (Figure 32-19).

THE LOWER EXTREMITY ARTERIAL SYSTEM

Common Iliac, External Iliac, Internal Iliac, Common Femoral, Deep Femoral, Popliteal, and Tibial Arteries

The lower extremity arterial system can be divided into three segments: aortoiliac (inflow), femoropopliteal (outflow), and tibioperoneal (run-off) (Figure 32-20).

The aortoiliac segment originates at the aortic bifurcation and terminates at the level of the inguinal ligament. The inflow segment of the lower extremity arterial tree is composed of the distal abdominal aorta, the common iliac, external iliac, and internal (hypogastric) iliac arteries. Arteries within this system supply the buttocks, pelvis, and thighs and are the second most common site for lower extremity arterial occlusive disease.

The femoropopliteal segment begins at the level of the inguinal ligament and ends at the trifurcation of the popliteal artery in the popliteal fossa behind the knee. The outflow segment is composed of the common femoral, deep femoral (profunda femoris), superficial femoral, and popliteal arteries. Arteries within this segment supply blood flow to the thighs and calves and

[handwritten: above the knee]

[handwritten: Femoral Pop Non-diabetes]

are the most common site for lower extremity atherosclerotic occlusive disease in the nondiabetic patient.

The tibioperoneal segment begins at the termination of the popliteal artery in the popliteal fossa and ends at the ankle, where the tibial arteries anastomose with the plantar and metatarsal arteries of the foot. The arteries within the run-off segment supply blood flow to the calves and feet. In patients with diabetes, the tibial arteries are the most common site for atherosclerotic disease.

[handwritten: Below the knee]

Sonographic Appearance of the Lower Extremity Peripheral Arterial Vessels

The abdominal aorta bifurcates into the common iliac arteries slightly left of midline at the level of the fourth lumbar vertebra. The common iliac arteries pass posterolaterally from their origin to the margin of the pelvis, where they divide opposite the last lumbar vertebra and the sacrum into the external and internal iliac arteries (Figure 32-21). The location of the aortic

[handwritten: causes DVT in left leg]

bifurcation is subject to variation as is the point of division of the common iliac arteries. On occasion, the common iliac artery may be absent, with the external and internal iliac arteries arising directly from the aorta.

The right common iliac artery lies inferior to the peritoneum, small intestine, and ureter. The common iliac veins and the psoas magnus muscle lie posteriorly with the inferior vena cava, sharing a lateral relationship.

The left common iliac artery lies posterior to the ureter and peritoneum and anterior to the left common iliac vein, an arrangement that may result in iliac deep vein thrombosis caused by extrinsic compression of the vein. Laterally, the left common iliac artery is bordered by the psoas magnus muscle.

The external iliac artery is larger than the internal iliac artery. The external iliac artery passes obliquely posterolateral to the inner border of the psoas muscle from the bifurcation of the common iliac to Poupart's ligament, where it enters the thigh and becomes the common femoral artery. The common and external iliac arteries are frequently difficult to image because of overlying bowel gas.

The common femoral artery originates posterolateral to Poupart's ligament, between the anterior superior spine of the ilium and the symphysis pubis, and courses down the medial aspect of the thigh through Scarpa's triangle as the superficial femoral artery, where it is contained in Hunter's canal (Figure 32-22). The superficial femoral artery terminates in the lower third of the thigh at the opening of the adductor magnus, where it becomes the popliteal artery. It is bordered on its medial side by the femoral vein (superficial femoral vein) and laterally by the adductor muscle. On rare occasions the superficial femoral artery may divide into two trunks below the origin of the profunda femoris, reuniting in the adductor canal to form the popliteal artery.

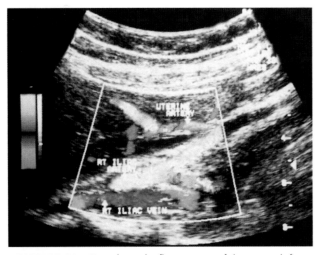

FIGURE 32-21 Doppler color-flow image of the aortic bifurcation. (Courtesy Philips Ultrasound.)

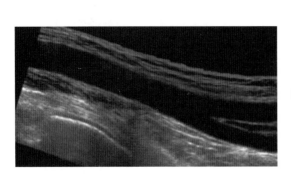

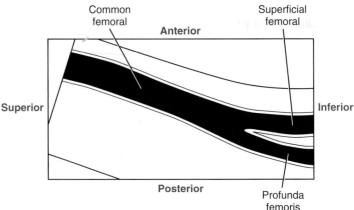

FIGURE 32-22 Long axis image of the common femoral artery to its bifurcation into the superficial femoral and profunda femoris arteries.

The deep femoral artery (profunda femoris) originates laterally from the common femoral artery at its bifurcation (Figure 32-23). It serves as the principal blood supply to the adductor, extensor, and flexor muscles and communicates with the external iliac arteries superiorly and the popliteal artery inferiorly.

The popliteal artery commences at the termination of the superficial femoral artery in Hunter's canal and passes obliquely behind the knee joint to the lower border of the femur, where it forms the tibioperoneal trunk (Figure 32-24). The trunk further divides into the anterior and posterior tibial arteries (Figure 32-25). It is bordered medially by the inner head of the gastrocnemius muscle and posteriorly by the popliteal vein. Occasionally, the popliteal artery divides prematurely into its branch vessels. The anterior tibial artery commences at the bifurcation of the popliteal artery and passes through the interosseous membrane to the deep part of the front of the leg, lying close to the inner side of the neck of the fibula. At the lower third of the limb, it lies on the tibia and on the anterior ligament of the ankle joint, where it moves superiorly to become the dorsalis pedis artery. The anterior tibial artery is accompanied by the anterior tibial veins that lie on each side of the artery.

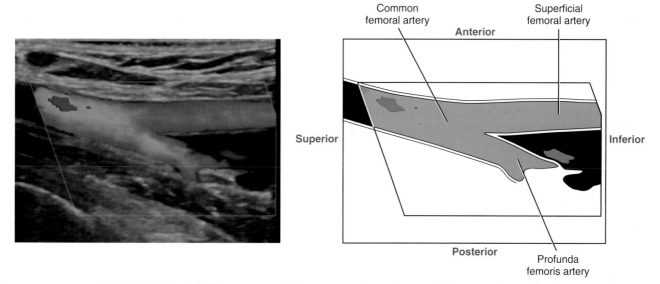

FIGURE 32-23 Color-flow image of the common femoral artery bifurcation. The profunda femoris artery originates laterally.

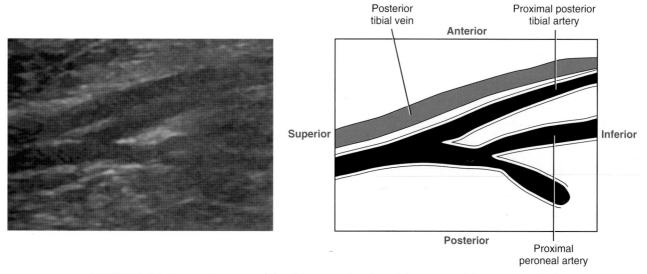

FIGURE 32-24 Long axis image of the tibioperoneal trunk and the origins of the posterior tibial and peroneal arteries.

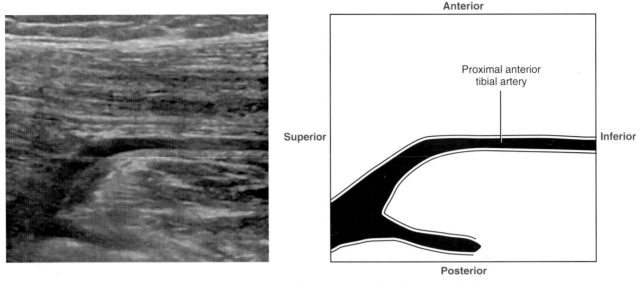

FIGURE 32-25 Long axis image of the anterior tibial and posterior tibial arteries.

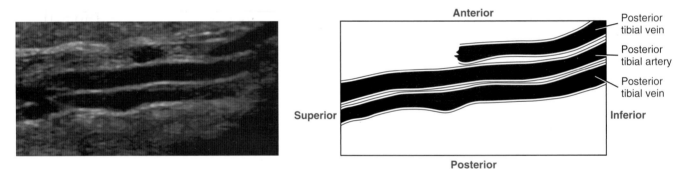

FIGURE 32-26 Long axis image of the posterior tibial artery surrounded by its companion tibial veins of the same name.

The posterior tibial artery originates between the tibia and fibula and extends obliquely downward along the medial (tibial) side of the leg, lying posterior to the deep transverse fascia. It terminates between the medial malleolus and the heel, where it divides into the medial and plantar arteries to supply the sole of the foot. It is accompanied by the two or more posterior tibial veins (Figure 32-26).

The peroneal artery lies along the posterolateral side of the fibula. It arises from the posterior tibial trunk about an inch below the border of the popliteus muscle, passing obliquely outward to the fibula. The peroneal artery supplies blood flow to the lateral lower extremity and the calcaneus (heel). The peroneal veins lie on either side of the artery.

The plantar arch, formed by branches of the dorsalis pedis and posterior tibial arteries, courses deeply, extending from the base of the fifth metatarsal to the proximal end of the first metatarsal space. The metatarsal and plantar branches carry blood to the skin, fascia, and muscles of the sole of the foot.

In the absence of disease the lumen of the peripheral arteries will be anechoic, with linear reflectivity apparent along both posterior and anterior walls of the vessels. Transverse pulsation of the arteries is notable and may become quite pronounced in tortuous segments of the lower extremity arterial tree.

Size of the Lower Extremity Arteries

Common iliac artery	1.20 cm
External iliac artery	0.79 cm
Common femoral artery	0.82 cm
Superficial femoral artery (proximal)	0.60 cm
Superficial femoral artery (distal)	0.54 cm
Popliteal artery	0.52 cm
Tibial arteries	0.45 cm

Hemodynamic Patterns in the Lower Extremity Arterial System

The pulsatile pressure wave that results from the pumping action of the heart is transmitted from the aortic root to the feet. During systole and left ventricular contraction, the walls of the aortic root expand, which creates a high-pressure wave. This wave is transmitted down the aorta and into the lower extremity arterial system. As the high-pressure wave travels peripherally, the lower extremity arterial walls also expand and contract in a pulsatile manner.

The resistance to blood flow in the small-diameter tibial arteries is greater than that in the wide-diameter aorta, resulting in a pressure gradient between the aorta and the distal tibial arteries. In the absence of flow-reducing arterial disease, systolic pressure is greater in the tibial arteries than in the abdominal aorta.

A secondary reflected pressure wave is created when the primary high-pressure wave from the aortic root meets the high resistance of the tibial arterial tree. The blood flow pattern to this high-resistance vascular bed is, therefore, multiphasic. There is forward flow in systole, then early reversed diastolic flow, and a forward diastolic flow component in vessels with normal arterial wall compliance.

Doppler Velocity Spectral Waveforms

A **triphasic Doppler spectral waveform** is normally found in arteries from the level of the distal abdominal aorta to the tibial arteries at the ankle (Figure 32-27). In healthy, young adults with normal elasticity of the vessel wall, an additional diastolic flow component may be recorded. Vessel wall compliance commonly decreases with advancing age, and the peak systolic forward velocity and peak diastolic forward velocity may diminish slightly. Reduced vessel wall compliance may result in a **biphasic Doppler spectral waveform** that lacks the forward diastolic flow component (Figure 32-28). Velocity waveforms recorded from peripheral arteries of women will generally demonstrate lower peak diastolic velocities than those from men of the same age.

The spectral bandwidth is narrow throughout systole and early diastole. Spectral broadening commonly occurs at bifurcations because of boundary layer

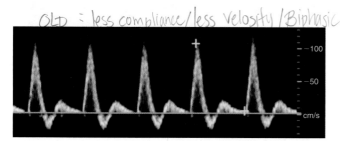

FIGURE 32-27 Doppler spectral waveform recorded from a lower extremity l artery. Note the triphasic pattern of flow.

separation and the presence of disturbed flow. In the absence of proximal disease, a systolic window and the reversed flow component will be present because peripheral resistance remains high.

Peak systolic velocity decreases in the normal lower extremity arterial tree from the central to the peripheral vessels (Figure 32-29). In the normal abdominal aorta, peak systolic velocity averages 90 cm/sec and decreases between the external iliac artery and the proximal superficial femoral artery, and again between the superficial

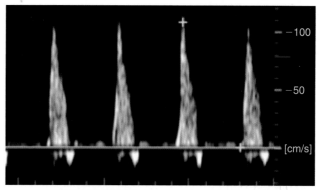

FIGURE 32-28 Biphasic Doppler spectral waveform recorded from a lower extremity artery.

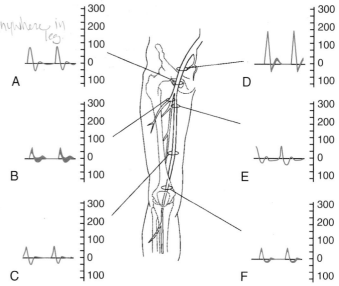

FIGURE 32-29 Normal Velocity Spectral Waveforms. A, Waveforms from the common femoral artery. B, Waveforms from the profunda femoris artery. C, Waveforms from the distal superficial femoral artery. D, Waveforms from the external iliac artery. E, Waveforms from the proximal superficial femoral artery. F, Waveforms from the popliteal artery. Note the decreases in peak systolic velocity between the external iliac artery and proximal superficial femoral artery and between the proximal superficial femoral artery and the popliteal vessel. (Redrawn from Neumyer MM, Thiele BL: Evaluation of lower extremity occlusive disease with Doppler ultrasound. In Taylor KJW, et al: *Clinical applications of Doppler ultrasound*, New York, 1988, Raven Press.)

femoral and popliteal arteries to average 60 cm/sec in the popliteal artery.

Indirect Physiologic Tests

Indirect physiologic test procedures indicate the presence of flow-limiting vascular disease by demonstrating blood pressure or volume changes distal to the site of disease. As noted, they have remained an integral part of vascular laboratory evaluations since the inception of noninvasive vascular testing. A thorough review of the various physiologic test procedures is beyond the scope of this chapter but is worthy of attention for sonographers and physicians who are employed in full-service vascular laboratories or facilities with a large population of diabetic patients.

When the internal diameter of a peripheral artery is narrowed by more than 50% to 60%, limb blood pressure decreases distal to the site of narrowing. The change in pressure can be detected by measuring the blood pressure proximal to the site of narrowing and comparing that to the blood pressure distal to that site. Normally, blood pressure at the ankle level should be equal to or slightly higher than systemic pressure, which is commonly measured at the brachial artery level. Given this, a pressure-reducing lesion in the lower extremity arterial tree is easily detected by comparing the patient's ankle pressure to the brachial pressure. In the absence of disease, the calculated ankle-brachial index (the ratio between the ankle pressure and the brachial pressure) should be 1.0 to 1.3. A value less than 1.0 suggests significant arterial compromise proximal to the ankle in the limb with the abnormal index (Table 32-2). The patient's presenting symptoms should be compared to the index as a means for determining the severity of arterial dysfunction.

For all patients suspected of compromised arterial flow to the lower extremity, it is important to determine if flow-limiting disease is present before performing the arterial sonographic examination. To accomplish this, brachial pressures are initially measured in both upper extremities. To ensure accurate pressure measurements, an appropriately sized blood pressure cuff must be used. Studies have demonstrated that the most accurate measurements are obtained when the width of the cuff bladder exceeds 20% of the diameter of the limb segment encompassed by the cuff. The cuff is wrapped snugly around the upper arm and a continuous-wave (CW) Doppler probe, usually 8 MHz, is used to sense arterial flow in the brachial artery. The cuff is then slowly inflated to a suprasystolic pressure to occlude the artery. When flow ceases, the cuff is slowly deflated (2 to 3 mm Hg/sec) until the arterial pulse signal is again detected. Record and retain the pressure for calculation of the ankle-brachial index (ABI). The measurement is repeated for the other arm. In a similar manner, blood pressures are measured for the posterior tibial and dorsalis pedis arteries of both lower extremities by placing an appropriately sized blood pressure cuff around each ankle and using a CW Doppler probe to sense blood flow sequentially in each of the tibial arteries. Record and retain the tibial artery pressures for both ankles. The ankle-brachial index is calculated for each limb by choosing the higher of the two tibial artery pressures and comparing that to the highest brachial pressure, as illustrated in Figure 32-30.

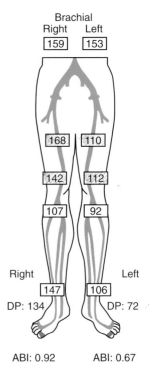

FIGURE 32-30 Lower extremity, indirect physiologic arterial study demonstrating segmental limb, ankle (dorsalis pedis and posterior tibial), and brachial artery blood pressures. Note the calculated ankle-brachial index using the highest tibial pressure on each side compared to the highest brachial artery pressure. *ABI,* Ankle brachial index; *DP,* dorsalis pedis.

■ ■ ■ **Table 32-2** Ankle-Brachial Index

Range	Finding
>1.3	Arterial calcification
1.0 to 1.3	Normal
0.9 to 1.0	Mild arterial compromise with only mild symptoms
0.5 to 0.9	Mild to moderate ischemia with mild to moderate claudication
0.3 to 0.5	Moderate to severe ischemia with severe claudication or rest pain
<0.3	Severe ischemia with rest pain or gangrene

THE LOWER EXTREMITY VENOUS SYSTEM

The veins of the lower extremity are divided into the deep, superficial, and perforating veins. The deep veins accompany the arteries and share the same names.

The Deep Venous System

The plantar digital veins and the dorsal digital veins become confluent and form four plantar metatarsal veins. The metatarsal veins are joined to the dorsal veins by perforating veins to form the deep plantar venous arch.

The normally paired anterior tibial veins arise in the dorsal venous arch and accompany the anterior tibial artery up the calf lying anterior to the tibia (Figure 32-31, *A*). The anterior tibial veins pass posteriorly from the anterior compartment of the leg to penetrate the interosseous membrane and course between the tibia and fibula, uniting with the common tibial and common peroneal trunks at the distal border of the popliteus muscle to form the popliteal vein.

The posterior tibial veins arise from the plantar venous arch of the foot. They accompany the posterior tibial artery through the leg, coursing posterior to the tibia, where they unite to form the common tibial trunk. The common tibial trunk and the common peroneal trunk converge to form the tibioperoneal trunk.

The peroneal veins arise medial to the lateral malleolus. These veins follow the medial surface of the fibula in the lower half of the calf and then course medially to form the common peroneal trunk in the upper third of the calf.

The tibial veins normally contain 6 to 12 **bicuspid venous valves**, which serve to promote unidirectional flow and regulate venous pressure in the distal lower extremity venous system.

The paired gastrocnemius veins drain the gastrocnemius muscles of the calf and become confluent with the popliteal vein in the popliteal fossa. They are accompanied by the popliteal artery along their course.

The popliteal vein extends cephalad to the medial aspect of the femur, lying 1 to 2 cm from the posterior surface of the distal femur, and then passes through the adductor hiatus to become the femoral vein (superficial femoral vein). The popliteal vein accompanies the popliteal artery lying within a fascial sheath. The popliteal vein normally courses posterior and superficial to the popliteal artery. At the distal popliteal fossa the vein lies slightly medial to the artery but crosses the artery laterally as it ascends into the proximal part of the fossa. The popliteal vein normally contains three to four valves.

The femoral vein (superficial femoral vein) is the continuation of the popliteal vein. It accompanies the superficial femoral artery as it courses up the medial aspect of the thigh to the level of the inguinal ligament. The femoral vein normally contains three to six valves along its course.

At the level of the inguinal ligament, the femoral vein becomes the common femoral vein. The common femoral vein lies within Scarpa's triangle medial to the common femoral artery. Normally, the common femoral vein contains three to five valves.

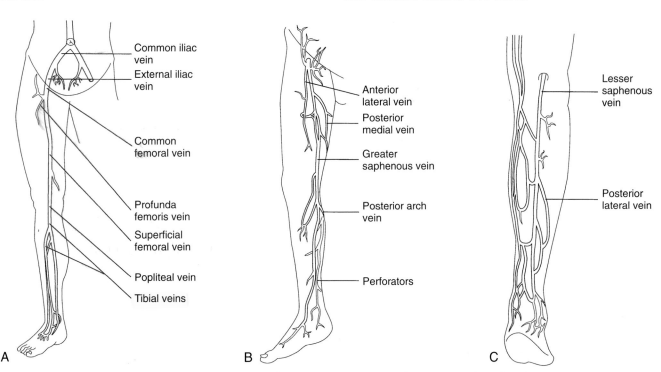

FIGURE 32-31   **A,** Lower extremity deep venous system. **B** and **C,** Great and small saphenous veins.

The external iliac vein is a continuation of the common femoral vein, accompanying the external iliac artery. It originates posterior to the inguinal ligament, ascending the pelvic brim to terminate anterior to the sacroiliac joint, where it becomes the common iliac vein. Occasionally, a single valve is found in the external iliac vein.

The internal iliac vein ascends the pelvis posteromedial to the internal iliac artery. It becomes confluent with the external iliac vein to form the common iliac vein.

The common iliac veins converge to form the inferior vena cava. The left common iliac vein courses posterior to the right iliac artery, accounting for a higher incidence of left lower extremity deep vein thrombosis and swelling. Normally, there are no valves in the common iliac veins.

Anatomic variations are common in the deep venous system. The most common anomalies include duplication of the popliteal and/or femoral veins, duplication of the distal segment of the femoral vein subsequently uniting to form a single vein in the mid to proximal thigh, and the presence of three or more tibial, popliteal, or femoral veins.

The Superficial Venous System

The major superficial veins of the lower limb are the great saphenous and the small saphenous veins (Figure 32-31, *B* and *C*). These veins lie in subcutaneous tissue and are superficial to the deep fascia.

The great saphenous vein arises from the medial aspect of the dorsal venous arch, continuing in the foot, and ascends in the ankle anteromedial to the medial malleolus. The vein most often courses 1 to 2 cm posterior to the medial border of the tibia. In approximately 4% of patients, the vein will course in a more posterior plane. It then crosses behind the medial condyle of the femur at the level of the knee. It courses up the medial aspect of the thigh to drain into the common femoral vein about 3.5 cm below the inguinal ligament, inferior and lateral to the pubic tubercle. The location of the confluence is variable; the superficial vein may empty into the deep system at the level of the femoral vein in the thigh or above the inguinal ligament, where it may join the deep system at the level of the iliac veins. There are usually four valves in the great saphenous vein in the lower leg and up to six valves in the thigh.

Most often (65% of patients), the thigh segment of the great saphenous vein is a single, continuous trunk with accessory medial and lateral branches originating in the groin. In 35% of patients the thigh segment is duplicated, with separate veins lying in the medial and lateral aspects of the limb. In the distal calf the posterior accessory great saphenous vein (posterior arch vein) becomes confluent with the main trunk. A single trunk is present in the calf in only 45% of patients. In a

significant number of patients the saphenous vein is duplicated below the knee, with the anterior branch being dominant.

The small saphenous vein begins at the lateral end of the dorsal venous arch and ascends in the ankle posterior to the lateral malleolus. This vein extends up the back of the calf to the distal popliteal fossa, where it perforates the deep fascia, passing between the heads of the gastrocnemius muscle, and drains into the popliteal vein. Like the great saphenous vein, the confluence with the deep venous system is variable. The small saphenous vein may empty into the popliteal vein, the femoral vein, or the inferior gluteal vein, or it may not have a confluence at all with the deep venous system but rather drain into the great saphenous vein in the thigh or at the level of the knee. The great and small saphenous veins may communicate through the cranial extension of the small saphenous vein (formerly termed the *vein of Giacomini*) in the proximal calf or via the posterior thigh circumflex vein.

The lateral arch vein is the primary tributary of the small saphenous vein. It courses upward along the lateral aspect of the calf to empty into the small saphenous vein just distal to the popliteal fossa. Perforating veins connect the lateral arch vein to the gastrocnemius or peroneal veins.

The Perforating Veins

The deep and superficial venous systems are connected by the perforating, or communicating, veins. In the calf there are eight groups of major perforating veins. These include the medial, lateral, and posterior perforators, with Cockett's I, II, and III having the greatest clinical significance. The posterior group of perforators connects the small saphenous vein with the great saphenous vein. The medial perforating veins connect the great saphenous vein (the posterior accessory great saphenous vein) with the posterior tibial veins, and the lateral perforators join the great saphenous vein with the anterior tibial and peroneal veins.

The Cockett's perforators lie in a defined area in the medial aspect of the distal calf and connect the posterior accessory great saphenous vein (posterior arch vein) with the posterior tibial veins. Cockett's I is located 7 to 8 cm superior to the medial malleolus, whereas Cockett's II and III are located, respectively, approximately 13.5 cm and 18.5 cm above the ankle.

In the proximal calf, Boyd's perforating veins connect the great saphenous vein to the posterior tibial veins.

The perforating veins of the thigh are also divided into medial, lateral, and posterior groups. There are up to six perforating veins in the medial thigh connecting the great saphenous vein with the femoral vein. Dodd's perforators, which are found along the medial aspect of the distal thigh, connect the great saphenous vein to the femoral and deep femoral veins and are the most important clinically. The Hunterian vein, a major perforating vein that connects the great saphenous vein to the femoral vein, is found in the mid-thigh approximately 15 cm above the knee.

Size of the Deep and Superficial Veins

Average Diameters of the Deep Veins

Tibial veins	Approximately 5 mm
Popliteal vein	0.9 to 1.5 cm
Femoral vein (superficial femoral vein)	0.9 to 1.0 cm
Common femoral vein	1.2 to 1.9 cm

Average Diameters of the Superficial Veins

Great saphenous vein	2 to 3 mm (calf)
	4 to 6 mm (thigh)
Small saphenous vein	4 to 7 mm

Sonographic Appearance of the Deep and Superficial Venous Systems

Every deep vein is accompanied by an artery that courses in close proximity. The common femoral vein lies midway between the pubis and the iliac spine at the level of the inguinal crease. It should be found medial to the common femoral artery and slightly deeper than this vessel. The lumen of the normal common femoral vein is anechoic, and the walls of the vein will coapt entirely with gentle transducer pressure applied to the anterior vein wall from the transverse image plane.

The great saphenous vein arises medially from the common femoral vein and courses superficially to the fascia of the thigh and calf to the dorsum of the foot.

The common femoral vein bifurcates into the femoral vein and the deep femoral vein (profunda femoris) about 2 to 4 cm distal to the confluence of the great saphenous vein. The profunda femoris vein courses laterally and deep to the femoral vein. It will lie in the same scan plane as the profunda femoris artery.

The femoral vein accompanies the superficial femoral artery, lying deep to this vessel and medial to the profunda femoris. Both the femoral vein and superficial femoral artery enter the adductor canal, crossing beneath the adductor fascia in the lower third of the thigh. The femoral vein is duplicated, over at least a short length, in 15% to 20% of patients.

The femoral vein becomes the popliteal vein at the level of the adductor canal. The vein will remain posterior to the popliteal artery; however, the vein is most easily interrogated from the popliteal fossa. From this image plane, the popliteal vein will appear superficial to its companion artery. The popliteal vein will be duplicated in approximately 35% of patients.

The small saphenous vein normally arises from the popliteal vein proximally at about mid-knee level. The vessel courses posterolaterally down the leg, terminating anterior to the lateral malleolus. The paired gastrocnemius veins are confluent with the distal segment of the popliteal vein and run parallel to the popliteal artery.

The popliteal vein can be imaged to the proximal calf, where it bifurcates into the anterior tibial trunk and the tibioperoneal trunk, which lies deep to the gastrocnemius and soleus muscles. At this point, the veins duplicate. For each tibial artery there are at least two tibial veins.

The anterior tibial veins can be imaged from the anterior aspect of the leg as they emerge after crossing the interosseous membrane. They remain on top of the membrane as they course down the leg to cross the region of the ankle.

The posterior tibial veins course superficially and can be imaged from the medial aspect of the calf from the proximal calf to the level of the medial malleolus.

The peroneal veins can also be imaged from the proximal calf level, lying deeper than the posterior tibial veins and adjacent to the fibula. From a lateral scan plane, the peroneal veins will lie superior to the posterior tibial veins.

Hemodynamic Patterns of the Lower Extremity Deep Venous System

Movement of blood in the lower extremity veins is influenced by respiratory variation, which causes changes in intraabdominal pressure, the calf muscle pump, and the presence of competent venous valves.

With inhalation, the diaphragm descends and the blood flow return from the lower extremities is impeded, *resisted.* resulting from an increase in intraabdominal pressure. With expiration, the diaphragm rises, intraabdominal pressure decreases, and venous return is possible.

In addition to respiratory variation, venous return is promoted by the calf muscle pump and competent venous valves. When a person is at rest, the energy for transport of venous blood from the legs to the heart is supplied by contraction of the left ventricle. This cardiac contraction alone is insufficient to move blood from the leg and is complemented by the calf muscle pump, which is activated with exercise. As much as 20% of the body's total blood volume may be pooled in the leg veins within 15 minutes of cessation of exercise.

During exercise, the cephalad movement of blood in the lower extremities is a complex function of the calf muscles and the venous valves. With each step taken during walking, there are periods of relaxation and contraction of the calf muscles. When the calf muscles are relaxed, the blood flows into the lower pressure deep venous system from the high-pressure superficial venous system. As the muscle contracts, the blood moves from the deep calf veins into the deep thigh veins. Valves in the deep veins prevent the flow of blood toward the feet, and the valves in the perforating veins prevent blood from flowing from the deep to the superficial system. The calf muscle pump helps to control the hydrostatic pressure in the leg veins by continuously pumping blood out of these veins. The venous pressure in the feet of an exercising adult will therefore usually be less than 25 mm Hg.

One of the most remarkable characteristics of veins is the capacity to undergo tremendous volume changes with little change in **transmural pressure** (Figure 32-32, *A*). The venous wall is about one-tenth as thick as the arterial wall, with little elastin present in the media of the vein. The percentage of smooth muscle

Pressure between 2 walls

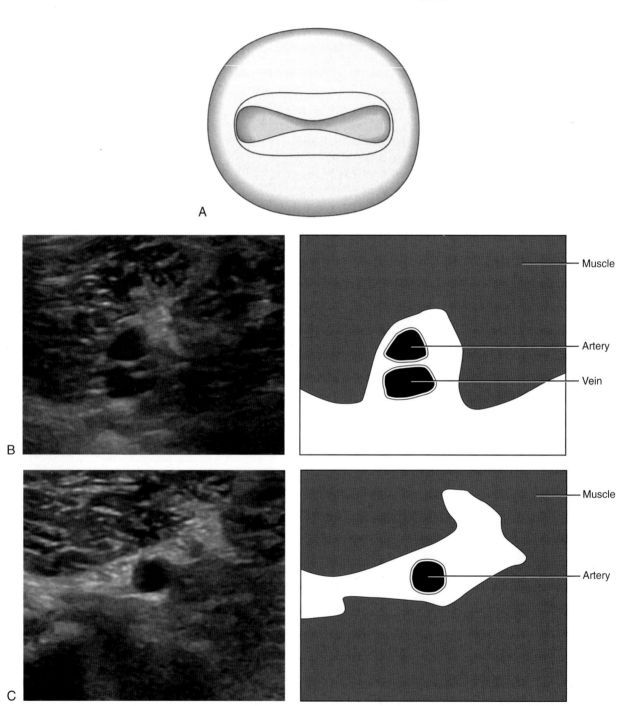

FIGURE 32-32 **A,** Short axis section of vein showing collapse of the venous wall with low transmural pressure. **B,** Transverse scanning plane image of axial sections of the superficial femoral artery and femoral vein. **C,** Transverse scanning plane image of axial sections of the superficial femoral artery and femoral vein demonstrating coaptation of the venous walls that occurs with gentle transducer pressure.

found in the wall of the media will vary depending on the location of the vein, with about 60% muscle being found in the veins of the foot—the veins subjected to the greatest hydrostatic pressure. The walls of the normal vein can be coapted with gentle transducer pressure during transverse imaging of the vein (Figures 32-32, *B* and *C*).

Doppler Spectral Analysis

Blood flow in the lower extremity veins is spontaneous and phasic with respiration, ceasing with inspiration and augmenting with expiration (Figure 32-33). Pulsatility of flow may be caused by increased central venous pressure due to fluid overload or tricuspid insufficiency or may be related to the proximity of the veins to the heart.

Flow can be augmented by compressing the limb below the level of the transducer (distally) and impeded by compression above the level of the transducer (proximally) (Figure 32-34). Valvular competence is confirmed by noting the absence of retrograde venous flow with proximal compression of the limb (Figure 32-35).

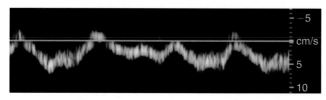

FIGURE 32-33 Doppler spectral waveform recorded from the normal common femoral vein. Note phasicity of flow, which varies with the respiratory cycle.

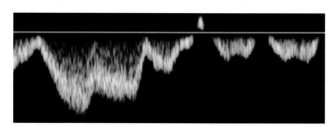

FIGURE 32-34 Doppler spectral waveform demonstrating augmentation of venous flow with manual compression of the limb proximal to the transducer position.

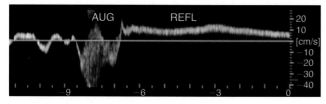

FIGURE 32-35 Doppler spectral waveform demonstrating venous augmentation when the limb is manually compressed distal to the transducer position. Flow is retrograde (refluxing) when the compression is released because the valve is incompetent. *AUG*, Augmentation; *REFL*, reflux.

A Valsalva maneuver often will enlarge a vein, dramatically aiding in identification and localization of the vessel.

Because they lie deep in the pelvis and are usually noncompressible, veins proximal to the inguinal ligament cannot be reliably studied using duplex technology alone. The addition of optimized color and power Doppler imaging to confirm luminal filling complements the examination procedure.

In general the flow characteristics should be examined in each limb and the symmetry of flow patterns compared with the opposite limb with regard to spontaneity, phasicity, augmentation, competence, and absence of pulsatility.

QUALITY ASSURANCE IN VASCULAR TECHNOLOGY

Vascular sonography allows us not only to recognize the presence of disease but also to determine the severity of the hemodynamic compromise. Initially, laboratories categorize disease severity based on criteria that are promoted nationally. Each laboratory must then internally validate the adopted criteria by comparing their test results to a recognized "gold standard." In the case of cerebrovascular and extremity arterial test procedures, this has historically involved comparison with arteriography. Most recently, magnetic resonance imaging and/or computed tomography angiography have been used as the standards for correlation of carotid and arterial noninvasive test results.

Measurements Used for Test Validation

Historically, for determination of severity of disease in the peripheral arteries, laboratories have used velocity measurement in the artery at the site of disease compared with the velocity of a proximal adjacent normal segment of the artery. For the extracranial internal carotid artery, laboratories historically used measurement of the diameter of residual lumen of the artery at the site of disease (usually within the carotid bulb) compared to the diameter of the bulb. More recently, determination of severity of internal carotid artery disease has been based on measurement of the diameter of the residual arterial lumen at the site of disease compared to the diameter of the more distal normal segment of the internal carotid artery. These data are then compared with velocities associated with each of the chosen categories of disease. The majority of vascular laboratories have established criteria based on **diameter reduction**, which in some laboratories may be complemented with area reduction, as their standard for diagnostic criteria. In the case of venous duplex examinations, venography served for many years as the gold standard, but in modern practice, clinical outcome or a same day, repeat, focused examination have been used as the means of choice for correlating the results of venous duplex examinations.

The following calculation is used for determination of the severity of peripheral arterial disease:

$$\% \text{ Luminal diameter reduction} = (1 \text{ residual diameter/original diameter}) \times 100$$

Given this, a diseased artery with a normal diameter of 8 mm and a 4 mm residual diameter would have a 50% stenosis.

$$\% \text{ Luminal diameter reduction} = (1 \text{ to } 4 \text{ mm/8 mm}) \times 100$$
$$= 1 \text{ to } 0.5 \times 100 = 50\% \text{ stenosis}$$

It is important to remember that the technique for determining diameter reduction for the extracranial internal carotid artery has changed in recent years as a result of the Asymptomatic Carotid Artery Stenosis (ACAS) study and the North American Symptomatic Carotid Endarterectomy Trial (NASCET). Currently, the diameter of the normal distal internal carotid artery lumen is used as the reference for comparison with the diameter of the residual arterial lumen at the site of disease. Using the example above, if an internal carotid artery has a residual lumen of 4 mm, and the diameter of the distal segment of the artery is also 4 mm, our measurement would be:

$$\% \text{ Luminal diameter reduction} = (1 - \text{residual/distal}) \times 100$$

If you look closely at this method of measurement, you can see how it would be possible to have disease with a resultant measurement of 0% stenosis or even a negative stenosis! Area reduction can be calculated from a single plane view or from two single plane views. When calculated from a single plane, the percent cross-sectional area reduction is:

$$(1 - \text{residual}^2/\text{original}^2) \times 100 = (1 - 4 \text{ mm}^2/8 \text{ mm}^2) \times 100$$
$$= (1 - 16/64) \times 100 = 75\% \text{ stenosis}$$

If the percentage of cross-sectional area reduction is calculated from two single plane views, the equation then becomes:

$$(1 - \text{residual}_1 \times \text{residual}_2/\text{original}_1 \times \text{original}_2) \times 100$$
$$(1 \text{ to } 2 \text{ mm} \times 4 \text{ mm/8 mm} \times 8 \text{ mm}) \times 100 = (1 - 8/64) \times 100$$
$$= 88\% \text{ stenosis}$$

Some laboratories attempt to use both diameter reduction and cross-sectional area reduction in hopes of achieving increased test sensitivity and optimization of the predictive values of noninvasive test procedures. It is important to recognize that a comparison of these methods of measurement requires an assumption that the lesion is uniform and circumferential, a feature rarely found with atherosclerotic disease. Careful study of the relationship between diameter and area reduction, as shown in Table 32-3, will reveal how

Table 32-3 Comparison of the Relationship Between Diameter Reduction and Area Reduction

Diameter Reduction	Area Reduction
10%	19%
20%	36%
30%	51%
40%	64%
50%	75%
60%	84%
70%	91%
80%	96%
90%	99%

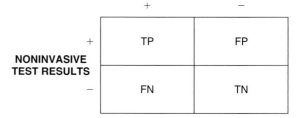

GOLD STANDARD RESULTS

	+	−
+	TP	FP
−	FN	TN

NONINVASIVE TEST RESULTS

FIGURE 32-36 Positive and negative noninvasive test results compared with the gold standard.

misunderstanding of the data and the nature of disease might lead to errors in diagnosis.

Statistical Correlation

Although the process of statistical correlation may seem quite complex, the steps are really straightforward. The first step in the validation process is to categorize the results of a noninvasive test as either positive or negative based on validated criteria. As an example, if you were evaluating the ability of cerebrovascular duplex scanning to detect ICA stenosis in the range 50% to 69% diameter reduction, a positive study would include only stenosis in that range, and a negative examination would include stenoses in all other categories and also normal arteries and those with total occlusions.

The next step is to compare (correlate) the individual test results with the "gold standard," using your chosen criteria for a positive or negative test result. Using the example described above, a positive carotid arteriogram would include only 50% to 69% diameter reducing stenoses, and negative test results would include all normals, all stenoses other than those in our chosen range, and all occlusions. The data are typically analyzed by using a 2 × 2 table as illustrated in Figure 32-36. The Chi-square table compares the positive and negative noninvasive test results with the gold standard.

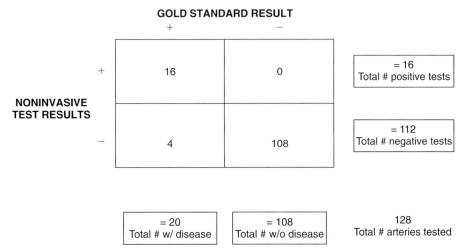

GOLD STANDARD RESULT

FIGURE 32-37 Example of positive and negative noninvasive test results compared with the gold standard.

Understanding the Assigned Values

True positive (TP) tests are those in which the noninvasive test is positive for the disease category in question, and the gold standard is also positive for the same severity of disease. In other words, if we use our example, the noninvasive test and the gold standard are in agreement that 50% to 69% stenosis is present.

True negative (TN) tests are those in which the noninvasive test is negative for our chosen category of disease and the gold standard is also negative. Using our example, the duplex scan and the gold standard both agree that the ICA does not have 50% to 69% stenosis.

False positive (FP) tests are those in which the noninvasive test is positive for the chosen category, but the gold standard is not in agreement. In other words, the duplex scan demonstrates 50% to 69% stenosis, but the gold standard indicates that the narrowing is only in a category with greater or less than 50% to 69% diameter reducing disease.

False negative (FN) tests are those in which the noninvasive test is negative for the chosen category of disease but the gold standard is positive for that degree of disease severity. Using our example, the duplex scan demonstrates less than 50% stenosis of the ICA, and the gold standard demonstrates 50% to 69% stenosis.

If we assume that the gold standard is always correct, then it is understood that TP and TN occur when the noninvasive test and the gold standard are in agreement and FP and FN occur when the noninvasive test and the gold standard are in disagreement.

Understanding the Columns and Rows

If we assign numerical values to our example, we can then determine the ability of our carotid duplex examination to detect stenosis in the category 50% to 69% diameter reduction. If we have 64 patients who

underwent carotid arteriography, we have a total of 128 ICAs to correlate with our gold standard. Of those 128 ICAs, duplex scanning showed 16 had stenosis in the category 50% to 69%, but the arteriogram showed 20 ICAs had that degree of stenosis (TP = 16). Therefore there must have been 0 FP. However, that leaves 4 that were FN (remember, the arteriogram said there were 20 arteries with the chosen category of disease severity, and the gold standard is assumed to be correct). The arteriogram and the ultrasound examination agreed that there were 108 ICAs that did not have disease in the category 50% to 69% diameter reduction (TN). If we fill these values into the 2 × 2 table, we can complete our analysis as shown in Figure 32-37.

Understanding the Calculations

Sensitivity is the ability of a noninvasive test procedure to detect disease when disease is present. Therefore the calculation indicates how "sensitive" a noninvasive test is in detecting the presence of disease. You should recall that the vascular laboratory test results are compared with the gold standard.

$$\text{Sensitivity} = \frac{TP}{TP + FN} \times 100$$

In our example above, sensitivity = (16/16 + 4) × 100 = 80%.

Specificity is the ability of a noninvasive test procedure to exclude disease when no disease is present. Therefore the calculation indicates how "specific" a noninvasive test is in determining when a patient is normal, or negative, for disease.

$$\text{Specificity} = \frac{TN}{TN + FP} \times 100$$

In our example, the specificity = (108/108 + 0) × 100 = 100%.

Positive predictive value (PPV) allows us to determine the likelihood that when the noninvasive test is positive, the gold standard will also be positive. In other words, the calculated PPV indicates the predictive capability of a positive test to identify patients with disease. You should note that this calculation takes into consideration only the "positive" tests.

$$PPV = \frac{TP}{TP + FP} \times 100$$

In our example, the PPV = (16/16 + 0) × 100 = 100%.

Negative predictive value (NPV) allows us to determine the likelihood that when the noninvasive test is negative, the gold standard will also be negative. In other words, the calculated NPV indicates the predictive ability of a negative test to identify patients without disease. You should note that calculation of the NPV takes into consideration only the "negative" tests.

$$NPV = \frac{TN}{TN + FN} \times 100$$

Using our example, the NPV = (108/108 + 4) × 100 = 96%.

Accuracy indicates the percentage (i.e., overall agreement) of all the noninvasive studies that were correctly identified when compared with the gold standard. You should note that the numerator in this calculation comprises the "true positives" and "true negatives" (the number of tests that were in total agreement with the gold standard), and the denominator is the total number of noninvasive studies submitted for correlation with the gold standard.

$$Accuracy = \frac{TP + TN}{TP + TN + FP + FN} \times 100$$

In our example, the accuracy of the noninvasive test for identification of carotid artery stenosis in the range of 40% to 59% would be represented as:

$$Accuracy = (16 + 108/16 + 108 + 0 + 4) \times 100 = 97\%$$

Prevalence is the incidence of disease in the total population of patients who were studied noninvasively. The calculation indicates when disease is truly present in the population. Therefore the numerator of the equation consists of the "true positives" (the number of times the noninvasive test agreed with the gold standard that disease was really present) and the "false negatives" (the number of times the gold standard identified disease in the chosen category of severity but the noninvasive test failed to identify it). Remember, we must assume that the gold standard is always correct.

$$Prevalence = \frac{TP + FN}{TP + TN + FP + FN} \times 100$$

In our example, prevalence = (16 + 4/16 + 108 + 0 + 4) × 100 = 16%.

SUMMARY

Noninvasive vascular diagnostic methods have shown tremendous advancement in recent decades with the development of sophisticated instrumentation and technology. As a result of enhanced imaging capabilities, sonography has become in many cases the procedure of choice for identification and evaluation of cerebrovascular, peripheral arterial, and venous disease. The laboratory staff must not only be skilled in the performance of each test but also be able to recognize the capabilities and limitations of each test procedure and understand the pathophysiology of vascular disease in order to provide the interpreting physician with an accurate study. The goal of the vascular diagnostic laboratory is to provide accurate, appropriate, cost-effective, noninvasive diagnostic procedures that will answer the following questions: Is vascular disease present? Where is it located? How severe is the vascular disorder? What are the therapeutic options? Has revascularization been successful?

REFERENCE CHARTS

■ ■ ■   ASSOCIATED PHYSICIANS

- **Vascular surgeon:** Specializes in the surgical and endovascular treatment of cerebrovascular, peripheral arterial, and venous disorders.
- **Cardiologist:** Specializes in the diagnosis and treatment of cardiac disease.
- **Neurologist:** Specializes in the diagnosis and treatment of cerebrovascular disorders.
- **Vascular/interventional radiologist:** Specializes in diagnosis, identification, localization, and endovascular treatment of cerebrovascular, peripheral arterial, and venous disorders. Treatment includes endovascular balloon dilatation (angioplasty), thrombectomy, embolectomy, atherectomy, percutaneous insertion of inferior vena cava filters, and stent placement.

■ ■ ■   COMMON DIAGNOSTIC TESTS

- **Vascular angiography:** A contrast medium is injected into an artery or vein, and radiographic films are taken at specific intervals to observe blood flow patterns in vessels and organ vasculature. Performed by interventional vascular radiologists and vascular surgeons assisted by radiologic technologists and interpreted by interventional vascular radiologists and vascular surgeons.
- **Computed tomography angiography:** A contrast medium is injected intravenously while x-ray data are acquired continuously during a single breath hold or as a bolus-tracking method. The acquired data are reconstructed and displayed as axial slices or in 3-dimensional format. Performed by interventional vascular radiologists and vascular surgeons with assistance by radiologic technologists and interpreted by interventional vascular radiologists and vascular surgeons.

- **Magnetic resonance angiography:** There are three types of magnetic resonance angiography (MRA). The first type is unenhanced, which uses no contrast agent. The second type, enhanced MRA, employs the contrast agent gadolinium and is not useful for imaging vessels less than 1 mm in diameter. The third type of MRA is referred to as phase-sensitive imaging. This method acquires paired images in either two or three directions. Each pair has a different sensitivity to flowing blood. The collected images are combined to create a 3-dimensional image. Performed and interpreted by interventional vascular radiologists.

■ ■ ■ LABORATORY VALUES

Nonapplicable.

■ ■ ■ NORMAL M-MODE MEASUREMENTS

Nonapplicable.

■ ■ ■ VASCULATURE

Nonapplicable.

■ ■ ■ AFFECTING CHEMICALS

Nonapplicable.

CHAPTER 33

3-D/4-D Sonography

CHERYL A. VANCE

Define three-dimensional (3-D) sonography.

Define four-dimensional (4-D) sonography.

Describe 3-D/4-D acquisition and display techniques.

Explain how to manipulate the volume data for simplified anatomic viewing.

Select the appropriate technology to demonstrate the anatomy of interest.

Identify examples of normal 3-D or 4-D anatomy.

Describe the clinical applications of 3-D and 4-D sonography.

Become familiar with some of the advanced 3-D/4-D features and technologies.

3-D (Three-Dimensional) Sonography — Acquisition and evaluation of static data created by stacking a series of two-dimensional (2-D) images into a volume data set. The volume data set can be rotated and manipulated to create optimal imaging planes.

4-D (Four-Dimensional) Sonography — Live acquisition of volume data sets. The fourth dimension is time. 4-D sonography is also known as *real-time 3-D ultrasound*.

Automatic Acquisition — Method requiring a dedicated 3-D/4-D transducer in which the elements within the transducer move to acquire a volume data set, regardless of whether the sonographer is moving the probe or holding it stationary.

Axis Dot — Also called the reference point. The axis dot is the point at which all 3 orthogonal planes intersect within the volume data set. It depicts the same anatomic point in all 3 dimensions.

Inversion Mode — Type of volume-rendering algorithm that displays anechoic structures or structures hypoechoic relative to adjacent anatomy as a solid object, giving the appearance of a cast or mold of the structure.

Manual Acquisition — Requires the sonographer to physically move the transducer across the region of interest.

Maximum Mode — Computer display of only the brightest intensity echoes within the volume data set. Used to assess fetal skeletal anatomy as well as pathology that appears hyperechoic relative to adjacent anatomy.

Minimum Mode — Computer display of only the lowest intensity echoes within the volume data set. Used to assess fluid-filled structures, such as vasculature, cystic areas, the fetal bladder, the stomach, and amniotic fluid.

Multiplanar Format/Display — Original acquisition plane plus two orthogonal planes are displayed simultaneously. Sagittal, transverse, and coronal planes are typically displayed, but any orthogonal variation may be displayed depending on the acquisition plane and post-processing manipulations.

Orthogonal Planes — Planes that are at right angles (90 degrees) to each other; typically displayed in sagittal, transverse and coronal planes.

Render Techniques — 3-D or 4-D display option that recreates the anatomy of interest from a volume data set. Rendering allows the user to select which echo information is emphasized and which echo information is reduced or removed from the display. One render feature option is to recreate the surface appearance of the anatomy. Another render feature recreates specified levels of echogenicity (i.e., hyperechoic) while ignoring other echogenicity levels (i.e., hypoechoic) of no interest.

Spatio-temporal Image Correlation (STIC) — 4-D feature that acquires and displays the fetal heart in a single moving, beating, continuous cycle. The 4-D fetal heart is able to be stored and manipulated to demonstrate any orthogonal plane necessary to evaluate the anatomy and physiology.

Thick Slice Imaging — Averaging multiple slices together within the volume data set to gain a "thicker slice" of displayed information and enhanced contrast resolution.

The thickness of the slice can be adjusted depending on the anatomy of interest. Also known as *volume contrast imaging*.

Tomographic Views — A format in which multiple slices within the same plane are displayed at varying depths (similar to traditional display methods seen in computed tomography and magnetic resonance imaging).

Volume Data Set — A series of 2-D image slices compiled to form a 3-D cube of data. This cube can be viewed not only from the original 2-D acquisition plane but also in any desired orthogonal plane.

Medical sonography is a progressive and ever-evolving diagnostic imaging modality. Spanning across its early features of A-mode and static B-mode to real-time two-dimensional (2-D) imaging with color- and pulsed-wave Doppler capabilities, sonography has now advanced even further by the use of three-dimensional (3-D) and four-dimensional (4-D) technologies. **3-D sonography** is the acquisition, reconstruction, and evaluation of volume data in multiple scanning planes. Most sonographers are familiar with basic 3-D capabilities through the emergence of 3-D fetal imaging (Figure 33-1). But keep in mind that obstetric imaging is only one of many uses for diagnostic 3-D sonography. Although 3-D is beneficial in obstetric scanning, it is also a valuable tool in the evaluation of gynecologic, abdominal, prostate, neonatal, small parts, musculoskeletal, and invasive sonographic procedures. New applications for 3-D sonography are continuously being identified. Any anatomy that is imaged using 2-D sonography may also be imaged using 3-D technologies.

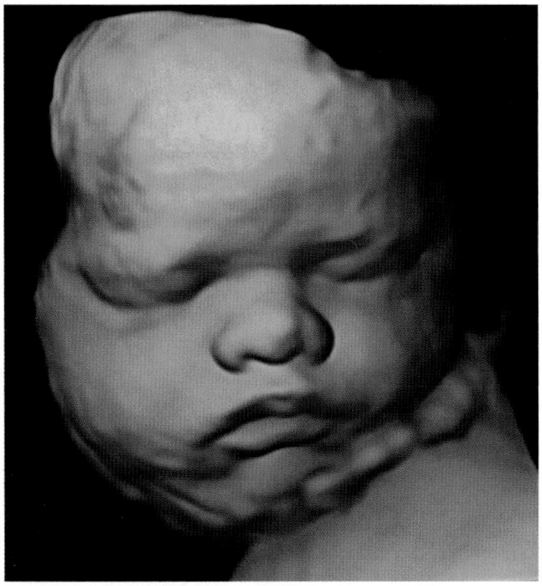

4-D sonography is simply "real-time" 3-D (time being the fourth dimension). It is available only with the **automatic acquisition** technique in which the elements within the probe continuously acquire, process, and display the 4-D image in real time. This method gives operators the advantage of observing 3-D volume information "in motion." It is particularly useful when imaging the heart (Figure 33-2).

Another advantage of 4-D volume imaging is to assist with needle guidance procedures. Using 4-D real-time multiplanar displays (explained later in the chapter), the operator can try to follow the needle, live, in all three dimensions rather than only using 2-D.

3-D sonography was first introduced in the late 1980s, and 4-D sonography appeared in the late 1990s. With the advent of faster processors and advances in ultrasound and transducer technology, 3-D/4-D sonography has become more widely accepted.

METHODS

The technologies behind 3-D/4-D sonography are diverse. Numerous companies are developing 3-D/4-D ultrasound—all using different technologies. Most higher-end ultrasound systems can be purchased with a 3-D/4-D option. In the past, companies designed offline computers that connected to existing ultrasound systems and converted 2-D ultrasound data into 3-D volume data sets (explained later in the chapter). Currently, most systems have their 3-D/4-D hardware and software integrated into the system. Dedicated 3-D/4-D ultrasound transducers provide the easiest, most accurate, and reproducible multiplanar images.

This variety in volume technology acquisition techniques may present a challenge to the sonographer as some methods are more difficult than others and the results of the various methods are different. This chapter will describe the more common methods to acquire volume data sets, simplify the manipulations to achieve the desired image, and address the variety of 3-D/4-D display options and available advanced features.

FIGURE 33-1   **3-D Surface Rendering of a Third Trimester Fetal Face.** A portion of the umbilical cord is seen below the fetal left cheek.

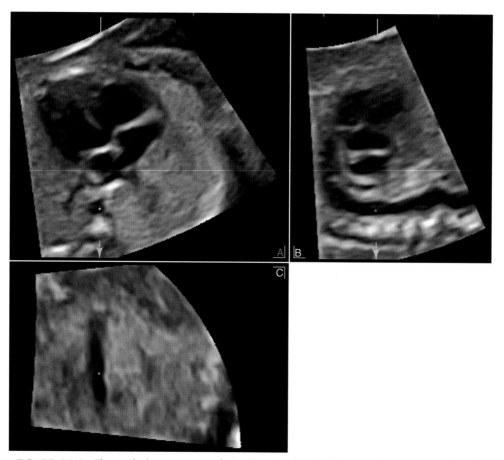

FIGURE 33-2 This multiplanar image of the four-chamber fetal heart (A-plane), ductal arch (B-plane), and descending aorta (C-plane) was reconstructed from a 4-D volume data set.

When the sonographer performs 3-D or 4-D sonography, the patient's anatomy is acquired as a volume data set. This volume data set is displayed on a flat screen, typically in a **multiplanar display/format**. With a multiplanar format the original acquisition plane plus the two **orthogonal planes** (planes that are at right angles [90 degrees] to each other; typically displayed in sagittal, transverse, and coronal planes) are displayed simultaneously on the screen. From this multiplanar display, the sonographer manipulates the data to display the anatomy of interest and then uses advanced system features to enhance various anatomy. Therefore, 3-D/4-D sonography can be divided into 3 basic steps: (1) volume acquisition, (2) volume manipulations, and (3) enhanced display features.

Step 1: Volume Acquisition

3-D/4-D sonography generates volumes of data, or **volume data sets**. To generate a volume data set, the system stacks a series of 2-D image slices together to form a cube of data. This cube can be viewed not only from the original 2-D acquisition plane but also in any desired orthogonal plane. As with 2-D imaging, the scan techniques used during 3-D/4-D imaging are also important. Adequate frame rates, optimal scan windows, reduction of image artifacts, and other 2-D imaging techniques are just as important in 3-D/4-D sonography. If the initial 3-D/4-D volume data set is acquired suboptimally, the resultant volume data set and any reconstructions will not be accurate and therefore will be of minimal use. Volume acquisitions can be categorized into 2 primary methods; manual acquisitions and automatic acquisitions.

The **manual acquisition** method requires the sonographer to physically move the transducer across the region of interest. This movement is best performed in either a steady sliding motion or a pivoting motion. The 2-D slices are stored in a cine loop and compressed into a 3-D volume data set. Because the method requires manual movement of the transducer, it is very operator dependent. The transducer must be moved a specific distance in a certain amount of time to acquire a quality volume data set. To compensate for the potential error related to manually moving the transducer, some manufacturers have developed positioning sensors that can be attached to the transducer. Once calibrated, the computer can more accurately estimate the movement of the transducer, resulting in a more accurate data set acquisition. These sensors are sometimes subject to interference from other equipment in the room and may not be the best solution for every department. 4-D volumes cannot be acquired using manual acquisition techniques. 4-D sonography must be acquired using automatic acquisition techniques with dedicated volume probe technologies.

Automatic acquisitions require dedicated 3-D/4-D transducers that have elements within the transducer that move to capture the volume data set. The 3-D/4-D transducers are often slightly larger than conventional transducers. Automatic volume transducers are currently available for almost all ultrasound applications, including transabdominal, transvaginal, transrectal, small parts, and neonatal. To acquire a volume data set, first optimize the 2-D image and then activate the 3-D or 4-D option on the system. Some newer systems will automatically display the volume information at this point. Older technology systems will produce a region of interest box first that needs to be placed over the anatomy of interest. When imaging in 3-D/4-D, the sonographer should consider the desired quality (resolution) and the volume angle (size of the data set in and out of axis planes). These are adjusted before initiating the acquisition in 3-D or they may be adjusted during the 4-D acquisition. As the quality and volume angle are increased, the length of time to complete the acquisition (3-D) is increased and volume rate is (4-D)

decreased. Volume rates are a factor if the patient is holding his or her breath or if the anatomy of interest is in motion (fetus, heart, etc.). After the pre-acquisition adjustments are made, the sonographer initiates the volume acquisition. With 3-D, the sonographer holds the transducer still over the anatomy of interest. When the 3-D acquisition begins, the elements within the transducer move automatically, acquiring the anatomy as a single volume data set. With 4-D, once the acquisition begins, the sonographer may move the transducer. Multiple volume data sets are acquired during 4-D acquisitions.

The resultant volume data sets can display the anatomy in a variety of ways depending on the system features. One of the most common is a 3-plane display. The 3 planes are typically referred to as the A-, B-, and C-planes. The A-plane represents the plane the initial acquisition was achieved from. The B-plane represents a 90-degree clockwise rotation of the A-plane. The C-plane represents a 90-degree forward rotation of the A-plane (Figure 33-3).

The intersection point of the three orthogonal planes is referred to as the **axis dot** or reference point. When the data set is manipulated, it revolves around this intersection. The axis dot is displayed in the same anatomy in all three planes (Figure 33-4). 2-D and volume measurements are also able to be accomplished on volume data sets (Figure 33-5).

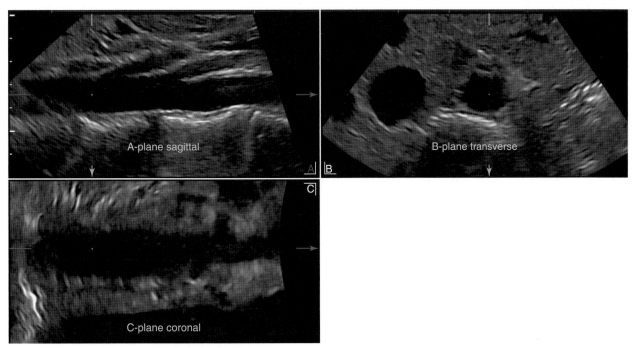

FIGURE 33-3 **Multiplanar Display of an Abdominal Aorta.** The A-plane represents the initial acquisition plane of the volume data set. The B-plane represents the A-plane rotated 90 degrees clockwise, resulting in an axial view of the aorta. The C-plane represents the A-plane rotated 90 degrees forward, resulting in a coronal plane, longitudinal view of the aorta.

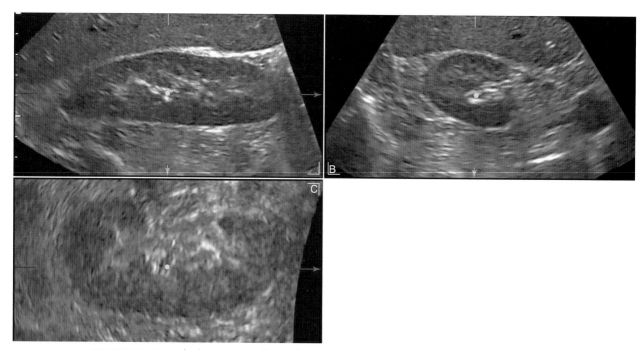

FIGURE 33-4 **Multiplanar View of a Right Kidney.** The axis dot (white dot) is the intersection point of all three planes. It is seen in the same renal vessel in all 3 planes.

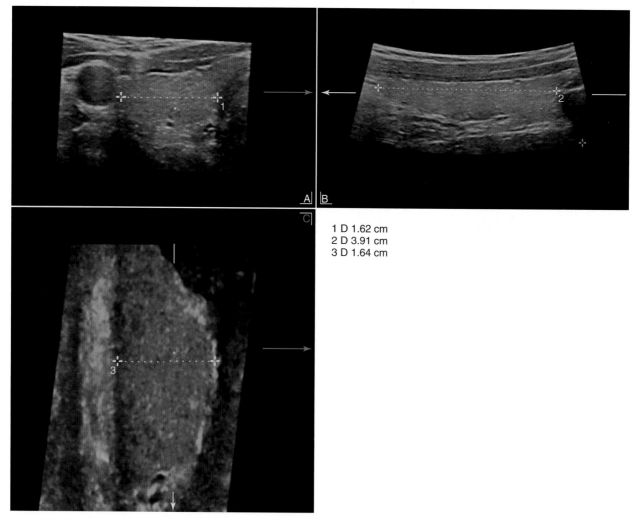

1 D 1.62 cm
2 D 3.91 cm
3 D 1.64 cm

FIGURE 33-5 3-D multiplanar view of a thyroid with measurements (A-plane = width, B-plane = length, C-plane = height). A blue tint was added to enhance the border definition.

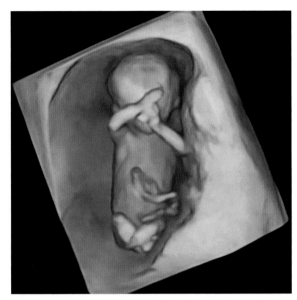

FIGURE 33-6 3-D rendering of a first trimester fetus with legs crossed and hands in front of face before any X-, Y-, or Z-manipulations.

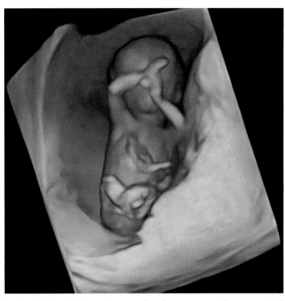

FIGURE 33-8 3-D rendering of a first trimester fetus rotated on the X-axis backward.

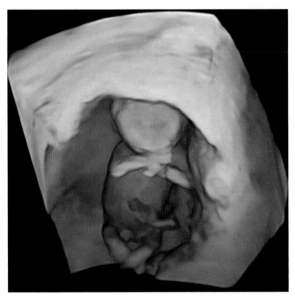

FIGURE 33-7 3-D rendering of a first trimester fetus rotated on the X-axis forward.

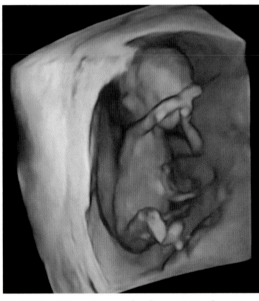

FIGURE 33-9 3-D rendering of a first trimester fetus rotated on the Y-axis to the observer's right.

Step 2: Volume Manipulations

After the volume data set is acquired, oftentimes it is necessary to realign the data set to view in standard orthogonal planes (sagittal, transverse, and coronal). By realigning the data set into standard orthogonal planes, the observer is more likely to recognize the atypical sonographic anatomic appearance (Figure 33-6).

Before manipulating the data set, it is first necessary to understand the X-, Y-, and Z-axis rotations. The X-axis rotation will roll the selected plane horizontally forward and backward (Figures 33-7 and 33-8). The Y-axis rotation will roll the selected plane vertically to the right or left (Figures 33-9 and 33-10). The Z-axis rotation will roll the selected plane horizontally clockwise or counterclockwise (Figures 33-11 and 33-12). In addition to X-, Y-, and Z-rotations, the data set may also be traversed along the active plane in a parallel manner (i.e., deeper or shallower within the active plane) (Figures 33-13 and 33-14).

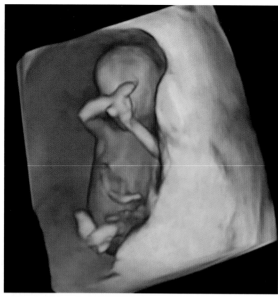

FIGURE 33-10   3-D rendering of a first trimester fetus rotated on the Y-axis to the observer's left.

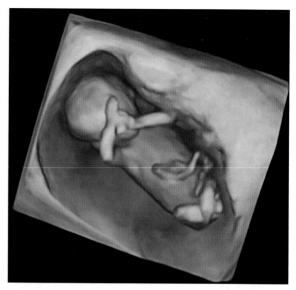

FIGURE 33-12   3-D rendering of a first trimester fetus rotated counterclockwise.

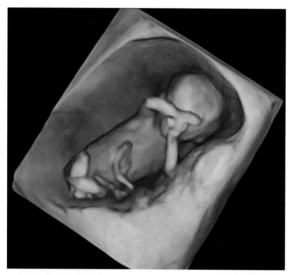

FIGURE 33-11   3-D rendering of a first trimester fetus rotated clockwise.

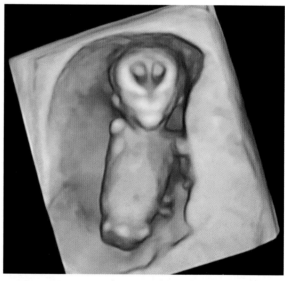

FIGURE 33-13   3-D rendering of a first trimester fetus with the depth adjusted deeper into the rendered image. Notice the arms and legs are not visible at this depth.

Aligning Data Sets Using the Z-Axis

Once the rotational planes are understood, the data set can be manipulated along the three orthogonal planes to achieve a more standard imaging plane. The "Z-technique" is a common method to align the volume data sets using primarily the Z-axis rotation. It was originally used to align the uterus to visualize the coronal plane. There are four simple steps involved when using the Z-axis to align volume data sets:

1. While in a multiplanar display, without the render feature activated, move the axis dot to a linear structure within the anatomy of interest (Figures 33-15 and 33-16).
2. Z-rotate the A-plane until the linear structure is either vertically or horizontally aligned (Figure 33-17).
3. Z-rotate the B-plane until the linear structure is either vertically or horizontally aligned (Figure 33-18).
4. Z-rotate the C-plane until the linear structure is either vertically or horizontally aligned (Figure 33-19).

Once all three planes have been aligned, the anatomy is easier to identify: the sagittal, transverse, and coronal uterus in this example.

The Z-technique can be used to align any data set. Focus on rotating at least two planes because the anatomy in the third plane is often spherical and not able to be aligned horizontally or vertically. Some landmarks commonly used as a focus point for placing the axis dot when using the Z-technique for nonuterine anatomy include:

- Vasculature (Carotid, Aorta, Inferior Vena Cava, Superior Mesenteric Artery, etc.)—Center of Vessel
- Neonatal Head—Falx
- Thyroid—Carotid or Midlobe Thyroid
- Gallbladder—Midbody
- Kidney—Echogenic Renal Sinus
- Uterine intrauterine device (IUD)—in IUD if visible or in Endometrial Stripe if IUD not visible
- Fetus
  - Brain—Falx
  - Upper Extremities—Radius or Ulna
  - Heart—Descending Aorta or Spine
  - Spine—Anterior Vertebral Body
  - Lower Extremities—Tibia or Fibula

Step 3: Enhanced Display Features

After the volume data set has been acquired and manipulated into the desired planes, the information can be displayed using several different system features depending on the anatomy of interest. The multiplanar format is useful to see the three orthogonal planes, but sometimes enhancing the volume information using other volume display features is necessary. Some of the more common display features include render techniques, tomographic imaging, and thick slice imaging.

Render techniques use algorithms to enhance the displayed anatomy. Most of us are probably familiar with the fetal face demonstrated with a surface render mode (Figure 33-20).

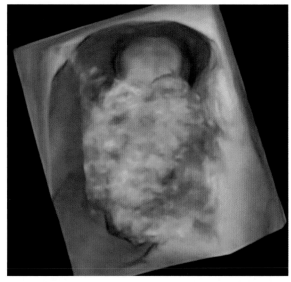

FIGURE 33-14 3-D rendering of a first trimester fetus with the depth adjusted shallower in the rendered image. Notice the uterine wall obscures most of the fetus at this depth selection.

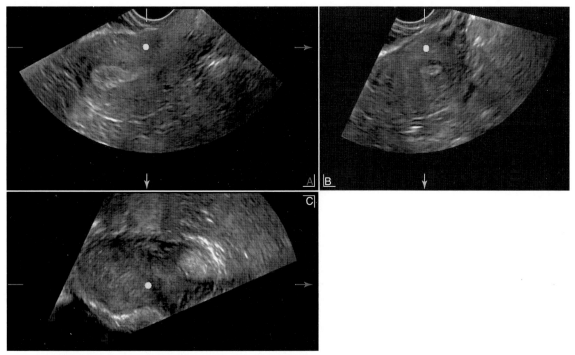

FIGURE 33-15 Notice that the white axis dot was initially located in the anterior uterine myometrium in all three planes.

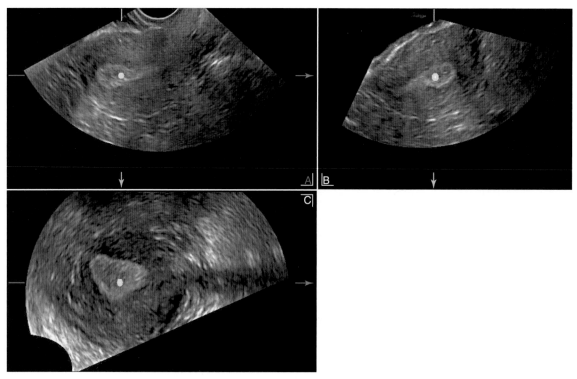

FIGURE 33-16 The axis dot has been moved from the anterior uterine myometrium to the endometrium, which is the "linear structure within the anatomy of interest" when imaging the uterine body.

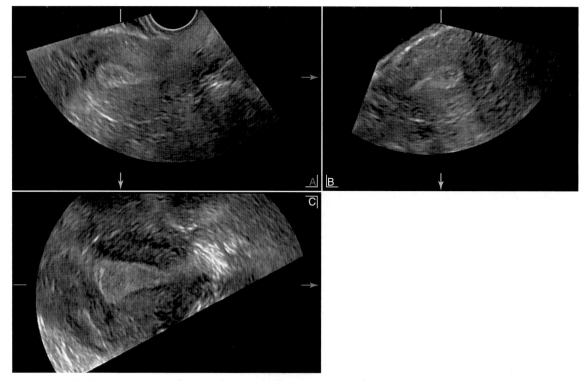

FIGURE 33-17 Once the axis dot is in the linear anatomy of interest, in this case the endometrium, the A-plane is rotated to align the structure (endometrial stripe) horizontally or vertically. In this case, the sonographer rotated the data set to make the endometrium horizontal.

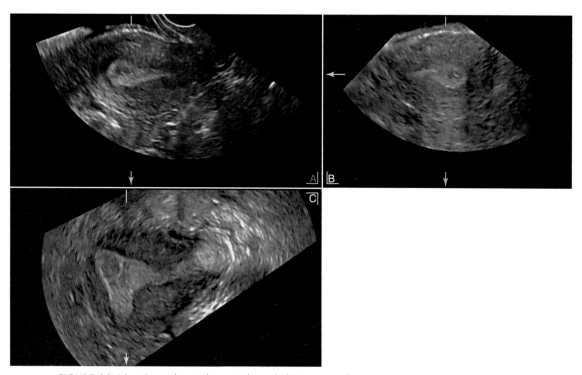

FIGURE 33-18 Once the A-plane is aligned, the sonographer activated the B-plane and rotated the linear structure (endometrial stripe) horizontally or vertically. In this case, the sonographer rotated the data set to make the endometrium horizontal.

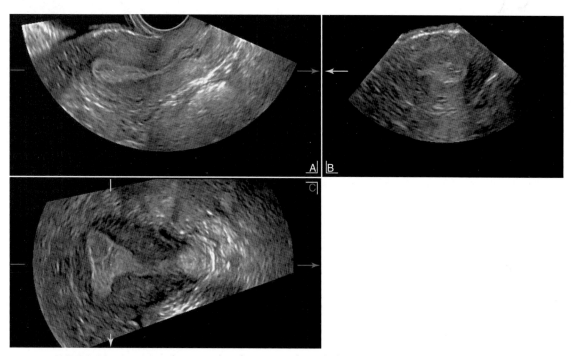

FIGURE 33-19 Once the A- and B-planes are aligned, the sonographer activated the C-plane and rotated the linear structure (endometrial stripe) horizontally or vertically. In this case, the sonographer rotated the data set to make the endometrium horizontal.

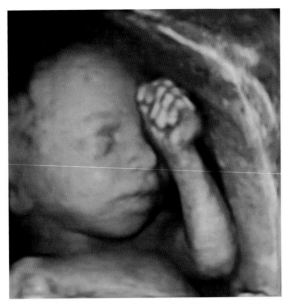

FIGURE 33-20   3-D rendering of a 27-week fetal face.

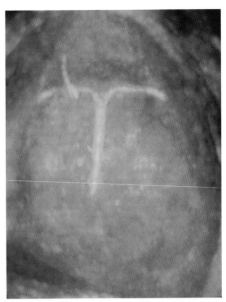

FIGURE 33-21   An intrauterine contraceptive device (IUD) is visualized using maximum render techniques to enhance the bright appearance of the IUD.

Surface rendering generates a surface perspective of the desired anatomy. This is a commonly used rendering mode, but there are other render modes that are often overlooked. For instance, the sonographer can select transparency rendering modes that display only the brightest intensity echoes within the volumes (instead of looking at the surface anatomy). This is called the **maximum mode**, or *maximum intensity projection.* Maximum mode can be used to visualize any anatomy or pathology that appears hyperechoic relative to adjacent anatomy, such as the fetal skeleton, hemangiomas, and intrauterine contraceptive devices (IUDs) (Figure 33-21).

In contrast to maximum mode, **minimum mode** rendering techniques emphasize the lowest intensity echoes within the volume. This is used to visualize fluid-filled structures, such as vasculature, cystic areas, the fetal bladder, and the stomach (Figure 33-22).

If rendering is not desired, the sonographer may choose to use a display option that resembles **tomographic views** similar to the display of computed tomographic (CT) or magnetic resonance (MR) images. This type of volumetric display can show parallel slices in an ultrasound volume at variable slice distances. Tomographic volume imaging is useful in application where the "bigger picture" is helpful including gynecology, abdominal organs, neonatal imaging, fetal brain, and fetal heart (Figure 33-23).

Another common display option is using a **thick slice imaging** technique. Rather than displaying a single slice from the volumetric planes, the system averages multiple slices together to gain a thicker slice and enhanced

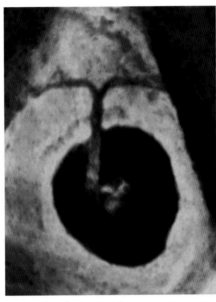

FIGURE 33-22   The shadowing from an intrauterine contraceptive device (IUD) and an early embryo inside the fluid-filled gestational sac are visualized using minimum render techniques to enhance the anechoic structures.

contrast resolution. The slice thickness can be adjusted depending on the anatomy of interest. Adjusting the slice thickness is often used when imaging thin endometriums, IUDs, abdominal organs, fetal spine, ribs, heart, and extremities (Figures 33-24 and 33-25).

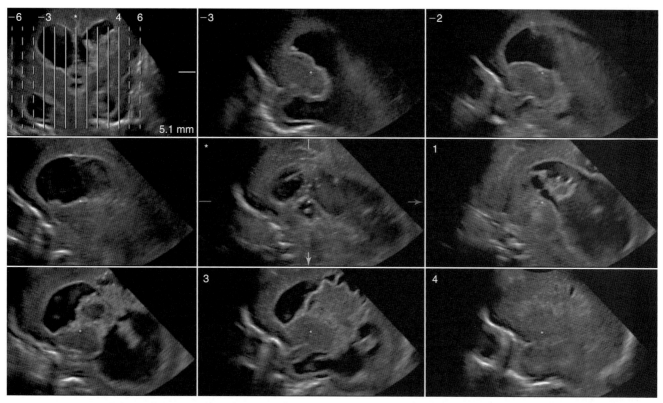

FIGURE 33-23 Tomographic view of longitudinal sections of the neonatal head demonstrating bilateral hydrocephalus.

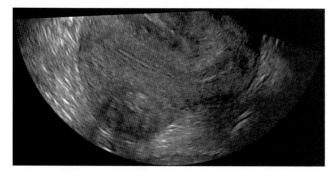

FIGURE 33-24 3-D image of a longitudinal section of the uterus with a posterior fibroid not using a thick slice.

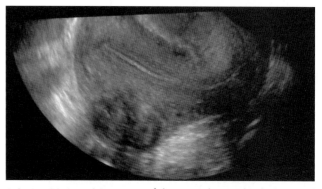

FIGURE 33-25 3-D image of the same longitudinal section of the uterus with a posterior fibroid using a slice thickness of 9.7 mm. Notice how the thicker slice makes the endometrium and the fibroid more prominent.

SONOGRAPHIC APPLICATIONS

There are many applications for 3-D/4-D ultrasound. Some uses discussed in this chapter include:

- Obstetrics
- Abdominal
- Urology
- Gynecology
- Small parts
- Pediatrics

Obstetrics

First trimester fetal evaluation using 3-D/4-D can be performed either transabdominally or transvaginally.

Early fetal anatomy is best demonstrated using the transvaginal technique. A 3-D/4-D surface rendering of a normal 10-week fetus is well demonstrated using the 3-D/4-D transvaginal probe shown in Figure 33-26.

Second and third trimester 3-D/4-D imaging is performed with abdominal transducers. 3-D/4-D evaluation on most fetal anatomy is easier to achieve in the second trimester. This can include evaluation of fetal cranial anatomy, fetal heart, or any other fetal structures. In the early second trimester, the fetal face does not have

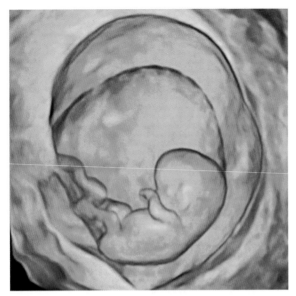

FIGURE 33-26 **A 3-D Surface Rendering of a 9-Week, 6-Day Fetus.** The amnion is visible within the gestational sac. The early fetal eye, ear, extremities, and umbilical cord are well demonstrated in this rendered image.

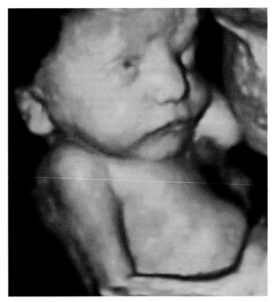

FIGURE 33-28 This 3-D rendering of a 30-week fetal face displays an open eye, an ear, and part of the fetus's right arm.

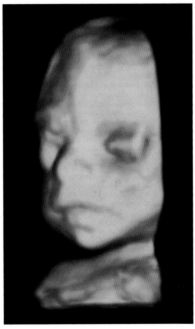

FIGURE 33-27 This 3-D rendering of the fetal face was taken at 22 weeks' gestational age.

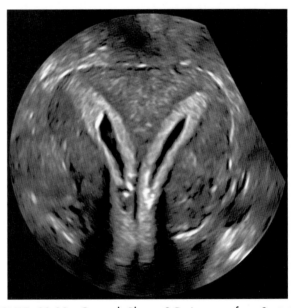

FIGURE 33-29 **Coronal Plane 3-D Image of a Septated Uterus.** The fluid in the endometrial cavity is from saline hysterosalpingography.

much fat and therefore may appear skeletal during facial renderings (Figure 33-27). Late second and early third trimester imaging often results in more pleasing fetal face renderings (Figure 33-28).

Gynecology
Using the endovaginal transducer, the non-gravid uterus can be evaluated with 3-D. In traditional endovaginal scanning the operator is limited in the image planes that can be acquired (sagittal and transverse). Using 3-D ultrasound, the coronal plane can be visualized. The coronal plane best demonstrates congenital malformations of the uterus. 3-D imaging can also be used during saline hysterosalpingography; by this method, the uterus is distended, a volume of the uterus is acquired, and more information is available than with 2-D ultrasound alone (Figure 33-29).

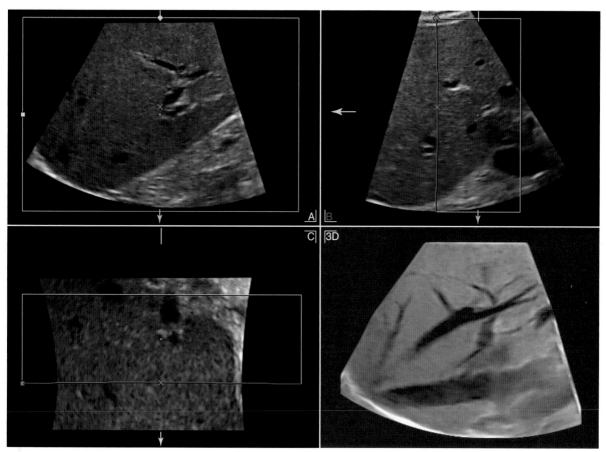

FIGURE 33-30   This 3-D liver volume demonstrates normal liver vasculature using minimum render techniques.

Abdominal

Volumetric abdominal imaging allows for a more complete evaluation of organ systems. 3-D can be used in serial examinations of tumors that require pre-treatment and post-treatment volumetric measuring. Additionally, disruption of vasculature caused by tumor growth can be easily documented using render techniques with or without color Doppler (Figures 33-30 and 33-31).

Small Parts

Using high-frequency linear transducers in a 3-D evaluation enhances visualization of small body parts such as the thyroid, breasts, and testicles. The appearance of breast masses can be better evaluated using the coronal plane, as demonstrated in Figure 33-32. Musculoskeletal structures can also be visualized.

Urology

Using the endorectal transducer, the prostate and seminal vesicles can be evaluated with 3-D. A single acquisition can yield more information than a lengthy examination, because all of the views (from coronal, transverse, and sagittal planes) can now be manipulated post exam. Transabdominal 3-D imaging with a full bladder can allow visualization of the bladder walls (Figures 33-33 and 33-34).

Pediatrics

With the introduction of high-frequency neonatal volumetric transducers, evaluation of the neonatal brain can be accomplished with a single volume acquisition as seen in Figure 33-35. This dramatically reduces the ultrasound scan time in the nursery, thereby reducing infectious transmission potentials, body temperature fluctuations, and disrupted rest for the newborn.

ADVANCED FEATURES

Beyond the basic render techniques, advanced render techniques are becoming more commonplace. Render color options now have more realistic shades, giving the anatomy a more skin tone appearance rather than the

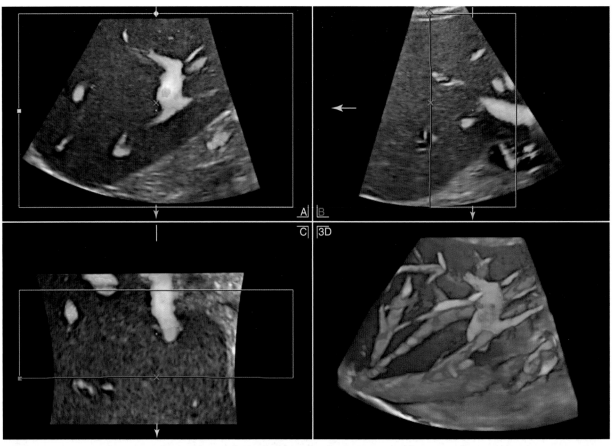

FIGURE 33-31   This 3-D liver volume demonstrates the same normal liver vasculature with color Doppler using a color render technique.

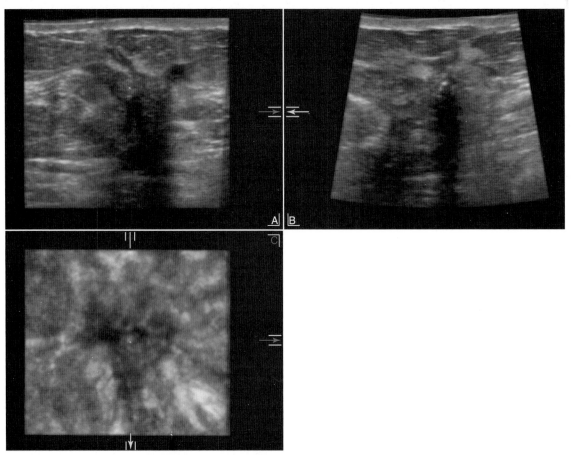

FIGURE 33-32   The A- and B-planes of this 3-D breast volume demonstrate a mass, but the C-plane demonstrates the spiculations of this cancer invading the surrounding breast tissues. The contrast resolution was enhanced by using a slice thickness of 1.0 mm.

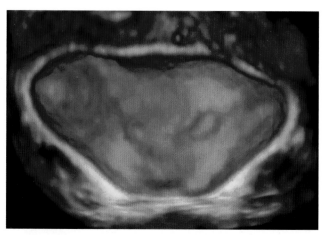

FIGURE 33-33   3-D surface rendering of the trigone region of the adult bladder.

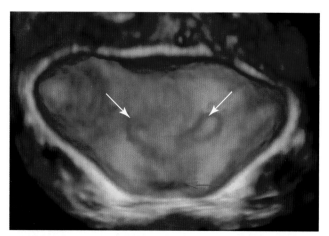

FIGURE 33-34   Both ureteral orifices *(white arrows)* and the internal urethral orifice *(green arrow)* are demonstrated.

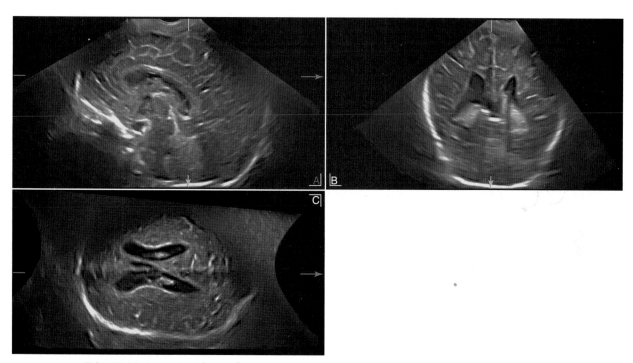

FIGURE 33-35   3-D volume of a neonatal head demonstrating all 3 planes (sagittal, coronal, and transverse) simultaneously.

traditional sepia coloring seen in the past. One render feature that has gained much acceptance recently is the ability to move a light source to visualize the anatomy better. The light source can be moved in any direction (360 degrees). This was first introduced in fetal imaging but can be useful on any anatomy when the render option is active (Figures 33-36 to 33-38).

Inversion mode is another type of volume rendering available. This rendering algorithm displays anechoic structures or structures hypoechoic relative to adjacent

anatomy as a solid object, giving the appearance of a cast or mold of the structure, as demonstrated in Figure 33-39).

As seen previously in the adult liver, 3-D/4-D acquisitions can be performed with color and power Doppler, allowing for enhanced visualization of the surrounding vasculature. This can be achieved with any structure, but it is especially beneficial in the evaluation of the fetal heart, placenta, adult liver, and any mass or tumor (Figure 33-40). When color is used during the 3-D/4-D

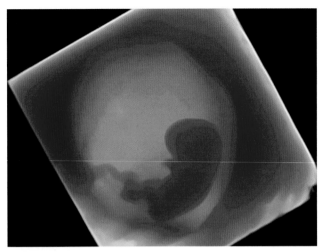

FIGURE 33-36 3-D realistic rendering of a first trimester fetus with the light source projecting from the back of the data set, giving the appearance of a live fetoscopic procedure.

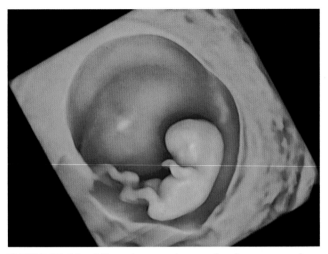

FIGURE 33-38 3-D realistic rendering of a first trimester fetus with the light source projecting from the front of the data set toward the left side of the fetal body. From this direction, the uterine wall behind the fetus and the amniotic sac are well visualized.

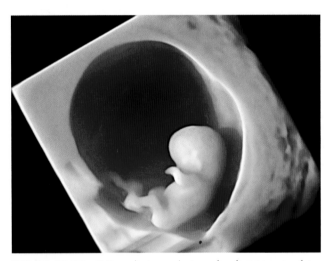

FIGURE 33-37 3-D realistic rendering of a first trimester fetus with the light source projecting from the side of the data set toward the anterior fetal body. The fetal left arm is more pronounced from this light source angle.

acquisition, color render techniques can be applied during post-processing.

3-D/4-D volume sonography continues to evolve. Some of the latest advances have centered on the automation of ultrasound. Automation allows certain structures to be identified, measured, and even manipulated by the ultrasound systems. One 3-D/4-D automation technology that may be encountered is designed to retrieve fetal heart images (outflow tracts, great vessels, etc.) from a four-chamber heart volume data set. The sonographer simply aligns the acquired four-chamber

heart to the system's heart graphics (Figures 33-41 to 33-43). Once the graphic is positioned appropriately, the system generates the various fetal heart images for the sonographer.

Another automation technology currently available counts and measures follicular volume measurements in a stimulated ovary. This 3-D tool is hoped to reduce exam time as well as create more accurate volume measurements (Figure 33-44). The sonographer captures a 3-D volume data set of the stimulated ovary and then selects the automated follicle feature. The system finds the anechoic follicles, color codes them, and calculates the volume for each follicle.

This technology has expanded to be used to calculate volumes of other irregularly shaped, fluid-filled structures. 3-D/4-D automated volume calculation features are helpful when monitoring hydrocephalus, ventricular systems, hydronephrosis, or any fluid-filled structure where a volume calculation would be performed (Figure 33-45). **Spatio-temporal image correlation (STIC)** is a technique that is valuable in the dynamic evaluation of the fetal heart. STIC uses 4-D technology to create a single, beating, continuous heart cycle that is able to be manipulated in all orthogonal planes. STIC combines multiple heart cycles into a single heart cycle volume that is able to be displayed in motion. The 4-D fetal heart can be stored for manipulations after the patient has left or after the fetus has moved to a less desirable scanning window. Figures 33-46 and 33-47 are taken from the same STIC volume data set but at different times within the fetal heart cycle.

New 3-D/4-D volume transducers are being introduced each year. The latest advancements are in the

Text continued on p. 656

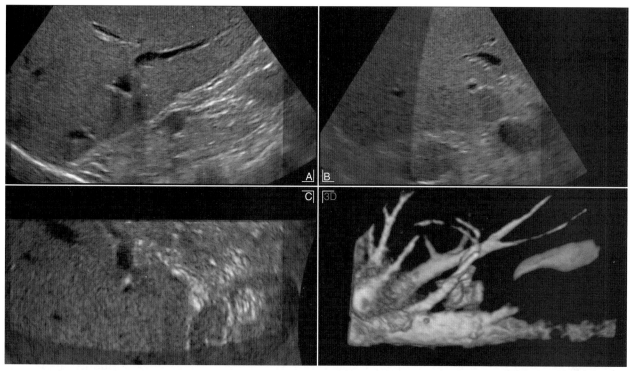

FIGURE 33-39 3-D liver, gallbladder, and right kidney volume data set rendered using inversion techniques. The anechoic liver vasculature and anechoic fluid-filled gallbladder are emphasized in the inversion rendering while the more echogenic anatomy is removed.

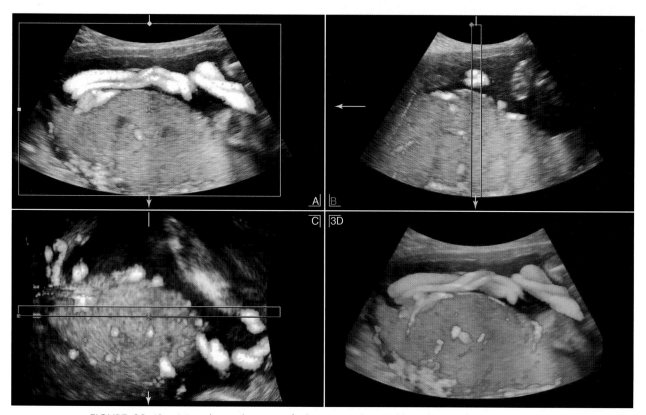

FIGURE 33-40 3-D volume data set of placenta with possible velamentous cord (abnormal insertion of the cord into the placenta). Color render techniques were used to enhance visualization of vasculature.

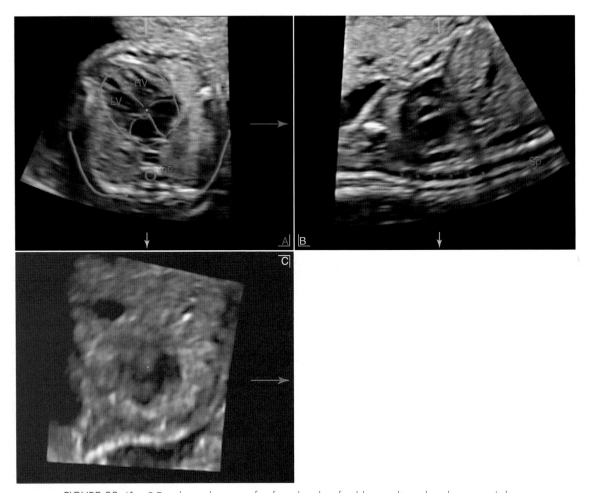

FIGURE 33-41 3-D volume data set of a four-chamber fetal heart aligned to the system's heart automation graphic.

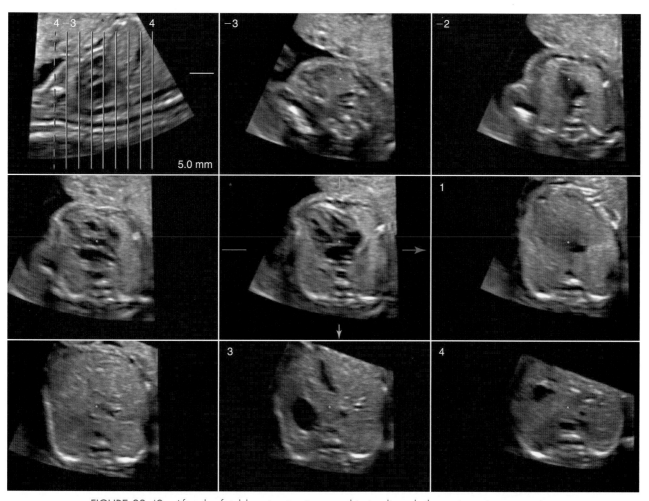

FIGURE 33-42   After the fetal heart animation graphic is aligned, the system gives a preview of the entire data set. In this example, the stomach, four-chamber heart, left outflow, and right outflow are visualized.

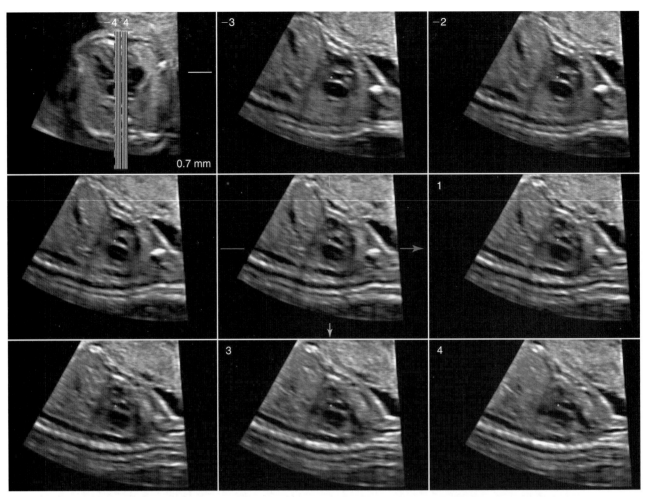

FIGURE 33-43 The heart automation feature automatically displays the following fetal heart structures: four-chamber heart, left and right outflow tracts, stomach, superior and inferior vena cava, and ductal and aortic arches. This image is displaying the system's ductal arch slices in a tomographic display format. Due to variations in fetal growth, not all of the tomographic slices will display the selected anatomy, but at least one slice should demonstrate it.

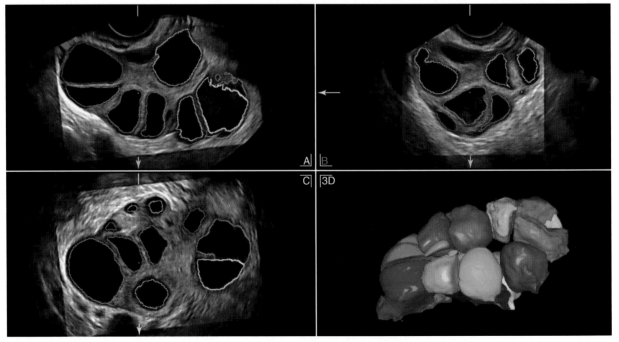

FIGURE 33-44 This simulated right ovary's follicles were assessed using 3-D automated technology. From the 3-D volume data set of the ovary, the system automatically color-coded, measured, and calculated follicular volumes and compiled the results for transfer into a worksheet/report.

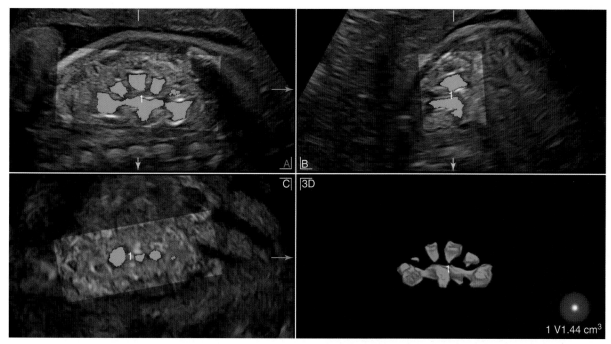

FIGURE 33-45 This fetus's renal dilation can be monitored using a 3-D automatic volume calculation feature. The system calculated a volume (1.44 cm³) of the fluid-filled areas selected within this fetal kidney. Serial measurements to determine if the dilatation is progressing or regressing would be easy to produce during later examinations on this same fetus.

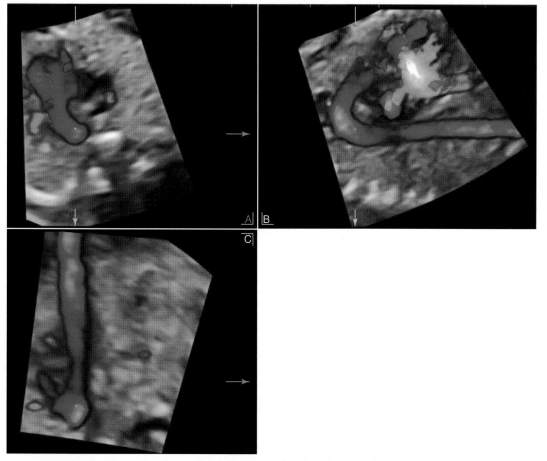

FIGURE 33-46 STIC volume data set acquired with color Doppler demonstrating the right outflow tract (A-plane), the aortic arch (B-plane), and the descending aorta (C-plane).

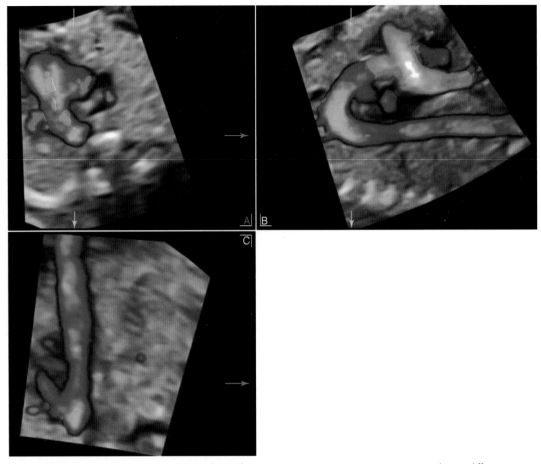

FIGURE 33-47 The same STIC volume data set as seen in Figure 33-46 captured at a different part of the fetal heart cycle. Notice the neck vessels of the aortic arch (B-plane) are demonstrating more color fill at this point in the heart cycle.

form of matrix array transducers. These volumetric transducers contain thousands of elements that can capture true real-time volumes and create live displays of multiple planes and 4-D rendering simultaneously while maintaining adequate resolution. Visualizing the live 4-D imaging orthogonal planes during the scanning process and the ability to make optimization adjustments during the live acquisition are invaluable tools for the sonographer. The reduction in postprocessing time alone makes this feature desirable.

SUMMARY

Clearly, 3-D/4-D imaging is beneficial in everyday practice. It enables manipulation of volume data to create the optimal imaging planes and ultimately may result in more accurate measurements. At this time, 3-D/4-D imaging does not replace the 2-D examination, but when used in conjunction with 2-D, it provides enhanced visualization and therefore more diagnostic information. Consequently, sonographers can have greater confidence in the studies they produce; likewise for sonologists in their diagnoses. In addition, the scanning time in applications such as transrectal, transvaginal, and neonatal exams can be greatly reduced while the image quality is also improved. 3-D/4-D scanning is an exciting, newly evolving area in sonography and will only improve as more applications are investigated and new aspects of the technology are introduced.

CHAPTER 34

Interventional and Intraoperative Ultrasound

BETTY BATES TEMPKIN

OBJECTIVES

Understand ultrasound-assisted interventional and intraoperative procedures.

■

KEY WORDS

Biopsy — Procedures to remove and examine tissue from the living body to determine an exact diagnosis.

Laparoscopic Surgery — Surgical exploration of the peritoneal cavity using a specialized endoscope.

Percutaneous Aspiration — Tissue obtained by applying suction to a needle inserted through the skin that is attached to a syringe.

Percutaneous Biopsy — Tissue obtained by a needle inserted through the skin.

■

Ultrasound is routinely used to assist certain interventional radiology cases and a number of various intraoperative procedures. Ultrasound-assisted interventional radiology cases generally include percutaneous needle-guided biopsies, aspirations, and drainage procedures. Ultrasound is used under these circumstances because the biopsy site can be easily located and the biopsy needle can be well visualized and tracked (Figure 34-1). Intraoperative ultrasound provides crucial information to surgeons that may influence their choice of surgical technique. Ultrasound is a timely way to precisely localize and characterize internal body structures. Because the transducer is in direct contact with the organ or vessel being examined, high-resolution images can be obtained that are not limited by overlying soft tissue, bone, or air. Scans are instantaneous, repeatable, multidimensional, and magnified at will.

ULTRASOUND-GUIDED INTERVENTION

Percutaneous Biopsies

Biopsy procedures are performed to remove and examine tissue from the living body to determine an exact diagnosis. Percutaneous biopsies obtain tissue samples by inserting a needle through the skin. Ultrasound is used during a percutaneous biopsy to determine accurate needle placement for tissue sampling. The biopsy site is scanned to determine the best point of needle entry with the shortest distance and least angle. To monitor the procedure, the transducer may or may not have to be in the sterile field. If it does, sterile couplant gel and a sterile sheath are usually used to cover the transducer. Some physicians, however, prefer that the transducer and cord be wiped down with alcohol instead because air bubbles can occur between the tip of the transducer and the sheath that adversely affect image quality.

Most chest tumors, abdominal organ masses, retroperitoneal lymph node masses, and gastrointestinal tumors can be percutaneously biopsied in lieu of surgical biopsy procedures. Chorionic villi sampling, musculoskeletal lesions, thyroid masses, and breast lesions can also be biopsied percutaneously (Figures 34-2 and 34-3).

Percutaneous Aspirations

Percutaneous aspirations obtain tissue samples by applying suction through a needle attached to a syringe. Ultrasound-guided percutaneous aspirations facilitate needle placement for fluid sampling or total evacuation of fluid. The technique is very similar to the percutaneous biopsy procedure. The site is scanned and the most

657

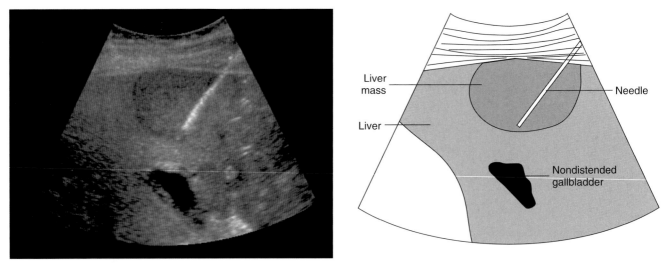

FIGURE 34-1 Ultrasound-guided, percutaneous biopsy of a liver mass. (Half-tone image courtesy Philips Medical Systems, Bothell, Washington.)

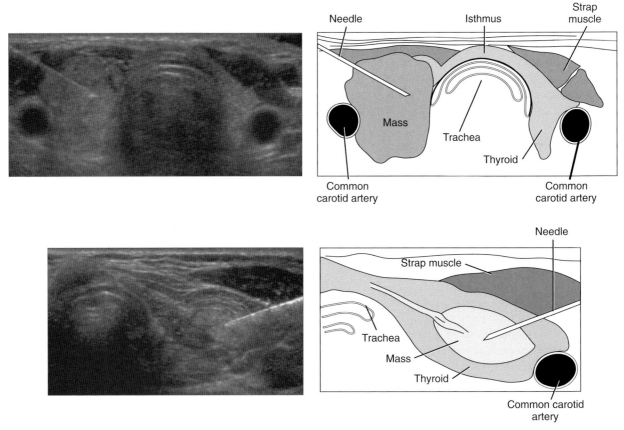

FIGURE 34-2 Ultrasound-guided, percutaneous biopsies of thyroid masses. (Half-tone images courtesy Philips Medical Systems, Bothell, Washington.)

direct entry determined. If monitored in the sterile field, sterile gel is used also as a sterile sheath or alcohol bath for the transducer and cord. Any change in shape or size of a fluid-filled structure can be seen on ultrasound while the needle tip is inserted and fluid is sampled or evacuated. Aspiration procedures may apply to percutaneous cholangiograms with biliary drainage, amniocentesis sampling of amniotic fluid, and various types of cyst aspirations such as pancreatic pseudocysts and renal cysts.

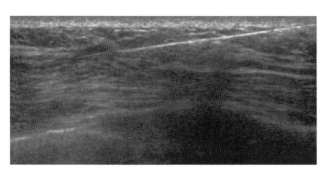

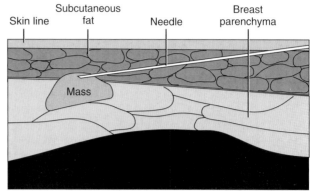

FIGURE 34-3 Ultrasound-guided, percutaneous breast mass biopsy. (Half-tone image courtesy Philips Medical Systems, Bothell, Washington.)

Percutaneous Drainage Procedures

Ultrasound-guided percutaneous drainages assist with needle and catheter placement for procedures that include abscess drainage, biliary drainage, and nephrostomy tube placement. Ultrasound is used to determine the entry site and monitors the placement of the needle and catheter. As with biopsies and aspirations, a sterile field is used. A radiologist performs these procedures, typically in interventional radiology suites equipped with fluoroscopy.

INTRAOPERATIVE ULTRASOUND

Intraoperative ultrasound is used to facilitate surgery. The technique can provide significant additional information to the surgeon at the time of the operation and may contribute to operative decision making and surgical planning.

Equipment and Transducers

Intraoperative ultrasound is best performed using routine mobile sonography equipment with dedicated transducers. Linear array probes have a small field of view with the best near-field definition, whereas sector probes give a larger field of view for small contact areas. Transducer choice depends on the structure(s) being imaged. Unlike conventional intraoperative sonography, laparoscopic surgery (surgical exploration of the peritoneal cavity using a specialized endoscope) assisted by ultrasound is performed using a flexible tip laparoscopic 5.0 to 7.5 MHz transducer.

Sterile Field Procedure

To maintain the sterile operative field, sterile cover sheaths or gas sterilization are options for the transducer. Sheaths should fit snugly over the transducer head to reduce tears and image artifacts. Acoustic gel is used as a couplant between the transducer tip and sheath cover but not as a scanning couplant. In most cases, natural surface moisture is sufficient to couple the transducer to

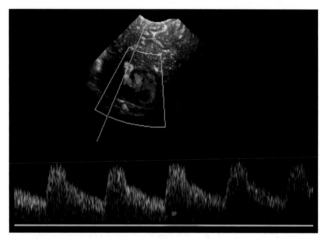

FIGURE 34-4 Color-flow Doppler intraoperative image of a brain aneurysm. (Courtesy Philips Medical Systems, Bothell, Washington.)

the target organ. If more moisture is required, warm sterile saline may be used to improve surface contact.

Because of potential contamination if cover sheaths tear, some authorities recommend presoaking transducers in alcohol for 30 minutes. Alternatively, ethylene oxide gas can be used to sterilize the transducer; however, this approach takes 24 hours, which limits the use of the transducer to once a day. Further, some equipment manufacturers do not recommend this method because it may ultimately damage the delicate outer coating of the transducer head.

Applications

Intraoperative ultrasound can be used for a variety of surgical applications:
- Neurosurgical uses of intraoperative ultrasound involve the brain and spinal cord (Figure 34-4).
- Intraabdominal applications have focused primarily on the liver, pancreas, and biliary tree (Figure 34-5, A to J).

Text continues on p. 666

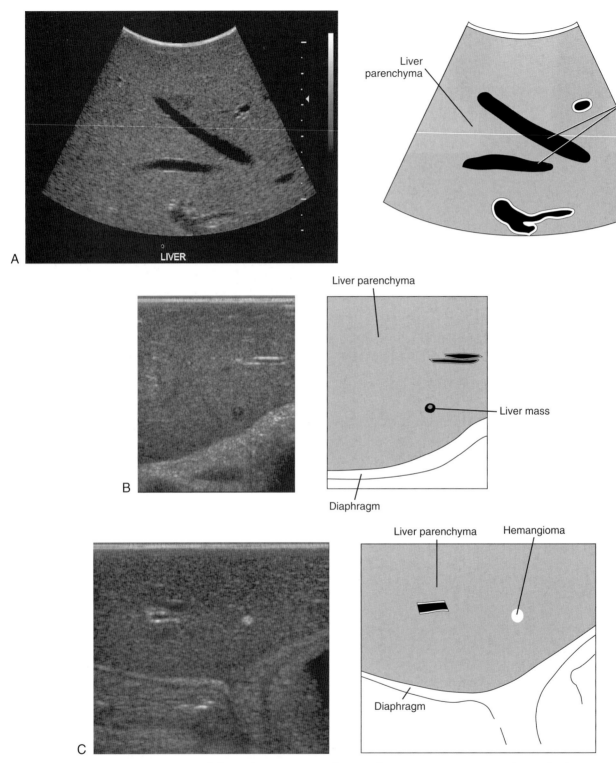

FIGURE 34-5 **Intraabdominal Intraoperative Ultrasound Images. A,** Intraoperative, longitudinal section of the normal liver. **B** and **C,** Transliver approach demonstrating small liver masses.

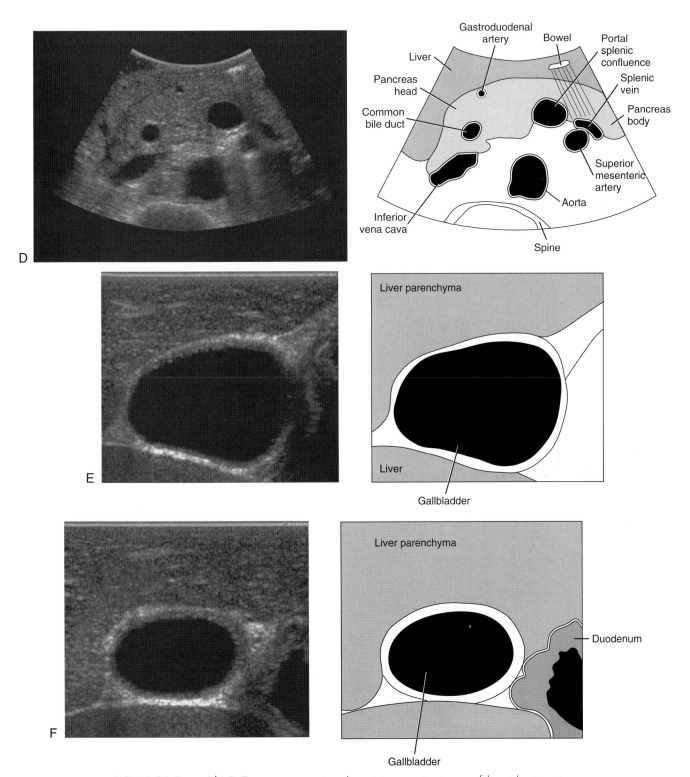

FIGURE 34-5, cont'd **D,** Transverse scanning plane, intraoperative image of the mid-epigastrium.
E and **F,** Axial gallbladder sections imaged intraoperatively. *Continued*

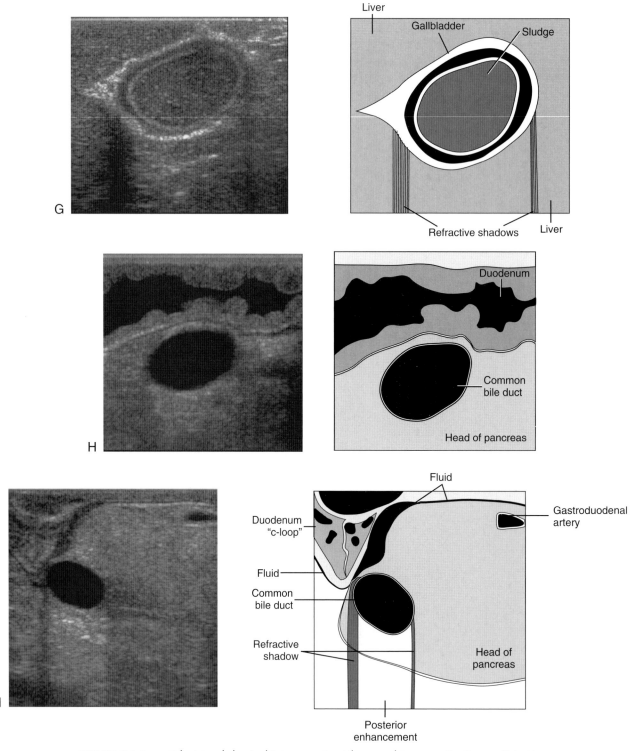

FIGURE 34-5, cont'd Intraabdominal Intraoperative Ultrasound Images. **G,** Trans-gallbladder approach showing a sludge-filled axial section. **H** and **I,** Intraoperative images showing the intimate relationship of the head of the pancreas, duodenum, common bile duct, and gastroduodenal artery.

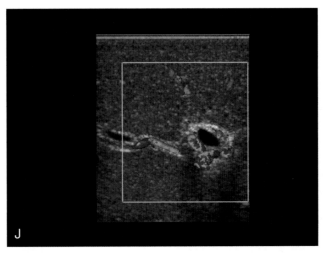

FIGURE 34-5, cont'd **J,** Color-flow Doppler, intraoperative image of the hepatic artery. (Courtesy Philips Medical Systems, Bothell, Washington.)

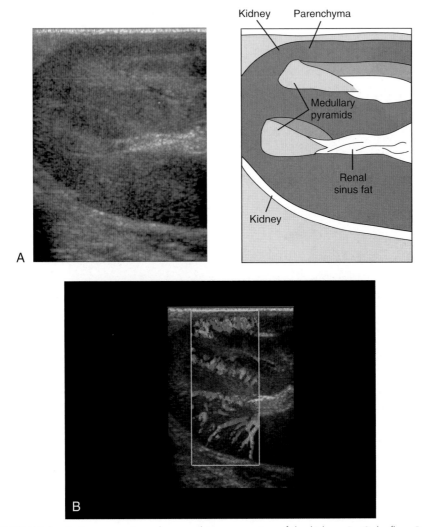

FIGURE 34-6 **A,** Intraoperative, ultrasound image section of the kidney. **B,** Color-flow Doppler of the same section. (Courtesy Philips Medical Systems, Bothell, Washington.)

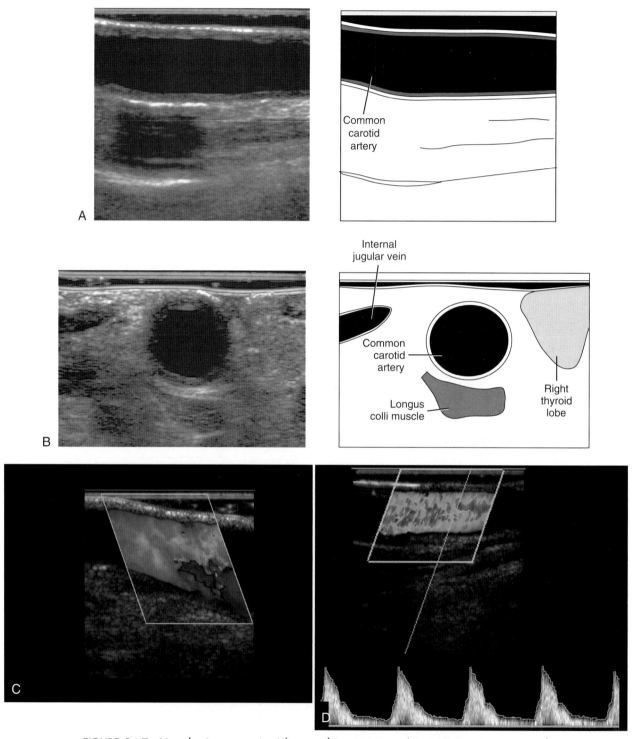

FIGURE 34-7 Vascular Intraoperative Ultrasound Images. A and B, Intraoperative images of longitudinal and axial sections of the internal common carotid artery. Note arterial wall detail. C and D, Intraoperative, color-flow Doppler images of longitudinal sections of the internal common carotid carotid artery.

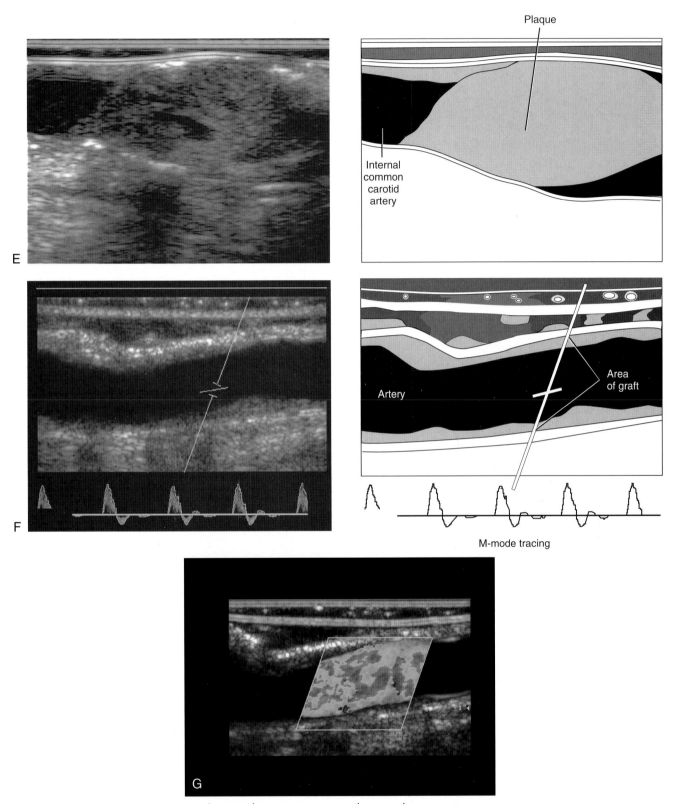

FIGURE 34-7, cont'd **Vascular Intraoperative Ultrasound Images. E,** Intraoperative image showing plaque inside the internal common carotid artery. **F,** Intraoperative image of an arterial graft. Shows Doppler tracing. **G,** Intraoperative, color-flow Doppler image demonstrating an arterial graft. Note arterial wall details. (Courtesy Philips Medical Systems, Bothell, Washington.)

- Evaluation of breast tumors.
- Evaluation of renal tumors (Figure 34-6).
- Vascular disorders (Figure 34-7, *A* to *G*).
- Endoluminal ultrasound is being used to evaluate vessels and grafts during vascular surgical procedures.
- Gynecologic diseases.
- Tumor ablation.

- Biopsies.
- Aspirations.
- Drainages.
- Laparoscopic ultrasound is used to identify and stage tumors, to detect retained biliary calculi in patients undergoing laparoscopic cholecystectomy, and to assist thoracoscopic procedures.

Index

A

Abdomen
  computed tomography of, 330
  fetal, 443, 443f–444f
  quadrant divisions of, 82f
  regional divisions of, 82f
Abdominal aorta, 158
  in abdominal layers, 68–69, 68f
  axial images of, 107–109, 107f–109f
  axial survey of, 100–103, 101f–103f
  bifurcation of, 99, 99f–100f
  branches of, 68–69, 68f, 161f–163f
  breathing technique when imaging, 97
  embryologic, 127–130, 128f
  laboratory values for, 155t, 156
  location of, 158, 162f–163f, 195
  longitudinal images of, 105–106, 105f–106f
  longitudinal survey of, 98–100
    bifurcation alternative for, 100b, 100f
    transabdominal anterior approach, 98–100, 98f–100f
  multiplanar display of, 637, 637f
  normal measurements for, 158b
  proximal portion of, 99, 99f, 164f
  scanning of, 95
    choosing transducer for, 96
    patient positioning for, 95–96, 96f
    patient preparation for, 95
    using transducer for, 96–97, 97f
  size of, 161
  sonographic appearance of, 163–168, 164f–170f. *see also* Aorta
Abdominal cavity, 48, 50, 50f
Abdominal circumference (AC)
  to determine gestational age, 443, 443f–444f
  in second and third trimesters, 446–447, 446b
Abdominal layers, 65–74
  abdominal aorta in, 68–69, 68f
  anterior muscle layer in, 74, 74f
  biliary tract in, 70–71, 70f
  gallbladder in, 70–71, 70f
  gastrointestinal tract in, 72–73, 72f
  inferior vena cava in, 67, 67f
  kidneys and adrenal glands in, 66, 66f
  liver in, 73–74, 73f
  pancreas in, 71–72, 71f
  portal venous system in, 69–70, 69f
  posterior muscle layer in, 65f
Abdominal plain film, 330
Abdominal vasculature
  arterial
    hemodynamic patterns of, 197–198, 198f
    location of, 193–197, 193f, 194t–195t
    normal measurements for, 197b
    sonographic appearance of, 197
  common diagnostic tests for, 205b
  normal measurements for, 192b
  venous
    hemodynamic patterns of, 203–204, 205f

Abdominal vasculature *(Continued)*
    location of, 199–200, 200f–205f, 201t–202t
    major branches of, 199, 200f
    normal measurements for, 200b
    size of, 200
    sonographic appearance of, 201–203
Abdominopelvic cavity, structures of, 82f
Abdominopelvic muscles, 344f
Abduction, 23
Absorption, 44
Accessory gastrointestinal (GI) organs
  defined, 125
  in embryologic development, 130–131
Accuracy, in vascular technology, 609, 632
Acini, 519
Acini cells, 249, 253–254
Acoustic enhancement, 89t–94t
Acoustic impedance, 89t–94t
Acoustic shadows, 89t–94t
Additional controls, 8, 13f–14f, 13t
Adenomas, parathyroid, 509
  detection of, 509, 512f–513f
  fine-needle aspiration/biopsy (FNAB) of, 516
  hypervascularization of, 509, 511f–512f
  lymph nodes distinguished from, 512
  measuring, 510f–511f
  mimicking of, 512
Adnexa, 341
Adrenal arteries, location of, 158, 159t–160t
Adrenal cortex, 266
Adrenal glands
  in abdominal layers, 66, 66f
  anatomy of, 290–292, 291f
  enlarged lesions of, 222–223
  fetal, 437, 437f
  functions of, 36t
  hormones secreted by, 36t, 290–292
  laboratory values for, 294
  location of, 267, 268t
  size of, 287–290
  sonographic appearance of, 287–290
  vasculature of, 292, 292f
Adrenal medulla, 266
Agenesis, of gallbladder, 246
Air, normal sonographic appearance of, 87t–89t, 88f
Alanine aminotransferase (ALT), 141, 144, 144t–145t
ALARA (as low as reasonably achievable), 89t–94t
Alcohol
  effect on pancreas of, 265b
  during pregnancy, 140b
Aldosterone hormone, 294
  defined, 266
  and renal function, 280, 280t
Alimentary canal, 44–46, 307–308, 309f, 310t–311t

Alkaline phosphatase (ALP), 144, 144t–145t
  in breast cancer, 528, 528b
  and liver damage, 144
Alpha cells, of pancreas, 249, 254–255, 255t
Alpha-fetoprotein (AFP), 448, 451
  during first trimester, 410, 410b
  in high-risk pregnancy, 455, 455b
  laboratory values for, 151, 152t
  in second and third trimesters, 446, 446b
Alphanumeric keyboard, 8–9, 9t
Alveoli
  mammary, 519, 521
  in respiratory system, 47
American Registry of Diagnostic Medical Sonography (ARDMS), 2
American Society of Echocardiography, 581, 592–593
Amniocentesis, 411, 448, 451
  in high-risk pregnancy, 455, 455b
  during second and third trimesters, 446, 446b
Amnion, 394, 398–399, 399f
  defined, 392
  during first trimester, 405–406, 406f
Amniotic cavity/sac, 398–399, 399f
  defined, 392
  during first trimester, 405–406, 406f
  normal sonographic appearance of, 87t–89t, 88
Amniotic fluid, 392
  AFP in, 451
  development of, 399–400
  during first trimester, 406
  during second and third trimesters, 415–416
Amniotic fluid index (AFI), 415–416, 449
  defined, 411
  in second and third trimesters, 446b, 447
Amniotic fluid volume (AFV), 399, 415–416
  in biophysical profile scoring, 449, 449t
  defined, 392, 411
Ampulla
  of uterine tube, 354–356, 357f
  of Vater, 44, 228, 232, 249
Amylase, 141, 146, 147t
Anal canal, in embryologic development, 135
Anatomical landmarks, identification of, 82f
Anatomy, sectional, 48
Andenohypophysis, 35
Anechoic, 89t–94t
Aneuploidy
  defined, 392
  fetal risk for, 408, 409f, 445
Aneurysm
  of brain, 659, 659f
  interatrial septal, 605, 607f
  sonographic identification of, 168
Angioblasts, 128
Angiography
  of abdominal vasculature, 205
  computed tomography, 205, 632
  of liver, 226, 226b
  magnetic resonance, 633
  of pancreas, 265

Page numbers followed by "*f*" indicate figures, "*t*" indicate tables, and "*b*" indicate boxes.